With Northwestern University
Medical School & Gary J. Martin, M.D.

The American Institute for
Preventive Medicine & Don R. Powell, Ph.D.

ALL NEW FAMILY MEDICAL GUIDE TO HEALTH & PREVENTION

PUBLICATIONS INTERNATIONAL, LTD.

Louis Weber, C.E.O.
Publications International, Ltd.
7373 North Cicero Avenue
Lincolnwood, Illinois 60646

Manufactured in U.S.A.

8 7 6 5 4 3 2 1

ISBN:0-7853-1229-3

Library of Congress Catalog Card Number: 95-72807

PART I
Consultants:

The American Institute for Preventive Medicine located in Farmington Hills, Michigan, is dedicated to helping people change to a healthier lifestyle through successful wellness programs, products, and publications. It works with over 5,000 hospitals, HMOs, corporations, and government agencies throughout North America. The Institute has been honored and recognized by the Department of Health and Human Services and the President's Council on Physical Fitness and Sports for its innovative health programs.

Don R. Powell, Ph.D., is the founder and President of the American Institute for Preventive Medicine. He is a licensed psychologist who earned his Ph.D. from the University of Michigan and taught in the University's Psychology Department. He is an authority on the design, marketing, and implementation of community and corporate health education programs. Dr. Powell has won numerous awards for his work in the field of health promotion and has appeared on hundreds of television and radio talk shows.

Elaine Frank, M.Ed., R.D., is Vice President of the American Institute for Preventive Medicine, a Registered Dietitian, and an instructor in the Department of Health and Physical Education at Henry Ford Community College.

Jeanette Karwan, R.D., is a Registered Dietitian and the Director for Product Development at the American Institute for Preventive Medicine.

Abe Gershonowicz, D.D.S., has been practicing general dentistry for 15 years in Sterling Heights, Michigan.

Terrence Higgins, M.S., is an exercise physiologist and the Fitness Program Director at Becton Dickinson Immunocytometry Systems in San Jose, California.

Contributing writers:

Brianna Politzer is a freelance writer specializing in health, fitness, nutrition, and technology. She has contributed to many consumer publications including *The Home Remedies Handbook, Women's Home Remedies Health Guide,* and *The Medical Book of Health Hints & Tips*. Ms. Politzer wrote the "Fitness," "Caring for Your Teeth and Gums," and "Keeping Tabs on Your Health" chapters.

Elaine Fantle Shimberg has written or contributed to numerous publications on various consumer health topics including stress, depression, teen pregnancy, and first aid. She has contributed articles to *Reader's Digest, Woman's Day, Glamour,* and *Seventeen.* Ms. Shimberg is a member of the American Medical Writer's Association and the National Association for Science Writers. Ms. Shimberg wrote the "Coping with Stress" and "Avoiding Potential Hazards" chapters.

Susan Male Smith, M.A., R.D., is a Registered Dietitian and nutrition consultant who specializes in consumer health writing. She is assistant editor of *Environmental Nutrition* newsletter and writes the "Food News" column in *Family Circle* magazine. Her writing has also appeared in *Redbook, McCall's, American Health,* and *Women's Health Advisor.* Ms. Smith wrote the "Food and Nutrition" and "Weight Control" chapters.

PART II

Northwestern University Medical School is located in Chicago, Illinois. The missions of the Northwestern University Medical School are education, research, and professional services, a major component of the latter being the delivery of high-quality patient care. The Medical School supports the overall mission of the University to achieve excellence in its scholarly and service programs and to participate in its framework for distinction. The provision of excellent medical education that builds on the foundation provided by the core academic disciplines is of the highest priority. The Medical School seeks to provide leadership in scientific discovery, intellectual inquiry and creativity, and innovative performance. Through its teaching, research, and professional service, the Medical School strives to achieve a leadership position in shaping health and research policy by encouraging faculty, staff, and student involvement at local and national levels.

Northwestern Medical Faculty Foundation is a premier multispecialty medical group consisting of health care professionals who are full-time faculty in the clinical departments of Northwestern University Medical School. The faculty members, jointly with a professional staff of administrative and clinical support personnel, are committed to providing exemplary medical care to patients in a sensitive and service-oriented environment. It is the Foundation's mission to support the teaching and research functions of the Northwestern University Medical School through a commitment to the Medical School's goals and objectives. Further, it is the Foundation's mission to create a health care delivery system in which innovation in patient care services, sound practice management techniques, and responsible allocation of resources are used to create an environment in which health care professionals can be educated and prepared for a changing health care environment and society's future medical needs. Within this environment, it is the Foundation's mission to support and facilitate the evolution of scientific endeavors from the laboratory to the direct delivery of patient care.

Gary J. Martin M.D., is Chief of the Division of General Internal Medicine at Northwestern University Medical School. He is an Associate Professor and is Board Certified in Internal Medicine and Cardiovascular Disease. He has provided primary care since 1984 as a member of the Northwestern Medical Faculty Foundation and as an attending physician at Northwestern Memorial Hospital of Chicago.

Contributors:

Martin J. Arron, M.D.
General Internal Medicine

Michelle Baer, M.D.
Obstetrics and Gynecology

Jennifer A. Bierman, M.D.
General Internal Medicine

Mark K. Bowen, M.D.
Orthopedics

Steven Brem, M.D.
Neurosurgery

Wade Bushman, M.D., Ph.D.
Urology

David Conley, M.D.
Otolaryngology

Thomas Corbridge, M.D.
Pulmonary Medicine

Therese A. Denecke, M.S., R.N., C.S., F.N.P.
Primary Care Nursing

Albert L. Ehle, M.D.
Neurology

Robert S. Feder, M.D.
Ophthalmology

David Fishman, M.D.
Gynecologic Oncology

Marilynn C. Frederiksen, M.D.
Obstretrics and Gynecology

William Friedrich, D.D.S.
Dentistry

Luther Gaston, M.D.
Obstretrics and Gynecology

Darren R. Gitelman, M.D.
Neurology

William J. Gradishar, M.D.
Medical Oncology

Zoran M. Grujic, M.D.
Neurology

Michael Haak, M.D.
Orthopedics

Nanci Fink Levine, M.D.
Obstretrics and Gynecology

John R. Lurain III, M.D.
Gynecologic Oncology

Michael T. Margolis, M.D.
Gynecology

Helen Gartner Martin, M.D.
Sleep Disorders and Pulmonary Medicine

Tacoma McKnight, M.D.
Obstretrics and Gynecology

Patricia Naughton, M.D.
Obstretrics and Gynecology

Gary A. Noskin, M.D.
Infectious Diseases

Harold J. Pelzer, M.D., D.D.S.
Otolaryngology

Robert V. Rege, M.D.
Surgery and Surgical Critical Care

Douglas Reifler, M.D.
General Internal Medicine

Jack M. Rozental, M.D., Ph.D.
Neurology

Frank R. Schmid, M.D.
Rheumatology

Arvydas D. Vanagunas, M.D.
Gastroenterology

Sybilann Williams, M.D.
Gynecologic Oncology

David T. Woodley, M.D.
Dermatology

PART III
Drug consultants:

Cheryl Nunn-Thompson, Pharm.D., BCPS, is assistant director of the Drug Information Center at the University of Illinois Hospital. She is a registered pharmacist and received her doctor of pharmacy degree at the University of Illinois, Chicago, where she is a faculty member in the College of Pharmacy.

Jan E. Markind, Pharm.D., is a drug information specialist at the University of Illinois Drug Information Center and an assistant professor in the College of Pharmacy at the University of Illinois Hospital. She received her doctor of pharmacy degree from the Philadelphia College of Pharmacy and Science.

Mary Lynn Moody, R.Ph., is director of the Drug Information Center at Michael Reese Hospital and a clinical assistant professor at the University of Illinois College of Pharmacy. She is past president of the Illinois Council of Hospital Pharmacists and a member of the American Society of Hospital Pharmacists.

Editorial assistants: Deborah A. Barnett, Pharm.D., and Toby Clark, M.Sc., Drug Information Center University of Illinois, Chicago

Picture Credits:

Bruce Ayres/Tony Stone Images: 157, 581; **Ron Chapple/FPG International:** 6

Illustrations: Yoshi Miyake

CONTENTS

PART I: PREVENTION

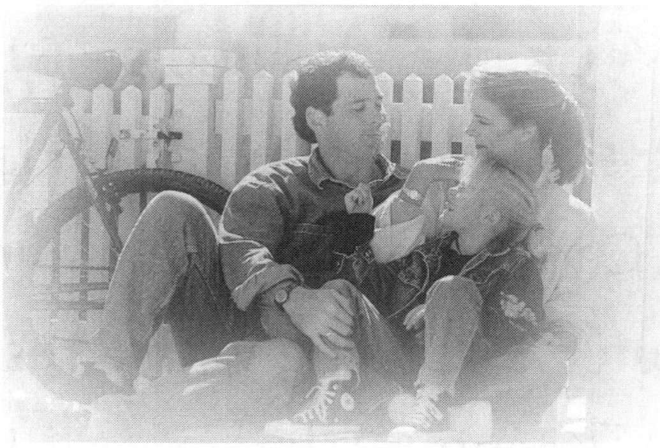

An ounce of prevention is worth a pound of cure, and herein are the basics of staying well. "Preventive health" and "wellness" are two catch-all terms you may hear a lot lately. Although they may sound like trendy 1990s jargon, the concepts behind them are among the most ancient in recorded history.

As far back as 3,000 B.C., cities on the Indian subcontinent were developing their own wellness and health-promotion programs—designing environmental-sanitation systems; constructing underground drains and public baths; creating their own mores of health-related conduct, hygiene, and dietary practices. The Greeks and Romans—as well as many societies since—also maintained a strong focus on preventive health.

Western societies, especially in the 19th and 20th centuries, have gone on a different health care tack. As a result of the development of powerful antibiotics and vaccines, we have come to assume that science would eventually be able to offer a cure for whatever ailed us. And while a great number of life-saving drugs have been developed, recent years have sobered us up a bit: We have learned that while science is powerful, nature usually holds the final trump card.

The reality is that the best medicine is prevention. Simple lifestyle changes can make the difference between health and illness (or life and death). True, some factors—such as family history or an accidental exposure to a virus—can't be changed, but a vast array of other important factors (including diet, exercise, drug and alcohol abuse, use of condoms during sexual intercourse) are completely under our control.

With the information in Part I, the wisdom to put it into practice, and a little good fortune, you and your family may never need Part II. We hope so.

FOOD AND NUTRITION

You are what you eat. Trite, but true. With the possible exception of quitting smoking, good nutrition is the single most important ingredient in the recipe for preventing disease. Unlike family history—which determines a lot of your risk, but which you can't change—the food you put into your body directly affects your health and is completely under your control.

Vitamin discoveries may be a part of history, but obscure minerals continue to be recognized for their contribution to health, and a whole new class of substances—phytochemicals—are being investigated for their role in preventing chronic diseases. We are no longer satisfied with the minimal amounts necessary to forestall nutrient deficiencies. We want to find out which nutrients will work for us. And longevity is not the only goal; modern nutrition addresses quality of life as well.

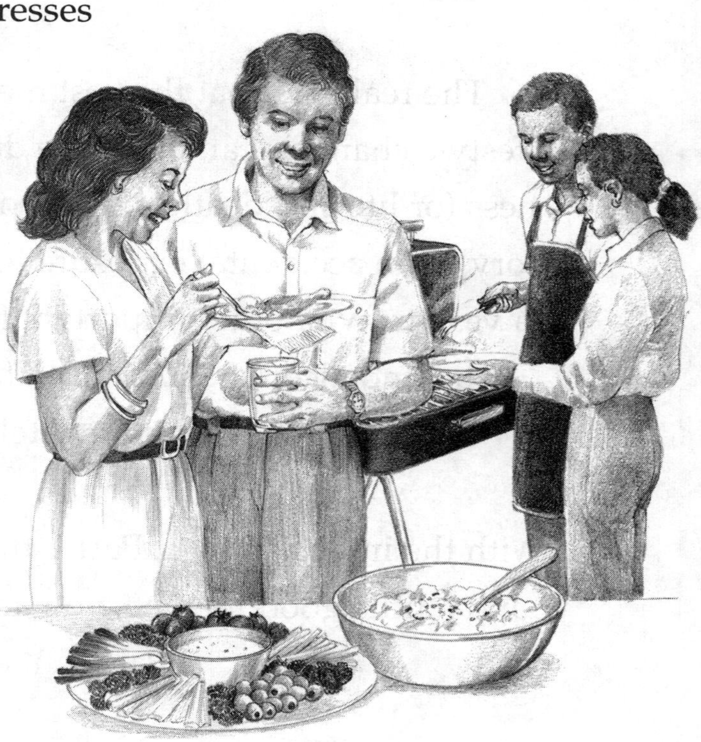

Experts tell us that half of all deaths are due to an unhealthy lifestyle, and that two thirds of those are related to diet. So there's a lot at stake when you cruise those supermarket aisles full of tantalizing come-ons and tempting choices. And while eating right won't guarantee you a long and healthy life, it certainly increases your odds.

NUTRIENTS

When you eat, you are ingesting substances that your body needs to build and repair tissues, to burn for fuel, and to use in the billions of chemical reactions that occur every second. These vital substances are called nutrients. When you think of nutrients, you may just think of vitamins and minerals, but you might be surprised at the wide spectrum of substances that you get from food. Before we even get to vitamins and minerals, here are the major nutrients.

WATER

It may not be as sexy as vitamin E or as trendy as beta-carotene, but water is the true nectar of the gods because it is so essential to life. Without it, you wouldn't live long—four or five days at most.

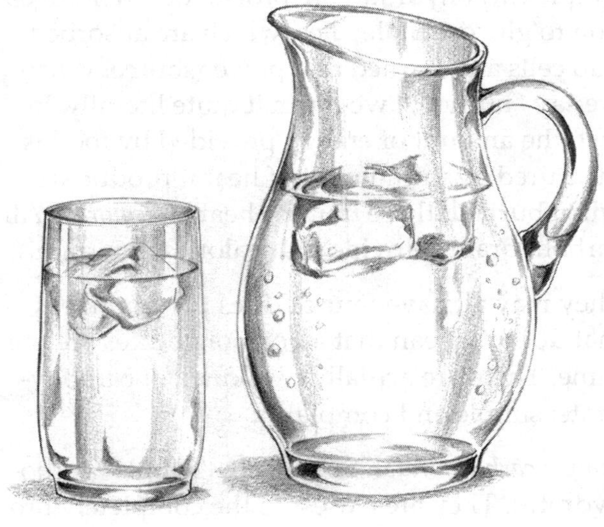

Every part of your body relies on water. Your blood, for example, is more than three-quarters water. Other body fluids, like saliva and digestive juices, are based on water, as is urine. You couldn't get rid of body wastes without it. Almost every chemical reaction in the body takes place in a water medium, and water also lubricates and protects the joints, organs, nose, and mouth. Most clever of all is how your temperature stays near that magical 98.6°F. Your body needs water so that when you get hot, you can sweat. The water you sweat off then evaporates on your skin, cooling you down. Without it, you'd suffer heatstroke.

Here's where most people get their water from:

- 28% drinking water
- 24% tea and coffee
- 9% vegetables
- 9% milk and dairy products
- 8% soft drinks
- 7% meat and eggs
- 6% fruits and juices
- 5% grains
- 2% alcoholic drinks

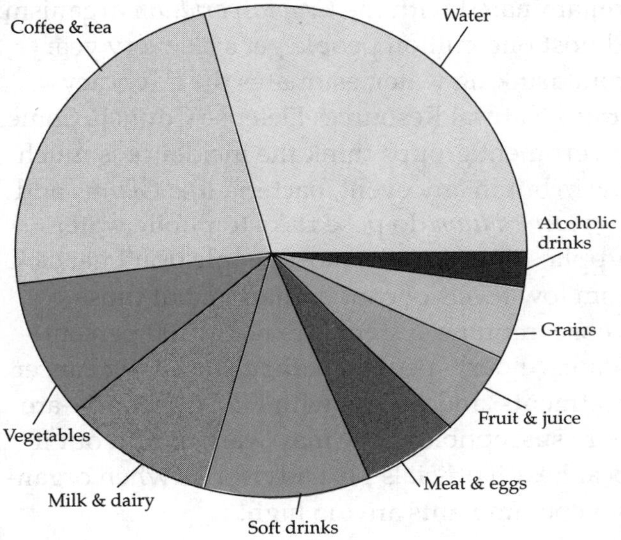

So how much do you need? Generally, you should drink six to eight cups of water a day. Although you can get by on less, drinking this much water is especially kind to your kidneys and colon, because it helps to flush toxins out of your body. When you drink a lot of water, the toxins can't hang around too long and cause damage to your kidneys or cancerous growths in the colon. In fact, drinking plenty of water may be the simplest of all disease-prevention tips.

Why not just drink when you're thirsty? Because your body's thirst-o-meter isn't very reliable. You should drink about three cups more than your thirst tells you to. And as you get older, your body loses the ability to tell when it's thirsty, making it doubly important to drink water even when you don't crave a cool drink.

Is your water safe? Milwaukee was not the place to be in 1993. Nearly 400,000 people were stricken with diarrhea and vomiting from drinking the public water, which had somehow been contaminated with the *Cryptosporidium* organism. Almost one million people get sick every year from drinking water, estimates the advocacy group Natural Resources Defense Council. Some government groups think the incidence is much lower, but in any event, bacteria like *Giardia* and *Cryptosporidium* do pose risks to public water supplies. Fortunately, most people don't get sick from low levels of contamination, but those whose immune systems are not at 100 percent—infants, elderly people, patients receiving cancer treatments, and people with HIV infection—are more susceptible. They may want to find out if local health officials post advisories when organism contaminants are too high.

Get the Lead Out

To minimize your exposure to lead:

- Let water run until cold before using.
- Let the first water drawn in the morning run for at least three minutes to flush the pipes; water that stands around all night contains significantly more lead leached from pipes, solder, and faucets.
- Never use hot water to reconstitute powdered baby formula or for cooking; hot water leaches more lead into the water.
- Don't boil water too long; it concentrates the same amount of lead into a smaller amount of water.

Organisms aren't the only problem, though. If your image of lead poisoning involves peeling paint in a rundown tenement, think again. Experts now warn that water is a significant source of lead—and not just in older houses. New faucets are particularly likely to leach lead into water. Exposure to lead is especially dangerous for pregnant women, infants, and young children, causing brain damage that results in learning difficulties. It can also injure the kidneys, nervous system, and red blood cells. (For more on water safety, see Chapter 4.)

CARBOHYDRATE

Poor misunderstood carbohydrate. It suffers from an image problem. Seems it got a bad rap years ago as a calorie-laden horror, and it hasn't been able to shake that reputation. The message may be getting through that fat is your biggest enemy, but unfortunately, "carbs" are still viewed with skepticism as well. Nothing could be further from reality.

Carbohydrates are your best friends. They are your body's preferred fuel. Both complex and simple carbohydrates are broken down in digestion to glucose molecules, which are absorbed into cells and burned as a power source. When we say "burned," we mean it quite literally. In fact, the amount of energy provided by food is measured by the amount of heat it produces when burned; these units of heat are *calories*. All carbohydrates provide four calories per gram.

They may all have four calories per gram, but that doesn't mean that all carbohydrates are the same. There are actually two kinds of carbohydrate: simple and complex.

Simple carbohydrates. Sugars are "simple" carbohydrates. They are closest to the completely broken down form that your body uses as fuel. In fact, glucose itself is the simplest sugar. So the body converts sugar directly into usable energy. Pure sugar foods, such as hard candies and soft drinks, raise your blood sugar level and your energy level temporarily—sometimes called a "sugar high." However, the levels quickly drop below what they were before, in a rebound effect. This has been dubbed the "sugar blues."

Sugar's reputation is truly battle scarred, but with very little reason. Sugar isn't quite the evil substance you may think it is. Its biggest fault is with the company it keeps; it is often found in foods with little or no nutritional value. Some of the charges leveled at sugar are baseless, some may be justified but haven't been proved, and a few are all too true. Here are some of the true and false charges:

- Sugar causes hyperactivity. False. Its reputation for creating sugar monsters—kids that eat sugar and go berserk—just isn't true. No well-designed scientific study has ever been able to prove a link between sugar and hyperactive behavior. Keep in mind that kids often overdo sweets at particularly exciting times of the year, such as birthdays and Halloween, when they're naturally wound up just from the excitement.

SUGAR-MONSTER MYTHS

The latest study on sugar and hyperactivity has been hailed as the most conclusive to date. Conducted at Vanderbilt University in Nashville, the study was particularly well designed to avoid the usual pitfalls. The children—and more important, their parents—didn't know which kids ate the sugar-laden foods; the food was eaten over the course of a day, not in one large dose; and the children chosen were those labeled by their parents as being hypersensitive to sugar. Still, the results showed no difference in behavior between the kids eating sugary foods and those who were unaware they were eating nonsugar foods.

- Sugar causes diabetes. False. Although there is a connection between sugar and diabetes, it is merely guilt by association. Diabetes is a hereditary disorder that appears when you lack insulin (type I) or you become insensitive to it later in life (type II). Can eating a lot of sugar cause this insensitivity? No, but being overweight can, and people who eat sugary sweets often gain weight—hence, the confusion.

- Sugar causes cavities. True, but it is hardly the worst offender. All carbohydrates can contribute to tooth decay. Complex carbohydrates, such as starches, can be just as much to blame for cavities as sugar, if not more so. The bacteria that cause decay are not picky about what they eat; starches that stick to your teeth provide plenty of food for bacteria. Surprisingly, one of the worst offenders is crackers. (For more on dental disease, see Chapter 5.)

Complex carbohydrates. Don't call them starches anymore. They're complex carbohydrates, and they're in the nutrition spotlight. Complex carbohydrates—found in bread, pasta, potatoes, rice, starchy vegetables, oatmeal, and dry beans—are the basis of a healthful diet (see the Food Guide Pyramid, page 33). These starches are better than the simple sugars for many reasons. One reason is that they are absorbed more slowly (good for blood sugar control), but their real advantage is that they are found in foods that contain many other nutrients. Unlike sugars, which are either by themselves providing empty calories or worse, paired with tons of fat, complex carbohydrates are found in grain products and vegetables that provide many important vitamins and minerals.

What's more, a diet based on complex carbohydrates has significant disease-prevention qualities. By getting the bulk of your calories from foods rich in complex carbohydrates, you decrease your risk of many diseases, including heart disease, high blood pressure, stroke, and certain types of cancer.

Fighting disease with fiber. A great deal of the credit for the preventive powers of complex carbohydrates goes to fiber—a certain type of complex carbohydrate found in whole grains, legumes, fruits, and vegetables. It seems strange that something your body rejects can be so important to your health, but that's just the case with fiber—the indigestible portion of carbohydrate. Your body can't break it down, so it passes right through and on out as waste. Yet to do without it is to invite trouble.

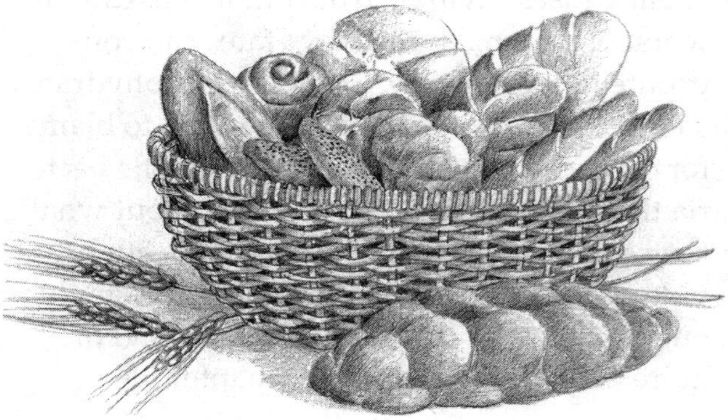

Without fiber, the other substances in your intestines would just sit there, fermenting and stagnating. Any toxins from food or created by bacteria would have that much more time to be in contact with your intestinal walls. It's this exposure that is thought to be at least one cause of colon cancer. Keeping things moving is a smart move that helps prevent other diseases and conditions as well: constipation, diverticular disease, hemorrhoids, and varicose veins. And the sticky properties of fiber keep diabetes, heart disease, and obesity at bay.

There are two types of fiber: soluble and insoluble. Insoluble fiber is the type that probably comes to mind when you think of fiber. It's found in the wheat bran that's in most bran cereals. The fact that it doesn't dissolve in water is what makes it so beneficial. Instead, it soaks up water like a sponge. This softens stool and increases its bulk, which puts pressure on the walls of the intestines and speeds the stool's movement through your body. If you make a regular habit of eating foods high in insoluble fiber, you can all but eliminate the worry of constipation and hemorrhoids, and it almost certainly decreases your risk of developing colon and rectal cancers.

Soluble fiber may not be as well known, but it's just as valuable. As soluble fiber dissolves in water, it forms gummy gels. These gels bind with substances you'd just as soon get rid of—like bile acids. Remember oat bran? Well, it was no silly craze. Oat bran is rich in soluble fiber, and by binding with bile acids, it helps lower blood levels of cholesterol. The higher your blood cholesterol level, the more it can help you. To make a difference, get in the habit of eating one or two low-fat oat-bran muffins or other foods high in soluble fiber every day.

By slowing the absorption of carbohydrates, soluble fiber also helps keep blood sugar on an even keel. Some people with diabetes are able to control blood sugar better by increasing the soluble fiber in their diet. For those battling the bulge, the extra bulk in the stomach and its delayed emptying help curb the appetite without adding calories. (For more on weight loss, see Chapter 2.)

How much is enough? Most Americans don't get even close to the recommended amount of fiber—20 to 35 grams per day. The average American gets about 10 to 15 grams per day. To boost your intake, make some simple adjustments in your daily diet:

- Switch to whole-wheat bread and whole-wheat pasta.
- Start your day with a bowl of bran cereal.
- Eat whole fruits instead of just drinking juice.
- Get two servings of vegetables at every meal.

Can you get too much? Yes, excessive fiber can interfere with mineral absorption, but you'd consistently have to take in more than 50 grams per day to be worried. Few people have that problem. A more common problem is that people increase their fiber intake too fast, resulting in gas, bloating, and intestinal discomfort. These gastrointestinal problems can be prevented by adding high-fiber foods gradually over six to eight weeks.

You must also be sure to drink enough water and other fluids, especially when you eat foods high in insoluble fiber. They soak up the available water in your intestines; if there isn't enough, you could end up with an intestinal blockage—rare, but serious.

PROTEIN

Protein is overrated. Although getting enough may be the difficulty in some areas of the world, it's rarely a problem in the United States. In fact, too much protein is our curse. Still, it is essential for growth, indeed for life itself. Protein is made up of amino acids that your body uses to make body tissue and vital enzymes. There are nine essential amino acids that you must get in your diet.

You need about 50 to 60 grams of protein per day, and that's not as much as it sounds. Consider this: A quarter pound of meat, cooked, provides about 20 grams of protein, and a glass of milk adds another 8 grams. Every slice of bread, or equivalent serving of starch, adds another 2 grams each. So you see how easy it is to get enough protein. Anyone who eats meat easily gets more than enough.

Do Athletes Need More Protein?

The image of football players eating steak for breakfast and Sylvester Stallone drinking raw eggs in *Rocky* has perpetuated a myth that athletes perform better the more protein they get. Not true. Although it may seem logical, protein does not help build muscles; exercise does. Extensive exercise requires extra carbohydrates, not protein. Although elite athletes may require more protein than weekend warriors, it is easily obtained from the extra food they eat to maintain their energy level. Protein powders and supplements are a waste of money, and single amino acids are potentially dangerous.

Too much of a good thing. Many people make the mistake of thinking you can never get too much protein. They associate protein with growth and assume more is better. They couldn't be more wrong. Once your body gets the amount of protein it needs, it converts the rest to energy, and if you already have enough energy, it is converted to fat. Obviously, this is not what you have in mind when you order the cottage cheese and hamburger diet plate!

Too much protein can also rob the body of its bone-strengthening calcium stores and has been implicated in osteoporosis. Although most people's kidneys can handle the job, eating excessive amounts of protein does put a strain on your kidneys, whose job it is to filter out the by-products of protein digestion.

Just as with sugar, protein's biggest problem is the company it keeps. Protein and fat just seem to go hand-in-hand. Think about it. High-protein foods are very frequently high-fat foods: meat, milk, cheese, and nuts. Fortunately, there is skim milk, new reduced-fat cheeses, and even leaner meats to choose, but nuts—there's no good solution there yet.

FAT

Fat is an ugly word—as descriptive as they come. We all know it's not our friend when we eat too much of it. If we could avoid it entirely it might make things easier, but fat is also essential to life. Linoleic and linolenic acids are essential fatty acids, and fat is needed for brain functioning and absorbing fat-soluble nutrients.

However, don't take those kind words as license to pig out on Ben & Jerry's New York Super Fudge Chunk. You need fat only in very small amounts, and as long as you include a small amount in your diet, you're probably getting plenty.

If you're the average American, more than one third of your calories come from fat—much more than called for. That's partly because fat, at nine calories per gram, provides more than twice the four calories per gram of either carbohydrate or protein. Research suggests that you'd do better if less than 30 percent of your calories came from fat. Perhaps much less.

Why this obsession with the percentage of calories from fat? Because it's hard to argue with a glut of studies indicating that if you lowered total fat, you could reduce your risk of several chronic diseases.

The road to heart disease. First and foremost among the health problems associated with too much fat

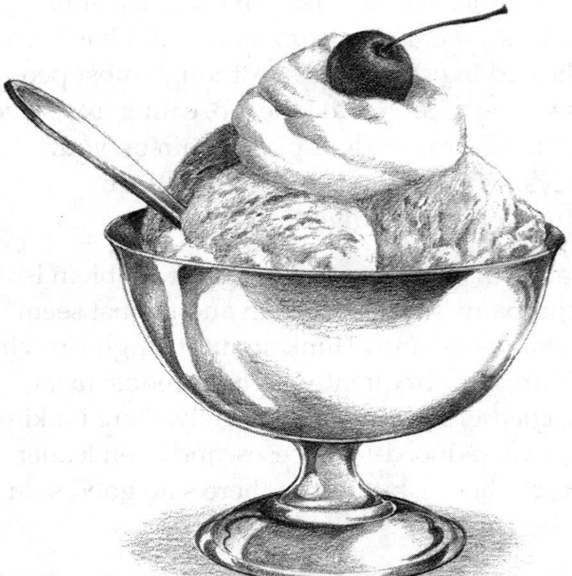

is heart disease—the leading killer of both men and women. The fat content of your diet is only one risk factor—family history, smoking, and exercise are others—but dietary fat plays a crucial role. And unlike family history, it's one you can control.

The relationship between dietary fat and heart disease risk may be very direct, but the mechanism is a little more complicated. If you want to understand how fat can increase your risk, you've got to look at the sometimes confusing topic of cholesterol.

Cholesterol is not a fat, although it falls into the lipid category. It is a waxy substance, found in all animal fats. Like fat, it leads a schizophrenic life: vilified, but essential to life. Cholesterol is needed to make vitamin D and the sex hormones, and is a key ingredient in the protective covering around nerves. The danger comes from the cholesterol circulating in your bloodstream. There, it can be attracted to any vulnerable spots along the walls of the arteries, where blood clots form and calcium also gathers. This *plaque*, as the deposit is called, continues to accumulate, narrowing arteries until blood can no longer flow through. If this happens to an artery in your heart, it's a heart attack; if it happens to an artery in your brain, it's a stroke.

Assessing Your Risk

When you have your blood cholesterol level checked, what do the numbers mean? The National Heart, Lung and Blood Institute gives the following guidelines for interpreting your cholesterol numbers:

Total Cholesterol	
Less than 200*	Desirable
200–239	Borderline-high risk
240 and over	High risk
LDL Cholesterol	
Less than 130	Desirable
130–159	Borderline-high risk
160 and over	High risk
HDL Cholesterol	
Less than 35	Increased risk
35–60	Acceptable
Over 60	Decreased risk

*Levels are shown in milligrams of cholesterol per deciliter of blood (mg/dL).

Cholesterol gets ferried around the bloodstream by substances called lipoproteins. There are different kinds—some better for you than others:

- Low-density lipoprotein (LDL) cholesterol is one form of the cholesterol found in your blood. LDL cholesterol has been dubbed the "bad" cholesterol. That's because LDLs carry cholesterol headed *to* your arteries.
- High-density lipoprotein (HDL) cholesterol is headed *away* from your arteries. Hence, HDL cholesterol is often called the "good" cholesterol.

The ratio of your total blood cholesterol level to your HDL cholesterol level is the most important factor in determining your risk of heart disease. As long as HDL cholesterol makes up enough of a portion of your total cholesterol level, you are not at increased risk.

If you're worried about cholesterol, you're not alone, but what can you do about it? It's logical to assume that if your blood cholesterol is high, then

NAMES AND FORMS	FUNCTIONS	DEFICIENCY (symptoms)	TOXICITY (symptoms)	FOOD SOURCES	PROTECTIVE AGAINST
MINERALS					
CALCIUM	Essential for strong bones and teeth; keeps heartbeat regular; needed for functioning of nerves and muscles; aids in blood clotting.	*Osteoporosis.* (Brittle bones, stress fractures of wrist and spinal column, "dowager's hump" of spine, back and leg pains.)	No specific toxicity levels, although excessive dietary calcium may interfere with the absorption of other minerals.	Milk and other dairy products, bok choy, broccoli, greens (not spinach), herring, fortified orange juice, salmon and sardines with the bones, soybeans.	*Osteoporosis.* *High blood pressure* worse in sodium-sensitive individuals if calcium intake is not adequate. *Colon cancer*, by binding with potential toxins.
CHROMIUM	Essential component of glucose tolerance factor, needed for insulin to work; maintains blood sugar levels.	Absolute deficiency is rare, but borderline deficiency may contribute to glucose intolerance. (Excessive thirst, frequent urination, weight loss, urinary tract infections.)	None known. Diabetics should take supplements only if monitored by a doctor.	Beef, whole-wheat or whole-grain breads and cereals, brewer's yeast, broccoli, American process cheese, chicken, liver, oysters, peanuts, prunes, wheat germ.	*Glucose intolerance* (can normalize some people's high blood sugar). *High blood cholesterol.*
COPPER	Essential for iron storage and connective tissue formation; aids red blood cell formation, nerve function, immune function, and cholesterol metabolism; component of the antioxidant enzyme superoxide dismutase.	*Menkes' "kinky hair"* (or *"steely hair")* *disease*—rare inherited inability to absorb copper. Deficiency only in infants fed exclusively milk or in people with kidney disease. (Anemia, brittle bones.)	*Wilson's disease*—rare inherited disorder that causes copper to accumulate in the liver, brain, and eyes.	Apricots, dried beans, whole-wheat and whole-grain breads and cereals, crab and lobster, liver, nuts, oysters, potatoes.	*Menkes' disease.* Possibly *cancer* and *heart disease.*
IODINE	Essential to the thyroid hormone for regulation of energy.	*Goiter* and *cretinism*—both rare in U.S. due to use of iodized salt. (Fatigue, weight gain, dry skin and hair, nervousness.)	*Goiter* and *Graves' disease*—rare in U.S.; more common in parts of Japan where seaweed is eaten.	Iodized salt, seaweed, seafood.	*Goiter.* *Cretinism* (mental retardation).
IRON	Essential part of hemoglobin needed to form red blood cells; needed as components of enzymes.	*Iron-deficiency anemia.* (Fatigue, listlessness, pallor, headache, tingling in hands and feet, irritability, shortness of breath, and cravings for nonfood items.)	*Iron toxicity* from supplements is the most common pediatric poisoning. *Hemochromatosis* is a hereditary disorder that causes irreversible damage. (Abdominal/joint pain, weight loss, fatigue.)	Dried apricots, dried beans, beef and pork, brewer's yeast, fortified cereals, liver, blackstrap molasses, oysters, green peas, prunes, raisins, tofu, wheat germ.	*Iron-deficiency anemia.*

NAMES AND FORMS	FUNCTIONS	DEFICIENCY (symptoms)	TOXICITY (symptoms)	FOOD SOURCES	PROTECTIVE AGAINST
MAGNESIUM					
	Essential for strong teeth and bones; balances body's acidity level; helps process carbohydrates, protein, and fats; helps regulate heartbeat.	Specific deficiency not known but suboptimal levels can cause trouble. (Brittle bones, nausea, high blood pressure, tremor, irregular heartbeat, muscle spasms and weakness, confusion.)	Rare. Only occurs with abuse of magnesium-containing laxatives, antacids, or supplements, or in those with kidney disease.	Almonds, avocados, bananas, dried beans, whole-wheat bread, cashews, lentils, oatmeal, peanut butter, spinach, tofu, wheat germ.	*Osteoporosis*, when teamed with calcium. Possibly *heart disease* and *high blood pressure*.
MOLYBDENUM					
	Activates enzymes.	None known.	Large amounts can cause gout symptoms and interfere with copper absorption.	Breads and cereals, milk, green leafy vegetables, legumes.	*Cancer* prevention suggested but not yet demonstrated.
PHOSPHORUS					
	Important for bone and tooth development, and the body's acidity balance.	None. Available in nearly all foods. (Appetite loss, bone pain, malaise, weakness.)	No frank toxicity, but excessive amounts in diet can be a problem if calcium and vitamin D intake are inadequate. Excessive amounts interfere with iron absorption.	Meat, poultry, fish, cereals and grains, green vegetables.	*Osteoporosis*, in combination with other minerals.
POTASSIUM					
	Essential for contraction of muscles, including the heart; needed to transmit nerve signals and regulate blood pressure.	Rarely caused by diet. (Loss of appetite, weakness, low blood pressure, drowsiness, irrational behavior, irregular heartbeat)	No specific toxicity in normal instances.	Apricots, bananas, dried beans, lentils, milk and cheese, meat, poultry, citrus fruits, potatoes, prunes, spinach, winter squash.	May help with *high blood pressure*. May reduce risk of *stroke*.
SELENIUM					
	Key component of antioxidant enzyme glutathione peroxidase and an enzyme that activates thyroid hormones; aids immune system functioning and heart health; promotes healthy sperm.	*Keshan's disease*—rare in U.S. (Muscle weakness and pain, heart abnormalities.)	Toxic at levels over 1 mg per day.	Whole-wheat and whole-grain breads and cereals, brewer's yeast, broccoli, carrots, cabbage, celery, seafood, liver, mushrooms, radishes.	As an antioxidant: *aging*, *cancer*, and *heart disease*.

NAMES AND FORMS	FUNCTIONS	DEFICIENCY (symptoms)	TOXICITY (symptoms)	FOOD SOURCES	PROTECTIVE AGAINST
SODIUM					
	Essential for regulation of fluid balance and acidity levels; needed for cell transportation.	None from diet. All foods and water contain sodium. Can occur from prolonged excessive sweating, chronic diarrhea, or in kidney disease.	Frank toxicity not a problem. (Fluid retention, high blood pressure—in susceptible individuals.)	Table salt, all foods—especially processed foods, smoked and processed meats, pickled foods, and condiments.	None.
ZINC					
	Essential for immune system functioning and wound healing; needed for development of bones and reproductive system; aids vision.	Frank deficiency rare in U.S., but borderline deficiency is common. (Halted growth and sexual development, infection, loss of appetite, altered taste and smell, scaly skin, depression, fatigue, diarrhea, delayed wound healing, low sperm count.)	Toxic symptoms start at amounts over 15 mg per day. Even relatively low levels can interfere with iron, selenium, and copper absorption and can reduce good HDLs and depress immune function.	Dried beans and peas, beef and pork, turkey, brewer's yeast, whole-wheat and whole-grain breads and cereals, crab and lobster, oysters, eggs, liver, wheat germ.	*Infection.* May reduce the severity and duration of the *common cold.* Promising results for *macular degeneration* and possibly *cataracts.*

can be deadly in greater quantities. The real trick is knowing which ones you need more of and which ones you should slow down on.

THOSE YOU MAY NEED MORE OF

If you're consuming "suboptimal" amounts of a nutrient, it's not good. You're not deficient—that is, you won't show disease symptoms—but you're taking in less than is thought to be the best for good health. The consequences of this aren't always clear, but the impact of less-than-desirable levels may accumulate over time, possibly leading to chronic health problems.

Nutrients are sexist. It's a fact. Men and women require most nutrients in similar amounts—men slightly more of some. Yet it's much easier for men to meet their needs, because they need and get more calories, on average, than women. And that means they get more nutrients, too. Women who are dieting have an even tougher time meeting nutrient needs, unless they take a supplement.

The following vitamins and minerals are ones that you may not be getting in adequate amounts. There are dietary solutions for most, but some nutrients are difficult to get in the average diet and may require supplementation. (For hints on how to get the proper nutrients in your diet, see pages 35–37.)

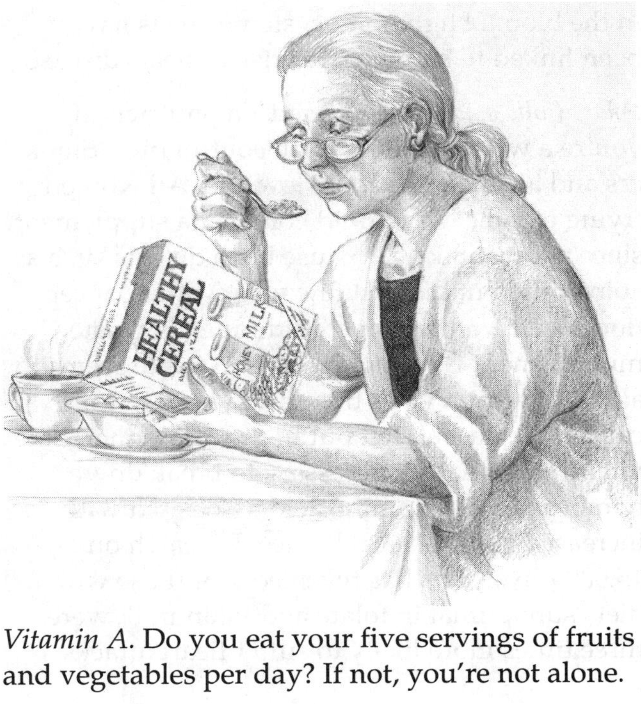

Vitamin A. Do you eat your five servings of fruits and vegetables per day? If not, you're not alone.

Surveys show that less than half of adult women meet the Recommended Dietary Allowance (RDA) for vitamin A, probably because they don't eat enough fruits and vegetables rich in beta-carotene—a precursor of vitamin A. Suboptimal intake could weaken your immune system.

Riboflavin. You don't drink milk either? Meet your counterparts: Only one half of adult women meet the RDA for this vitamin. If you're included in this poor showing, it may be because you're not including enough dairy products and enriched grains in your daily diet.

Vitamin B_6. Again, it's women who are at greatest risk for not meeting their needs for this vitamin. The average intake is just over 50 percent of the RDA. Women on birth control pills seem to need more than average. Some men may fall short too, as may seniors of both sexes. If you fit into any of these groups, your all-important immune system may suffer for it. In studies, supplements of vitamin B_6 have been shown to boost immune function in seniors.

Vitamin B_6 may do much more than simply keep your immune system up and running. Exciting new research has identified that vitamin B_6 protects the body from a build-up of homocysteine in the blood. High homocysteine levels have been linked to an increased risk of heart disease.

Folate (folic acid). This is a red-flag nutrient if you're a woman taking birth control pills. Smokers and alcoholics may be low, too. All women trying to conceive should consider a supplement, since a low intake can cause birth defects such as spina bifida in the first few weeks after conception. Even women not considering pregnancy might benefit from the protection folate seems to afford against a virus that can cause cervical cancer. Men aren't left out in the cold either. Like vitamin B_6, folate is necessary to break down homocysteine, an amino acid associated with increased risk of heart disease. Research on 15,000 physicians has revealed that those with diets suboptimal in folate and vitamin B_6 were three times more likely to suffer heart attacks than those whose diets were adequate in the two nutrients.

Vitamin C. Such an easy-to-get nutrient shouldn't be in this category, but certain groups of people don't get enough, particularly those who skimp on vegetables and fruits. Smokers typically have low blood levels of vitamin C, because their needs are twice those of nonsmokers.

Calcium. The trend toward drinking soft drinks instead of milk with meals is having an effect. Less than a quarter of adult women and less than half of young children meet the RDA for calcium. That sounds bad enough, but it's really worse. The RDA's 800-milligram recommendation for adults is seriously outdated and may not be enough in the long run. This prompted the National Institutes of Health to issue new recommendations—much higher than the RDA. If you want to keep up with the new recommended levels, it may mean supplements, because now all adults are urged to get 1,000 to 1,500 milligrams of calcium, about the same as teenagers. In postmenopausal women, a recent study found that those who took a daily supplement of 1,000 milligrams of calcium reduced their bone loss by 43 percent.

Copper. No one is yet certain about the cost of ignoring this seldom-noticed mineral. Some studies have linked low copper levels to arthritis, high blood sugar, heart disease, and high cholesterol. If you're typical, you are not getting even close to the RDA for copper. And if you take megadoses of vitamin C (1,500 milligrams per day or more) you could be disrupting copper absorption and contributing to a copper insufficiency.

Chromium. Talk about a deficit. A government chromium researcher estimates 90 percent of Americans get less than the minimum recommendation of 50 micrograms per day. So the new focus on chromium is deserved, but misdirected. Its value is not in weight loss but in blood sugar regulation. The rise in blood sugar that comes with age may not be inevitable, but a result of inadequate chromium in the diet, as chromium is needed for insulin to work.

Adequate chromium may even help keep cholesterol levels in check. A 1994 report found that people with diabetes who received chromium lowered their triglyceride levels by 17 percent, significantly reducing their heart disease risk. Your first step toward adequate chromium nutrition is to cut down on the sugar content of your diet, which can rob the body of chromium.

The Chromium Connection

Could diabetes be a simple matter of a nutrient deficiency? Probably not by itself, but some researchers are convinced that an inadequate chromium intake coupled with excessive sugar in the diet can trigger diabetes in susceptible individuals. The mineral chromium is essential to insulin functioning, and a high-sugar diet can, by stimulating insulin, actually hasten the body's depletion of chromium. Thus, less chromium is left for insulin to use—a classic catch-22. The proliferation of high-fructose corn syrup in foods, especially in soft drinks, is worrisome because it adds to our sugar load and presumably to our need for chromium.

Iron. Remember those old Geritol ads? Well, forget them. They gave a generation the wrong impression that older women needed more iron. It's just the opposite. Women in their childbearing years who are menstruating and losing iron monthly are at risk for anemia. Less than one fifth of them meet the RDA for iron. Children are also susceptible, especially toddlers, preschoolers, and adolescents who are growing rapidly and whose diets are typically lacking in iron. Athletes and vegans (strict vegetarians) should also be on the lookout.

Fatigue doesn't always signal anemia, and anemia isn't always due to an iron deficiency, so any suspicion should be checked out by your doctor, who can run the appropriate tests. To boost iron absorption, drink orange juice (or another good vitamin C source) when you eat meat. Avoid drinking coffee or tea at mealtimes and never at the same time you take a supplement that contains iron.

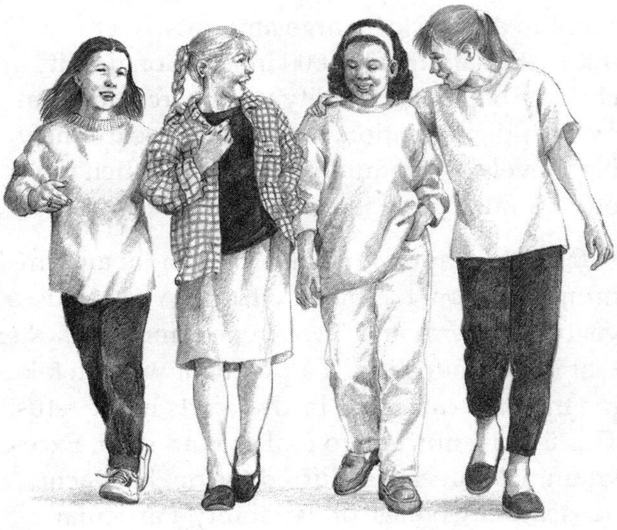

Magnesium. Three out of four people do not meet the RDA for magnesium. This has implications for many growth and repair jobs in the body, but it can also contribute to osteoporosis. Calcium gives bones their strength; magnesium makes them elastic—just as important for resisting breakage.

Zinc. If you're not a big meat eater you might be short on zinc, unless you happen to like oysters. Just six medium Eastern oysters will give you five to six times the RDA. Otherwise, you probably get only about half what's recommended. You need zinc for literally hundreds of enzymes that trigger important reactions in the body. The lower levels of zinc that come with age may be one reason for an increase in infections in older people. Seniors given zinc supplements show improved immune response.

However, caution is in order here. Too much zinc can also impair the immune system as well as cause a copper deficiency and lower blood levels of the beneficial HDL cholesterol. If you take a multivitamin-mineral supplement, be sure it contains 15 to 30 milligrams of zinc. Avoid supplements with a megadose of zinc.

THOSE YOU SHOULDN'T OVERDO

Vitamin A. Don't make the mistake of substituting preformed vitamin A (called retinol) for beta-carotene in the hopes of preventing disease. Vitamin A is toxic in large amounts, over 50,000 international units (20,000 international units in children). Though toxicity usually results from oversupplementation, liver contains extremely high levels of vitamin A; eating too much too often is not a good idea.

Although vitamin A is vital to eyesight and immune function, too much vitamin A also causes vision problems and a weakened immune system that invites infection. If a pregnant woman takes too much, it can cause birth defects in the fetus. This is *not* a nutrient to fool around with. Excess vitamin A can cause blurred vision, headaches, nausea, achy bones, or irritability. Particular caution for seniors: As you age, your liver is less able to remove vitamin A from the bloodstream, making toxicity a bigger worry. Supplements with preformed vitamin A should not contain more than the RDA. If you feel that you need a vitamin A supplement, it's best to take beta-carotene, which can be converted to vitamin A in the body.

Vitamin D. This is another nutrient that demands respect. Toxic levels are only five times the RDA. Children are particularly susceptible to a toxic reaction to vitamin D, which causes blood calcium levels to soar—a dangerous condition. Seniors often don't get enough vitamin D. They are not in the sun a lot, and when they are outside, their skin requires more time to convert vitamin D to its active form. Often, they don't drink much milk either. If this describes you, ask your doctor about taking a combination calcium–vitamin D supplement, or a multivitamin-mineral supplement. Just be sure you take only one of these options and that the amounts don't exceed 100 percent of the RDA.

Niacin. As its nicotinic acid alter ego, this B vitamin becomes powerful enough to lower high cholesterol levels. Unfortunately, those who are prescribed such high doses (over 1,000 milligrams) often pay the price. The megadoses cause nicotinic acid flush—an immediate redness and swelling of the face and neck, often accompanied by itching, headache, and nausea. This side effect lessens with use. Heartbeat abnormalities are more serious. People with diabetes are advised to stay away from high doses of nicotinic acid because it can raise blood sugar to dangerous levels.

Vitamin B_6. This nutrient was once thought to be immune to toxicity. It took until the 1980s, when it became popular to take vitamin B_6 supplements in ever larger amounts, to discover the upper limit of its safety. Here's what caused it to finally lose its cachet: nerve damage from doses as low as 500 milligrams a day, more commonly from amounts over 2,000 milligrams. Fortunately, the damage is reversible if the supplements are stopped at the first sign of tingly or numb extremities or trouble walking.

The Scandal in Our Milk Supply

When was the last time you saw a child with the unmistakable bowed legs of rickets? Probably in the 1930s, before the government mandated the fortification of milk with vitamin D. However, faith in that solution has been shaken by several recent studies showing milk fortification to be unreliable. The latest study found that 80 percent of milk samples from around the United States and Canada contained nowhere near the amount of vitamin D their labels claimed—14 percent of them had *none*! More worrisome was the finding that four milk samples were dangerously overfortified. It was eight cases of vitamin D toxicity that prompted the initial investigation.

What to do? Chances are, your milk is providing you with some, but try not to rely on it for all your vitamin D needs. Expose your unprotected hands and face to sun (skip midday, however) for at least 15 minutes two or three times a week. In northern areas in winter, however, this won't do much, especially if you're older. So a supplement containing no more than 10 micrograms (400 international units) of vitamin D may be in order.

What about getting too much vitamin D? Should you stop drinking milk? No, the odds are in your favor. However, even though it's unlikely you'd get toxic amounts of vitamin D from your milk, be prepared to recognize the symptoms: nausea and vomiting, abdominal pain, and excessive urination.

Iron. Like vitamin A, this Jekyll-and-Hyde nutrient is on both lists. Many people don't get enough, but too much can be dangerous, too. You hear a lot more about having iron-poor blood than you do about iron overload (or hemochromatosis), which can develop in people who inherit a gene that causes the body to absorb too much iron. This potentially fatal condition threatens a surprisingly large number of people—1 in every 250—mostly men and postmenopausal women, because their iron needs are lowest. They are best off avoiding supplements with iron.

Iron's Dark Side

For those susceptible to iron-overload disease (about 1 in 250 people), there is little warning before iron builds up so much it causes irreversible damage to the heart and liver and triggers diabetes, arthritis, and impotence. What symptoms there are show up late, including fatigue (which might be mistaken for iron deficiency), abdominal pain, achy joints, and a bronze skin tone.

The only way to identify whether you have an impending problem is to test your blood levels of serum iron, total iron-binding capacity, and percent transferrin saturation. If suspicious, serum ferritin is then checked as well. Because this is an inherited disease, anyone with an affected relative must be tested. The only treatment is frequent blood donation.

Iron supplements also threaten children; they are the leading cause of accidental pediatric poisoning. It takes only five tablets of high-potency iron to kill a child under age six. Childproof caps are a must, though recent cases have been caused by caps left off or not tightened. Don't overlook grandparents' homes, where caution may be less vigilant and accidents more likely. (For more on poison safety, see Chapter 4.)

ANTIOXIDANTS TO THE RESCUE

If you haven't heard of antioxidants by now, you're just not paying attention. They're *the* hot topic in disease prevention. Antioxidants aren't new, however. They've been around all the time; we just weren't smart enough to appreciate them. Now we know they're like secret service nutrients that fight against a form of biological damage called oxidation—a chemical reaction that occurs when oxygen latches onto substances that have left themselves exposed to attack.

With oxidation come the inevitable party crashers—free radicals—that do harm to whatever cells are in their way. This destruction escalates into chain reactions that eventually can even alter the genetic makeup of cells. Scientists now think free radicals are formed by pollution, cigarette smoke, even sunlight. It's been said that we have never needed antioxidant protection more than we do now.

In addition to their regular duty, several nutrients act as antioxidants. The best-known of these are vitamins C and E and beta-carotene (though beta-carotene's primary benefits may not stem from its antioxidant role). In addition, selenium and copper are essential components of enzymes needed for antioxidants. Other nutrients now being credited with antioxidant properties include riboflavin, magnesium, manganese, zinc, and another carotenoid called lycopene.

We know antioxidants work to prevent certain reactions from taking place, but what proof do we have that antioxidants really prevent disease? Although research has suggested tantalizing connections, there is still disagreement over just how important antioxidants are.

Some researchers say antioxidant nutrients not only protect against chronic diseases like cancer and heart disease, but also boost immune function and combat aging, which may simply be the body's response to repeated assaults by free radicals. Others disagree, but there's little doubt that antioxidants are beneficial to health to some degree. And some conditions we've traditionally associated with aging may not necessarily be inevitable.

Vitamin E, in particular, has shown the strongest results in protection against heart disease, most likely by preventing the formation of the more

Anti-Rust Protection

Oxidation may sound exotic, but you encounter it every day. Whenever anything metal rusts, that's an oxidation reaction. An oil that turns rancid is another example, as is an apple cut open and left in the open air—the brown you see is the result of oxidation.

How do you prevent the apple from turning brown? As any beginning cook knows, you dip it in lemon juice. And what magical ingredient does lemon juice possess? Vitamin C. Aha! So vitamin C must be an antioxidant. There are others, too. And just as you wouldn't want a car without any anti-rust protection, you wouldn't want to go through life without antioxidant protection. Fortunately, the antioxidant nutrients are there. The question is whether you get enough of them.

dangerous oxidized form of LDL cholesterol. Vitamin C appears to be a jack-of-all-trades, with links to lower rates of cancer, heart disease, and cataracts. Beta-carotene, on the other hand, has been riding a roller-coaster of evidence as to whether it protects against certain cancers and heart disease (see "The Study That Rocked the Nutrition World"). Despite mostly strong research results, particularly with lung cancer, some are skeptical of beta-carotene's role because most of the evidence came out of studies with fruits and vegetables, not simply beta-carotene supplements. It has become increasingly clear that other substances in fruits and vegetables may be just as important. (See discussion of phytochemicals, pages 31–32.)

TO SUPPLEMENT OR NOT?

That truly *is* the question these days. Although nutritionists like to insist on "food first," that isn't necessarily the end of the story. With smart supplementation, you may be able to make a good diet better or at least provide a measure of insurance against a deficit, but don't expect supplements to do too much.

Supplements, by definition, are there to *supplement* a diet, not substitute for it. Pills can't provide you with the disease-fighting phytochemicals that are in foods. Moreover, they certainly can't make a high-fat, low-fiber diet a healthy one. Downing single nutrients in large amounts can be risky because of the interactions among nutrients. That's why a multivitamin-mineral supplement may be best for most people, with exceptions for certain key nutrients.

The Study That Rocked the Nutrition World

For most, the news went in one ear and out the other. But for nutritionists, the news in 1994 that a major study found antioxidants did *not* protect against cancer was akin to heresy. The six-year study of male smokers in Finland found no protection from lung cancer for those taking vitamin E, beta-carotene, or both. Almost inconceivably, the beta-carotene group suffered *more* lung cancer, and the vitamin E group suffered more bleeding-type strokes. Not exactly what was expected.

But hold on just a minute. There are many caveats here. For one, these were heavy smokers, who may have already done too much damage to be repaired by just six years of antioxidants. And the vitamin E dose (50 milligrams) was not in the 100- to 400-milligram range considered by many to be protective.

The findings of *more* cancer are disturbing, but even the researchers consider it a statistical fluke. The stroke finding is not totally unexpected, considering that vitamin E can thin the blood.

Overall, it simply means that we don't have all the answers yet. It may mean that these antioxidants have no impact on lung cancer but might on other cancers, or it may well prove that the beneficial substance in fruits and vegetables is something other than beta-carotene. That argues against supplements and for eating more fruits and vegetables. You can't argue with that.

Who might benefit from supplements? You'll notice that unless they fall into one of the special categories listed, men as a group are noticeably absent from this roster. However, men who do not eat a balanced diet and are worried about their nutritional status certainly might also benefit from a multivitamin-mineral supplement. They're best off seeking out one of the new for-

When to Take Supplements

Even the experts don't agree on when to take supplements. That's because some nutrients are best absorbed with food (most vitamins) and some are best absorbed on an empty stomach (most minerals). You could alternate, of course, to give each a fair chance, but most nutritionists think it doesn't make that much difference when you take them. What about morning or night? It makes little difference. Just choose which time of day is easier for you to remember, and stick with it.

mulas especially formulated for men that contain no iron.

◆ *Infants* need a source of iron when they reach the age of six months. Breast milk provides very little, and by this time, their body stores are depleted. Fortified cereal or formula fills the bill. A fluoride supplement is also recommended, to prevent dental decay.

◆ *Children* usually get what they need from their diet. If their eating habits tend toward long jags or if they are vegetarians, a multivitamin-mineral supplement can provide insurance.

◆ *Pregnant women and women planning to conceive* are good candidates for a multivitamin-mineral supplement. It's wise to be sure your nutrient levels are optimal *before* becoming pregnant. This is particularly important in the case of folate, as low levels are linked to birth defects that occur in the first few weeks after conception—often before a woman even knows she is pregnant. It's also important to meet your body's increased need for the vitamins B_6, C, and D and the minerals calcium, copper, iron, and zinc.

◆ *Breast-feeding women* are also candidates. Although their increased nutrient requirements can largely be met by the extra food needed to meet their increased calorie needs, a supplement can help insure against depletion of the vitamins B_6, C, and D, and the minerals calcium, magnesium, and zinc. Calcium needs may dictate a separate supplement.

◆ *Vegans and children who are vegetarians* may not get all the nutrients their bodies need. Most vegetarians are no more likely to need a supplement than anyone else, but the exceptions may be growing children and adult vegans (who also shun dairy and eggs in addition to meat, fish, and poultry). They may need other sources of vitamin B_{12}, vitamin D, calcium, iron, and zinc.

◆ *Seniors* over 50 need more of some nutrients and less of others, so they shouldn't pop pills indiscriminately. They need more folate and vitamins B_6, B_{12}, and D, though the body may have its own mechanisms for filling the B_{12} and folate gaps. Some also think it's wise for seniors to up their intake of the antioxidant vitamins C and E and beta-carotene. Postmenopausal women almost certainly need a calcium supplement. Based on the latest National Institutes of Health recommendations, women in this group require 1,000 to 1,500 milligrams per day.

Guidelines for Savvy Supplementing. Once you've decided whether or not you want to supplement, you have to choose from the rows upon rows of vitamins, minerals, and scads of other more questionable substances thrown in-between. It can be daunting, but don't be swayed by clever advertising or scare tactics. Strict rules govern what's allowed on supplement labels, but not what's printed in promotional literature displayed nearby. Wild claims made in places other than the label are suspect. Here are some helpful tips to guide you through the maze of supplements:

◆ Check the supplement for which nutrients are present. Key nutrients to look for include vitamin B_6, folate, magnesium, and zinc. Consider it a plus if the supplement contains some of the less popular, but no less important, minerals like boron, chromium, copper, and manganese.

◆ Choose a supplement with close to 100 percent of the RDA for most nutrients listed. Up to 250

Supplement Labeling

In 1994, the government passed legislation covering the labeling of dietary supplements. Despite a concerted campaign by the supplement industry to portray the Food and Drug Administration as champing at the bit to break into homes and seize supplements out of unsuspecting hands, no such scenario was ever going to happen.

Instead, the new "pill bill" allows for specific health claims on the label, and even general statements of a nutrient's role in the body. Literature will be allowed to be displayed, but must be balanced and truthful.

The new rules will require expiration dates on all supplements. New ingredients will require safety testing but not any assurance that they work. Nor will any existing supplement or ingredient require testing for safety or effectiveness. It seems buyer beware will still be the order of the day, even in 1997, when all this becomes mandatory.

percent for water-soluble vitamins (C and the B complex) is OK. Avoid those that contain unbalanced amounts of key nutrients, since many of them work together.

- Don't fall victim to tunnel vision—looking to single supplements for each individual nutrient. A multivitamin-mineral supplement embraces more nutrients than you could swallow with single supplements, and you're less likely to have an imbalance of nutrients that creates the opportunity for large doses of one nutrient to interfere with the absorption of another nutrient.
- Don't look to a multivitamin-mineral supplement to provide you with any significant calcium or magnesium. If much of either is added, it simply makes too large a pill to swallow. Instead, calcium is one case when a single supplement makes sense. Choose calcium alone, or a calcium–vitamin D combo (*if* you aren't also taking a multivitamin with vitamin D). Look to food sources such as tuna and wheat germ to boost your magnesium intake.
- Try to choose a calcium supplement with smaller doses (500 or 600 milligrams) that you can take two or three times during the day; spreading out the doses improves absorption and lessens the likelihood of constipation.
- Don't choose a calcium supplement made of bone meal or dolomite. Though some tests show them to be safe, others reveal the presence of lead and other toxic metals. Choose calcium carbonate or calcium citrate supplements over calcium gluconate ones. There is more available calcium in them.
- Look for a multivitamin-mineral supplement *without* iron if you're a man or a postmenopausal woman. You probably do not need the extra iron, and there is a small chance it could be harmful if you've inherited the gene for iron-overload disease.

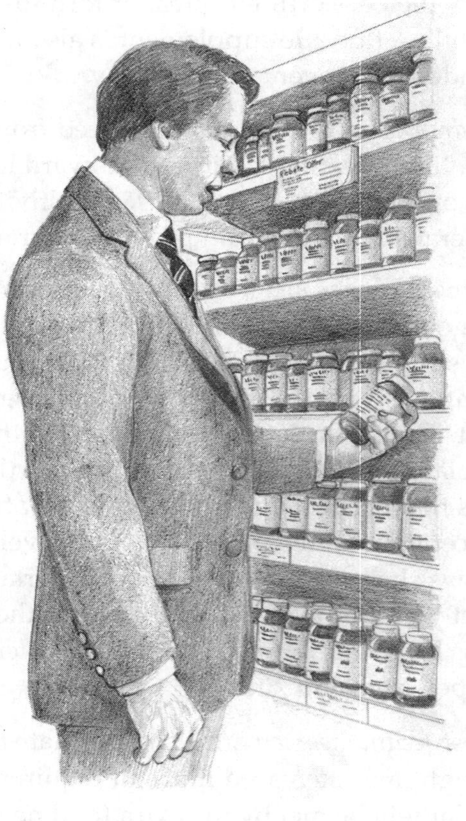

- Look for a multivitamin-mineral supplement with beta-carotene as its vitamin A source; it's safer than vitamin A as retinol. Be aware, however, that supplements that boast "with beta-carotene" often lump it together with vitamin A on the label, making it impossible to tell how much beta-carotene you're actually getting.

- Choose a supplement with an expiration date. Vitamins and minerals can deteriorate over time, losing their effectiveness. Vitamin A is notorious for this. Deterioration happens sooner if you keep them in the humidity of the bathroom. Find a drier place.

- Don't waste money on supplements that contain numerous unrecognized nutrients, such as lecithin, pangamic acid (sometimes misrepresented as "vitamin B_{15}"), choline, orotic acid, rutin, and other made-up vitamins ("vitamin B_{17}" or "vitamin U"). Some of these are required by other animals but not humans, some are made in the body, and some are simply nonessential nontoxic substances. They aren't harmful, but too many of them can add unnecessary bulk, making a supplement harder to swallow.

- Don't pay extra for inconsequential attributes, such as "natural," "chelated," or "time-release." Vitamins E and C may be more potent in their natural forms, but the difference is not significant. Some, like folate, are actually better absorbed in their synthetic form. Time-release is primarily a gimmick. In the case of calcium, time your own release by spacing out your doses. As for niacin, the time-release form of nicotinic acid is dangerous, as it can be toxic to the liver. Even claims of "no sugar or starch" are meaningless; starch in a supplement can actually improve nutrient absorption.

- Don't assume a brand name and higher price are any indication of quality. Although some generic and no-name brands may not dissolve as well as name brands, generally what you see on the label is what you get. Some private-label brands are identical to name brands but are less than half the price.

- Err on the side of caution if you decide to take antioxidant supplements. You should be able to glean benefits without any risks by taking 250 milligrams of vitamin C, 100 international units of vitamin E, and 3 to 6 milligrams of beta-carotene.

- Don't use supplements as an excuse to eat a poor diet. Don't let yourself develop a false sense of security that you're "covered."

WHOLE FOODS AND PHYTOCHEMICALS

Just when we thought we knew it all, along come phytochemicals to prove that we don't. Our parents and grandparents witnessed vitamin discoveries in the first half of this century. The next generation came of age when more and more minerals were being recognized for their importance. Now, our children and grandchildren will explore the myriad of mysterious phytochemicals in foods.

The word *phytochemicals* refers to protective compounds found in plants. They are neither vitamins nor minerals, for they are not essential to life, but they may hold the key to optimal health. Genistein in soy foods, polyphenols in tea, psoralens in celery, sulforaphane in broccoli, allylic sulfides in garlic, and ellagic acid in strawberries—these are just a few of the exciting discoveries of the past few years.

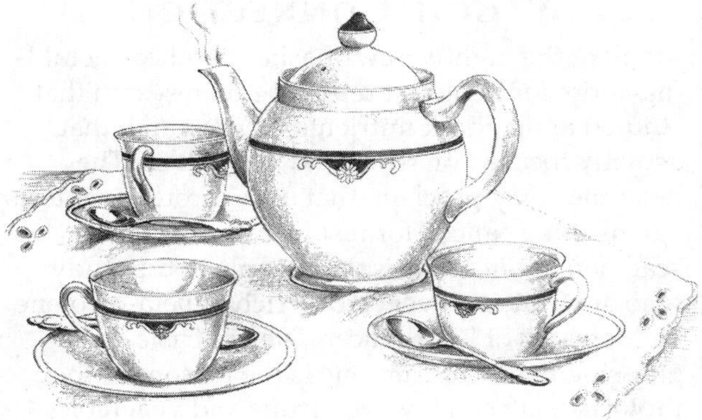

Scientists are busy trying to identify these and other phytochemicals and to discover just what they do. The task is daunting. In an orange alone, it's been estimated there are 150 phytochemicals that provide various benefits, such as cancer prevention, cholesterol-lowering properties, and heart disease protection. Some researchers have futuristic notions of isolating some of these chemicals and then concentrating them into a single super-duper protective cocktail. However, it's premature to be so optimistic.

To benefit from phytochemicals, you need only to start eating more fruits and vegetables. You've probably heard the call to eat five servings per day. That's just the beginning. The real goal, say experts, is to eat five to nine servings of fruits and vegetables a day. Until now, researchers have focused on the beta-carotene and fiber in fruits and vegetables as the reason for their protective effect, but maybe that's not all there is to it. Maybe there's something else they have in common. Enter phytochemicals.

Carotenoids, other than beta-carotene, have begun to receive more attention. A lot of the same foods rich in beta-carotene are rich in other carotenoids that appear to have anticancer effects as well. Lycopene is one of the most promising. A study just out of Italy suggests that people who eat a lot of tomatoes may have less risk of cancers of the gastrointestinal tract. Tomatoes are rich in lycopene.

The Fruit and Veggie Connection

Many of the nightly news flashes you hear heralding antioxidants aren't reporting on research that studied antioxidant nutrients, but research that actually focused on fruits and vegetables. The headlines may proclaim that beta-carotene protects against lung cancer, for instance, but all the researchers *really* know is that people in the study who ate fruits and vegetables rich in beta-carotene had less risk of lung cancer. They're basically guessing that beta-carotene is the reason for the protective effect. However, fruits and vegetables are also rich in other carotenoids and phytochemicals we don't even know about. Even if we did, it might be the particular mix of phytochemicals in those foods that's protective. So why not just eat more fruits and vegetables? Why not, indeed.

Of course, tomatoes are rich in vitamin C, also. So, which is it? Maybe both; maybe neither; maybe fiber is part of the equation as well; and maybe the protective effect works only when these substances are all combined in the exact way they are in tomatoes. Perhaps the idea of extracting out "the good stuff" is naive. Of course, if you just eat more fruits and vegetables, it won't matter. That way, you can cash in on the benefits from all the phytochemicals—known and unknown.

GUIDELINES

Okay, let's get down to business. All these facts and figures probably have you yearning for some simple directions. Several health and governmental organizations have put together recommendations to help you implement the research in nutrition and actually start putting the science to work for you.

DIETARY GUIDELINES

Although there are many guidelines for healthy eating, the simplest and most comprehensive are what's known as the Dietary Guidelines for Americans, which are issued and periodically revised by the U.S. Department of Agriculture (USDA) and the U.S. Department of Health and Human Services. Think of these seven directions as the seven wonders of the nutrition world.

Eat a variety of foods. This may seem obvious, but it's probably the most important prevention tip you can remember. No one food is perfect. No one food has it all. You can be assured of obtaining the best possible array of nutrients, getting the most important of the yet unknown phytochemicals, and avoiding too much of a single natural toxin by eating the widest variety of whole foods you can.

Maintain a healthy weight. Notice this doesn't say "ideal" weight. That's because what's healthy for one person might not work for another. You probably know what weight feels best for you. If you're overweight, try to lose; obesity is a risk factor for many serious diseases, such as high blood pressure, heart disease, stroke, cancer, and diabetes. (For more on weight control, see Chapter 2.)

Choose a diet low in fat, saturated fat, and cholesterol. Cutting down on fat and saturated fat can help you prevent heart disease, stroke, high blood pressure, diabetes, and probably certain cancers. Cutting back on cholesterol is just a bonus. Only certain people are sensitive to its effects, and if you cut the other two, cholesterol usually takes care of itself.

Choose a diet with plenty of vegetables, fruits, and grain products. Follow this advice and you'll find it easier to eat a low-fat diet, because complex carbohydrates are what should be replacing the fat in your diet. If you take this advice to heart, you'll automatically take care of your fiber needs, too. Besides, you can't get those all-important disease-preventing phytochemicals if you don't eat fruits and vegetables.

Use sugars only in moderation. Although not the villain it's rumored to be, it's no saint either. A diet filled with sugary foods is likely to be high in fat and short on nutrients. It's not good for your teeth and may rob you of chromium.

Use salt and sodium only in moderation. Again, its reputation exceeds reality. Most people don't have a problem with sodium, but because we don't know who among us is the one person in ten whose blood pressure is sensitive to it, it's recommended that everyone take it easy with the salt shaker. Avoiding processed foods as much as possible also helps.

If you drink alcoholic beverages, do so in moderation. This is a controversial one. No one wants to advocate a drinking habit, because there are those who cannot handle it, but it's true that many studies have shown one drink per day can be good for your heart. Red wine may be best of all, because of the extra phytochemicals it contains. However, alcohol carries calories with no nutrients, so moderation more than makes sense. In excess, it can damage the liver; in pregnant women, it is a time-bomb waiting to go off; and combining it with medications is dangerous.

FOOD GUIDE PYRAMID

Forget the Four Food Groups you probably had drilled into you as a kid. The new look is triangular. For an at-a-glance look at good nutrition, check out the USDA Food Guide Pyramid.

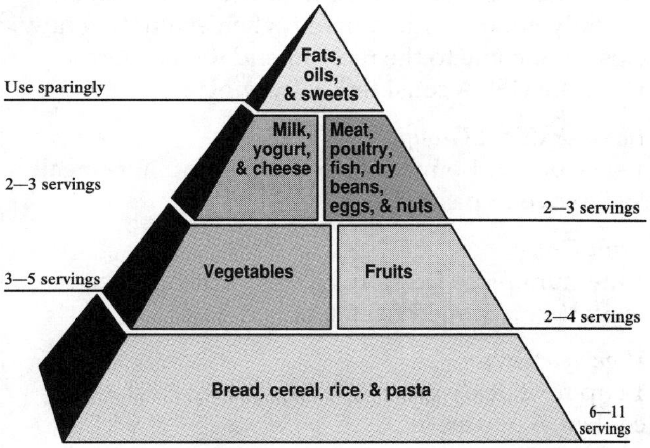

How does it work? Build your diet from the base up; it should be as bottom-heavy as the pyramid is. That is, base your diet on whole grains and cereals, heavily supplemented with fruits and vegetables. Relegate protein sources to a backseat role. You can include meat, but skip half-pound portions; think of meat as a condiment, not the centerpiece of your meal. Finally, fats, oils, and sweets can top off a healthy diet, if kept to a minimum.

There are some problems with this pyramid as the paragon of a healthy diet. Lumping legumes and nuts in with meats and eggs does the former an injustice. The nonanimal protein sources are healthier than meat, poultry, and fish; they have less saturated fat and more fiber. Also, nowhere on the pyramid does it indicate that your choices from the meat and milk groups should be low-fat choices—lean meats, skim milk, and low-fat yogurt.

Still, the pyramid does convey the concept of proportion that earlier guides did not. That's the biggest change Americans need to make to convert the average diet into a healthful, preventive

A Serving By Any Other Name

If you seem daunted by the 6 to 11 servings recommended for the bottom layer of the Pyramid, don't be. Often, what you eat at one sitting may constitute two or three pyramid servings. When it comes to counting servings of fruits and vegetables, however, most people overestimate what they eat. Be brutally honest with yourself when evaluating how close you come to the recommendations. Here's what the USDA considers a "serving":

Bread & Cereal Group
1 slice bread; 1 ounce cold cereal; ½ cup hot cereal; ½ cup rice or pasta

Fruit Group
1 medium piece fresh fruit; ½ cup cut-up fresh fruit; ½ cup canned fruit; 6 ounces juice

Vegetable Group
1 cup fresh leafy greens; ½ cup cut-up fresh or cooked; 6 ounces juice

Meat, Poultry, and Legume Group
2–3 ounces meat, poultry, or fish (½ cup cooked legumes, 1 egg, or 2 tablespoons peanut butter count as 1 ounce of meat)

Milk Group
1 cup milk or yogurt; 1½ ounces cheese (2 ounces if processed)

one. Right now, the average American eats according to a decidedly top-heavy pyramid.

MEDITERRANEAN DIET PYRAMID

Not everyone is enthralled with the USDA pyramid. Its biggest drawback is that it continues to promote the traditional American way of eating. As an alternative, another pyramid was jointly devised and endorsed by the World Health Organization, Harvard School of Public Health, and Oldways Preservation & Exchange Trust (a private nonprofit organization). This one banks on the notion that the traditional Mediterranean way of eating is protective against heart disease and other chronic diseases. (Modern Mediterranean diets, on the other hand, are not so healthy, having adopted many of the pitfalls that mar our own eating.)

You'll notice the base of the pyramid is pretty much the same, except that some other grain

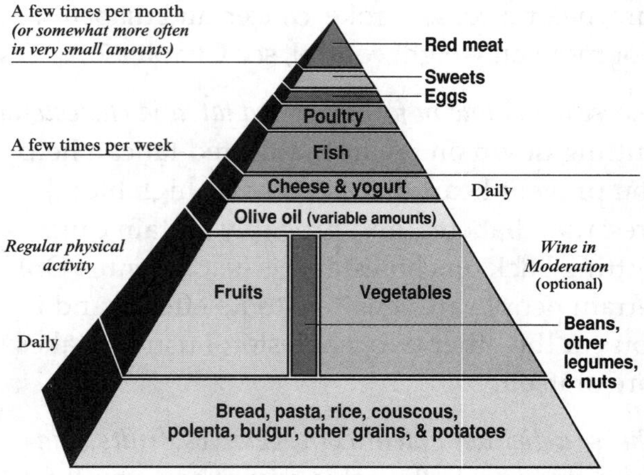

© 1994 Oldways Preservation & Exchange Trust

dishes such as bulgur, couscous, and polenta are also emphasized. In addition, legumes and nuts are given their rightful place nearer the base of the pyramid.

However, it's the top half that differs so drastically from the USDA pyramid. It heavily promotes olive oil as the fat of choice. It favors cheese over meats, and ranks fish, poultry, and eggs in that order. How this guide really parts company with the USDA original is by rating red meat even less desirable than sweets. It also breaks ground by advocating regular exercise and wine in moderation.

Some have criticized this pyramid because it doesn't reduce overall fat. However, the design is based on population studies showing that people from the Mediterranean ring of countries—Greece, southern Italy, Turkey, Spain, Morocco, and southern France—suffer less heart disease, despite eating a diet higher in fat than Americans eat. While the monounsaturated fat in olive oil and nuts may be responsible, the fact is, no one knows what the magic ingredient is. A recent study fingered tomatoes as being protective.

Perhaps what's important is not just the types of foods eaten, but the way food is eaten in the traditional Mediterranean style—slowly, in the company of family and friends, with red wine. Whatever it is, it is delicious and certainly worth trying in the name of prevention.

MEAL PLANNING

Even the guidelines, which are supposed to help us, can be a little daunting when it comes right down to deciding what to cook for dinner tonight and what to buy at the supermarket. Planning smart menus and shopping wisely are crucial links in the good nutrition chain. The government's recent mandate of standardized labels can help, as can a few fat-cutting menu ideas and cooking techniques.

FOOD LABELING

Don't you hate it? You're all set to enjoy a gooey, rich chocolate bar, and there it is, staring you in the face—the new food label. Even when you have no desire to know, those "Nutrition Facts" can't be ignored. Most nutritionists think that means we've come a long way, and indeed, we have.

Most of us, when we aren't sneaking a candy bar or splurging on ice cream, are grateful for whatever information we can get about what we eat, because we really do want to eat right. Though the new labels are easier to understand than before, they can still be confusing, partly because of what they *don't* reveal.

You may have noticed that the new food labels, which made their debut in May 1994, are now on more than 90 percent of packaged foods. But besides being mandatory, the focus has changed. Before, the emphasis was on vitamin content, reflecting the concern with nutrient deficiencies in the first half of this century. Now, however, we're more worried about diseases of excess, in particular heart disease and cancer. So the new food labels reveal less about vitamins and much more about fat content.

What's in an acronym? Scratch the acronym USRDA from your vocabulary. It's history. Labels now use the Daily Value (DV) as the standard. The actual numbers are still the same, but the name and the way it is used has changed.

The percentage of the Daily Value (%DV) listed on the label for each nutrient shows a food's relative contribution of nutrients to a 2,000-calorie diet, but don't get fooled by this seemingly simple concept. If you eat less than 2,000 calories, like many women, your DVs are really lower, making the %DVs in a food higher for you than what's shown on the label. For men and

QUICK GUIDE TO LABEL READING

Here's a survival guide for at-a-glance label reading as you're rushing through the aisles.

- Check the DVs. In general, a %DV under 5 indicates the food is low in that nutrient. A %DV over 20 is high. Look for high %DVs for vitamins, minerals, and fiber, but low %DVs for fat, saturated fat, cholesterol, and sodium.
- Check for grams of fat. It's easier to interpret than %DV for fat, especially if you know your maximum fat grams. Compare *Calories From Fat* or *Fat Calories* to Calories, to see just how much of the total calories are from fat.
- Check for fiber. Don't forget to consider this when comparing foods. If you're confused by labels proclaiming "high in fiber" or "whole grain," check this value to get the real story. Your aim is 20 to 35 grams per day.
- Check the serving size. Be sure the calories and fat listed are for the amount you usually eat; if not, do some quick math in your head (if you eat double the amount listed, then double all the numbers). If you're comparing foods, be sure you're comparing equal serving sizes.
- Check the ingredient list. It's not part of the "Nutrition Facts" label, but it's still a treasure trove of information on what's in a product. Remember, whatever is present in the greatest quantity is listed first, then on down in order of weight. If crackers, for instance, are labeled "with whole wheat," check the ingredient list. If whole wheat is listed far down the label, you can be sure there isn't much of it in the product. And if partially hydrogenated oils are present, then *trans* fats are too.

athletes, who probably eat more than 2,000 calories, their DVs are higher, so the %DVs in a food are really lower. Clear as mud, right?

To make matters worse, in most cases (for example, vitamins, minerals, and fiber) the higher the %DV, the better. However, for fat, cholesterol, and sodium, you want a low %DV. Don't make the mistake of thinking a food with 25%DV for fat is a nutritional bargain because it's under 30%. Truth is, it has nothing to do with the 30 percent that refers to fat as a percent of calories. The %DV for fat on a label refers to how much of your daily total of fat this one food contributes. A %DV of 25 means that this particular food provides one quarter of your fat allowance for a whole day. That's a lot of fat for one food.

If you want to avoid the %DV confusion, just check out the grams of fat. It's listed in regular type right next to the boldface words *Total Fat*—easy to miss unless you look for it. It tells you all you really need to know. If you want, you can also check out the number of calories from fat after *Calories from Fat* (on smaller packages, it may be listed as *Fat Calories*).

Supermarket schizophrenia. If all this is too confusing, don't worry. You don't even need to understand it, if all you want to do is compare foods. Just compare numbers, but be careful what you're comparing. Although serving sizes are supposedly standardized now, the government's idea of a serving size may not be yours. Worse, some foods have schizophrenic serving sizes; they're different depending on the version of the food. Be especially careful of diet or "light" foods—their serving size is often twice what the regular version of the food is. For example, a serving size of regular bread is considered one slice, but light bread must use a serving size of two slices, even though you wouldn't necessarily eat any more of the light bread than regular bread.

Health claims become legit. It was novel—and even shocking to some—ten years ago, when Kellogg first aired its All-Bran ads that linked a high-fiber diet with less risk of "certain types of cancer." It was ground-breaking, and not technically legal at the time, because it made a health claim for a food. However, the Food and Drug Administration (FDA) tolerated it, and more followed, for better or worse.

Now, finally, there are guidelines that allow for seven specific health claims linking diet and disease to appear on food labels that link specific nutrients with specific diseases. The following pairings of nutrients with health claims are the only ones now allowed on food labels:

- Dietary fat with increased risk of cancer
- Dietary saturated fat and cholesterol with increased risk of heart disease
- Sodium with increased risk of high blood pressure
- Fruits and vegetables with reduced risk of cancer
- The fiber in fruits, vegetables, and grains with reduced risk of cancer
- The soluble fiber in fruits, vegetables, and grains with reduced risk of heart disease
- Calcium with reduced risk of osteoporosis

Reading between the lines. One thing the new labels will not tell you directly is how many *trans* fatty acids there are in a food. (These are unsaturated fats that have been transformed through hydrogenation into a foreign, and some say harmful, form.) You may be able to figure it out, however, for those foods that list saturated fat and unsaturated fat (poly- or mono-) as well as total fat.

Even though *trans* fats are unsaturated, they act like saturated fats in the body, so the FDA does not allow them to be included in the unsaturated fat total listed on the label. They're not counted as saturated fats either. So if the grams of saturated fat plus the grams of unsaturated fat do not add up to the grams of total fat listed, the difference is roughly the amount of *trans* fats.

If the necessary information isn't there, or you don't feel like being a sleuth, check the ingredi-

Why Light Became Right.

Did you notice the big name change? Some companies, instead of reformulating their products, simply renamed their products this past year. That's because they couldn't meet strict new definitions. For example, Pringles' *Light* Potato Chips apparently didn't have one-third fewer calories than the regular potato chips, so they mysteriously became *Right* Potato Chips.

Here are some of the more common descriptive words that now have specific definitions:

- *Reduced*—contains 25 percent less than the regular product. (*Reduced fat* means 25 percent less fat than the regular version.)
- *Light* (including *lite*)—contains less than one third of the calories of the regular version, or half the fat (if 50 percent or more of the calories come from fat).
- *Free* (including *without, no,* and *zero*)—meaning depends on the specific claim: *Calorie-free* means less than 5 calories per serving; *Sugar-free* means less than 0.5 grams per serving; and *Fat-free* means less than 0.5 grams per serving.
- *Low* (including *little* and *few*)—meaning depends on the specific claim: *Low-fat* means 3 grams or less per serving; *Low-sodium* means less than 140 milligrams per serving; and *Low cholesterol* means less than 20 milligrams per serving.
- *High*—contains 20 percent or more of the DV for that nutrient. (*High-fiber* means 5 grams or more per serving.)
- *Lean* (for meats)—Less than 10 grams fat *plus* less than 4.5 grams saturated fat *plus* less than 95 milligrams cholesterol per 3½-ounce serving.
- *Extra lean* (for meats)—Less than 5 grams fat *plus* less than 2 grams saturated fat *plus* less than 95 milligrams cholesterol per 3½-ounce serving.

ent label. If partially hydrogenated fats are listed, then the product contains *trans* fatty acids, and the closer it is to the beginning of the list, the more there is in the food.

Good news for food-allergy sufferers. Companies now have to be more specific in their ingredient lists, making life easier for people who are allergic to certain ingredients and must ferret out foods containing them. For example, companies can no longer list protein hydrolysates as "flavorings." They must be listed by name, such as hydrolyzed wheat gluten or hydrolyzed casein. Color additives must also be listed by name, such as yellow dye #5 (tartrazine).

The juice truth. Companies must now 'fess up to the percentage of juice in their juice products. However, it's easy to be fooled if you don't check the ingredient list and nutrition label. A juice can be labeled as 100 percent juice but contain mostly "filler" juices—white grape juice, apple juice, or pear juice—which provide little nutrition and, in the case of apple juice, can even trigger diarrhea. Check the ingredient list to know what you're getting. Then check the nutrition facts to see what nutrients, if any, are present.

CUTTING BACK ON FAT

By now, you've realized that cutting back on the fat you eat is one of the most important changes you can make in your diet if you want to prevent chronic diseases like heart disease and cancer. But how?

Start slowly. Don't try to cut back all at once; it won't work. A good example is milk. Don't try to switch from whole milk to skim milk in one fell swoop. You'll gag. Instead, switch to two percent milk first and stay with it until you get used to it, even if it takes months. Then switch to one percent milk and allow yourself even more time to get used to it. Finally, make the switch to skim milk. You may notice the difference, but you won't mind it, because you've allowed yourself to get used to a low-fat taste. This is a switch worth making, especially if you drink a lot of milk.

Cutting Fat? Start with Milk

Type of Milk	Fat (*grams*)*	Calories*
Whole (3.3 percent fat)	8.2	150
2 percent fat	4.7	121
1 percent fat	2.6	102
Skim	0.4	86

*Values are for an 8-ounce serving.

Counting all grams. You hear a lot about keeping your fat intake to less than 30 percent of calories, but does it mean every food you eat has to be less than 30 percent fat? Not at all. It means your overall diet—as it averages out over three days, or even a week—should be less than 30 percent calories from fat. Some days can be over, if other days are under. Of course, some meals will be over, and others under. It makes sense, then, that some foods will be way over, because other foods are practically fat-free.

The easiest way to keep track of all this is to count the number of fat grams you eat. You don't need to do it forever, just long enough so you have an idea of the fat content of foods and when you're close to going overboard. If you consistently eat about the same number of calories, you just need to find out your fat gram limit once (see "Instant Maximum Fat Gram Calculator"). Then, no more calculations, just simple counting.

Instant Maximum Fat Gram Calculator

Rather than going through the contortions and calculations of figuring what the upper limit of your daily fat budget is, use this quick chart. The maximums listed here represent how many grams of fat make 30 percent of the corresponding daily calorie intake. The numbers are rounded off, but the slight differences don't really matter; it would be almost impossible to follow a diet that precise.

Calories per Day	Maximum Fat Grams per Day
1,200	40
1,500	50
1,800	60
2,000	67
2,500	83

Remember, however, that this number is the *maximum* grams of fat allowed per day, on average, if your goal is 30 percent of calories from fat. Ideally, you might want to aim for even less.

Tips for trimming fat. To reduce the number of fat grams that you eat, try some of the following fat-cutting hints.

- Trim all meats of visible fat.
- Buy lean cuts: those with *round* or *loin* in the name (sirloin, tenderloin, top round).
- Choose *select* or *choice* grade cuts, not *prime*, and save one third to one half the fat.
- Include more fish and poultry (without skin) in place of meat.
- Cut back on added fats: margarine, mayonnaise, and salad dressings. Regular margarine has the same amount of fat and calories as butter; it's just less saturated.
- Switch to a diet margarine and reduced-fat or fat-free mayonnaise and salad dressings to truly save fat grams.
- Cook in nonstick pots and pans, using no added fat. Remember, each tablespoon of butter or margarine you throw in the sauté pan adds about 12 grams of fat, and each tablespoon of oil adds 14 grams of fat. You can also use vegetable sprays such as Pam, or try sautéing with broth, soup stock, or juice.

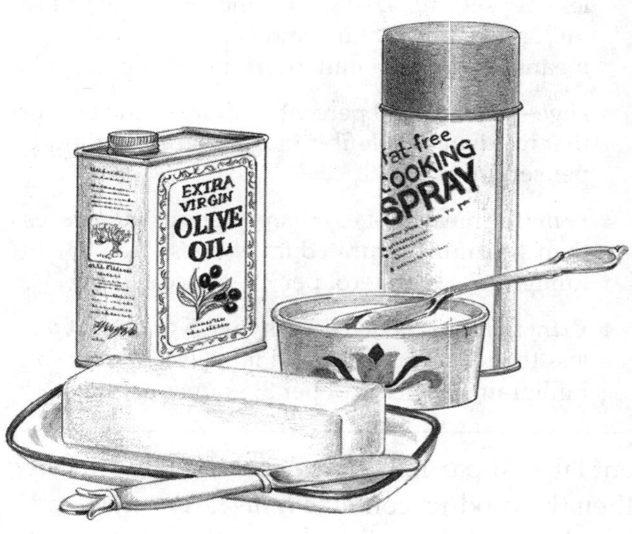

- Switch to low-fat or nonfat dairy products. Experiment with reduced-fat cheeses; some brands are better than others. Substitute low-fat yogurt for sour cream, or try a fat-free sour cream.

- If you're unsure of the fat in breads, crackers, and muffins, use the napkin test: Let the product sit on a napkin or paper towel for an hour or so; if it leaves a grease stain, there's too much fat in it.
- Snack smart. Munch on pretzels instead of potato chips. Don't dip. Buy low-fat tortilla chips, and dip in salsa instead.
- Have your salad at the end of your meal. It may take away your desire for rich desserts. If not, try fruit for a satisfyingly sweet dessert.
- At restaurants—especially fast-food joints—beware breaded and fried items. Ask for sauces to be served on the side or not at all.
- Beware the fat traps at salad bars. Steer clear of cold salads such as potato, macaroni, tuna, and coleslaw; they're usually loaded with mayonnaise.
- Don't automatically reach for fat-free foods in the supermarket. For only a gram or two of fat, reduced-fat foods often have much more flavor, making you much more likely to switch permanently.

FITTING IN FIBER

Upping your intake of fiber can be easier than you think, and you already know the benefits can be great (reduced risk of heart disease and cancer to name only two). Boosting your fiber intake can go hand-in-hand with cutting back the fat, as long as you do it right. Here are some tips for filling up with fiber.

- Switch to the whole-grain version of the foods you normally eat: brown rice instead of white rice; potatoes with the skin instead of peeled; whole-wheat bread instead of white bread; whole-wheat or lupin pasta instead of semolina pasta; whole-wheat or buckwheat pancakes instead of regular; bran muffins instead of blueberry muffins; Graham crackers instead of buttery crackers; and so on. Then try adding new grains: barley, millet, triticale, and quinoa for extra fiber and pizzazz.

FIBER SAFETY HINTS TO REMEMBER

- Don't double your fiber intake overnight. It takes time for your body to adjust. If you go too fast, your intestines will react, and you'll have to cut back. So go slow.
- Be sure to increase your fluid intake along with your fiber. Too much bran without enough water can be dangerous.
- Experiment. If one high-fiber food doesn't agree with you, it doesn't mean they'll all give you trouble. If beans give you too much gas, try lentils.
- If gas is a real problem, try Beano, a product that breaks down some of the fiber for you. There's some disagreement as to how well it works, but it's worth a try.

- Start your day with bran—either a cereal or a muffin (if it's not too high in fat). You could be a third of the way to your daily goal if you choose your cereal wisely.
- Slice up dried apricots, prunes, or other fruits to add to your cereal; dried fruits are an excellent source of fiber.
- Opt for the whole fruit instead of juice whenever you can. Juicing removes most of the fiber, especially if the juice is pulp-free.
- Fruits with seeds are a powerhouse of fiber; raspberries and blackberries are the richest in fiber, but strawberries, blueberries, figs, and elderberries are chock full.
- Top your sandwiches with spinach instead of lettuce; add tomato, avocado, or sweet peppers. Use your imagination, but get some fiber-filled veggies in there.
- Find new ways to add vegetables: Add lightly steamed vegetables to spaghetti sauce, layer vegetables in your casseroles, or add vegetable purees to soups, sauces, and casseroles when cut-up veggies won't work.
- Top your salads with lentils, chick peas, green peas, and florets of broccoli.

◆ Add wheat germ into any baked product you make: cookies, brownies, muffins, quick breads, and especially pancakes. You can replace one half to one cup of flour with wheat germ (you may need to add a little extra liquid, though, and don't replace more than half of the flour).

DIETS FOR SPECIAL NEEDS

If your doctor has placed you on a special diet, don't feel singled out. If you are following a diet prescribed for heart disease, high blood pressure, or diabetes, in particular, you may need to pay more attention to planning your meals, but the advice for you is basically the same advice we all would be wise to follow.

We can't, of course, provide specific diet plans here, as they need to be individualized for particular circumstances. If you have special needs, seek out a registered dietitian (R.D.) to help you plan your meals; your doctor can help you find one. Here is some information to get you started, though.

Cholesterol-lowering diet. People refer to this diet as a "low-cholesterol diet," but that's a misnomer. Although a diet to combat heart disease usually is low in dietary cholesterol, that's not the focus. The aim is to lower levels of blood cholesterol. A cholesterol-lowering diet starts by limiting total fat (to 30 percent or less of total calories), with special emphasis on limiting saturated fat (to 8 to 10 percent of total calories). It also limits dietary cholesterol to less than 300 milligrams per day.

Saturated fats are anathema to those with heart disease, because saturated fats have a direct effect on blood cholesterol—even more of an effect than the cholesterol you eat. Saturated fats come mainly from animal foods such as meat, poultry, and dairy products. Important exceptions include the so-called tropical oils—coconut oil, palm oil, and palm kernel oil—which are vegetable oils but loaded with saturated fat. (See "Smart Alternatives to Foods with Saturated Fat" for examples of how simple changes can make a big difference.)

Besides substitutions, though, there are other heart-saving hints. Eat more fiber, particularly soluble fiber (found in oat bran, legumes, and fruits). And don't overlook garlic. Research suggests it can raise blood levels of HDL cholesterol and lower blood levels of LDL cholesterol. It may also thin the blood so that it's less likely to clot and build up as plaque on your artery walls. Here are other suggestions:

Meat

◆ Choose lean cuts of red meats—loin, round, tenderloin. Avoid organ meats.

◆ Trim all visible fat before cooking.

◆ Broil, boil, bake, or roast. Don't fry.

◆ Choose poultry. Opt for light over dark meat. Remove the skin.

◆ Choose low-fat processed meats (check label for grams of fat).

Dairy

◆ Drink skim or one percent milk or low-fat buttermilk.

◆ Choose nonfat or low-fat yogurt and cottage cheese.

◆ Limit hard and processed cheese to part-skim or reduced-fat varieties.

Breads

◆ Avoid croissants and fat-laden muffins (use the napkin test on page 39).

◆ Buy reduced-fat or low-fat crackers.

◆ Limit commercial baked goods and mixes. Bake your own.

Soups

◆ Make cream soups with skim or one percent milk.

◆ Remove any fat that rises to the surface after cooling.

Vegetables

◆ Eat them without added butter, margarine, or cheese sauces.

SMART ALTERNATIVES TO FOODS WITH SATURATED FAT

Substitutions are one way to cut back on fat without having to limit your food choices. Try these lower-fat alternatives to save yourself some fat grams.

INSTEAD OF	EAT	SAVE
Butter	**Diet margarine**	**6 grams/tablespoon**
Whole milk	**Skim milk**	**5 grams/cup**
Cheddar cheese	**Reduced-fat cheese**	**5 grams/ounce**
Sour cream	**Low-fat yogurt**	**1.5 grams/tablespoon**
Ground beef—80% lean	**Ground beef—90% lean**	**6 grams/3 ounces**
Beef—prime rib (trimmed of fat)	**Beef—eye of round**	**8 grams/3 ounces**
Chicken breast with skin	**Chicken breast, skinless**	**2 grams/3 ounces**
Chicken thigh, skinless	**Chicken breast, skinless**	**2 grams/3 ounces**
Pork—rib roast	**Pork—tenderloin**	**7 grams/3 ounces**
Premium ice cream (16% butterfat)	**Ice milk or low-fat ice cream (5% butterfat)**	**9 grams/cup**

Desserts

- Choose ice milk, low-fat ice cream, sherbet, fruit ice, Popsicles, or sorbet over regular or premium ice cream.
- Choose angel food cake, ginger snaps, graham crackers, Fig Newtons, animal crackers, or other low-fat cookies. Avoid commercial pastries. Home-baked cakes made with egg whites instead of whole eggs and vegetable oil are also lower fat.
- Use cocoa powder in baking instead of milk chocolate.

Fats/Oils

- Choose a diet tub margarine over stick margarine or butter (liquid vegetable oil should be listed first in the ingredients).
- Use vegetable oil (olive or canola preferred) in baked goods and homemade salad dressings.
- Purchase fat-free salad dressings.

Other foods can remain the same. For example, most whole-grain breads, cereal, fruit, and juices have no significant restrictions.

Low-sodium diet. This is a diet usually prescribed for people with high blood pressure. Not everyone is sensitive to salt or sodium, but it's considered prudent for everyone with high blood pressure to watch their sodium intake.

Though cutting back on salt can help, weight loss is actually the number one dietary step to take to lower blood pressure. (For more information on weight control, see Chapter 2.) Other steps include eating more fruits and vegetables to increase your potassium and fiber intake. Getting enough calcium may also be important, but that's more controversial and may only be true for some people, just like sodium.

The National Heart, Lung and Blood Institute recommends a daily sodium intake below 2,500 milligrams (about the amount in ¼ teaspoon of salt). Here's how to meet that goal:

- Check labels for salt and sodium in any form.
- Whenever you can, cook from scratch; limit your use of mixes, which are usually loaded with sodium. Remember, the more packaged and processed a food is, the more likely it is to have sodium added. Plain oats that you cook yourself, for example, have no salt, but instant oatmeal is full of it.
- Stay away from pickled, cured, or smoked foods. Especially high in sodium are luncheon meats, salami, and hot dogs.

- Soups are notoriously high in sodium. Look for reduced-sodium varieties; they taste much better than sodium-free. Better yet, for low-sodium and economical meals to last a while, make your own soups in large quantities and freeze them.
- Avoid packaged vegetables in sauce. Squirt on lemon juice for flavor.
- One of the biggest hidden sources of sodium is condiments. Ketchup, mayonnaise, and dressings are big culprits. Use them only in moderation. Other infamous salt hoarders include sauerkraut, pickles, soy sauce, bouillon, olives, and tomato juice.
- Find herbs and spices you like to substitute for the salt flavor you miss. Hot sauce can make you forget salt rather quickly (read the label to make sure it has no added salt; some brands do). Freshly ground pepper works well too.

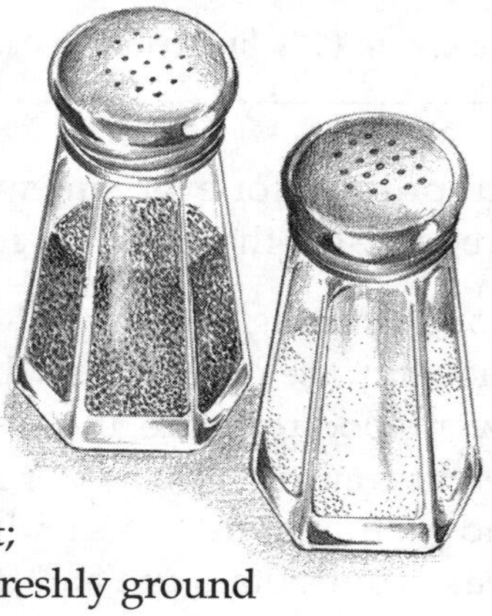

Halt the Salt; Spice Up Your Life

Over time, your taste buds learn to prefer less salt, but when you first cut back, you'll probably miss it. You can minimize the trauma to your taste buds by giving them something else to savor. Try these specialized blends you mix yourself:

Poultry blend: lovage, marjoram, sage

Vegetable blend: basil, parsley, savory

Salad blend: basil, lovage, parsley, tarragon

Italian blend: basil, marjoram, oregano, rosemary, sage, savory, thyme

French blend: chervil, chives, parsley, tarragon

Barbecue blend: cumin, garlic, hot pepper, oregano

FOOD SAFETY

Although these days most of us are concerned with fat and fiber more than we are with poisoning and pesticides, it is important not to forget that food can affect our health in more ways than one. After all, we eat the stuff. Fortunately, many of the problems that tainted food presents can be prevented by careful selection, handling, and preparation.

FOOD-BORNE ILLNESS

So, you think food-borne illness—or "food poisoning" as it's commonly but incorrectly called—is a relatively minor occurrence with relatively minor consequences? Think again. There are about six million cases of food-borne illness in the United States each year. That's not even counting all the cases wrongly attributed to the nebulous "stomach flu." Far from being innocuous, food-borne illnesses land many people in the hospital; some even die. The effects of food-borne illness can be long-lasting. Some fish-borne diseases can leave a victim with nerve damage. Reactive arthritis is an allergic-type reaction that has long-lasting effects on joints.

Unfortunately, these days, food-borne illnesses are only getting deadlier. New organisms are cropping up, minor players are becoming major players, and eating hamburgers at a fast-food restaurant has taken on an air of Russian roulette.

But it doesn't have to be this way. Prevention is the name of the game with food-borne illnesses. The solution lies in how often and how well you wash your hands and utensils, how you store your food, and how you cook it.

Fish gone bad. Many of the forms of food-borne illness that are on the rise originate in fish. They're not well known, but they can be deadly.

The Major Offenders

ILLNESS/ORGANISM	ONSET/SYMPTOMS	TRANSMISSION	FOOD SOURCE
Botulism ***Clostridium botulinum***	4–36 hours after eating. Double vision, trouble speaking, swallowing, breathing.	Organism produces dangerous toxin only when no air is available, e.g. in cans. Beware bulging cans.	Usual culprits: foods canned improperly at home, especially low-acid foods—corn, green beans, mushrooms, beets. Also in restaurant food left out (sautéed onions, soups) and foods preserved in oil (chopped garlic).
Clostridium perfringens	12 hours after eating. Mild, brief symptoms: abdominal pain, diarrhea.	Needs time to grow in food before it will cause illness, then needs time to grow in intestines before producing spores that release toxin.	Food cooked and kept warm a long time—often at picnics and pot-luck suppers. Needs protein-containing foods: meats, gravies, soups.
Listeriosis ***Listeria monocytogenes***	Days to weeks after eating. Fever, diarrhea, headache. Can cause conjunctivitis, miscarriage, meningitis.	Not common. Can be fatal, especially in young, old, or immunodepressed people. Not killed by refrigerator temperatures.	Soft cheeses, pâté, raw milk, uncooked poultry.
Campylobacter enteritis ***Campylobacter jejuni***	2–5 days after eating. Fever, cramps, bloody diarrhea.	Can cause illness even if food is not left out, allowing organism to grow. Increasingly common, but easily killed by cooking.	Raw poultry, raw hamburger, milk, mushrooms.
Escherichia coli ***(E. coli)*** Deadly form—0157:H7	Few hours to 1 week after eating. Watery or bloody diarrhea. 0157 form can cause severe infections, kidney failure, and death.	Also transmitted by personal contact, especially through feces. Children are very susceptible to severe effects.	Undercooked meat, especially ground beef; raw milk.
Salmonella	6–72 hours after eating. Fever, headache, cramps, nausea, diarrhea.	Organism doesn't need time to grow, but symptoms will occur sooner if more bacteria are present. Easily prevented by proper refrigeration and cooking. Dangerous in immunodepressed, young, and old people.	Raw poultry, meat, fish, and dairy products; eggs.
Staph ***Staphylococcus aureus***	½ hour to 4 hours after eating. Severe but brief symptoms: explosive diarrhea, cramps, vomiting. Often mistaken for the flu.	Food contaminated easily by cut hands, skin infections, nasal secretions, boils, and acne, but must be left unrefrigerated for some time for organism to grow enough to cause illness. Very common.	Protein foods: meats, poultry, egg products, tuna fish or chicken salad, cream pastries.

Many involve toxins that can't be detected and aren't killed by refrigeration or cooking. You can protect yourself by not eating raw fish or fish pulled from questionable waters, but the only foolproof prevention is to avoid eating susceptible fish. Here's a sampling:

- Anasakiasis has symptoms (fever, nausea, diarrhea, and vomiting) that don't appear for a week, so diagnosis is often missed. It's not common, but it is a risk whenever you eat raw fish. The organism's larva can penetrate the stomach lining, causing severe pain that mimics an ulcer. Cooking and freezing will kill the organism (ask for sushi made from frozen fish).
- Paralytic shellfish poisoning causes an immediate burning sensation of mouth and extremities, nausea, vomiting, and diarrhea and can lead to muscle weakness and paralysis. The neurotoxic form may take hours to appear, but it is milder. The illness is caused by toxins formed in mollusks—mussels, clams, scallops—off the Pacific, New England, and Florida coasts.
- Ciguatera poisoning causes the typical nausea, vomiting, and diarrhea that starts 6 to 12 hours after eating, but it is followed by slowed heart rate, low blood pressure, severe itching, a characteristic temperature reversal (cold feels hot and vice versa), and tingling and numbness of extremities. These symptoms can last for days or months. Caused by toxins produced by algae and passed on to bottom-dwelling predator fish, such as amberjack, red snapper, and sea bass, caught near reefs in Florida, Hawaii, and the Caribbean, it is not destroyed by cooking.
- Scombroid poisoning is an immediate reaction to a toxin produced by bacteria in fish that hasn't been refrigerated properly. It causes flushing, burning of the throat, itching, nausea, cramps, and vomiting and can lead to dangerously low blood pressure and difficulty breathing.

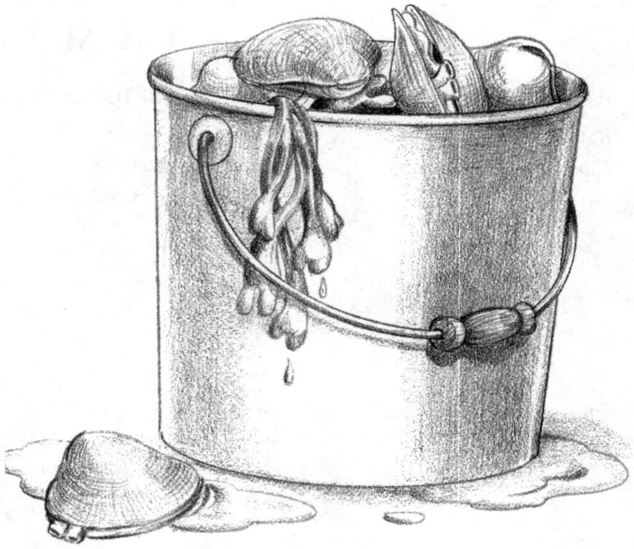

- Vibrio poisoning is characterized by explosive, watery, or bloody diarrhea. The form found in raw oysters is the most dangerous and can cause fatal wound infections, but any poorly refrigerated shellfish, especially shrimp and mollusks, are risky.

Food storage and preparation. It's much easier to head off a food-borne illness than it is to suffer through it. Here are some prevention tips:

- The maxim of food-borne illness prevention: Keep cold foods cold and hot foods hot. Bacteria grow best at temperatures between 40°F and 140°F. Don't let food sit at room temperature for more than two hours—the longer it sits, the more organisms build up in the food.
- Using hot, soapy water, wash your hands and all utensils that touch raw meats and poultry. When you grill, never put cooked food back on a platter that held raw meat or poultry.
- Don't thaw at room temperature. Plan ahead so you have enough time to defrost meat in the refrigerator. If you can't, thaw the meat in a closed plastic bag in a sink of cold water that you change every half-hour.
- Cook hamburgers until the juices run clear and the meat is no longer pink in the middle. Save your predilection for rare meat for steaks;

they're less likely to be contaminated in the interior.

◆ Don't eat foods with visible mold, unless it is a hard cheese. Even then, cut around it with a generous margin. Don't sniff mold or stick your nose into a bag of moldy food. Throw the bags away.

◆ All eggs should be refrigerated. Even hard-boiled eggs should not be left out for more than two hours; boiling them destroys their protective coating, so they are even more likely to go bad than raw eggs.

◆ Realize you run a risk of salmonella if you eat raw eggs. That includes foods made with raw eggs like homemade eggnog, fresh Caesar salad dressing, fresh Hollandaise sauce, homemade French vanilla ice cream, and homemade mayonnaise. Everyone should steer clear of these, especially the very young, the very old, and those with compromised immune systems.

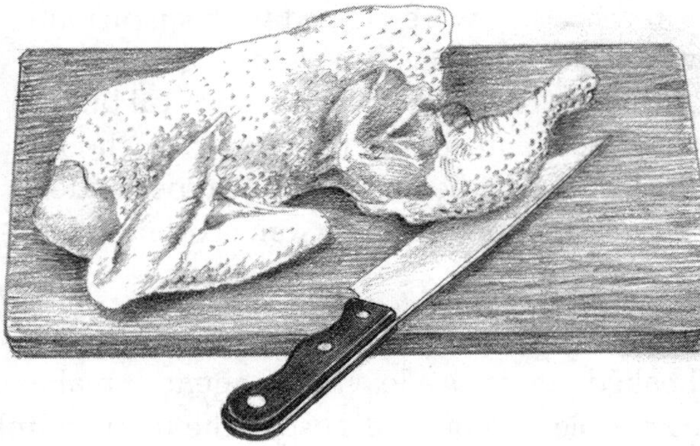

◆ Use a wooden cutting board; research shows it may resist bacterial contamination. Wash it with hot, soapy water. Wash plastic cutting boards in the dishwasher to remove fat that clings to them. Replace both when scarred or splintered.

◆ Don't store easily perishable foods—such as milk—in the refrigerator door; it doesn't stay as cold as the interior of the refrigerator.

◆ Do not drink straight from the milk carton; germs from your mouth will contaminate the contents.

◆ Don't reuse leftover marinade; it's contaminated from the raw meat or poultry.

◆ Eat or freeze fish and shellfish within one day of purchase.

◆ Discard any clams or mussels that do not close tightly when tapped before cooking. Steer clear of any that don't open after cooking.

◆ Avoid raw milk. It has been linked to numerous outbreaks of food-borne illness, with serious outcomes.

◆ Throw out soft cheeses after a week; they can harbor *Listeria* organisms.

◆ Store whole-wheat flour and brown rice in the refrigerator to discourage rancidity and bug infestation.

◆ Don't cook your Thanksgiving turkey by the slow low-temperature method—the meat will not get hot enough to kill bacteria.

◆ Never stuff a turkey the night before. And always remove the stuffing immediately after removing it from the oven. A turkey cavity provides just the right temperature for bacterial growth.

NATURAL TOXINS

Many people worry about what we add to the foods we eat. While it's hard to argue against natural and organic, it's not always clear what that means. The word *natural* had a lot of cachet in the 1970s. It was perceived as referring to foods with no additives or added sugar. In reality, it meant little, and it still means little. There is no legal definition of the word *natural*. Perhaps that's because foods in their natural state contain many chemicals—both good and bad. For instance, butter and sugar are natural, but you don't see anyone willing to hawk them as health foods.

To signify a diet based on real foods in their natural state, we prefer the term *whole foods*. However, not even all whole foods are always good for you. There are literally tens of thousands of toxins found naturally in foods—by some estimates more than 10,000 times the number of man-made pesticides.

Aflatoxin. For the most part people don't worry about natural toxins because they can't do anything about them. That's not entirely true. A good example is aflatoxin, one of the more pervasive toxins. It's a known carcinogen in animals and most likely in humans too. It's produced by molds that grow on peanuts, corn, and other nuts and grains that sit in warm, humid silos. There are government limits on the amount of aflatoxin that can end up in the peanut butter. Most experts believe it is way too high. Fortunately, most peanut butter falls far below this limit, but fresh-ground peanut butters sold in health food stores tested rather high by Consumer's Union a few years ago. Name brands fared much better.

How can you avoid aflatoxin? You can't entirely. Even Consumer's Union concedes that eating peanut butter once every ten days poses a seven times higher risk of cancer than most pesticides, but you can reduce the risk.

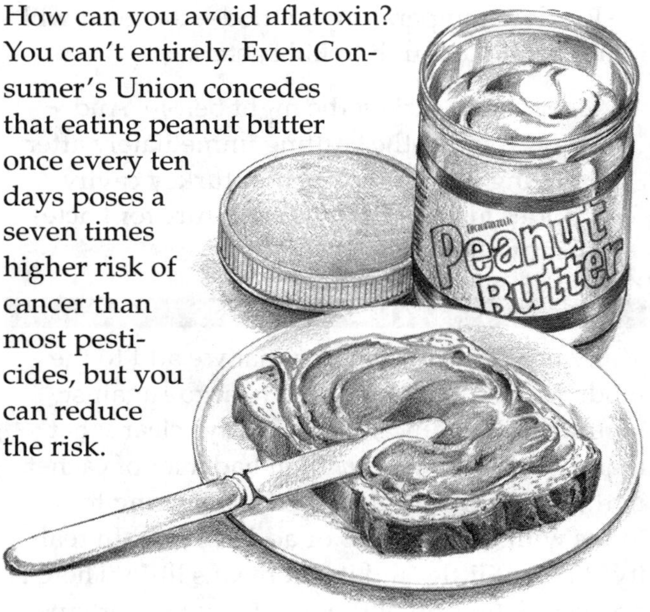

Don't eat peanut butter every day, or look for a mail-order brand (Walnut Acres is one) that is very low in aflatoxin levels. If you eat fresh peanuts in the shell, reject any that look dark, shriveled, discolored, or soft, and if any nut or grain looks moldy or discolored, throw it out.

Solanine. Another natural toxin, solanine, is found in some potatoes. Your mother told you not to eat potatoes with a green tinge and to throw away sprouted potatoes, and she was right.

Hydrazines. Mushrooms, when eaten raw, are a source of potentially cancer-causing hydrazines. Because they're inactivated when cooked, this is a case where cooked is better than raw.

Psoralens. Produced in moldy celery, this relatively mild natural toxin can give you a skin rash when you're in the sun—a reaction called photosensitivity.

There are many, many more natural toxins. You can't avoid them all. Simply eat a varied diet, without overdoing any one particular food. That way, one toxin cannot build up and hurt you. By spreading out your food choices you are, in effect, hedging your bets.

FOOD ADDITIVES

With all the research centered on fruits and vegetables these days, whole foods are finding a more mainstream audience than natural foods did in the 1960s and '70s. That was when additives reigned but were viewed with suspicion. Now, we know better. Some additives are helpful; some are harmful; some are harmful but too helpful to be banned. For the most part, though, additives are not the major problem pesticides are. Here's the lowdown on some common additives.

Aluminum compounds. You see these in breads and baked goods as a leavening agent. It makes some people nervous, because of the reputed link between aluminum and Alzheimer disease. However, that link is generally disregarded, and even if legitimate, you get much more aluminum from the environment, antacids, and buffered aspirin.

BHA & BHT. The preservatives BHA (butylated hydroxyanisole) and BHT (butylated hydroxytoluene) protect against rancidity in many foods, including powdered drink mixes, cereals, instant potatoes, and shortenings. The two are often vilified in the same breath, although only BHT has been linked to cancer. Hold on before you panic, though. Studies show it can both *cause* and *prevent* cancer in animals, depending on the circumstances. The effect in humans is only speculative; indeed, many scientists feel it is safe. There's actually no evidence that BHA causes cancer. In fact, just the opposite may be true: BHA may have some of the same benefits as antioxidant nutrients.

Food dyes. Talk about controversy! Some dyes seem perfectly safe, but others have an all-too-deserved tattered image. Maraschino cherries seem to bear the brunt of all this, as red dyes continually cause concern. The latest in red dye fiascoes was with red dye #3. In 1989, it was banned in cosmetics such as lipstick, but inexplicably not in foods. The FDA may yet take action on this front. Yellow dye #5, also called tartrazine, is another infamous coloring. For most people it is harmless, but a small number of people are allergic to it. That's not surprising since it's related to salicylic acid, otherwise known as aspirin. Fortunately for those who are allergic, manufacturers must now clearly state its presence on the label, not just list it under "artificial colors."

Gums. These aren't the chewing variety, but natural-source gums, which are valued for their ability to thicken foods, prevent separation of ingredients, and improve the consistency of texture in foods like pudding, ice cream, salad dressings, and baked goods. Commonly used gums include carrageenan (from seaweed known as Irish Moss), guar gum, gum tragacanth, gum arabic, locust bean gum, and xanthan gum. They improve what the food industry likes to call "mouth feel." Many are not only safe, but as soluble fibers, are beneficial to health. Guar gum has been shown to lower blood cholesterol levels.

Modified food starch. This garnered a bad rap years ago when baby foods were castigated for containing it. It's not that it's a dangerous additive, or at least it's never been proved to be. The problem is when it takes the place of more nutritious ingredients. The chemically modified corn or tapioca starch is indigestible, so it has no calories, and babies need all the nutritious calories they can get. It prevents caking and clumping in puddings, spaghetti sauce, and toddler foods, but it is no longer included in baby foods.

Mono- and diglycerides. These are really fats (related to triglycerides) added to give a smoother texture to foods, but they rarely add many calories to a product because they're used in very small amounts.

Nitrites (sodium nitrite). This is one of the few additives known to be harmful. It's added to processed luncheon meats like bologna and salami, as well as to hot dogs, bacon, and other cured meats. It does have a useful purpose: preventing the growth of the deadly *Clostridium botulinum* bacteria (the organisms that cause botulism). It also gives these meats their characteristic pink color. The problem is that the nitrite converts to cancer-causing nitrosamines in your body. Manufacturers have cut back to half the amount of nitrites used. Still, it's best not to get any nitrites, or at the very least, be sure to have a vitamin C–containing food along with nitrite-containing foods, for antioxidant protection.

Sulfites (sodium sulfite, bisulfite, metabisulfite). These are not used as extensively as they were ten years ago, but are still used to prevent browning of foods such as golden raisins, dried apricots, french fries, shrimp, dried potatoes, and salad-bar items. They are often added to wine in addition to the sulfite that is produced naturally in wine. For most people, sulfites are not a problem, but for those who are allergic to it, even a small amount can be life threatening. Since 1988, all foods that have added sulfites must be clearly labeled.

PESTICIDES

The alar scare in apples brought it all home—the fear that what we are spraying on our food to deter insects and organisms is poisoning us as well. Sometimes, it's not even in the name of preserving crops from damage, but merely to make produce look better. The fault for that lies exclusively with us. Yes, us. It is consumers who will only buy the best-looking produce, with no worm holes, torn leaves, green in their oranges, or less than perfectly shiny red apples; we drive the demand for such pesticides.

The organic revolution. "Natural" may be a slowly dying concept, but "organic" is just hitting its stride. It's becoming establishment, now that it's entering the supermarket. Fortunately, certification organizations have aided the difficult task of knowing what's organic and what's not. Even the government has attempted to enter the fray (see "Can You Believe 'Organic' on a Label").

With reports of the numbers of pesticides lurking on your fruits and vegetables, and the revelation that washing and even peeling won't get rid of all of it, the simple solution seems to be stop eating fruits and vegetables. Bad move. If there's one thing *everyone* agrees on, it's that you should *not* stop eating fruits and vegetables. The disease prevention benefits they offer far outweigh any risks they pose from the pesticides they harbor.

The best advice is to eat a wide variety of both fruits and vegetables. This cuts down on your exposure to any one pesticide. Heed the following tips for further protection:

- Wash all fruits and vegetables; scrub with a vegetable brush (not raspberries, of course). Use a very dilute solution of dishwashing liquid in water.
- If you can afford only a few of your vegetable purchases to be organic, make it the root vegetables you buy, like carrots, rutabagas, and turnips. They accumulate more pesticides than others when grown conventionally. Otherwise, trim an inch off the root end; that's where most of the pesticides concentrate.
- Peel your produce, especially if waxed, as apples, cukes, and eggplants often are. You'll lose some fiber, of course, but not most of it, and though some pesticides penetrate into the interior, you'll be rid of whatever remains on the peel. (The nonabsorbable wax itself is considered harmless, but it's usually mixed with a fungicide you'd rather avoid.)
- In the same vein, discard the outer leaves of leafy vegetables.
- Buy locally whenever possible; waxes are less likely to be used.
- West-coast grown produce usually requires less fungicide than produce grown in the humid East.
- Avoid imported produce as much as possible; it's typically higher in pesticide residues.

Can You Believe "Organic" on a Label?

In 1993, the Food and Drug Administration proposed new labeling regulations for foods labeled organic. It would require that 95 percent of the ingredients be organic. Those with less than that but more than 50 percent organic ingredients would be able to say "made with organic corn," for example. Those with less than 50 percent would be able to list ingredients as organic in the ingredient list but not refer to them on the label. However, none of that has happened. The proposal remains in limbo, waiting for the U.S. Department of Agriculture to decide what it wants "organic" to mean for fresh produce.

In the meantime, it's buyer beware. Your best bet is to look for a "certified organic" designation from one of several organizations. Reputable groups include: California Certified Organic Farmers, Farm Verified Organics, Organic Crop Improvement Association, and Organic Growers and Buyers Association. While standards may differ, a certified organic label usually means food that's grown without the use of chemicals on land not sprayed with pesticides for three years.

WEIGHT CONTROL

If you're like many Americans, you can identify with the popular lament, "I'm too short for my weight." If only we could grow taller! Instead, many of us spend a lifetime trying to diet our way into a size 5.

Call it a national obsession or an American rite of passage. Struggling to lose weight is a way of life for too many of us. The latest figures from the National Center for Health Statistics, though, say that one third of us are still overweight—that's 58 million overweight American adults. Something is obviously wrong here. We're dieting more, but all we're losing is our self-esteem, along with any sense of what a reasonable weight is.

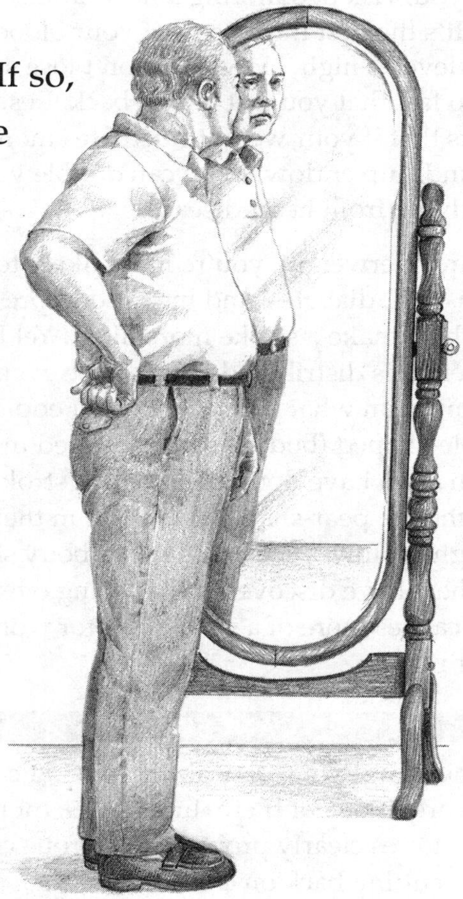

Could it be that dieting is the problem? If so, focusing on weight *loss* is not necessarily the answer. Weight *control* through healthful eating and exercising is. With few exceptions, if people concentrated less on the latest diet fad and more on eating right and staying fit, the weight would take care of itself. Everyone would not automatically be thin, but we'd settle in at a comfortable, reasonable weight that's meant for us. We'd also be the healthier for it, physically and mentally.

IMPORTANCE OF WEIGHT CONTROL

Fad diets may not be the answer, but there's no denying that excess pounds are not healthy. Being overweight increases your risk of numerous diseases and conditions. Obesity is linked to five of the ten leading causes of death in the United States.

HEART DISEASE AND STROKE

Here's a strong incentive for everyone who is overweight: Losing weight can immediately reduce your risk of suffering a heart attack or stroke. It's the first thing to do if your blood cholesterol level is high. However, don't lose so much so fast that you just gain it back. Research suggests that if your weight fluctuates more than ten pounds, up *or* down, you can double your risk of dying from heart disease.

If you are overweight, you're more likely to have heart disease, diabetes, and high blood pressure, all of which make a stroke more likely. Yet how your weight is distributed seems to be even more important than what your weight is. People who are apple-shaped (body fat concentrated in their stomach area) have double the risk of stroke than those who are pear-shaped (body fat in their hips and thighs). However, regardless of body shape, researchers have discovered that being overweight carries more of a stroke risk for women than for men.

CANCER

Of all the things we worry about causing cancer, calories aren't one of them. In animals, though, excess calories clearly promote cancerous cells, whereas cutting back on calories can quell some cancers. If this proves true for humans as well, it presents a quandary, because you can't just stop eating. You can avoid excessive weight gain, however, which could be fueling a low-simmering tumor you may not know you have.

Some of the controversy surrounding fat's connection to cancer, particularly breast cancer, involves whether the real culprit is fat or calories. No one is sure yet. Cancer of the endometrium—the lining of the uterus—is more common in women who are overweight. A similar link may exist between being overweight and cancers of the cervix, breast, ovaries, colon, gallbladder, kidney, prostate, and thyroid.

HIGH BLOOD PRESSURE

Here's another strong weight connection. It's as simple as this: If you are overweight, you are more likely to develop high blood pressure. If your blood pressure is high, losing weight is the single most important diet-related change you can make to lower it.

Many people cut back on salt but not on calories. Big mistake. Research indicates that for many folks, losing just five pounds can be enough to keep blood pressure under control, maybe even enough to avoid medication. Not surprisingly, the more overweight you are, the bigger the benefit losing weight is for your blood pressure.

DIABETES

Diabetes boasts the strongest weight–disease link. Being overweight doesn't cause diabetes, but it can trigger the disease to appear later in life in those with a family history of the disease.

Diabetes that appears in adulthood (type II) is the result of cells that have lost their ability to respond to insulin. This lack of memory for insulin apparently builds up over time, and the repeated insult of excess calories seems to speed up the process. The good news is that if you have a family history of diabetes but are careful to keep your weight under control, you may prevent, or delay, the disease from appearing.

The big guns you need to do battle against developing diabetes are weight control and physical activity. We're not even talking enormous weight loss. Recent research indicates that a 10- to 20-pound weight loss in the average overweight person who is at risk for diabetes may be enough to stave off the illness. Massively obese individuals might have to lose a great deal more to accomplish this, but they don't necessarily have to reach their ideal weight.

Controlling your weight can also help keep blood sugar levels on an even keel if you already have diabetes. Studies suggest that losing just five to ten percent of your weight can improve blood sugar levels. It will probably help triglyceride levels as well.

THE YO-YO MYTH

The idea is not just to *lose* weight, but to keep it off. This is easier said than done. Still, things are not as bleak as they seemed a few years ago, when experts had us so in fear of yo-yo dieting—the cycling of weight up and down—that people were scared to lose any weight at all.

Now, the truth is out. The National Institutes of Health (NIH) recently concluded that there is no convincing evidence that weight cycling increases body fat or that it decreases metabolic rate, supposedly making it harder and harder to lose the weight each successive time. What might very well happen, the experts concede, is that repeated losses and gains make it psychologically harder to lose the weight again.

However, the NIH noted that being very overweight does indeed increase the risk of disease and death, which more than offsets any consequences of weight cycling. So don't let the fear of gaining the weight back keep you from losing it to begin with. Besides, those who benefit most from weight loss—the very obese—are the least likely to suffer any yo-yo effects.

OTHER RISKS

If you have arthritis and are overweight, surely you know how much of a problem the extra weight is on your joints. One study found that losing more than 11 pounds cut in half the risk of developing osteoarthritis of the knees. Even gout, a type of arthritis, responds to weight loss with fewer attacks. Similarly, people with lower back problems, the biggest cause of missed work days, can relieve the strain on their backs by losing weight. Lastly, gallbladder disease is much more common among overweight women than in any other group.

PREFERRED WEIGHT

Are you fated to be fat? Is anyone? The surprising and discouraging answer may be yes, in a way. However, even though you may have a genetic predisposition to being heavy, that doesn't mean it is inevitable. You can fight your genes, at least to some degree.

YOUR FAMILY LEGACY

You inherit your eye color and personality from Mom and Dad. Why should your body type and metabolism be any different? It's not. Studies with identical twins reared apart show that they end up with similar body weights and fat distribution no matter how different the environments in which they grew up. Experts estimate that, on average, your genes dictate about one quarter of what your weight turns out to be. For some people, genes are even more important; for others, they carry little weight.

Before you try to lose weight, you should know what your genetic predisposition is, so you don't have a ridiculously unrealistic notion of what's possible. How do you know what your genes have planned for you? Look around—especially at your parents. Check out your grandparents and siblings, too. Chances are, if they're all round and plump, you're not likely to be thin and svelte. You can still be a healthy weight, but it'll be harder for you than other people. You'd probably be smart to revise your model-thin goal. It might save you from the vicious yo-yo merry-go-round. Just aim to be healthy. The upper end of your recommended weight range may be what your genes have planned for you, and that weight can be a healthy goal.

WHAT EXPERTS SAY YOU SHOULD WEIGH

Those infamous Metropolitan Life height and weight tables—you either love them or hate them, depending, of course, on what they say about you. They've been called *ideal* weights and *desirable* weights, and now they aren't labeled anything for fear of offending someone. We like the term *preferred* weight or *reasonable* weight. Whatever they're called, remember, the weights in the Metropolitan tables are simply data gathered from insured customers and compared to mortality data. In fact, because they include smokers and people with cancer—both of whom tend to weigh less and die sooner—the statistics are skewed to imply that heavier weights are healthier.

Perhaps the table released with the 1990 revision of the Dietary Guidelines is better? Think again. This table is even more generous with the amount of weight and the size of the range given. There's only one chart of numbers for both men and women. It seems the lower end of the ranges apply more to women and the upper end of the ranges apply mostly to men.

THE EASY WEIGH

There are quicker, easier, and maybe even more accurate ways to determine your preferred weight. Here's a method dietitians have been using for years to give them a rough idea of someone's desirable body weight:

Women:

Allow 100 lbs. for first 5 feet of height.

Add 5 lbs. for every additional inch over that.

Men:

Allow 106 lbs. for first 5 feet of height.

Add 6 lbs. for every additional inch over that.

If you are particularly small-boned, subtract 10 percent; if you are large-boned, add 10 percent. There, now wasn't that easy?

Then there's the Gerontology Research Center in Washington, D.C., which advocates its own age-adjusted tables that allow increasing weight—almost ten pounds—for each decade of life after 35 years of age. It claims this matches survival statistics. It certainly goes along with the natural tendency to put on pounds with age.

A recent Harvard study, however, criticizes all these tables of desirable weights for their ever-upward trend every time they are revised. The researchers believe the practice is encouraging obesity. Their data show that women are at much lower risk for heart disease if they weigh less than the U.S. average weight.

So, to consult the tables, or not? If so, which one—the Metropolitan Life table, the much-criticized Dietary Guidelines table, or the controversial Gerontology Research Center age-adjusted table? Look at them all, but take the numbers with a large grain of salt; everyone differs in what is right for them. Besides these three, there is also an easy method for figuring it out yourself (see "The Easy Weigh").

BODY FAT

Let's face it. You don't really care what the scale says, do you? What you care about is how you look: those rolls of fat that curl over your waistband, the post-baby belly that won't go away, or the double chin you've acquired with age. What you care about then, is how over*fat* you are, not how over*weight*.

ARE YOU OVERWEIGHT OR OVERFAT?

Knowing just your weight really isn't enough. There's evidence that how much body fat you have and how it's distributed is what matters most to your health. The experts use something called body mass index (BMI) to estimate the amount of body fat. It takes your weight *and* height into account by using a formula. We've simplified it a bit for you here, though you still probably need a calculator.

To calculate your BMI:

- Multiply your weight (in pounds) by 700.
- Divide this number by your height (in inches).
- Divide this number by your height (in inches), again.

Of course, this number probably means nothing to you, but it does to researchers. Here's how to interpret what your BMI means:

- 20 to 25—normal (associated with least disease risk)
- 26 to 30—overweight (low to moderate disease risk)
- over 30—obese (moderate to high risk)
- over 40—massive obesity (very high risk)

ARE YOU A PEAR OR AN APPLE?

This is a useful clue to how susceptible you are to heart disease. It turns out that abdominal fat—that typical "spare tire" or "beer gut" you see around men's middles—is much more dangerous than the bottom-heavy hip and thigh fat you see on women. "Apples," it seems, are more susceptible to heart disease than "pears."

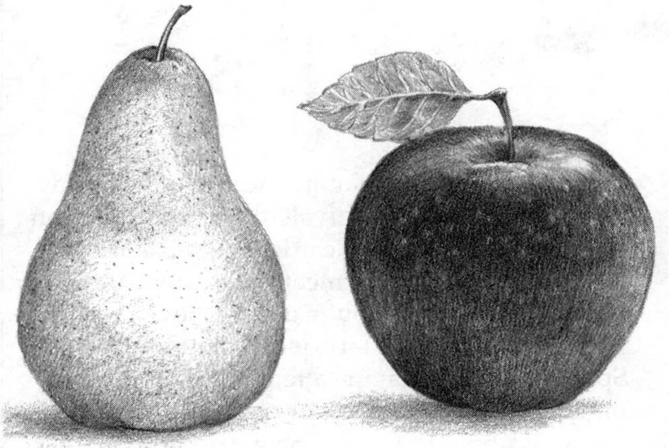

Experts have turned this apples versus pears scenario into another calculation called waist-to-hip ratio. This one is simple; to calculate waist-to-hip ratio:

- Take your waist measurement (at its smallest point).
- Take your hip measurement (at its widest point).
- Divide your waist measurement by your hip measurement.

The result of your waist-to-hip ratio is easy to interpret: For men, a ratio less than 0.95 is desirable; for women, less then 0.80 is desirable

LOSING EXCESS WEIGHT

If you're a veteran of the grapefruit diet and the low-carb diet and the rice diet, you know that the motivation to turn to fad diets like these often comes from a specific result you have in mind.

Do any of these motivations sound familiar?

- "I want to lose ten pounds before my high school reunion."
- "I have to lose the weight I gained when I was pregnant."
- "If only I could get rid of this beer belly."

However, losing weight for a specific event or dress size just invites a temporary dieter's attitude. You need to think lifetime changes for a healthier, happier existence. To do that, you need to be sure you are ready for the change in lifestyle it requires. Otherwise, you'll be on that yo-yo string forever, bouncing up and down between weights.

ARE YOU READY TO LOSE?

You might not be, you know. Perhaps that possibility has never occurred to you, but if you aren't committed to changing your eating habits, you will not be successful. And we don't mean changing them for just four weeks, or eight weeks, or even eight months. If you want to lose the weight, keep it off, and improve your health, you can't approach weight loss as a "diet." It's really embarking on a new way of eating for life. So, before you attempt to amend your habits, be sure you know what your incentive is and what your goals are, and gather family and friends for support. You will need it.

To know if you're ready to lose, take this tell-the-truth quiz: *true* or *false?*

- I have not recently had any major life upheavals, such as moving, changing jobs, having a baby, getting divorced.
- My family supports me in my desire to lose weight.
- I'm losing weight not for someone else's sake, but because *I* want to.
- I will be satisfied losing only one to two pounds per week.
- I will not give up if my weight levels off for a while.
- I am willing to read labels on every food I eat.
- I am willing to make time to be physically active every day.
- I am convinced that being overweight is bad for my health.
- I am convinced that losing weight will improve my health.

Did you answer *true* to all of the statements? If so, congratulations, you're probably ready to tackle that excess weight. If not, consider that this might not be the best time for you to try to lose weight. Wait until you're ready.

HOW MANY CALORIES DO YOU NEED?

We almost hate to bring this topic up, because counting calories tends to bring out a dieter's mentality. You should, however, have a general idea of your calorie needs, but don't feel you need to stick to a strict calorie level. Allotting a rigid number for each day is likely to make you obsessed with calories and eventually feeling deprived. A healthy diet may vary up and down 500 calories from day to day, but averages out for the week. So, chill on the calorie counting.

YOUR SECRET WEAPON: PORTION CONTROL

Whether it's high-fat foods or complex carbohydrates, your key to keeping slim is keeping portions moderate. There's a trend these days toward humongous servings. It only makes sense that this adds up to a humongous weight problem.

Researchers have discovered that dieters who thought they weren't losing weight because they had a "slow metabolism" were really eating double what they thought. Retrain your eyes to recognize what a reasonable portion is. How do you do that?

- First use technology. To get used to what sensible portions are, try measuring your food for a week. Weigh meat portions, or if you don't have a scale, carefully figure the portions from the weight listed on the package. Measure the amount of rice or pasta you put on a plate. It only takes a week to really train your eye.

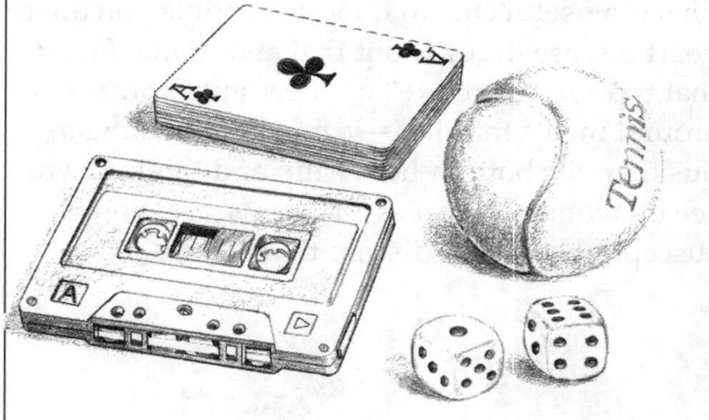

- Then use imagery: Imagine the size of everyday household items as equivalent to certain portion sizes of food. A deck of cards is the size of a three-ounce portion of meat. The palm of your hand works also. If you're a music lover, perhaps imagining a cassette tape works better for you. Sports fans can imagine a tennis ball as one cup of mashed potatoes, rice, or pasta. An ounce of cheese is about the size of a pair of dice. You get the idea.
- Finally, try trickery: Use a smaller plate. Smaller portions will still look like a full plate of food.

In general, to lose one pound of fat per week, you need to cut back 3500 calories, or 500 calories per day. So, once you know how many calories you need to maintain your weight, just subtract 500 and that's your average daily total. To lose two pounds per week, you'd have to cut back 1,000 calories per day. For most people, that's probably too low. Experts advise not going below 1,200 calories per day for women, 1,600 calories per day for men. Even at these levels, it's hard to get all the vitamins and minerals you need, so consider a multivitamin-mineral supplement for insurance.

Your everyday, no-activity needs—the calories you need just to keep breathing and thinking—are called your basal, or resting, metabolic needs. This amount is surprisingly high. Above that, add the calories your body needs to sustain your activity level, and then you have your daily calorie requirements. You can estimate your calorie needs with a simple formula:

- Multiply your weight (in pounds) by ten.
- Add 300 calories if you're an inactive couch potato (*tsk, tsk*).
- Add 500 calories if you're moderately active (you walk, play a little tennis, take the stairs instead of the elevator).
- Add 700 calories if you're active (you regularly work-out).

Remember, this is just to maintain your weight. If you want to lose, you have to subtract 500 or 1,000 calories a day. Better yet, forget the calorie-counting; just watch your fat and exercise, exercise, exercise.

CUTTING FAT VS. CUTTING CALORIES

A calorie is a calorie is a calorie, right? Wrong. A calorie from fat is more likely to end up on your thighs than a calorie from carbohydrate or protein, say researchers. It's *so* important, in fact, that counting fat grams can be as effective for weight loss as counting calories—maybe even more because low-fat foods are often very filling foods. (For more on cutting fat from the diet, see Chapter 1.)

Counting calories can have some unwanted consequences. That constant scorecard of calories and lists of taboo foods only create a feeling of deprivation and desperation. This can eat away at you until you give in to the urge and end up bingeing. That's definitely not healthy.

If you keep a close eye on your fat intake, however, you are practically guaranteed to lose weight. The secret is to replace high-fat foods with high-fiber foods—complex carbohydrates like fresh fruits and vegetables. You still can't go to town on starches, sugars, and other foods. They can also be fattening, of course, if you eat enough. Calories do still count, even though you're not counting them.

EXERCISE, EXERCISE, EXERCISE

You can't underestimate how important this component of a weight-control program is, but its value is not necessarily what you might think. Although exercising burns calories, it takes a lot of laps in the pool to burn off even one glazed doughnut.

The truth is that exercising, by itself, will not pare many pounds, and dieting with no increase in activity is destined for failure. However, when you pair a cut in fat and calories with an increase in activity level, both become more effective. Exercising also has a residual effect by increasing your metabolic rate for a time, even after you stop the activity. It also increases your muscle mass, which will increase your resting metabolic rate and hence your calorie-burning capacity generally. All this means that the well-exercised body burns more calories even when it is at rest.

Let's face it: We've become a stagnant society. It's no wonder more of us are overweight than ever before. Study after study has examined the habits of obese people and discovered they are invariably sedentary. We're talking couch potatoes. It's no coincidence that what many of us do on that couch is watch TV. Several studies have confirmed a link between what people weigh and how much television they watch. This is especially true for kids.

On the other hand, one study has found that thin people tend to fidget more, expending anywhere from 100 to 800 calories on "spontaneous activity" alone. The solution, then, is simply to get moving. A half-hour of aerobic exercise every other day would be nice, but it doesn't have to be that formal. Just GET MOVING! For trimming pounds and maintaining weight loss, it's probably better to do moderate activity every day, such as a brisk walk, rather than intense activity every other day. Speed is not that important; being active for a certain number of minutes per day is.

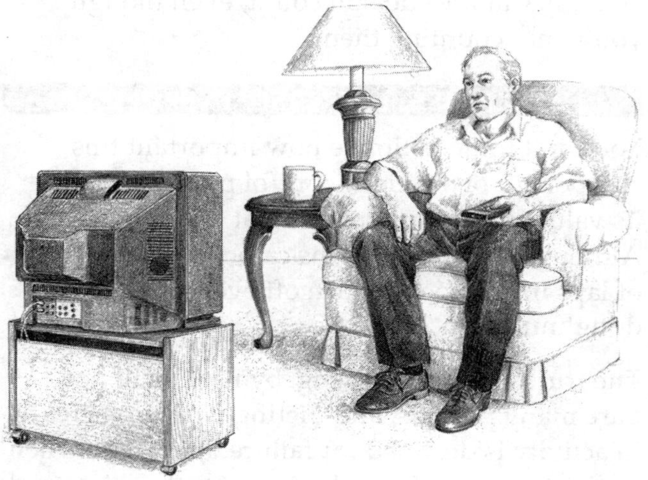

If you don't like to run, jog, bike, swim, or do any other specific activity, then just walk everywhere you can. Take the stairs instead of the elevator. Work in your garden. Park far away from the mall entrance and the supermarket. Open your garage door yourself. (For other hints on getting more exercise, see Chapter 3.)

THE REAL TRICK: KEEPING IT OFF

Okay, so you're ready to lose weight. You've calculated your BMI and waist-to-hip ratio, you've faced up to your risk factors for disease, and you've made the decision to become more physically active. You've come up with a realistic goal for yourself. What's next?

You need to think about more than just how to lose the weight. You need to consider whether the method you use to lose will help or hinder you in the long run. Simply put, to keep weight off successfully, you need to take it off the right way to begin with.

Let's face it, anyone can lose weight. That's not particularly difficult. The reason everyone struggles so much is because they can't keep the weight off. If you truly want to succeed in the weight-loss game, work a little harder at maintaining the lost weight than at the actual losing of the weight.

Suggestions for how to maintain your weight have more to do with how to lose it right in the first place. Here are some tips:

- Set short-term goals for yourself. Don't try to achieve a large weight loss all at once.
- Compensate yourself with nonfood rewards, such as a movie or a day off from work or chores, as you reach each goal.
- Keep a food diary: what you eat, how much, what time of day, your mood at the time, your activity at the time, your company. Reviewing these entries will help you pinpoint your problem areas, whether they are eating junk food, eating too-large portions, nighttime eating, eating from stress, eating from boredom, eating alone, or eating with friends.
- Plan for small relapses. You can learn from them. What's not OK is viewing a splurge as total failure and simply giving in to every whim—"blowing the diet." If you allow a small treat every day, you'll be less likely to feel deprived and less likely to give up.
- Don't panic when your weight plateaus. This is normal. If you keep at it, you will start to lose again. Have faith.
- Be flexible in your expectations and goals. You may need to revise what you think is realistic. If necessary, reevaluate the methods you have chosen.

Survival Guide to Dining Out

- Order à la carte. That way you can order just what you want. Request one or two appetizers to be served as your entree.
- Ask for a half serving. If they'll only cook it all, have them doggy-bag the other half without even serving it (it circumvents the temptation to eat it all).
- Beware the salad-bar trap. It may seem healthy, but it isn't if you choose mayo-laden salads or end up with a salad swimming in oil. Check to be sure there's diet dressing, or bring your own. Stick with greens and fresh veggies.
- Don't attack the free bread, especially if there's butter on the table. It's difficult to know when to stop. If you must munch, go for breadsticks. And you can always ask the waitstaff to remove the butter so you're not tempted.
- Remember, alcohol packs almost as many calories as fat, and they're empty calories at that. If you get stuck at the bar waiting for your table, order a white wine spritzer or just mineral water (lucky for you, that's considered chic these days).
- Don't deny yourself dessert if you really want it, but consider splitting it with someone and consider the fruit option.
- At fast-food joints, shun all special sauces and super-huge "value" meals—they may be a value for your pocketbook but not your waistline.
- Ask for sauces and dressings to be served on the side. That way, you control the portion.
- Watch out for hidden calories. Chicken and veal may sound low in fat, but they're not if they're coated with breading and fried in oil. You're better off with a lean steak.
- Beware these give-away descriptors that signal fatty food ahead:

Alfredo	Crispy
Au gratin	Escalloped
Batter-dipped	Flaky
Béarnaise	Hollandaise
Béchamel	Parmigiana
Breaded	Tempura

- Think less in terms of a *diet* than of a life-long maintenance of your reasonable weight—a healthy weight.
- Think of your weight-loss program as more of a retraining of eating habits for life instead of an unrealistic, temporary fad diet. Then there will be no difficult transition because you'll already have new eating strategies you can live with.
- If you lose weight slowly in the first place, maintenance will be a much easier task.

AIDS, PLANS, AND PROGRAMS

There's a new diet or weight-loss product every minute just waiting to sucker you in. Why? Because it's big business, that's why. Americans spend $3 billion on commercial diet programs alone, and that probably pales in comparison to what the shysters and hucksters rake in.

DIET AIDS

In 1992, the Food and Drug Administration (FDA) attempted to clean house by prohibiting over 100 weight-loss ingredients from being listed as "active ingredients" in over-the-counter products. These ingredients were singled out because there's no proof that they do anything. The substances, including alcohol, caffeine, vitamin C, and grapefruit extract, still remain in many products, however.

There's no point in throwing away money on ineffective diet methods, and you certainly don't want to throw away your health by using dangerous substances or following questionable practices. Here's a rundown on some diet aids to avoid:

Chromium picolinate. This is *the* hot supplement right now, based on the fact that chromium is needed for building muscle and burning fat.

However, it's not the magic fat-burning pill that some ads suggest. A few studies found it improved the muscle-building effects of exercise. Theoretically, the more muscle you have, the more calories you burn, but there's little evidence that this makes much practical difference in weight-loss efforts. Besides, it would also have to accompany a dedicated exercise program anyway, and if you're that dedicated in the first place, you don't really need a pill. On the good side, chromium picolinate is a well-absorbed source of chromium, a mineral most of us probably don't get enough of.

Ma huang (ephedra). This Chinese herb is widely used in diet aids and nonprescription cold and asthma remedies (as ephedrine, the active ingredient in the plant, or pseudoephedrine). This widespread use creates potential problems from inadvertent overdosing. Ephedrine is a potent stimulant similar to amphetamines. It gives you a nervous high, blunting your appetite. However, it is not safe for those with heart conditions, high blood pressure, diabetes, or thyroid disease. For most people, small amounts are safe, but too much of it can make anyone's heart race and blood pressure soar. Because herbal products like ma huang are not standardized in the amount they contain, they are best avoided.

Laxatives (senna). Many "natural" weight-loss products live up to their promise to help you lose weight only because their main ingredient is a diuretic or a laxative—both of which cause temporary water loss. Senna, for example, is present in many herbal preparations and so-called herbal "dieter's teas." It's a potent cathartic used in numerous over-the-counter laxatives. Long-term abuse of laxatives can ruin your intestinal tone and will not help with long-term weight loss.

Herbal teas. These are gaining in popularity to the dismay of herbal experts who say their ingredients are untested and not standardized, leaving the door open for fraud and health risks. Common ingredients in the teas promoted for weight loss include: ginseng, locust plant, papaya, buchu leaves, and juniper berries.

Amino acids (carnitine). This popular amino acid supplement and others, such as arginine, ornithine, lysine, and methionine, are said to enhance the burning of fat. Although amino acid levels in the blood do rise, researchers can find no increase in the rate of body-fat burning. In addition, amino acids have calories; supplementing with them means supplementing your calorie intake, too.

Lecithin. This fatty substance has been touted for weight loss forever, it seems, but it's no more useful now than it was years ago when it was introduced.

PPA (phenylpropanolamine hydrochloride). This is a popular ingredient in many over-the-counter diet aids from prominent drug companies, but its usefulness is much more modest than many people perceive it to be. Research shows that PPA, an appetite suppressant, can improve weight loss by an extra half pound per week, *if* coupled with a low-calorie diet. The FDA has approved it for 12 weeks at a time, but products containing it must carry warnings on their labels that shouldn't be dismissed.

DIET PLANS

Liquid protein diets (very-low-calorie diets, protein-sparing modified fasts). These are no longer in their heyday, thanks to Oprah. She caused sales to soar when she unveiled herself on TV in size 8 jeans, after a liquid diet. However, the tide turned when she zoomed back up past her previous weight, revealing the pitfall of this method—you usually don't maintain the weight loss.

The liquids provide from 300 to 800 calories per day, with very little carbohydrate. The extra protein they contain supposedly prevents muscle loss and promotes fat breakdown for energy. Early powdered versions of these diets were dangerous because they provided too little carbohydrate, poor quality protein, and inadequate nutrients. The revamped liquid diets that first appeared in the late 1980s are safer than the earlier versions, but they still work best when followed under a doctor's care.

The biggest problem with these liquid protein diets, however, is that they don't work in the long run because they don't teach you how to eat real food in the real world. As soon as you return to reality, your weight balloons back up.

Low-carbohydrate diets (Stillman Diet, Atkin's Diet, Scarsdale Diet). These diets have been around a long time, but still crop up under different names. They are all modified ketogenic diets, which severely restrict carbohydrates to induce ketosis, forcing the body to break down fat for energy. Thus, you lose fat, or so the theory goes. However, ketosis has consequences. By-products called ketones build up in the blood and can create a dangerous acid–alkaline imbalance. Unbeknownst to the dieter, much of the actual weight loss is water, because the body is trying to get rid of the ketones through the urine. Weight regain is usually rapid.

Food combining (Fit for Life Diet, Beverly Hills Diet). The theory of food combining has been around for over 100 years, although it has gotten more popular in the past decade. The diet claims that proteins and carbohydrates are digested by different enzymes, and if eaten together will destroy each other's enzymes and create toxins, making us fat. The diet imposes severe restrictions on fruit—it must be eaten alone, and at certain times of the day. Moreover, meat can't be combined with grains.

The truth? Most foods contain both carbohydrates and proteins, making it impossible not to combine the two. The touted enzymes in fruits and vegetables can't survive our stomach's strong acid environment, so are of little use to us.

The diet isn't inherently dangerous if a variety of foods are eaten, but the silly restrictions are unnecessary and make an unbalanced diet more likely. Besides, there's no proof it'll help you lose weight, unless you cut back on food because you're too scared to combine anything.

Grapefruit diet. Everyone has heard this one—that grapefruit actually burns calories, or that it has negative calories because it takes so much energy to chew and digest. Hogwash! There's nothing wrong with eating grapefruit, but this and other one-food diets—rice, banana, potato—are nutritionally unsound. By eliminating certain groups of foods, these diets limit your access to a variety of nutrients.

LOSING WEIGHT THE PROGRAM WAY

There are plenty of diet programs you can join to lose weight. These recently endured their own form of government scrutiny when the Federal Trade Commission demanded that they put up or shut up. Weight-loss claims made in advertising must now be backed up by scientific studies, or disclaimers must be used. The trouble is most companies are unwilling to divulge long-term success rates. Short-term results are often much more flattering.

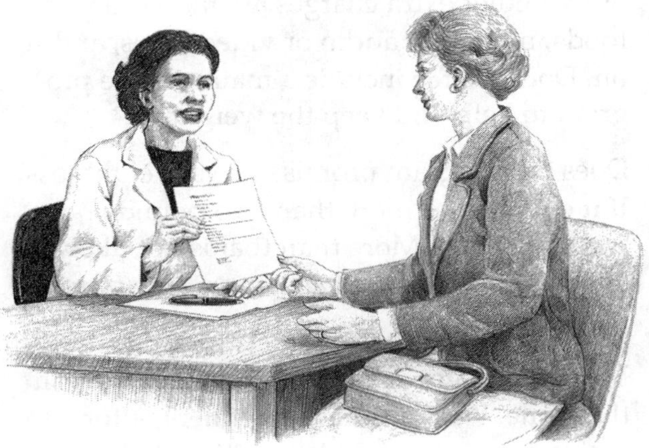

Commercial weight-loss programs have kept up with the times, however. They continually evolve, embracing current dietary recommendations like keeping fat intake low and fiber intake high. Most encourage exercise and behavior change and offer counselor or group support.

Before plunking down your hard-earned bucks, be sure you know what you're paying for. Review the following considerations in light of your needs and safety:

- Is the diet plan a sound, balanced program? Are all the major food groups represented? If not, it might not be nutritionally adequate.

- Are you comfortable with the type of program? Groups offer much needed support, but if you are uncomfortable in such a setting, one-on-one counseling may be better for you.
- Will the demands of the program fit in with your lifestyle? Can you attend regular meetings? If there are special foods, can you eat them easily at work or when you travel?
- If the program has foods that you can purchase, what do they cost, and how do they taste? Sample the cuisine before you sign up. Be sure there is enough variety so you won't get bored. Be extra cautious if the plan requires you to purchase their food; it is simply a way for them to make more money. Their food has no special low-calorie properties.
- Do you know the total cost? Be sure you find out whether extra charges are tacked on for foods, meetings, audio or video tapes, and so on. Does the fee include a maintenance program to help you keep the weight off?
- Does the program promise rapid weight loss? If it encourages more than two pounds per week, be wary. More than that is not likely to stay off and may indicate an unsafe approach.
- Does the program promote physical activity? You need to get in the exercise habit early in the game. Without this component, efforts to maintain your weight loss will probably fail.
- Is there a registered dietitian (R.D.) on staff? If so, ask to talk with him or her about the safety of the program, its nutritional quality, and its track record for successful weight loss. Ask for one-year *and* five-year follow-up statistics. You may not get them, but it's more than reasonable to expect to see them before you join.

The choice among programs, and even within programs, these days is enormous. If you are interested in the program approach, be sure to shop around. If one approach is not your cup of tea, try another. Perhaps this entire route is not for you. You may do better on your own, simply revamping your dietary habits and increasing your activity level. Here are brief synopses of some programs competing for your business.

Diet Center features one-to-one counseling with nonprofessional former clients. It focuses on body composition, not weight. Daily visits to the center are encouraged to keep you focused on the goal but could make you feel tied down. You get your choice of supermarket foods or prepackaged cuisine. There is no group support.

Jenny Craig offers weekly one-to-one counseling with a nonprofessional and periodic support groups. It combines its own prepackaged cuisine with store-bought foods for some variety.

Nutri/System has one-to-one or group counseling available. It uses its own portion-controlled prepackaged foods in a rigid diet plan. There are no decisions to make, but you must eventually return to supermarket foods.

Optifast is a medically supervised program that includes professional consultations with doctors, registered dietitians, and registered nurses. The program uses liquid meal replacements at first, and then you slowly make a transition to prepackaged foods. The daily calorie intake is lower than that of most programs, ranging from 800 to 1,200 calories. This program offers quick weight loss, but you must relearn how to eat normal foods without gaining it all back.

Overeater's Anonymous is a nonprofit support group, similar in approach to Alcoholics Anonymous. It is not a diet program; it is merely for group support.

TOPS (Take Off Pounds Sensibly) is another nonprofit support group. Participants meet and weigh in weekly. No specific diet is recommended.

Weight Watchers is a flexible diet and healthy lifestyle program with weekly meetings and weigh-ins. Participants choose between the program's own cuisine, supermarket foods, or both. A well-balanced diet is continually presented in new ways, as in its current fat and fiber program.

FITNESS

There's a lot of talk about fitness these days—most of it emanating from the mouths of muscular, oiled-up models as they strut across our television screens in skimpy bikinis and bike shorts.

But what does it really mean to be fit? Does it require the kind of perfection shown in these ever-present health club and diet-shake commercials? Is it truly attainable for the average Joe (or Josephine) who puts in eight hours at the office and then comes home to face a hungry spouse and demanding children?

Fortunately, becoming fit doesn't mean eating a perfect diet or looking like a model. The word "fitness" simply means "being fit." Fit for what? For ordinary activity—walking, carrying children, running for the bus, stretching to reach something on the top shelf. It means feeling energetic, maintaining a healthy weight, and taking care of your body so it can fight off the diseases associated with inactivity, such as cardiovascular disease, diabetes, osteoporosis, and some cancers.

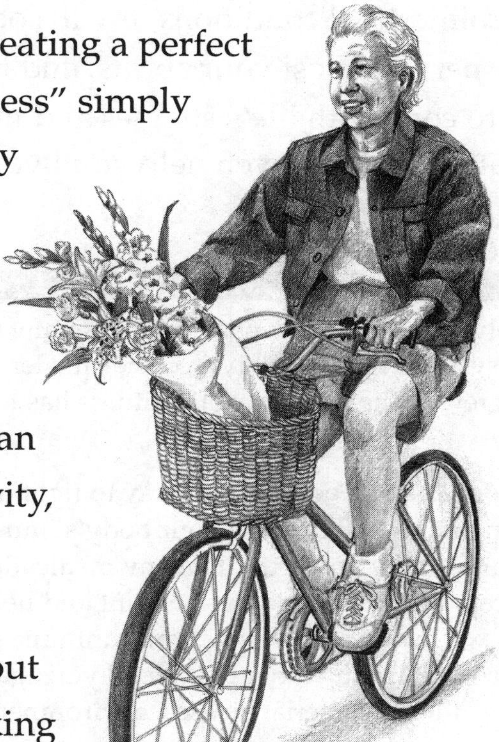

Can you attain this type of fitness without spending endless hours in the gym or drinking fiber-laden, artificial chocolate-flavor milk shakes? You bet you can, and it's not as hard as you think.

THE BENEFITS OF FITNESS

Getting your body into shape (and keeping it there) will do a lot more for you than simply help you look great in your favorite jeans. It will decrease your risk of developing diseases and incurring injuries. It will strengthen your bones, muscles, ligaments, and tendons, making them less vulnerable to degenerative diseases (such as osteoporosis). It may alleviate chronic pain and certain gastrointestinal conditions. It will soothe your nerves, boost your spirits, and help you to cope with life's stresses and minor irritations. It may even help you live longer.

FIGHTING OFF ILLNESS

Simply put, regular exercise protects many of the vital systems in your body from harm. Here are just a few of the many benefits fitness has to offer:

Immunity. You have a built-in way to fight off degeneration and disease. Your body's immune system is more powerful than any medication you can take. Keeping your body fit and healthy is an excellent way to rev up your immune system, so that it can vigilantly defend you against the assaults of bacteria, viruses, environmental toxins, and time.

Weight control. One of the health benefits of fitness is the maintenance of a healthy ratio of fat to muscle. Why is this so important? Muscle is the prime determinant of your metabolism, meaning that the rate that you convert calories to energy (instead of storing them as fat) is linked to the proportion of lean mass (bones, skin, organs, connective tissue, and muscle) that you have on your body. In other words, the more muscle mass you have, the faster you burn calories and the less likely you are to be overweight.

Too little muscle leads to a slowed metabolism, which can result in the accumulation of excess body fat and, eventually, obesity. Obesity has been linked with many dangerous health conditions, including high blood pressure, arteriosclerosis (hardening of the arteries—a factor in strokes and heart disease), diabetes, chronic back and knee pain, and heart problems.

Improving your body composition can reverse or prevent many of these problems. Studies have shown that when an obese person loses even a modest amount of fat, his or her blood pressure drops, circulation improves, blood-sugar levels begin to return to normal, and some forms of chronic pain start to fade away. There is no medication in the world with a track record that can compare to these benefits. As you already know from Chapter 2, fitness plays an integral role in the weight-loss equation.

EXERCISE IMPROVES PROGNOSIS FOR ELDERLY HEART PATIENTS

Exercise not only makes you look better and feel better, but it may even restore activity and energy to elderly patients with heart trouble, according to researchers at the University of Maryland Medical Center.

In that study, investigators found that after a three-month program of aerobic training, their ten elderly subjects with congestive heart failure were able to walk an average of twice as fast and 120 percent farther than they could at the outset of the project. Some were able to take up activities again that had long been out of their reach, including driving and shopping.

In the past, elderly patients with congestive heart failure were told to remain inactive. Such inactivity usually led to increased weakness and, in turn, even less activity. Death often followed quickly. The new study raises hope that exercise can restore quality of life to patients whose hearts are slowly failing.

Preventing heart disease. Perhaps the most significant benefit of increasing your fitness level is the effect it can have on your risk of heart disease. Heart disease is the nation's number one killer, but fitness is a great way to fight back.

Your cardiovascular system needs exercise as much as the rest of your body does, and a little regular exercise will strengthen your heart muscle, in addition to the muscles that show when you're wearing a bathing suit.

Aerobic exercise, such as walking, jogging, and biking, increases your heart's endurance by forcing it to pump increased amounts of blood and oxygen through your body for extended periods of time (20 minutes or more). It has also been shown to raise the level of high-density lipoprotein (HDL) cholesterol—the heart-healthy type of cholesterol—in your blood. High levels of HDL have been shown to reduce the risk of heart attacks. Lastly, aerobic exercise has been shown to help reduce high blood pressure, a primary cause of life-threatening conditions such as strokes.

Anaerobic exercise—weight training and stop-and-start sports such as tennis and basketball—is also beneficial to your heart. This type of exercise causes a sudden (but short-lived) demand for extra oxygen. Over time, regular anaerobic exercise can help the heart and your other muscles become stronger.

Protecting you against osteoporosis. You've probably heard about how important your calcium intake is in protecting you against osteoporosis—a debilitating, degenerative disease that causes the bones to weaken and become more porous over time. However, exercise is just as important in maintaining the health of your bones.

Weight-bearing exercise, such as walking and jogging, has long been established as an effective way to protect against loss of bone density. More recently, researchers have discovered that weight training incurs similar benefits. When you force your bones to carry more weight on a regular basis, they respond by retaining more of the minerals that keep them sturdy and strong.

DECREASING YOUR RISK OF INJURY

Improving your fitness has another unexpected side effect: It may help protect you against injury. There are several reasons for this:

Weak and inflexible muscles lead to injury. When muscles are deconditioned, tight, or out of balance with opposing muscle groups, the risk of injury is greatly increased. For example, sedentary office workers who spend many hours a day at a desk commonly end up with tight back muscles and weakened abdominal muscles. Because the abdominal muscles and the back muscles support the spine together, an imbalance often results in injuries that can cause chronic low- or middle-back pain. By increasing your muscles' strength and range of motion, you decrease your likelihood of these types of injuries.

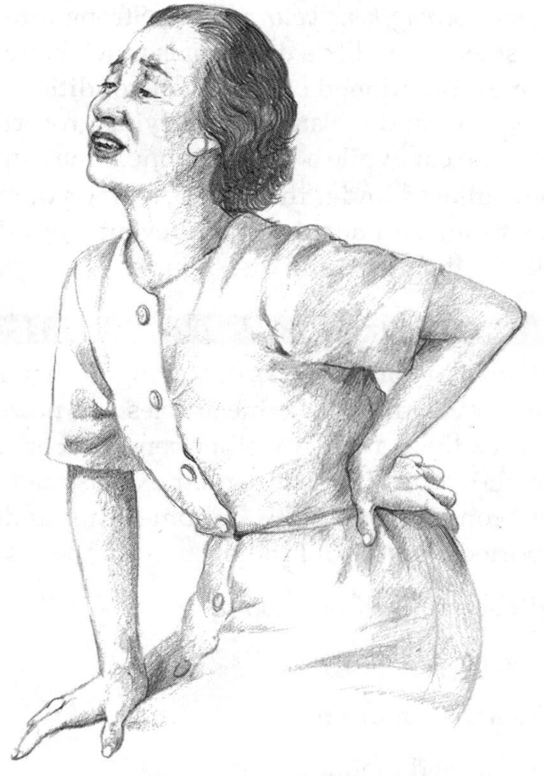

Exercise increases agility. "Practice makes perfect," the old adage reminds us. When it comes to exercise, this maxim certainly holds true. Why is this important when it comes to preventing injury? It stands to reason that if you practice a sport consistently, you are much less likely to be injured while doing it (beginning step aerobics students are always tripping over their steps).

Also, the time you devote to exercise may make you more movement-conscious, increasing your coordination, thereby making you less likely to lose your balance. You improve your ability to know where each body part is in space (called *kinesthetics*). Well-tuned kinesthetics may help you recover from tripping over a curb before you sprain your ankle.

Exercise keeps your bones strong. As noted earlier, weight-bearing exercise and strength training both help to maintain bone density. Lower-density bones often suffer injuries, such as stress fractures, hip fractures, and so on. By attending to the health of your bones, you may avoid many complications later on.

Exercise strengthens your muscles. Strong muscles can stand up to life's daily trials much better than deconditioned ones. A well-conditioned back can stand the stress of carrying groceries from the car, while a deconditioned one can become injured under the load. Keeping your muscles strong and healthy may prevent painful muscle, ligament, and disk injuries.

THE UNEXPECTED BENEFITS OF EXERCISE

While many of the perks of staying in shape are often covered in magazine articles and news reports, there are many other benefits. For example, did you know that regular exercise can prevent constipation? Here are some other under-reported benefits of fitness:

- Relief from chronic joint pain
- Increased energy
- Relief from insomnia
- Improved mood
- Enhanced self-image
- Increased sex drive
- Increased alertness and job performance
- Stress relief

THE FIVE COMPONENTS OF FITNESS

Fitness can mean different things to different people. After all, the marathon runner, the ballerina, and the weight lifter are all fit, but their individual abilities are not interchangeable. There are five basic areas that combine to make up overall physical fitness. Here is a breakdown of the five essential components.

MUSCULAR STRENGTH

Muscular strength is the force that a muscle or a muscle group can exert when it contracts. For example, when you pick up a shopping bag, you

The Sixth Component of Fitness

There is another component of fitness that is rarely discussed by aerobics instructors or physical education teachers: Emotional fitness.

Contemporary research is constantly revealing new and potent links between the mind and the body. In other words, your emotional state may be related to certain physical symptoms. The reverse is also true: Physical conditions (such as pain or illness) may affect your emotional well-being.

The jury is still out on the extent of the connection. However, until researchers come up with definite answers, you'd do well to take steps to maintain your emotional fitness along with your physical fitness.

While regular exercise helps the body become fit, taking measures to combat stress in your life can help you become emotionally fit. Try working in a brief meditation with your stretching routine, or taking a walk in the woods instead of on the treadmill at the gym. Who knows: A little quiet, stress-free time may benefit your body, as well!

are contracting the biceps muscles and exerting a force on the bag against gravity. Muscular strength assists you whenever you make a move. It is required in all aspects of life. Without it, you would feel weak and lethargic, unable to walk, stand, sit, or perform simple everyday tasks.

MUSCULAR ENDURANCE

Muscular endurance is the length of time you can continually exert muscular force or the number of contractions the muscle can withstand before becoming fatigued. Walking is a test of muscular endurance, as is standing for long periods, gardening, cleaning, writing, and so on.

CARDIOVASCULAR ENDURANCE

Cardiovascular endurance, also called aerobic fitness, is a measure of your heart's stamina. It is a function of the heart-lung system and its ability to deliver blood and oxygen to the muscles during ongoing exercise. This is arguably the most important component of fitness. All of the other systems of the body also require a well-tuned circulatory system. To maintain a high energy level, to prevent disease, and to enjoy a high quality of life, this system must be taxed on a regular basis.

FLEXIBILITY

Flexibility is a measure of your joints' range of motion. Adequate flexibility allows you to reach for your seat belt or sit cross-legged comfortably. It also gives you more mobility and helps to prevent injury. Lower-back and hamstring (back of the leg) flexibility is particularly important, since tightness in these areas is associated with lower-back pain and injury. Although it is often overlooked, flexibility is one of the most important components of fitness.

BODY COMPOSITION

Body composition is the ratio of lean body mass (muscles, bones, nerve tissue, skin, and organs) to fat. Lean tissue is metabolically active, meaning that it uses plenty of fuel for activity. Fat is not. Too much fat can inhibit your performance during exercise by putting additional stress on your muscles and joints. It also puts strain on the heart, forcing it to work harder to carry the extra load.

Because muscle is more dense than fat (it takes up less space for a given weight), it is more important to measure body composition than body weight when evaluating fitness. In other words, a five-foot, two-inch, 175-pound male body builder could be considered overweight, if evaluated on body weight alone. However, consideration of his muscle-to-fat ratio would make it obvious that the extra weight was muscle, not fat.

A desirable amount of body fat is between 8 and 15 percent for men and between 15 and 22 percent for women. Above 24 percent for men and above 33 percent for women is considered obese.

MEASURING YOUR BODY FAT

Your weight on the scale is not as important as the percentage of your body composed of fat. How do you measure the amount of fat on your body? There are a few methods:

- Hydrostatic (underwater) weighing, which is done by trained personnel at some health clubs. This is thought to be the most accurate method of body-fat measurement.
- Skinfold-caliper testing, which relies on a device that pinches and measures the amount of fat directly below the skin. This method is most accurate when conducted by trained personnel. (You can, however, purchase a caliper and instruction booklet for use at home.)
- Bioelectric impedance analysis, which uses a device that estimates the total amount of water in the body and, from there, gives an estimate of the percentage of body fat. Of the three methods, this is thought to be the most imprecise.

Fitness, then, is a combination of all of the above components. A fit person is strong, can perform physical tasks for reasonable lengths of time, is flexible enough to move comfortably and avoid injury, and has a healthy ratio of fat to muscle.

Any fitness program must target each of these areas to be truly beneficial. In other words, you cannot be considered totally fit if you can bench press 150 pounds but are unable to walk a mile briskly without becoming short of breath.

Fortunately, it doesn't take hours and hours in the gym to get from here to there. And when you consider the benefits that getting in shape can offer, chances are that you'll be happy to put in the modest investment of time that it does require.

SETTING YOUR FITNESS GOALS

To get started on your road to fitness, you have to be pointed in the right direction. Knowing where you are now and where you want to be can give you a realistic picture of the fitness program that's right for you. First, we'll start with where you are now, and then we'll take it from there.

WHAT'S YOUR FITNESS LEVEL?

The following quiz will help you make an informal evaluation of your fitness level in each of the five areas. Although there are more scientific tests for rating your fitness level (see "The Bent-Knee Sit-Up Test," page 67), this test should help you get at least a preliminary idea of how fit you are and where you could stand some improvement.

Choose the statement in each of the following categories that best describes you. When you have finished, score your answers. (Note: If you have an injury or a physical handicap, the scoring system may not realistically assess your fitness level.)

Muscular Strength

a) I lift weights regularly and feel that I am stronger than my peers.
b) I have no problem lifting bags of groceries and other heavy items that I encounter daily.
c) I have no problem lifting light objects, but cannot lift anything as heavy as a bag of groceries.
d) I often feel weak or experience pain when I try to lift even light objects.

Muscular Endurance

a) I can window shop or walk at a leisurely pace for hours without tiring.
b) I can walk a mile or two without my legs getting too tired.
c) I'm good for a walk around the block, but more than that, and my body starts to ache.
d) A trip around the grocery store leaves me tired and in pain.

Cardiovascular Endurance

a) I can run a mile without stopping or becoming overly winded.
b) I can walk a mile at a brisk pace without stopping or becoming overly winded.
c) Running 100 yards for the bus leaves me red-faced and panting for minutes afterward.
d) When I walk to the corner, I become so out of breath that I must stop and rest.

Flexibility

a) With my legs together, I can bend from the waist and put my palms flat on the floor.
b) With my legs together, I can bend from the waist and touch my ankles.
c) With my legs together, I can bend from the waist and touch my shins.
d) I cannot bend very far without experiencing pain.

Body Composition

a) I am quite lean and muscular.
b) I'm thin, but have little muscle tone.
c) I have a bit of a spare tire around my middle, or I can pinch several inches of fat on the inside of my thighs.
d) I have little muscle tone and am more than 20 percent over my ideal weight.

The Bent-Knee Sit-Up Test

As noted earlier, muscular endurance is a measure of how many times a set of muscles can contract before becoming fatigued. If you'd like to try rating yourself more scientifically in this area, try an old standard: the two-minute, bent-knee sit-up test.

- Lie on your back with your feet flat on the floor and your knees bent. Your heels should be 12 to 18 inches from your buttocks.
- Clasp your hands firmly behind the back of your head. If you like, have someone hold your feet on the ground.
- Contract your abdominal muscles, and, keeping your hands behind your head, sit up until your elbows reach or pass your knees, then return to the starting position.

Repeat the exercise (counting the number of repetitions you perform) for a timed period of two minutes. Evaluate your result with the following scoring chart:

Rating	Men	Women
Outstanding	79–91	64–72
Excellent	68–78	57–63
Very Good	60–67	50–56
Average	51–59	45–49
Below Average	42–50	39–44
Poor	33–41	33–38
Very Poor	32 or below	32 or below

Give yourself three points for every *a* that you circle, two points for each *b*, one point for each *c*, and zero points for each *d*.

If your score was 12–15, give yourself a pat on the back—you're in excellent shape. You probably exercise regularly and eat a healthy, low-fat diet. Keep up the good work. If you had a low score in any one area, consider shifting your focus a bit to make the necessary improvements.

If your score was 9–12, you're probably in adequate shape for daily life and at lower risk for certain diseases, such as high blood pressure and heart disease. If you answered *c* or *d* in any area, you know where you need more work.

If your score was 5–9, this is your wake-up call. Chances are, your muscles—including your heart—are weak, your limbs are inflexible, and you have an undesirable ratio of fat to muscle. If you don't make some changes in your lifestyle, you could be setting yourself up for health problems down the road. Make a plan to become more active, and gradually increase activity as your fitness improves. A daily walk and some gentle stretching might be a good start.

If your score was under 5, there is no need to panic, but your score indicates that you are in poor physical condition. Consult your physician for a thorough examination, and ask for advice on beginning a fitness routine that is appropriate for your age and your fitness level.

FOCUSED GOALS AND STRATEGIES

Now that you've got a good idea of how fit you are and where you need improvement, it's time to set some goals. A goal-oriented approach may motivate you by helping you focus on milestones and mark your progress.

To start, think about what you've learned about your present fitness level. Did you find, for example, that you have excellent cardiovascular endurance, but that you can't touch your toes? Or perhaps you're sufficiently limber, but you can't run even one lap around the block without

Exercise Vocabulary: Aerobic vs. Anaerobic

Fitness lingo is becoming more and more confusing these days. And if it seems as though everyone else in your aerobics class is hip to the "in" vocabulary but you, take heart: Here's some help.

For starters, here's a quick overview of two of the most commonly used words in fitness-speak: aerobic and anaerobic. An aerobic exercise is a repetitive motion using large muscle groups that elevates the pulse to between 55 and 85 percent of its maximum rate and holds it there for at least 20 minutes. In so doing, the activity exercises the cardiovascular (heart-lung) system.

The following is a list of activities that, when performed at the appropriate intensity level for 20 minutes or more, constitute an aerobic workout:

- Walking (at a brisk pace)
- Jogging
- Running
- Bicycling (stationary or moving)
- Stair climbing
- Aerobic dance
- Step aerobics
- Swimming
- Cross-country skiing
- Rowing
- In-line skating

Anaerobic activities require large amounts of oxygen in quick bursts. Because of the high oxygen demand it places on the heart, anaerobic exercise cannot be sustained continuously for 20 minutes. These activities do not directly burn fat (although they do increase caloric expenditure while they are performed).

The following is a list of anaerobic activities:

- Weight training
- Push-ups
- Chin-ups (pull-ups)
- Any exercise, when performed at an intensity that leaves the participant gasping for air, or unable to sustain the activity for at least 20 minutes

stopping to rest. Then again, maybe it's the fact that you can't close your favorite jeans that's got you raring to make changes.

Make a list of the fitness categories in which you'd like to improve, as well as a list of the areas that you're happy with. Then, start to formulate some goals (see "Setting Realistic Goals," page 69). Rank these goals in order of the importance you place on them. Lastly, if you like, write down a list of rewards that you plan to give yourself once you reach your goals. This list may help you stay motivated.

Once you've identified your goals, you need to know the strategies for achieving them. See if any of these goals are similar to the ones that you have in mind:

To shed fat. You'll need to focus on fat-burning (aerobic) exercise, in addition to strength training, which boosts your metabolism and firms up your whole body. Make sure to integrate three to five long (30 to 45 minutes or more) sessions of moderate-intensity aerobic exercise into your weekly fitness regimen. In addition, work in two to three strength-training sessions of a half-hour to an hour in duration.

Of course, you'll also have to modify your eating habits (see Chapter 2). Make sure your diet doesn't drop too low in calories, though, or you may end up slowing down your metabolism, which will, in turn, slow your progress. A low-fat diet that consists of several small meals per day—instead of three large meals—is probably your best bet for building muscle and keeping your metabolic fires burning.

Lastly, make sure you don't get too hung up on the numbers on the scale. After all, your exercise program will likely result in a loss of fat but a gain in muscle, and muscle weighs more than fat. Remember, too, that effective weight-loss programs are slow and steady. Instead of weight, concentrate on your measurements and your clothing sizes. The general idea is to get smaller in the right places; getting lighter is only a side effect.

Setting Realistic Goals

A common road to fitness self-sabotage is setting unrealistic goals. Creating goals that are impossible to achieve is the easiest way to justify giving up on your plans. (After all, you've already failed, so what's the use in continuing to strive?)

Some examples of unrealistic goals are:

- To have a body like Kim Basinger's when you're five-foot-two and come from a family of muscular, stocky football players.
- To have a body like Arnold Schwarzenegger when you've always been as rangy as Jim Carrey.
- To lose 15 pounds in a month. Unless you're planning on investing in liposuction, losing that much weight that fast is neither possible nor healthy.
- To enter a body-building contest in two months when you've never lifted anything heavier than your television's remote.

To be effective, goals should be both realistic and specific. They should reflect small steps that can be achieved in discrete amounts of time. The following are examples of realistic, specific goals:

- To lose a pound a week
- To go down a clothing size in four months
- To be able to run a mile without stopping
- To be able to complete the hardest aerobics class at your club by the end of the year
- To be working out four times a week by the end of six months
- To be able to bench press 20 pounds more than you can now by your next birthday

To get stronger or to build muscle mass and definition. Put the focus on weight training. You'll need to concentrate on lifting progressively heavier amounts of weight for relatively few sets of repetitions. The basic formula is to start off, after warm-up, with a weight that you can lift for one set of 12 repetitions. By the second set, you should be struggling to complete 10 reps. By the third and final set, you should be able to complete no more than 8 reps. Rest one or two minutes between sets. When you can lift the weight for three full sets of 12 repetitions, it's time to move up to a heavier weight. (For a more detailed program of this type of weight training, see pages 79–83.)

A few words of warning: Weights are potentially dangerous objects when used without adequate warm-up or proper form. Make sure you don't push yourself too hard at first and that you've mastered proper form before challenging yourself to move up to higher weights. Otherwise, you may be setting yourself up for injury. If you choose to use a weight that you can lift for less than eight reps, always use a spotter—a training partner or trainer who stands over you while you lift, ready to help you in case you run out of steam or start to lose control of the weight. Also, never compromise proper technique in an attempt to squeeze out an extra repetition or two. (For more training tips, see the strength-training and toning sections of this chapter, beginning on page 77.)

To tone your muscles. Toning your muscles, like building muscle mass, requires resistance training. Toning generally requires a lighter resistance but more repetitions and shorter rest intervals than strength and muscle-mass training. Depending on your goals and the equipment you have available, you may choose to use your own body weight as resistance (as you do when you perform leg lifts, for example). You may also choose another type of resistance, such as the elastic tubing sold at most sporting-goods stores.

As with building muscle mass, you'll want to integrate at least two or three sessions of toning exercise per week. And don't skip the aerobics—those newly toned muscles won't show if they're hidden under a thick layer of fat. (For more toning tips, see the strength-training and toning sections of this chapter, beginning on page 77.)

To improve your cardiovascular endurance. Perhaps you'd like to be able to walk longer, bike longer, run longer, shop longer, or make love longer. Whatever your motivation, if your goal is to increase your body's ability to endure long periods of aerobic exercise, you'll need to devote three to five exercise sessions a week to gradually adding time and intensity to your workouts. There are several different ways to accomplish this:

- Tack an extra minute on to your workout each time you exercise. After a 5- to 10-minute warmup, start with a basic 20-minute aerobic workout (walking, jogging, biking, skating, stepping, or whatever you prefer). Make it 21 minutes for your next session, 22 for the third, and so on. Psychologically, one minute feels insignificant, but by the end of three months—if you work out three times per week—you'll have added 36 minutes to your workout time!
- Try interval training. Interval training is a technique used by many different types of athletes, including sprinters, basketball players, football players, race walkers, and swimmers. The basic idea is to alternate periods of moderate-intensity exercise with short intervals (one to three minutes) of high-intensity exercise. Interval training will help increase your cardiovascular capacity and strengthen your heart. Over time, this can be of assistance in improving your endurance.

  Here's a sample interval-training walking program that can be substituted for your regular workout once or twice per week: Start with a ten-minute warmup, then begin alternating five minutes of brisk walking with two minutes of jogging. Continue for the amount of time that you usually work out. End with a ten-minute walking cool down.

  When your two-minute jogs begin to feel like a piece of cake, increase them to three minutes. By the time you can alternate five minutes of walking with five minutes of jogging, your heart will already be much stronger.

  At this point, you can stop the interval program for a while and tack extra time onto your regular workout. Chances are, you'll find that your endurance has increased tremendously. Because of the higher intensity, you should limit interval training to one or two times per week. Even elite athletes have slow easy sessions. Overdoing it can lead to strain and injury.
- Cross-train. If you feel that your endurance level has plateaued, you might try integrating different exercise activities into your workout schedule. The reason is that over time, your body becomes accustomed to the demands of the same old routine. Adding new and different types of exercise will work different muscle groups and challenge you in new ways. It may also help to alleviate exercise boredom and burnout.
- Increase the frequency of your workouts. If you've been working out twice a week, make it three times. If you've been coasting along at three, make it four. The more you exercise, the healthier and stronger your heart will get. If you like, try adding two additional sessions per week until you become accustomed to it. Then drop one session and add extra time onto the remaining workouts.

Endorphins: The Runner's High

You've probably heard talk of a mysterious phenomenon called "the runner's high," a state of euphoria and well-being experienced by veteran runners. In fact, these fleet-footed athletes often cite the runner's high as the root of their devotion to the sport.

But what is the truth about runner's high? Can a jog around the block (or a half-hour on the stair climber) really lift your spirits? Or is this phenomenon simply an advertising gimmick promoted by the fitness industry?

Surprise! It's no fairy tale. Aerobic exercise promotes the release of endorphins—chemicals produced by the brain that cause feelings of pleasure and well-being. While you may not experience an endorphin rush the first time you take an aerobics class, you'll probably get a taste of the runner's high after a few weeks.

So it's true: A little sweat really can make your day.

To improve your flexibility. Instead of just stretching as a warm-up and cool-down before and after your regular workouts, try adding one or two 20-minute stretching sessions to your routine every week. Stretching can be a wonderful way to boost your energy level first thing in the morning or to unwind after a hard day. If you don't know very much about stretching, refer to the flexibility-enhancing routine in this chapter (see pages 83–84).

If you're looking for a way to make stretching more interesting, consider trying yoga. Formerly thought of as the domain of hippies and new-age flunkies, yoga is now recognized by the mainstream as a great way to stretch, relax, and rejuvenate. Several fitness gurus—Jane Fonda and Kathy Smith among them—have released yoga workouts within the last couple of years. Check out the selection in your local library and video store.

To boost your energy level. There are many reasons for sagging energy levels, including stress, sleep deprivation, pregnancy, and physical illness. Even though a lack of exercise is not usually a cause of fatigue, it can be an excellent antidote. Even if you feel fatigued before starting, your energy level will be vastly improved by a moderate exercise session.

If you are suffering from a physical problem, check with your doctor before you embark upon a new exercise program. However, most people (even pregnant women) can benefit from a progressive walking program that starts off with 15-minute sessions at a moderate pace and progresses to a four-day-a-week, 30- to 45-minute brisk walking program. (For more on pregnancy and exercise, see pages 85–86.)

You may feel even more tired than usual during the first week or two of a new exercise program. However, after that, chances are your energy levels—and your mood—will begin to pick up. You may even find that you start sleeping better at night and feeling more rested and alert during the day.

Want To Be 25 Years Younger? Get Physical!

We often consider physical decline to be an inevitable part of aging, but new research is showing that the onset of many conditions—such as weight gain, flabbiness, osteoporosis, and decreased mobility—can be reversed or prevented through regular exercise, including cardiovascular conditioning and strength training.

Americans usually grow more sedentary as they age. This lack of activity results in a decline in aerobic capacity, which leads to a further decrease in mobility over time. It also causes the average American to lose about 6.6 percent of his lean-body mass per decade. This loss is associated with a slowed metabolism, an increase in body fat, and a rise in blood pressure—all risk factors for serious illnesses.

A regular exercise program can prevent these common ills. In fact, according to researchers from the National Institute on Aging, by improving your physical fitness, you can reverse up to the equivalent of 20 to 25 years of aging.

To improve your overall health. Maybe you aren't focused on losing enough fat to become a model, running five miles, or doing splits. Perhaps you'd just like to do the minimum of exercise that you need to do to boost your fitness to a level that will benefit your overall health. This is a reasonable goal.

The minimalist approach is simple. It is based on the current recommendations endorsed by most medical associations. It consists of:

- Three 20-minute aerobic sessions per week
- Two strength-training sessions per week
- Five- to ten-minute stretching sessions before and after each aerobic or strength-training workout

Following this schedule won't prepare you to run a 10K road race, but chances are, you'll shed some fat, gain some muscle, tone up, and start to feel better. Perhaps at that point, you'll be encouraged by your results and become a true exercise convert!

CARDIOVASCULAR CONDITIONING

We invite you to think of the following section as your own personal cardiovascular-training encyclopedia. By the time you've finished reading it, you will know everything you need to know to start work on improving your cardiovascular capacity and endurance.

If you faithfully follow the principles outlined in this section, you will develop superlative agility and speed, lungs and legs of steel, and a body that will have your entire neighborhood green with envy. Well, almost. Aerobic activities are those that can be sustained at a specific rate of intensity for at least 20 minutes at a time. There are good reasons for this type of workout:

- It allows the heart and lungs to supply oxygen to the muscles at the rate they require it without building up an oxygen debt.
- It strengthens the heart by requiring it to pump large volumes of blood.
- It temporarily elevates the metabolism and burns fat.
- It encourages the release of endorphins, natural substances within the body that produce a pleasurable sensation, such as the so-called "runner's high."
- It permits you to exercise continuously without feeling distressed, allowing you to enjoy your exercise routine.

FIGURING YOUR TARGET HEART RATE

The target aerobic heart rate—the zone where you can expect to experience the benefits of a good cardiovascular workout—is usually considered to be between 55 and 85 percent of your maximum pulse rate. Beginning exercisers, pregnant women, and people with health problems should stay at the lower end of the zone; more advanced exercisers and athletes can push to the top of the zone.

The following are two easy and relatively accurate ways to determine your aerobic target heart-

YOUR TARGET HEART RATE

The following chart shows the target aerobic training zone as a factor of age, using the Maximal Heart-Rate Formula. To find your appropriate aerobic training zone (in pulse beats per minute), simply examine the row after your age range. At the peak of exercise, your pulse should be between the first and last numbers in the row or roughly 55 to 85 percent of your maximal heart rate.

Age (*years*)	Percentage of Maximal Heart Rate						
	55%	60%	65%	70%	75%	80%	85%
20–25	109	119	128	138	148	158	168
26–30	106	115	125	134	144	154	163
31–35	103	112	122	131	140	150	159
36–40	100	109	118	127	137	146	155
41–45	97	106	115	124	133	142	150
46–50	95	103	112	120	129	138	146
51–55	92	100	109	117	125	134	142
56–60	90	97	105	113	122	130	138
61–65	86	94	103	110	118	126	133
66–70	84	91	99	106	114	122	129

rate zone: the Karvonen Formula, which is the more scientific of the two, and the Maximal Heart-Rate Formula, which is the more popular.

The Karvonen Formula:

1) Calculate your maximum heart rate. Maximum heart rate is the highest heart rate that a person can attain during vigorous exercise. Although the only way to accurately assess maximum heart rate is a medically supervised test that monitors the heart, you can estimate your maximum heart rate by subtracting your age from 220. (This formula is based on the knowledge that a baby's maximum heart rate is approximately 220 beats per minute and that it decreases by about one beat per year).

2) Determine your resting pulse rate. Resting pulse is best measured first thing in the morning, before you get out of bed. The pulse should be taken either for 30 seconds and multiplied by two, or for a full 60 seconds (see page 74 for how to take your pulse). For the most accurate determination of resting pulse, take your pulse on three consecutive mornings, then average the readings.

3) Calculate your heart-rate reserve by subtracting your resting heart rate from your maximum heart rate. This number is the greatest number of beats your heart can vary from total rest to maximum exertion.

4) Determine your target heart-rate range. To establish the range, you will need to complete the following formula twice—one using the lower end of the intensity range (55 percent), the other with the higher end of the range (85 percent). This formula determines the target heart rate as a percentage of the target heart-rate reserve, plus the resting heart rate:

- Multiply the heart-rate reserve by 0.55. Add the resting heart rate. This number is the lower end of your target zone.
- Multiply the heart-rate reserve by 0.85. Add the resting heart rate. This number is the upper end of your target zone.

The Maximal Heart-Rate Formula (also see "Your Target Heart Rate," page 72):

1) Calculate your maximum heart rate (see step #1 under The Karvonen Formula).

2) Multiply your maximum heart rate by 0.55. This is the lower end of your training zone.

3) Multiply your maximum heart rate by 0.85. This is the upper end of your training zone.

Other methods: There are two other less complex, but still useful, methods of assessing whether you are working to the proper level of aerobic intensity: the Perceived-Exertion Scale and the Talk Test. Here's how to use them.

- Perceived-Exertion Scale: At the peak of your exercise period, rate how hard you feel you are working on a scale between 0 and 10:

  0—Nothing

  ½—Very, very light (barely noticeable)

  1—Very light

  2—Light (weak)

  3—Moderate

  4—Somewhat hard

  5—Heavy (strong)

  6—Heavy

  7—Very heavy

  8—Very heavy

  9—Very heavy

  10—Very, very heavy (almost the maximum you can possibly do)

  When you assess your exertion, combine all sensations of physical stress, effort, and fatigue. Concentrate on your total inner feeling of exertion, not on one factor such as leg pain or shortness of breath. You should be working at a level somewhere between four and six, which corresponds, roughly, to about 55 to 80 percent of maximum heart rate.

◆ Talk Test: Throughout your exercise period, check the signals your body is sending you. You should be able to answer affirmatively to the following questions:

Can you breathe comfortably, deeply, and rhythmically?

Could you carry on a short conversation while exercising at this level?

If you are gasping for breath or cannot talk, you should slow down and reduce your intensity. This method is best when used in conjunction with taking your pulse or with the Perceived-Exertion Scale.

WARNING!

Medication for your heart or blood pressure can affect your heart rate, thus making intensity monitoring difficult. If you take this kind of medication, the Perceived-Exertion Scale is probably the most appropriate. Check with your doctor before embarking on your exercise program.

TAKING YOUR PULSE

If you've chosen to use the Maximal Heart-Rate Formula (or the Target Heart Rate Chart on page 72) to monitor your intensity level as you perform aerobic exercise, you'll need to learn the proper way to take your pulse. The count you'll use is based on the average number of pulses in a full minute. However, since your pulse rate drops very rapidly when you stop moving, it is best to take the pulse for no longer than ten seconds, then multiply by the appropriate factor to calculate a full minute's pulse rate. For example, you can take your pulse for six seconds and multiply by ten, or take your pulse for ten seconds and multiply by six. (Under six seconds is not recommended, since the time is too short to count accurately.)

Never try to take your pulse with your thumb, since it has a pulse of its own. Also, when you start counting, count the first beat as "zero," not as "one."

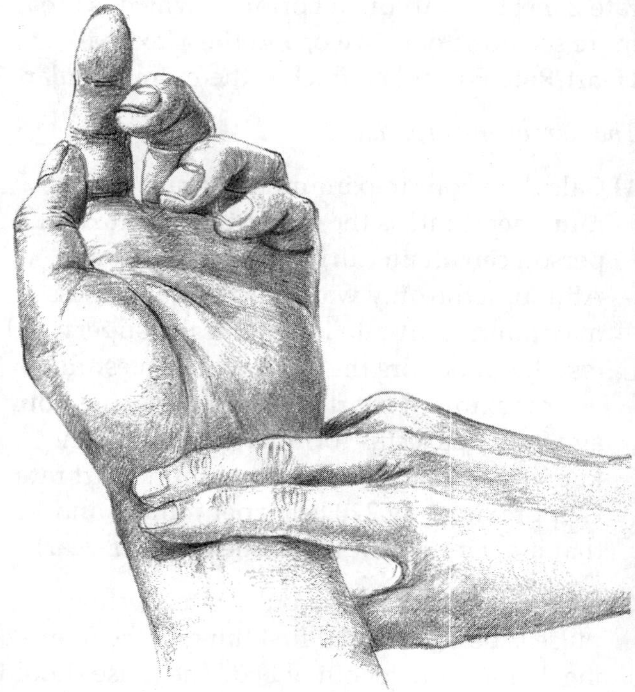

You can take your pulse at one of the following four locations:

◆ The wrist. Take the index and middle finger and place them on the radial artery of the wrist (the artery in line with the thumb). Press down lightly to feel the pulse.

◆ The temple. Use the index and middle finger to press down lightly in front of the upper part of the ear, above the cheekbone.

◆ The neck. Gently place the index and middle finger on the carotid artery, which is located on the neck, just to the side of the throat. Never press hard at this location, since excess pressure can cause a reflex action that slows the heart rate down.

◆ The chest. Place the heel of the hand over the left side of the chest, fingers pointing in the direction of the shoulder.

Wireless heart-rate monitors can give you an accurate, continuous readout of your heart rate. These devices can be found in sporting-goods, running, and bicycle shops for about $100.

THE RIGHT AEROBIC EXERCISE

Next, it's time to choose the aerobic exercise that will fit with your life. Many considerations should be included in the decision because choosing the right exercise is crucial. If you don't like the routine, if it's too difficult, if it's inconvenient to start—if anything isn't quite right, then you're starting off on the wrong foot, and your fitness program could be doomed. You need to find an exercise that's safe, convenient, and enjoyable. After all, no exercise program is going to help you if you can't get yourself to do it.

The main idea is to use large muscle groups to increase your energy output and your heart rate for a continuous, extended period. The considerations that follow can help you determine how your personality, your fitness level, and the options available in your environment can lead to the proper selection of the aerobic activities that suit you.

Your environment

- If you have access to a gym, you can take advantage of the many types of equipment it has to offer. Cardiovascular equipment, such as rowing machines, stair-climbers, exercise bikes, and treadmills, offers potentially great fitness benefits. Cross-training on different equipment can keep your motivation high, reduce your chances of injury, and give your body a well-rounded workout.
- Access in your community to a swimming pool is a great fitness opportunity for some people. Swimming or even just walking though water offers a good aerobic workout that is easy on sore joints. You may find that the fun of swimming helps you stick with it.
- Are aerobics classes (step, low-impact, cardiofunk, Jazzercise, slide, and so on) offered in your area? The chance to participate in a well-controlled class with other people may strike your fancy.
- If you live in an area where you can spend time outside, walking, hiking, running, in-line skating, and cycling are all viable options. If the weather is reasonably good for most of the year in your area and you enjoy exploring your neighborhood, the out-of-doors offers many pleasant distractions that can make a long walk something to look forward to.

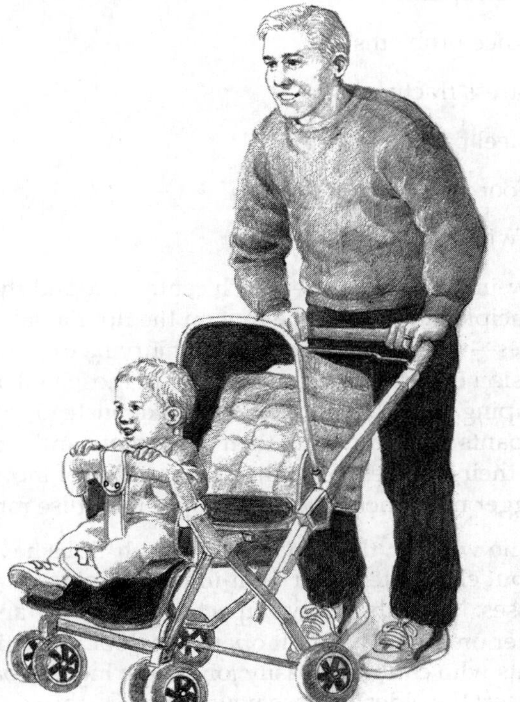

- If you have small children at home or can't often leave the house by yourself, it may seem difficult to find a good aerobic activity, but there are plenty of options. Exercise videos, walking (with a stroller, if necessary), or home exercise equipment are all possibilities.

Your experience level

- If you're new to fitness, instruction in the form of a trainer at a gym or in an exercise class will help ensure that you get a safe and effective workout. An instructor can also help you safely increase the intensity and duration of your exercise as your fitness improves.
- Do you want to learn a new activity or sport, or do you want to continue with an activity or sport that you know well? If you have some experience in the sport of your choice, go to it.

High-Impact Aerobics: A Dangerous Proposition

With aerobic dance's rise in popularity has come an accompanying rise in the number of injuries caused by the sport, including:

- Shin splints
- Knee problems
- Stress fractures
- Heel pain
- Foot pain
- Twisted ankles

Low-impact aerobics—which centers around the principle of keeping one foot on the floor at all times—virtually eliminates the injury factor. This version of aerobic dance cuts out all those violent jumping jacks, bounces, and the like. Instead, participants focus on using their arms more and working their muscles through a larger range of motion. (Bigger movements help to elevate the pulse rate.)

It's no wonder, then, that some health clubs have all but eliminated their high-impact aerobics classes: Not only is low-impact exercise safer and easier on the body, but it opens the door to participants who could not easily join in the high-impact classes: the elderly, those new to fitness, the severely overweight, and those with joint problems.

However, if you're primed for a change to something new, consider taking exercise classes or joining a gym that has good, certified instructors.

Your health

- Are you pregnant or have you recently given birth? Exercise during pregnancy and after can be perfectly safe and beneficial to the mother—provided that appropriate exercises are chosen and that the activities are performed correctly. If you are pregnant or have recently given birth (especially if you're new to fitness), you're probably best off joining a pregnancy or postpartum exercise group. There are also several good pregnancy and postpartum exercise videos on the market. (See page 85 for more information.)

Low-Impact Exercise: A Varied Array of Options

High-impact exercise, such as running and high-impact aerobics, can be tough on your body. But if the idea of performing one of the traditional forms of low-impact exercise—stationary cycling, walking, rowing, cross-country skiing, or swimming—leaves you cold, try one of the following popular alternatives. All provide a respectable cardiovascular workout, without over-stressing your joints:

- Step aerobics. In this sport, instructors lead participants through a variety of arm and leg movements while stepping up and down on a bench of varying height.
- Slide aerobics. This sport involves wearing nylon booties over athletic shoes and sliding back and forth on slick plastic while listening to music.
- Stair climbing. A variety of different machines enable participants to raise their pulse rates by stepping, climbing, or jogging on pedals.
- Cross-country ski machines. These machines give participants the low-impact, calorie-burning power of cross-country skiing.
- Aerobic Boxing. This new incarnation of aerobic dance combines traditional boxing moves (jabs, upper-cuts, blocks, and so on) with more customary aerobics moves. Your local video store probably has a large selection of tapes.

- If you have any chronic health problem, you should definitely consult your physician before beginning any exercise program. After a thorough physical examination, ask the doctor about the types of exercise that you can safely participate in. Also ask about types of exercise that may favorably affect your condition.
- If you suffer from any joint problems, or if you have any old injuries, you'll need to choose activities that can improve your condition or, at least, won't cause your condition to deteriorate. Low-impact exercises will probably be your best bet (ask your physician which type he or she prefers you to try).
- If you are a beginning exerciser age 50 or older, consult your physician before beginning an exercise program. If you get a clean bill of

health, consider starting out with walking, stationary cycling, low-impact aerobics, or swimming. These activities, when performed correctly, can provide a safe, gentle cardiovascular workout.

- If you are severely overweight, consult your physician before choosing an exercise program. When you get the green light, consider starting out with low-impact activities. Running, jogging, and high-impact aerobics may put too much stress on your joints.

Your personal preferences

- Are you very self-disciplined, or do you find that you are more motivated by participating in a group? If you just can't get motivated on your own, consider taking exercise classes or joining a gym that has good instruction.
- If you're more of a self-motivator, consider outdoor activities, swimming, exercise videos, or home exercise equipment.
- If you can't put up with the loud rock and roll, disco, or rap music played in many aerobics classes and gyms, you might be happier running, walking, in-line skating, or cycling alone with a portable stereo and headphones. Books on tape are another option for the quieter exerciser. (Be aware, though, that for safety reasons, cycling with headphones on is illegal in some areas.)

STRENGTH TRAINING AND TONING

You have no desire to be an elite athlete or a bodybuilder. Why should you incorporate strength training into your fitness regimen? It's easy to overlook the benefits that strength training has to offer, but improving your muscle strength and muscle tone will aid you in a variety of ways.

Here's what you'll have to look forward to:

- A toned, more attractive physique
- Decreased chance of injury
- Greater stamina in everyday activities
- A higher metabolism (Muscle burns more calories than fat, even when the body is at rest.)
- Better body composition (an improved ratio of lean tissue to fat)
- Improvement in or maintenance of bone density (a way to prevent osteoporosis and fractures)

A common mistake is to assume that by lifting weights, you will inadvertently build bulky muscles. In fact, body builders have to work very hard (through exercise *and* diet) to achieve that sinewy, rippled look—there's nothing inadvertent about it! In addition, muscle takes up much less room than fat. Therefore, if you stay the same weight and add muscle mass, you will automatically lose inches, not add them. (If you want to gain weight and add muscle mass, you will have to lift moderately heavy weights, perform many sets, exercise every muscle group, work out for many hours, and add extra protein and low-fat calories to your diet.)

Here is the difference between a routine that is designed to tone the muscles and one that is designed to add muscle mass: A mass-building or strength workout uses very heavy weights, lifted through fewer repetitions but more sets than are incorporated into a toning workout. The amount of weight is increased as soon as the muscle can withstand it. A toning routine, on the other hand, uses relatively light weights, no weights, or elastic tubing lifted through many repetitions but fewer sets. As the muscles get stronger, more repetitions are added.

While it's a valid goal to want a strong, muscular physique, most of us simply want a leaner, toned

The Amateur's Guide to Muscle Anatomy

Before embarking on a strength-training or toning program, it is helpful to familiarize yourself with the major muscle groups that you'll be working. Although there are many more muscles in the body than are listed here, the following is a lexicon of terms that you're likely to hear in an exercise class or around the gym. The scientific name of the muscle group is listed first. The more common, weight-room terms (where appropriate) are enclosed in parenthesis.

Biceps brachii ("biceps" or "bis") are two muscles that originate at the front of the shoulder and upper arm and attach below the elbow. The belly of the muscle is in the front of the upper arm.

Deltoids ("delts") are three muscles: the anterior deltoid (at the front of the shoulder), the posterior deltoid (at the back of the shoulder), and the medial deltoid (along the side of the shoulder). In the weight room, these muscles are often lumped together.

Gastrocnemius ("calves" or "calf muscle") is the large muscle at the upper portion of the calf.

Gluteus maximus, medius, and *minimus* ("gluteals" or "glutes") are more commonly referred to as the buttocks and are actually three separate muscles.

Hamstrings are the muscle group made up of the biceps femoris, the semitendinosus, and the semimembranosus, all of which run down the back of the thigh.

Latissimus dorsi ("lats") give your upper back width above the waist. They pull the arms down when you do a pull-up.

Obliques ("waist") are the muscles that make up the waist, on either side of the trunk, below the latissimus dorsi.

Pectorals ("pecs") are three muscles that run diagonally from 1) the shoulder toward the chest, 2) straight across from the shoulder joint toward the chest, and 3) along the collarbone toward the chest.

Quadriceps ("quads") run down the front of the thigh from the hip joint down to just above the knee.

Rectus abdominis ("abdominal" or "abs") is the muscle that extends from the diaphragm down to the pelvis.

Rhomboids are two separate muscles: the major and the minor. They are located between the shoulder blades. They are covered by another muscle, so they are hard to see or feel.

Trapezius ("traps") are three muscles: the upper, the middle, and the lower. However, when you hear the name of this muscle group tossed around in the weight room, it usually refers to the upper trapezius, which spans the area between the top of the shoulder and the side of the neck.

Triceps ("tris") are usually called by their proper name. They are opposite the biceps. The center of the back of the upper arm is where they are most easily felt, but they run from the shoulder down to the elbow.

look. If that is your intention, you should perform a routine based on the principles mentioned above for a toning and strengthening routine.

GUIDELINES FOR TRAINING

If you belong to a gym, you'd be well-advised to ask for strength-training tips from a credentialed instructor. There are also many strength-training videos on the market. However, if you've decided to go it alone, you must be extra careful to avoid injury from improper technique and to insure that you are getting the optimum benefit from your workout. First, we'll cover some basic guidelines for this type of training, regardless of the specific exercises you choose. Then, we'll get into designing a safe and effective strength-training program for use at home. Here are a couple of tips to make your workouts safer and more effective:

- Choose the right weight. If you are using weights or bands, you'll have to do a little bit of trial and error to figure out how much weight (or what size band) to start out with. A general guideline for strength training is that you should be able to complete at least two sets of at least eight controlled repetitions with the weight you choose. If you can't, it's too heavy. Likewise, if you can comfortably do more than three sets of 12 repetitions, it's time to move up to a heavier weight.

For toning exercises, shoot for two sets of 15 to 20 repetitions, whichever you prefer. The weight or band width you choose should leave you struggling a bit by the end of your last set.

- Always warm up by performing 15 reps with only 50 to 75 percent of your usual working weight.
- Alternate your training schedule. If you want to train every day, you should work your upper body one day and your lower body the next. Always allow muscle groups one day of rest in between workouts. If you want to work out every other day, you can train the whole body during each session.
- Breathe properly. With all strength-training exercises, you should exhale as you contract the muscle or lift the weight. Inhale as you relax the muscle or lower the weight. Don't hold your breath.
- Pay attention to good form. Control your weights or bands while lifting **and** lowering them. Go slowly; never jerk the weights up or let them drop too quickly.
- Don't lock your joints. While performing strength-training exercises, take care that you never lock your knees or elbows. Instead, always bend them slightly to prevent repetitive-strain injuries.

The exercises in the following sections are intended only for those who are in good health and who are not pregnant. If you have chronic health problems or any reason to believe that you should not be performing these exercises, consult your doctor before starting a strength-training or toning program.

Some of the exercises in this section require the use of handheld dumbbells, wrist weights, or ankle weights. If you're just beginning, or if you haven't yet bought dumbbells, you can start out using small cantaloupes or large soup cans. You can also use light wrist or ankle weights, rubber bands, or elastic tubing as resistance for the toning modifications given.

Fitness Gadgetry: Magic Bullets or Snake Oil?

The Abdominizer. The ThighMaster. Plastic body suits. Complicated-looking cable setups that hang from your door frame and promise to make you fit "in just five minutes a day." What's the truth behind these hyped-up widgets? Will they help you get fit faster, or just deplete your bank account?

One rule of thumb you can use when evaluating such purchases is: If it seems too good to be true, it probably is. If there were a mystical machine that helped "inches disappear like magic," we'd probably all have perfect bodies by now (and we don't).

The bottom line is—any product that promises results without a substantial investment of time and effort is, at best, a bogus way to capitalize on consumers' naïveté. There's only one prescription for a great body: regular exercise, a healthy diet, and tenacity.

TONING THE UPPER BODY

Now that you have the general guidelines for strength training and toning down, you're ready to move on to the specific exercises. First, we'll start with the upper body. Unless otherwise noted, each exercise should be performed for three sets of 8 to 12 repetitions (for strength training) or two sets of 15 to 20 repetitions (with lighter weights for toning). The exercises given are performed with weights. Toning and rubber-band modifications are noted with an asterisk (*). If no toning modification is given, follow the exercise as written, using a lighter weight (or no weight).

Biceps curl. Sit on the edge of a stool or bench or stand with the knees slightly bent, about hip-distance apart. Hold one weight in each hand and extend the arms down the front of your thighs with the inner forearms facing outward. Without moving the upper arms, slowly lift the weights for four counts, until they are almost touching your upper arms. At the peak of the movement, contract the biceps muscles and hold for two counts. Slowly lower the weights to the starting position to the count of four.

*Toning modification: From a standing position, with a rubber band anchored under your feet, grasp the band with both hands (use an underhand grip). Keeping your elbows firmly anchored to either side of your waist, curl the band up, until your fists touch your chest. Pause, then slowly lower.

Triceps kickback. Stand with your knees bent, feet about hip-distance apart. Lean slightly forward, take a weight in each hand and hold them right next to your hips. Elbows should be bent and held closely to your sides. Without moving your upper arms or your elbows, straighten the arms and extend the weights as high as you can in back of you to the count of four. Contract the triceps and hold for two counts. Slowly lower the weights to the count of four. (Some find it more comfortable to do this exercise one arm at a time. The resting arm can be placed on the knee to assist in supporting the upper back.)

Front raise. This exercise tones the anterior deltoid, at the front of the shoulder. Stand with the knees slightly bent, feet about hip-distance apart. Hold a weight in each hand, with the arms extended down the front of the thighs, inner wrists facing forward and the elbows slightly bent. Slowly raise the weights to shoulder level, to a count of four. Hold for two counts, then slowly lower to the starting position, again, to the count of four. (Again, this exercise can be performed one arm at a time.)

*Toning modification: Stand with a rubber band anchored under the soles of your feet. Grasp the band with both hands, using an overhand grip. Straighten (but don't lock) the elbows and slowly raise your arms up to shoulder level. Hold, then slowly lower.

Lateral raise. This exercise tones the middle deltoid at the side of the shoulder. Hold a weight in each hand, with the arms extended down the sides of the thighs, inner wrists facing outward, and elbows slightly bent. Slowly raise the weights to shoulder level, to a count of four. Hold for two counts, then slowly lower to the starting position, again, to the count of four.

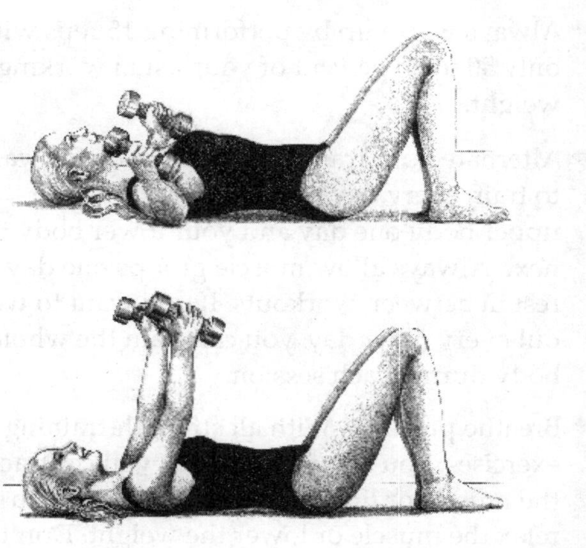

Chest fly. This exercise tones the pectoralis major muscles. Lie on a weight bench or on the floor. Hold a weight in each hand, arms extended out to the sides at chest level, the insides of the forearms facing up toward the ceiling. The arms should remain rigid throughout the exercise, although the elbows should be slightly bent (not locked). Slowly bring the weights together (over your chest) to the count of four. Hold for two counts, then slowly lower to the starting position, again, to the count of four.

ABDOMINAL TRAINING

Unlike other types of resistance training, abdominal exercises can (and should) be performed every day. Remember, toned abdominals not only make you look better, but they improve your posture and help prevent back injury. To increase the intensity of the following exercises, try performing them slower or try adding repetitions or a few sets of pulses (small, rapid lifts from the upright position, without lowering to the floor in between).

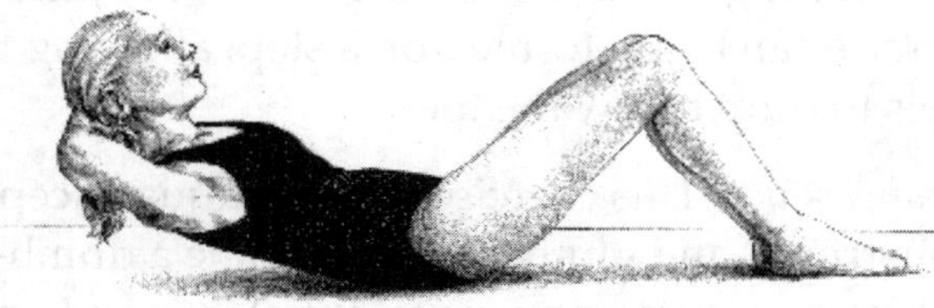

Abdominal crunch. This exercise tones the upper portion of the rectus abdominis. Lie on your back, with your knees bent, feet on the floor, slightly closer than hip-distance apart. Lace your fingers behind your neck, holding the elbows straight out to the sides. Keep your chin up by looking directly up toward the ceiling. Holding this position, curl your upper body up toward the knees, keeping the lower back firmly pressed into the floor. As you lift, simultaneously contract the abdominal muscles and curl the pelvis up and toward the navel. Lower shoulders and pelvis to starting position. At the peak of the crunch, the shoulders and back should form no more than about a 45-degree angle with the floor (don't come up all the way to your knees). This exercise can be performed for a slow 24 repetitions (two counts up, two counts down).

Oblique crunch. This exercise tones the oblique muscles at the sides of the waist. Lie on the floor in the same position as for the abdominal crunch, except rest the outside of one ankle against the opposite thigh, with the knee pointing out from the body. Keep your fingers laced behind your neck. One shoulder—the one on the same side of the body as the leg that's resting against the other thigh—stays on the ground, while you curl the abdomen and the opposite shoulder up toward the knee. Lower to the starting position. As with the abdominal crunches, oblique crunches can be performed for a slow 24 repetitions (two counts up, two counts down). After one set is completed, switch sides and repeat the exercise crunching the other way.

Reverse crunch. This exercise tones the lower portion of the rectus abdominis. Lie on the floor, with your arms at your sides or with your hands under your hips (the latter position helps to support the lower back). Hold your legs up so the thighs are perpendicular to your body, and cross your legs at the knee, allowing your lower legs and feet to hang loosely. In a slow, controlled motion, lift the buttocks and lower back off the floor while contracting the lower abdominal muscles. Slowly lower to the starting position. Complete as many repetitions as you can without compromising proper form. Gradually build to three sets of eight repetitions.

TONING THE LOWER BODY

Handheld dumbbells and ankle weights (where noted) will increase the intensity of these exercises. If you do not own any weights, wear your heaviest athletic shoes during the leg lifts and "butt-busters" (their weight will add intensity).

Again, before trying these exercises, be sure that you have read the section on general guidelines for strength training (pages 78–79). Unless otherwise noted, each exercise should be performed for three sets of 8 to 12 repetitions (for strength training) or four sets of 12 to 15 repetitions (with lighter weights or bands, for toning). Toning and rubber-band modifications are noted with an asterisk (*). If no toning modification is given, toning can be accomplished by following the exercise with a lighter weight (or no weight).

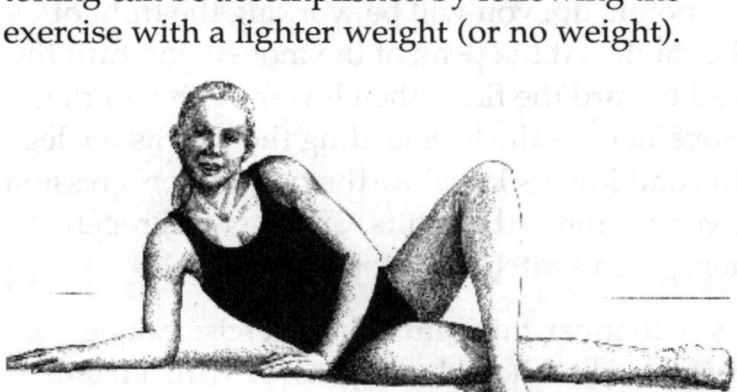

Inner-thigh lift. Lie on your side, propping yourself up on one elbow. Bend the top leg and place it in front of the bottom leg, with the foot on the floor, and the knee pointed up. Check your alignment to be sure that your bottom leg is lined up with your hip, your waist, and your shoulder. Extend the bottom leg out straight, with the inner thigh facing the ceiling and the ankle bent. Using the inner-thigh muscles, lift the bottom leg toward the ceiling. At the peak of the movement, contract the inner-thigh muscle. Lower the leg slowly. Follow the training progression below. (Don't worry if you can't do the whole routine at first. Simply do as many sets as you can and gradually work up to the whole progression.)

- Complete three sets of eight full repetitions—two counts up, hold for two counts, down in two counts (a total of six counts for one rep).
- Complete two sets of eight repetitions—three small pulses up, down in one count.
- Complete one set of eight small pulses.

Complete all repetitions, then switch to the other side. To increase intensity, add extra sets of pulses at the end. For strengthening, this exercise can be performed with ankle weights, or with a handheld weight placed on top of the working thigh.

Outer-thigh lift. Lie on one side, propped up on one elbow. Check to be sure your bottom leg, hip, and shoulder are all in alignment. Extend your top leg, with the ankle bent and the heel rotated toward the ceiling. Lift the leg, making sure to keep the heel pointing toward the ceiling (if your toe points up, you will be working the front of the thigh). At the peak of the movement, turn the heel toward the floor, then lower. (Think of the movement as the heel leading the way as the leg lifts and lowers.) Follow the training progression given for inner-thigh lifts. Complete all repetitions, then switch to the other side.

As with inner-thigh lifts, this exercise can be performed with ankle weights, or with a handheld weight placed on the working thigh.

*Toning modification: Place a rubber band around both ankles.

Calf raise. This exercise tones and develops the gastrocnemius muscles. Stand with one hand against a wall for balance, feet hip-distance apart. Rise onto your toes, hold for one count, then lower. Repeat for three sets of eight repetitions. For strengthening, this exercise may be performed with weights held on the shoulders. To work through a more full range of motion, the exercise can be preformed on a step, allowing the heels to drop below the toes.

Parallel squat. This exercise tones the quadriceps, hamstrings, and gluteal muscles. Take a dumbbell (or a soup can or a cantaloupe) in each hand. Stand with feet a little closer than hip-distance apart, knees slightly bent. Hold the weights on the shoulders or at the top of each thigh. Look up slightly to maintain the curve in your lower back. Squat down by sitting back, as though you were lowering yourself into a chair. To avoid knee stress, make sure that your weight is firmly in your heels. Lower yourself until your thighs are parallel with the floor. Do not squat too low (your knees should never go farther forward than your toes). Contract your buttocks, and press up to the starting position. Perform each repetition to a count of eight (four counts up, four counts down). Safety tip: If you feel pain in your knees, or if they grind or click excessively, try this exercise without weights. If you still feel pain, skip this exercise altogether.

Wide-leg squat. This exercise also tones the quadriceps, hamstrings, gluteal, and inner-thigh muscles. Assume a wide stance, with the toes pointing outward. Follow the procedure for parallel squats, above. Again, your knees should never come out further than your toes. If you feel excessive strain in your knees, try these squats without the weights. If you still feel pain, skip this exercise altogether.

Butt buster. This exercise tones the gluteals and hamstrings. Kneel on the floor with the hands clasped together and the elbows and forearms on the floor, supporting you. Extend one leg straight out behind you, foot flexed, heel to the ceiling. Lift the leg while simultaneously contracting the

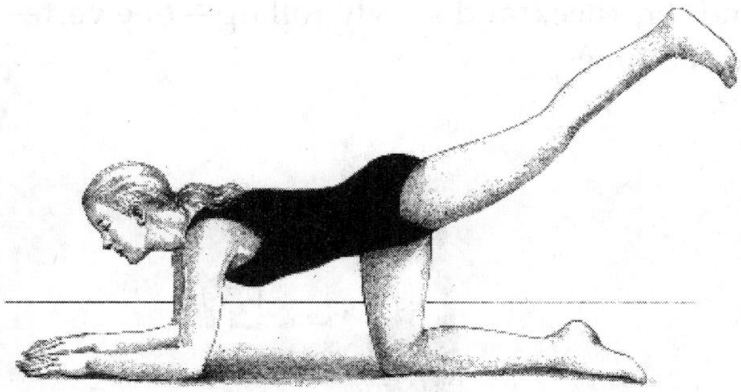

buttocks. Do not lift too high, or you will place strain on the lower back (the back should not arch excessively during this exercise). Lower almost to the floor, without touching. Repeat the exercise for three sets of eight slow repetitions. To add intensity, follow the training sequence described for inner-thigh lifts. This exercise may be performed with ankle weights.

ENHANCING YOUR FLEXIBILITY

As mentioned previously, flexibility is important in preventing injury, during both athletic and everyday activities. As such, you should make stretching a permanent part of your exercise routine. Most fitness associations recommend that you perform stretching exercises before and after a strength-training or aerobic workout.

As a general guideline, stretch only as far as is comfortable. You should feel tension, but never push a stretch to the point of pain. Also, you should never bounce while stretching. "Ballistic stretching," as this is called, can injure your connective tissue. A good way to ensure that you're not stretching too far is to breathe slowly and rhythmically during the stretch; when you stretch too far, you have a tendency to hold your breath. One final safety tip: During pregnancy, joints loosen and become lax. To avoid connective-tissue injury, pregnant women should take extra care not to overstretch muscles.

The following stretches should be performed in sequence. Before beginning, warm up the muscles with five minutes of very low-intensity marching, walking, stair-climbing, or any other aerobic activity.

Shoulder loosener. Stand with the knees slightly bent, feet hip-distance apart. Shrug the shoulders, pulling them up toward the ears, then lowering. Repeat four times. Slowly circle the shoulders backward for eight counts, then forward for eight counts.

Neck loosener. Gently cock the head to the right. Hold for a count of eight. Repeat on the left side. Look as far to the right as you can, while still holding your shoulders square. Hold for a count of eight. Repeat on the left side. Gently roll the head from shoulder to shoulder, pulling the head close to the chest. Do not roll the head to the back. Repeat eight times.

Waist stretch. Assume a wide stance, bending the knees. Rest your right elbow on your right thigh for balance and extend the left arm diagonally up and toward the right, in line with the ear. Hold for a few counts; breathe in; then exhale deeply, allowing your body to relax even further into the stretch. Keep your head up and don't bend too far forward at the waist. Hold for a slow count of eight, then repeat on the left side.

Standing back stretch. Stand with your feet hip-distance apart, knees bent. Put one hand on each knee. Arch your back toward the ceiling (keep your abdominal muscles tight), hold for a slow count of four, then release, allowing your back to arch only slightly. Repeat three times.

Note: If this stretch puts too much strain on your back, skip it.

Runner's lunge. Assume a wide stance, then turn to your right, bending your right knee and keeping your left leg straight (but don't lock your knee). Place both hands on the floor and stretch forward, checking to make sure that your knee never juts out past your toes. Press the left knee toward the floor, feeling the stretch in the front of the upper thigh. Hold for a count of eight, then proceed to the hamstring stretch described below. After performing both stretches on the right, repeat both on the left.

Modified runner's lunge. If the position of the runner's lunge is too difficult for you, either because you can't reach the floor, or because it puts too much strain on your back, perform the stretch from a standing position, with both hands on the right knee. Hold for a count of eight, then proceed to the modified hamstring stretch. After performing both modified stretches on the right, repeat both on the left.

Hamstring stretch. From the runner's lunge position, walk the back leg in a couple of steps, then bend it. Straighten out the front leg (but don't lock the knee). Pull the toes off the floor, until they are pointing toward the ceiling. Hold for a count of eight. When you have finished this stretch with the first leg, walk the back leg up to the front leg. Place one hand on each knee, keeping the knees bent, and slowly roll up—one vertebra at a time. Perform the runner's lunge and hamstring stretch with the other leg. Then, without rolling up, proceed directly to the calf stretch described below.

Modified hamstring stretch. From the modified runner's lunge position, walk the back leg forward a couple of steps. Perform the stretch as described above, but place one hand on the upper thigh of each leg. Repeat both modified stretches on the other leg, then proceed to the modified calf stretch.

Calf stretch. From the hamstring-stretch position, walk both legs back until you feel a stretch down the back of the legs. Press the heels into the floor, slowly alternating between left and right for a count of four on each side. Then press both heels into the floor and hold for a count of eight. After you have finished, walk your hands back to your legs, place a hand on each knee, bend the knees, and slowly roll up—one vertebra at a time.

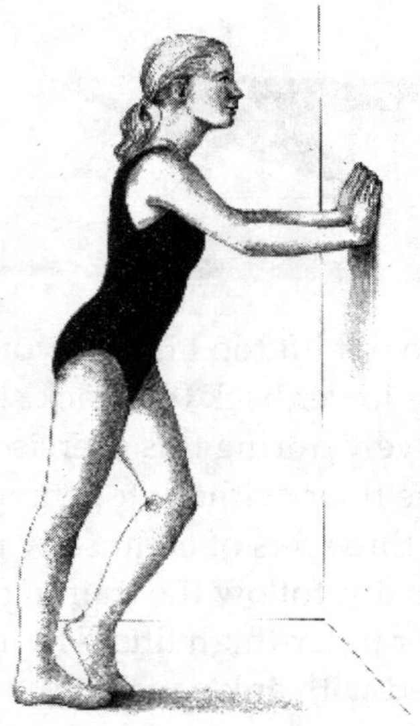

Modified calf stretch. Lean against a wall with your arms out straight (but don't lock the elbows), and your palms on the wall. Walk your legs out behind you until you feel a stretch down the back of the legs. Press the heels into the floor, alternating between the left and right for a count of four on each side. Then press both heels into the floor and hold for a count of eight.

EXERCISE SAFETY

THE PERFECT WORKOUT

Cardiovascular conditioning, strength training, and flexibility are all important parts of fitness. However, there is more to a safe and effective workout than elevating your heartbeat, lifting a few weights, and touching your toes. The following guidelines can serve as the blueprint for a textbook-perfect workout.

Warm-up. Start every exercise session—whether it be an aerobic workout, a strength-training workout, even a stretching routine—with a five- to ten-minute warm-up. You can march, walk briskly, jump rope, dance—whatever you like—as long as it gets your blood flowing and warms up your muscles. Just a short warm-up can help in preventing injury during athletic activities.

Stretching. A routine that stretches all of the major muscle groups, such as the routine mentioned above, further loosens up the muscles. If not properly stretched out, muscles and other connective tissue such as ligaments and tendons can tear or pull when a strong action is suddenly demanded of them. So, take the time to stretch properly—without bouncing or overstretching to the point of pain—and you will improve your overall flexibility and help prevent needless injuries.

The main event. If you are planning a strength-training or aerobic workout, go to it. During an aerobic workout, check your aerobic intensity. At the peak of your exercise, check your pulse to be sure it's in your target training zone. If it's too high, ease up a bit; if it's too low, pick up the pace. (See pages 72–74 for more on proper intensity level and target heart rate.)

Cool-down. The cool-down is the opposite of the warm-up. It's a chance to allow your pulse rate and blood pressure to return to normal and, in the case of a strength-training workout, to relax the muscles that you've been working. It should consist of 5 to 15 minutes of progressively slower walking, stationary cycling, or any other gentle aerobic activity. It can be tempting to just stop and flop after an intense bout of exercise, but resist the temptation and bring it down slowly.

Stretching. This final stretch is thought to prevent soreness after exercising. It prevents the muscles from tightening and cramping. By giving your body this chance to cool down further, you end the workout on a placid note. This is also the best time to improve your flexibility because your muscles are warm and pliable.

EXERCISE DURING PREGNANCY

There's no need to drop your fitness routine during pregnancy. In fact, appropriate types of exercise can help you stay energized; sleep better; preserve your aerobic fitness (important when you're lugging around a chubby eight-month-old); alleviate back pain; prevent constipation, hemorrhoids, and varicose veins; and prepare your body for the rigors of childbirth. However, you may have to modify your normal routine. Be sure that any workout you plan during your pregnancy follows the safety guidelines put forth by the American College of Obstetrics and Gynecology:

- Regular, consistent exercise is preferable to intermittent activity. Shoot for three to five workout sessions per week.
- Put competitive activities on hold until a couple months after the baby is born.
- Do not exercise in hot, humid weather, or while you are feverish.
- Avoid all forms of high-impact exercise. Exercise on a wooden or tightly carpeted floor.
- Avoid deep knee bends.
- Stretch only to the point of gentle tension, never beyond.
- Warm up the muscles with at least five minutes of slow walking or another low-intensity aerobic activity before performing vigorous exercise.
- Perform gentle stretches after vigorous exercise. Again, do not stretch to the point of maximum resistance.
- Rise from the floor slowly and gradually to avoid large drops in blood pressure.
- Drink plenty of water before, during, and after exercise. Every 15 to 20 minutes you should get at least six ounces of water.
- If you have been sedentary before your pregnancy, only engage in low-intensity activities, such as walking, and increase your activity level very slowly and gradually.
- Stop exercising and consult your physician if you develop any unusual symptoms.
- After the fourth month of pregnancy, do not perform any exercise that requires you to lie on your back. Avoid abdominal exercises in the supine position.

Sports Drinks: Are They Really Necessary?

There are plenty of sports drinks on the market whose manufacturers claim that they boost energy and performance or that they replace essential minerals that are lost through sweating. Do these (often expensive) drinks deliver what they promise? Or is water a sufficient rehydrater?

Most sports drinks contain electrolytes, a fancy term for the minerals sodium and potassium. Fitness experts say that although you lose a certain amount of electrolytes through sweating, the amount of these substances contained in your next meal will usually be more than adequate to replace what you've lost.

Sports drinks also contain varying amounts of calories in the form of sugar (often noted on labels as high-fructose corn sweetener or sucrose). If shedding some of that excess fat is one of your fitness goals, these are probably unwanted calories.

Water is the best and most easily absorbed fluid. It is exactly what your body wants, and it contains no calories. Drink plenty of plain old water before, during, and after exercise.

- Avoid exercises that might cause a temporary rise in blood pressure. Such exercises include push-ups, pull-ups, and lifting heavy weights. (Ask your physician if it is safe for you to use light weights.)
- Make sure that you are consuming enough calories to make up for those you burn during your workouts.
- Periodically monitor your temperature before and during exercise. It should not rise more than one degree Fahrenheit. Excessive body heat may cause harm to the developing fetus. Avoid exercise in warm water. Cool-water exercises, though, may help regulate your core temperature.
- The Perceived-Exertion Scale may be more suitable than heart rate for monitoring maternal exercise intensity (see page 73).

STAYING MOTIVATED

Just as you can learn how to do a perfect abdominal crunch, you can also learn methods to help you stick to your weekly exercise schedule. Here are a few of the tried-and-true:

Use the buddy system. An exercise partner can be a great way to inject some fun into what could easily turn into a monotonous routine. If you've got plans for a lunchtime jog with a friend, you're less likely to cop out when the noon hour rolls around (and the burger joint beckons).

Participate in local athletic events. Cycling trips, race-walks, and road races can all be ways to make exercise more exciting. A dose of friendly competition may inspire you to reach new fitness heights.

Keep a journal of your progress. Each day that you work out, jot down what you did, and how long you did it for. If improving your body composition is your goal, write down your weight and body measurements once a month. When you get discouraged or feel like quitting, flip through this journal to remind you of how much progress you've made.

Commit yourself to six weeks. If you can stick to your workout schedule for six weeks—performing at least three sessions of aerobic exercise and two strength-training workouts per week—you are virtually guaranteed to see some improvement in your fitness level. Seeing this progress might be just the kick you need to keep you going back for more.

AVOIDING POTENTIAL HAZARDS

You've probably heard the expression, "It's a jungle out there." While it's true that the world can be a hazardous place, knowledge, some advance planning, and a little common sense can help reduce the number of dangers in our lives.

Your well-being can be jeopardized by three major types of hazards: 1) accidents, especially among children and the elderly; 2) ill-advised health choices; and 3) ignorance, which prevents early diagnosis and control of various illnesses.

Eighteenth century French author, Voltaire, said this about health: "Everyone should be his own physician." This chapter deals with ways in which you can be your own physician by learning to take responsibility for your health, recognizing and avoiding threats to your well-being, and making lifestyle choices that promote good health, thereby giving you more control over your quality of life. Even if it is a jungle out there, you can be prepared to survive it.

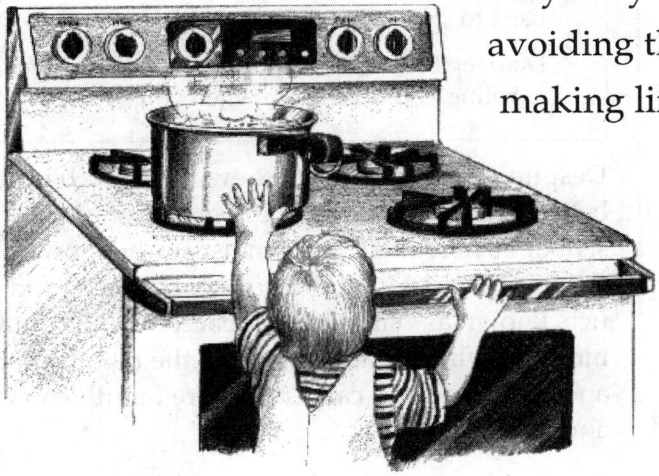

HAZARDOUS SUBSTANCES

In our environment, there are, unfortunately, dangerous substances. Our bodies are tough in many ways, but we are no match for some chemicals. Some of these substances are difficult to avoid, but the strange thing is that some of the most dangerous chemicals are ones we choose to come in contact with.

SMOKING AND CHEWING TOBACCO

Would you spend $900 to $1,000 a year to shorten your life span by increasing your risk of heart disease, arthritis, asthma, high blood pressure, stroke, emphysema, and cancer? That's just what you're doing when you smoke.

A smoker has ten times the chance of getting lung cancer as a nonsmoker does and twice the chance of heart disease. Women who take birth control pills and smoke have ten times the chance of having a heart attack as a nonsmoker and 20 times the chance of having a stroke. One out of seven deaths in America is caused by smoking. Cigarette smoking kills more people than AIDS, heroin, cocaine, alcohol, car accidents, fire, and murder combined.

You may also be harming your children's health by exposing them to "second-hand" or "passive" smoke. The children of those who smoke are more likely to suffer from respiratory disorders and allergies, sustain hearing defects, have high cholesterol, and miss more days of school because of illness than children of nonsmokers. As babies, they are also more likely to die from sudden infant death syndrome. Recent studies have shown that a pregnant woman's smoking can cause premature birth and low birth weight and affect her child's lung function well into adulthood.

TIPS TO HELP YOU GIVE UP SMOKING

- List the reasons you are motivated to stop smoking.
- Select a specific day on which you plan to stop smoking.
- Plan pleasurable activities for that day in places where smoking is not permitted.
- Throw out all cigarettes, matches, and ashtrays.
- Avoid friends, places, and situations associated with smoking.
- Recognize that withdrawal symptoms such as headaches, increased appetite, and irritability are only short-term problems.
- Take a walk or practice relaxation techniques when you crave a cigarette.
- Drink six to eight glasses of water a day to clean the nicotine out of your system.
- Plan for low-calorie snacks such as air-popped popcorn, carrots, celery, and fruit.
- Reward yourself each day you don't smoke.
- Set up a "ciggy" bank. Each day you don't smoke, set aside the amount of money you used to spend on cigarettes.
- Do deep breathing to replace the inhaling and exhaling you used to do when you smoked.

Despite popular opinion, chewing tobacco is no better. It is estimated that 20 percent of high school boys regularly use moist snuff, known as "dip," and chewing tobacco, two tobacco products known as "smokeless tobacco." Both contain nicotine, which is absorbed into the bloodstream and can cause oral cancers, severe mouth sores, and gum disease.

Even with supportive friends and family, smokers often need the additional help found at a clinic or in a smoking-cessation group. Some programs combine nicotine chewing gum or the nicotine skin patch with group therapy. Others rely on positive thinking, substitute behaviors, self-rewards, and the buddy system. Look in your telephone book under "Smokers Information and Treatment Centers" or contact your local office of the American Lung Association, the American Heart Association, or the American Cancer Society.

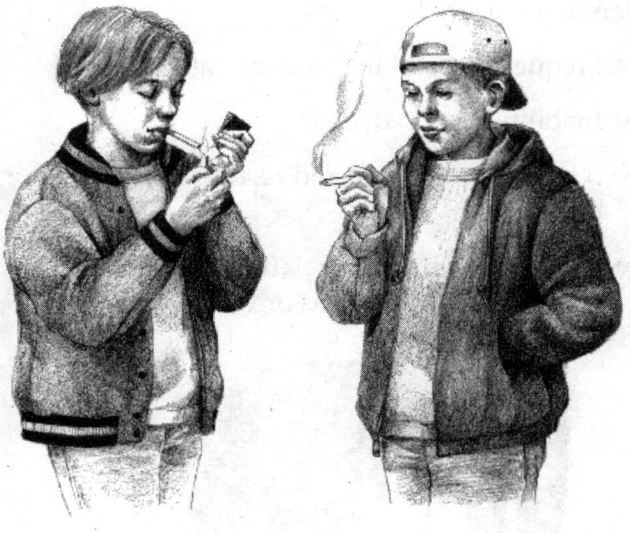

Some people find success in quitting their smoking habit through hypnosis. Check with your local medical association for names of psychiatrists and other professionals trained in this type of treatment.

ALCOHOL

Various research studies estimate that more than 100 million Americans drink alcohol. About 10 percent of those who drink have alcohol problems that have a negative effect on their lives and the lives of their families. Alcohol can adversely affect your health in many different ways. The drug itself (and it *is* a drug) can damage body tissue; its intoxicating effects can create dangerous situations, and its addictive qualities can destroy lives.

Alcohol and health. Heavy drinking can cause cirrhosis of the liver, which means that the liver is unable to filter toxins from the blood properly. Alcohol also widens the blood vessels, which causes the skin to flush, allowing heat to escape from the body. When delicate blood vessels in the nose enlarge from alcohol intake, it may trigger substantial nosebleeds. Chronic use of alcohol can cause malnutrition, promote memory loss, and depress antibody production in the body, which impairs the immune system, making the drinker more susceptible to infection and disease. Alcohol upsets your digestive system, produces impotence in men, and when used by pregnant women, increases the possibility of birth defects.

Alcohol and accidents. Many who drink say that they enjoy doing so because it is "relaxing" or because it gives them a confidence boost. But alcohol is a depressant. What many drinkers describe as a reduction of tension is actually the dulling of senses, which leads to a loss of inhibition, slowness in reaction time, and for many, dangerous aggressive tendencies.

Alcohol and driving is a deadly combination, whether you are driving a motor vehicle or a boat. Statistics show that more than half of fatal boating accidents are due to alcohol. After a few drinks, a person tends to lose inhibitions and is willing to take more risks. Visual acuity is adversely affected and reaction time slows. For this reason, the National Safe Boating Council offers the same advice as the National Safety Council: Don't drink and drive; always have a designated driver behind the wheel.

Automobiles and boats are not the only safety concern, either. All sorts of seemingly simple tasks, such as crossing the street or going down stairs, are much more dangerous when performed by someone whose judgment and coordination are impaired by alcohol. Research shows that people who drink tend to have injuries more and to die from these injuries more than those who drink moderately or not at all.

Alcoholism. Alcohol is a drug, and individuals can become both physically and emotionally dependent upon it. Many people become addicted to alcohol when they use it to forget their problems; to overcome a loss of a person, a pet, a job, health, or status; or to gain false courage. The use

How to Be a Responsible Drinker

- Know your limit and stick to it.
- Don't make drinking your primary activity.
- Always have food available to eat while you're drinking.
- Don't drink fast. Savor your drink and sip it.
- Dilute wine with water or ice.
- Don't let others freshen up your drink; you can't judge how much alcohol you're actually consuming.
- Don't consume drinks when you are unsure of what's in them.
- Don't try to keep up with other drinkers.
- Don't use alcohol to relax; instead, exercise, meditate, or use other relaxation techniques.
- Don't drink if you're taking medications unless you know *specifically* that the combination mixes safely.
- Never urge someone to have an alcoholic drink.
- NEVER drink and drive.

of alcohol can destroy friendships, sever family relationships, and threaten job security.

Nearly five million children—some as young as nine or ten—suffer from drinking problems. It's estimated that about nine percent of adult American men and four percent of adult American women are alcoholics. Recent studies reveal that anywhere from 700,000 to more than 7 million of our nation's alcoholics are over the age of 55.

There are different types of alcoholics. The most obvious is the person who can't stop tossing down drinks, staggers around with slurred speech, and eventually falls down and blacks out with no memory of what occurred. There is also the secret drinker, the one we call the "functional alcoholic," who holds down a job and fulfills responsibilities, but who needs alcohol to "get by." Other alcoholics feel they don't need to drink, but when they do, they may binge, lose control, and undergo a personality change, turning mean and often physically or verbally abusive.

These are some warning signs to help you recognize when you or someone you know has a problem with alcohol:

- Frequently drinking to intoxication
- Inability to stop drinking
- Nausea, headaches, and restlessness when not drinking
- Behavioral problems relating to drinking in social or work relations or with the law

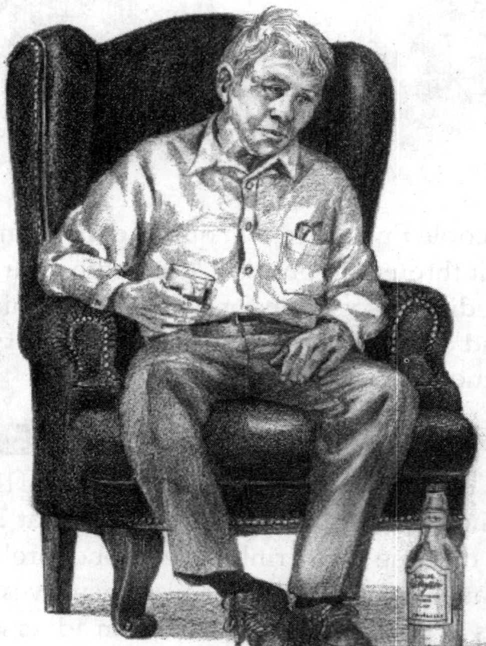

Today people are far more aware of alcoholism and its effect on the entire family. Organizations such as Alcoholics Anonymous, Al-Anon, and Alateen are among the best-known sources for help, although it is difficult for young children of alcoholics to get to meetings without their parents' support. The telephone numbers for Alcoholics Anonymous affiliates are in your local directory. In addition, many communities, churches, and synagogues sponsor support groups for alcoholics and their families. There is a Children of Alcoholics Foundation for adults still struggling with memories of their parents' alcoholism. Psychiatrists, psychologists, trained social workers, and other medical professionals can work with those battling alcoholism, either as their own demon or that of a loved one. There are also in-patient treatment clinics, crises centers, alcohol support help lines, and even computer bulletin board support groups. But before any of this expertise can be of help, the alcoholic must admit to him or herself that a problem with alcohol exists.

Detecting Problem Drinking Among the Elderly

Many of the symptoms of alcoholism are problems typically attributed to old age, such as insomnia, poor concentration, and depression. Alcoholism in the elderly is particularly serious because many of them are on numerous medications that, when combined with alcohol, can be deadly. In addition, the warning signs of problem drinking in the elderly are more subtle than in a younger drinker. They include:

- Increased indications of self-neglect or letting the house or apartment become cluttered and dirty if the person has typically been neat
- Confusion over simple things such as time of day, surroundings, and people
- Repeated falls and accidents around the home
- Drinking small amounts of alcohol on a daily basis

If you suspect that alcoholism is a problem for an older person that you know, convince them to seek help. Alcoholics Anonymous addresses all age groups.

ILLEGAL DRUGS

Illegal drugs are substances that are either illegal in themselves, such as heroin, or legal prescription drugs that are sold without a prescription. Like alcohol, illegal drugs can be harmful in several ways. To some extent, the government controls alcohol quality and distribution, but there are no governmental safeguards to insure quality control of illegal drugs. They may be "cut" (diluted or mixed with other ingredients) to stretch profits—a procedure that is seldom done in sterile laboratory environments, but rather in dirty warehouses, garages, and other unsuitable locations. Because the contents of these drugs are often unknown and unidentified, the user is at risk, especially when mixing illegal drugs or taking them with alcohol.

Different drugs have different damaging effects on the body. Drugs that are smoked are often worse for your respiratory tract than even cigarettes; narcotics can damage your nervous system and lead to overdose; and intravenous drug use puts you at risk for diseases such as hepatitis and AIDS.

According to the C. E. Mendez Foundation, a drug education program for children in Tampa, Florida, an addict's life span is shortened by 15 to 20 years due to the dangers of drug overdose, interaction of drugs with alcohol, malnutrition, and use of shared and contaminated needles. According to the Annenberg Washington Program, more than 50 percent of the domestic violence in America is associated with drug abuse. Drug users are involved in 10 to 15 percent of our highway fatalities.

If you or a family member has a problem with drugs, there are many programs available to help, such as Narcotics Anonymous. Check your local telephone book or contact your state agency for drug abuse prevention; there is a national hotline run by the National Institute on Drug Abuse at 1-800-662-HELP. There are also numerous well-known drug abuse rehabilitation centers such as the Betty Ford Clinic and others.

Illegal drugs pose a threat to the health of children and all of society. Being well informed is the first step in combating the problem. The list of popular "street drugs," as illegal drugs are sometimes known, changes from time to time. These are some of the most common:

Marijuana, also called "grass," "reefer," "weed," and "pot," comes from the cannabis sativa plant and is smoked either in a hand-rolled cigarette called a "joint," in pipes, or in water pipes called "bongs." Chronic use of this drug can make an individual psychologically dependent on it, although it is not addictive in a physical sense. Chronic use may cause decreased blood supply to the heart and damage to the lungs and pulmonary system. A loss of attention and motivation, impaired reaction time, and altered perception are also reputed effects of the drug.

Hallucinogens, also known as "psychedelics," are drugs that produce an altered state of mind including profound distortions of the senses as well as direction, time, and distance. Hallucinations can conjure up frightening scenes, which have led some users to injure themselves. The most common hallucinogens are lysergic acid diethylamide (LSD), mescaline, peyote, phencyclidine (PCP, or "angel dust"), and psilocybin mushrooms.

Sedatives, also referred to as "downers," "barbs," "red devils," "blue devils," and "yellows" are barbiturates used medically as tranquilizers and sleeping aids. These drugs are highly addictive, and when misused or used in conjunction with alcohol, they can be fatal. Barbiturate overdose is a factor in close to one third of all reported drug-related deaths, including suicide and accidental drug poisoning.

Stimulants, also called "uppers," "pep pills,"or "speed," are drugs that increase energy and were once used as diet aids to reduce hunger. They are addictive and can be a difficult habit to break. Stimulants produce an initial high, which can be followed by violent and dangerous behavior. Depending on the dose and the individual's overall health, users may suffer from heart attacks, seizures, strokes, and personality changes.

Cocaine, a stimulant, is a white powder that is typically ingested by inhaling or "snorting," usually through a straw into the nose, although it also can be injected directly into a vein. After conversion back to its base form, cocaine, then called "crack," can be smoked. Cocaine, also called "coke," "blow," and "nose candy," is one of the most popular and dangerous drugs on the street. It is highly addictive, especially in the smokable crack form, and has been known to cause sudden cardiac arrest in some users.

Narcotics, such as morphine and codeine, are used medically to alleviate pain and to help patients sleep. However, they can be extremely addictive. On the street, drug users find they require ever-larger doses of these drugs to prevent painful and unpleasant withdrawal symptoms. Heroin, a popular street drug known as

MONITORING THE FUTURE STUDY ON DRUG ABUSE

Since 1975, the Monitoring the Future Study has measured the extent of drug use among high school seniors. Among the graduating class of 1993, 42.9 percent of students had used an illicit drug by the time they reached their senior year of high school, up from 40.7 percent in the class of 1992, but still far below the peak of 65.6 percent in 1981. Here are the numbers for specific drugs.

Lifetime prevalence of drug abuse, 1993: Monitoring the Future Study

	8th graders	10th graders	12th graders
Marijuana	12.6 percent	24.4 percent	35.3 percent
Cocaine	2.9	3.6	6.1
Inhalants	19.4	17.5	17.4
LSD	3.5	6.2	10.3
Alcohol	67.1	80.8	87.0
Cigarettes	45.3	56.3	61.9

Information released by the National Institute on Drug Abuse

Tips for Taking Medications

All medications have side effects, and many of them can interact dangerously with other medications. Regardless of what kind of medication you're taking, be sure to take these precautionary steps:

- Ask for information concerning side effects when you get a new prescription.
- Carry a card in your wallet listing all medications—both prescription and over-the-counter—that you are presently taking.
- Always check with your physician before taking any new medication. If you have more than one doctor—and many people do—each may be prescribing for you without knowledge of your other drugs. Let every one of your doctors know about all the medication you are taking.
- If you drink alcohol, ask if it is safe to drink and how much is OK while taking a particular medication.
- If you're not sure of the names of, or the reasons you take, some of your prescriptions, put all the bottles in a bag and bring them to your doctor.
- Use the same pharmacy for all your prescriptions, and ask the pharmacist to record your medicines on the computer.
- Make a chart noting how often you are to take each medication, when (before meals or after), what it's called, and what it's for.
- Always check the label before you take any medication.
- Never take any medicine in the dark; be sure it's what you think it is.
- Record the time you take your medication to prevent forgetting and taking it again. Ask your physician or pharmacist for instructions if you miss a dose.
- Don't stop taking your medication when you begin to feel better; complete the total prescription if your doctor told you to do so.
- Keep medications in a dry and secure place, not in the bathroom medicine cabinet.
- Throw away old medications as they may deteriorate with age.

"junk" or "smack" is sniffed or injected into the body. It has no medicinal value. Narcotics most often abused include morphine, heroin, codeine, and the prescription drugs hydromorphone (Dilaudid), meperidine (Demerol), Darvon, Percodan, and Percocet.

Inhalants are a particular problem for children. These substances can be inhaled through the nose or "huffed" by mouth. Many of these inhalants—such as paint thinner, glue, spray paint, nail polish remover, and aerosol sprays—are household products and, therefore, easily obtained. Although these substances, along with amyl nitrate and butyl nitrate, may appear harmless, they're not. The immediate effects of inhalants include nausea, nosebleeds, coughing, lack of coordination, loss of judgment, and sometimes even "sudden sniffing death," a form of acute cardiac arrest. The more serious long-term effects of inhalants include breathing difficulties, headaches, kidney and liver damage, vomiting, and impaired reflexes. Some of these chemicals can coat lung tissue, causing severe or even fatal pneumonia. Inhalants are addictive, and users suffer painful withdrawal symptoms when they try to stop using them.

PRESCRIPTION DRUGS

There is a false security in the assumption that a drug prescribed by a doctor is "safe." All prescription drugs have side effects, and interactions with other medications, foods, and beverages are always a possibility. So, even though it comes from a doctor, you still need to be careful. Individuals taking antidepressants known as monoamine oxidase inhibitors (MAOIs), for example, must avoid aged cheese, yogurt, and several other foods that contain large amounts of tyramine, which can severely elevate blood pressure. Blood pressure prescription drugs, some tranquilizers, and numerous over-the-counter preparations such as cold medications and antihistamines can make men temporarily impotent and cause women to lose their interest in sex. Other drugs can cause nausea, drowsiness, confusion, and irregular heartbeat. The elderly, most of whom take an average of 6.5 pills each day, are particularly vulnerable because they tend to metabolize drugs more slowly, which means the substance stays in their system longer and may build up to combine with other medications.

SUBSTANCES IN FOOD

Caffeine. Coffee, tea, cola drinks, chocolate, and some prescription and over-the-counter medications (such as Midol Extra-Strength, Dexatrim, and Excedrin Extra-Strength) contain caffeine, which stimulates the nervous system. Caffeine is also a diuretic, which means it stimulates urination. Many women have found relief from fibrocystic breast pain and premenstrual syndrome by excluding caffeine products from their diet. Omitting caffeine may also reduce anxiety.

Food additives. Many convenience food products contain potentially dangerous chemicals used to give them a longer shelf life. Even fresh produce, meat, fish, poultry, and bakery products are often treated with preservatives or dyes to enhance their appearance and salability. For those with allergies to these chemicals, eating can be a dangerous act, as these additives can trigger asthma attacks, gastrointestinal upsets, or even life-threatening anaphylactic shock. (For more on food additives, see Chapter 1.)

Pesticides. Much of our produce is sprayed with pesticides. Imported products may contain more than domestic ones, because imports are not subject to rulings by the U.S. Food and Drug Administration. Always wash fruits and vegetables before eating. (For more on pesticides in food, see Chapter 1.)

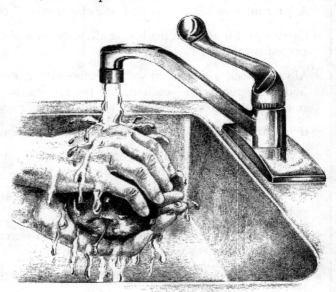

Food-borne illness. Much of what is often considered to be the flu is actually food poisoning, or food-borne illness. Symptoms of food-borne illness may range from stomach cramps, diarrhea, fever, and vomiting that lasts for a few days to severe dehydration, kidney failure, and even death. Those most vulnerable to the bacteria that causes food-borne illness are pregnant women, the elderly, those with compromised immune systems such as individuals undergoing chemotherapy or those with HIV infection, chronic liver disease, or diabetes. (For more on food-borne illness, see Chapter 1.)

SUBSTANCES IN THE ENVIRONMENT

Lead. Before World War II, most homes were painted with lead paint. In fact, about 75 percent of all homes built before 1980 have lead-based paint. In 1978, the United States banned lead paint for interior use, but many non-lead paints were then used to cover older walls that still contained traces of lead. Sanding off this bottom coat of paint releases lead dust that is highly toxic. In addition, many ceramic-glazed and antique dishes contain lead, as do some older painted wooden and metal toys. Older homes may have lead pipes that can seep lead into the family's drinking water. This is especially serious in families with infants when tap water is used to make the formula. Traces of lead may also be in the soil of the yard where children play.

According to the Centers for Disease Control and Prevention in Atlanta, an estimated 10 to 15 percent of preschoolers in the United States are affected by lead poisoning. These youngsters are at greater risk because they have more hand-to-mouth exposure, have less body mass, and are growing at a faster rate than adults. Children don't even have to eat dirt or paint chips to be harmed by the lead. Unfortunately, lead dust is absorbed by the body. Minor traces of lead in the body can cause extreme fatigue, headaches, mental confusion, learning disabilities, behavioral problems, and vague aches and pains. According to the American Lead Consultants, even low levels of exposure to lead can cause a four- to six-point drop in a child's IQ. But higher amounts of lead poisoning can have even more drastic effects, including damage to the brain, kidneys, and nervous system, especially in young children and fetuses. It also can be fatal.

If you think your house may have lead paint, contact your local health department or your state or county agriculture agency, or call the National Lead Information Center at 1-800-424-LEAD. Although wiping windowsills frequently and vacuuming often can reduce some of the danger of lead dust, experts say it is vital to remove it entirely to prevent the possibility of lead poisoning. In many states, if you are aware of the presence of lead paint in a house you are renting or selling, you are required to disclose that information to potential renters and purchasers.

Radon. In our zeal to build air-tight buildings for more efficient heating and cooling since the energy crunch of the 1970s, we've sealed ourselves into boxes where we are prey to a deadly gas known as radon. Radon is a colorless, odorless, tasteless, naturally occurring radioactive gas produced by the decay of uranium in rocks, soil, and building materials. This gas may be lurking beneath your home, your office, or your child's school and can creep inside through cracks and seams in the building. The Environmental Protection Agency (EPA) estimates that radon may be the second leading cause of lung cancer, ranking just after cigarette smoking. Radon is responsible for causing anywhere from 7,000 to 30,000 of the 140,000 cases of lung cancer annually in the United States. According to a recent Swedish study, those at greatest risk of developing lung cancer from radon were smokers living in homes with high radon levels.

Radon levels are measured by picocuries of radiation per liter of air (pCi/L). Although no level of radon is considered safe, the EPA has established anything in excess of 4 pCi/L as a health hazard, estimating that living in a home with this level of radon carries the same risk of developing lung cancer as smoking ten cigarettes a day. In homes with levels higher than 4 pCi/L, the EPA suggests that steps should be taken to reduce the amount.

Before buying a home or to check levels in your present home, test for radon by using a radon detection kit, called a "charcoal canister," available at most major hardware stores for $15 to $25. Start with the basement, as that is closest to the ground and has more potential for seepage. The EPA recommends that all homes below the third floor be tested, as radon tends to dissipate as it moves upward.

For more information about radon, contact your local chapter of the American Lung Association or your area's EPA. Call the EPA's radon hotline at 1-800-767-7236. Ask for their free booklet, "Home Buyer's and Seller's Guide to Radon."

Asbestos. Asbestos is a mineral fiber that has been in use since ancient times. It was used as insulation in one quarter of all homes, hospitals, and office buildings built from 1920 to 1970. Self-contained asbestos is safe. As the fibers age, however, they disintegrate, forming a fine dust. This dust from the asbestos fibers can cause serious respiratory problems, including cancer. Children are more vulnerable to the effects of the asbestos dust because of their size. In 1973, the EPA banned the use of asbestos as insulation for schools. Sixteen years later, the ban was extended to forbid the production and sale of asbestos products by 1997.

If you live in an older house or apartment building or work in an older office building, ask your local environmental control agency for an asbestos inspection. If it is discovered, do not try to remove it yourself. Have a reputable and knowledgeable technician remove it.

Formaldehyde. Experts estimate that most of us spend 90 percent of our time inside our homes and offices. Many of these buildings are sealed boxes with windows that either cannot open or are not open due to air conditioning and heating considerations. In essence, we breathe recycled air most of our day.

Formaldehyde is found in insulation, fiberboard, paneling, carpeting, and fabrics and is used in window treatment and upholstery. Although formaldehyde insulation is no longer used in new construction, it may be present in older homes, places of business, or schools.

You probably remember the smell of formaldehyde coming from your frog specimen in high school biology class. It bothered your mucous membranes then, and it can have the same effect in its present uses. Gases from this chemical can also cause dizziness, nausea, fatigue, and other symptoms. Check with an environmental specialist especially if your surroundings contain a number of synthetic products with formaldehyde as their base.

Water quality. Although it may be difficult to think of water as a potential hazard, pollution has made this situation a reality. While many travelers worry about the quality of drinking water when they venture abroad, they also need to concern themselves with the safety of drinking water at home. Our drinking water has become polluted by industrial wastes, pesticides, lead, and bacteria.

A home water-filtering system can help screen out many of the pollutants in tap water, but not all of them. Bottled water, which Americans now drink at an average annual rate of eight gallons per person, also isn't 100 percent safe. Today's Food and Drug Administration requirements only specify that bottled water be as safe as water that comes out of the tap.

How to Determine if Your Drinking Water is Safe

- Avoid drinking water if it looks, smells, or tastes "funny."
- Read the label on bottled water to determine whether the water is merely bottled tap water or is really "mineral water," "spring water," or "purified water."
- Ask your local water department for an up-to-date report of its contaminant analysis. They are required to furnish it promptly to any citizen requesting it.
- If your drinking water comes from a well, have it analyzed at regular times. The Environmental Protection Agency can refer you to a qualified laboratory.

Don't just worry about drinking water either. Be careful about the water you swim or boat in also. Swimming in polluted water can be dangerous. You can absorb the contaminants through your skin, nose, and eyes, and some water is bound to get swallowed.

Allergens. More than 40 million Americans suffer from some form of allergy. For some, the allergy symptoms may be no more than a runny nose, itching eyes, or a slightly annoying skin rash, but for others, allergies can pose a serious health hazard causing unrelenting vomiting and diarrhea, severe asthma attacks that make it difficult to breathe, or hives and swelling of throat tissues.

In some cases, an allergic reaction can become so severe that the person suffers from anaphylactic shock. Although most of us with allergies will never have to deal with a life-threatening attack, the nuisance and expense of simply run-of-the-mill sniffling and itching is enough to make us take action.

Because a complete cure is not in the offing, the best strategy is to minimize exposure to the offending triggers. Here are some tips on how to reduce your risk from allergens:

- Avoid carpeting wherever possible; instead, use wood or linoleum.
- Don't store things under the bed because they collect dust.
- Omit heavy curtains, draperies, venetian blinds, and upholstered furniture.
- Keep pets out of the bedroom area; if you don't have a pet, don't get one.
- Don't use feather pillows or duvets.
- Vacuum your mattress often because it contains dust mites.
- Wash blankets and pillows every two weeks in hot water.
- Encase your mattress, pillow, and box spring in plastic coverings.
- Keep bedrooms uncluttered to cut down on dust accumulation.
- Remove books from your bedroom because they attract mold spores.
- Eliminate houseplants and flowers because they drop pollen, and the wet potting soil invites mold.
- Exercise inside when the air quality is bad or the pollen count is high.
- Invest in a vacuum cleaner that holds dust in a cup or airtight bag, rather than the kind that recycles air through a cloth or paper container.
- Keep windows closed at night.
- Change your heating and air-conditioning filter monthly to reduce the dust and mold accumulation.
- Avoid using chemical cleaning agents in aerosol containers because they are easily inhaled. Instead use natural cleaning materials such as baking soda or vinegar.
- See an environmental physician or allergist for possible allergy shots.
- If you are severely allergic to shellfish, peanut oil, corn, or other food products, make sure to read the ingredients lists on food labels carefully. Ask about the recipes and ingredients of food items that do not have labels, such as those at a restaurant or other people's homes. Remember that even smelling or touching these foods can produce an allergic reaction in some individuals.
- Wear a medical ID bracelet if you have a severe allergy to a food.
- If your child has an allergy, be sure to inform teachers and camp counselors.
- Watch out for dyes and chemical additives such as sulfites, monosodium glutamate (MSG), nitrates, and nitrites that may trigger allergies.

HAZARDOUS SITUATIONS

Although we don't usually think of them as such, accidents are a major health hazard. Accidents rank in the top five leading causes of death, killing approximately 100,000 people a year in the United States. What's worse is that most accidents are preventable if everyone would simply use common sense.

POISON

Each year thousands of people die from accidental poisoning, many of them children. Children, especially those under five years of age, learn by exploring and investigating their world. Unfortunately, what they see and reach for often ends up in their mouths. For example, when babies are in the crawling stage, they can find drain cleaners and dishwasher detergent under the sink. As soon as they become toddlers, they can grab furniture polish and medicines in purses on beds. When they start to climb, they can drag a chair over to a tall dresser or high cabinet and get into perfume, medicine, and other potential poisons. The substance doesn't even have to taste good; children will eat and drink almost anything. Moreover, substances do not have to be swallowed to be toxic. They can also be inhaled or absorbed by the skin.

Almost 90 percent of poison exposures are accidental and, therefore, preventable. Insecticides, including those used domestically, are a common form of accidental poisoning because they often are purchased in large quantities and may be stored open and unprotected in cupboards, making them easily obtained by toddlers.

Iron pills are one of the most common causes of accidental poisoning deaths in toddlers. Vitamin and mineral supplements may seem harmless, but in large doses, some are dangerous, and it does not take very much to be a large dose for a toddler. (For more on vitamin toxicity, see Chapter 1.) Birth control pills, alcohol, vitamins, tranquilizers, nail polish remover, pesticides, plant fertilizer, and hobby chemicals such as glue, enamel paint, ink, paint thinner, and photography liquids are all potentially poisonous if ingested by a child.

The key to preventing accidental poisoning is simple: Don't allow your children to have access to any potentially toxic substances. That doesn't mean merely telling them that this cabinet is not for children or that these items are "poisons." It means locking cabinets and heeding labels when they say "keep out of reach of children." Make sure your children know what is off limits, but also make sure that there is more in their way than simply your rule. Here are some important safety tips for adults and adults with children:

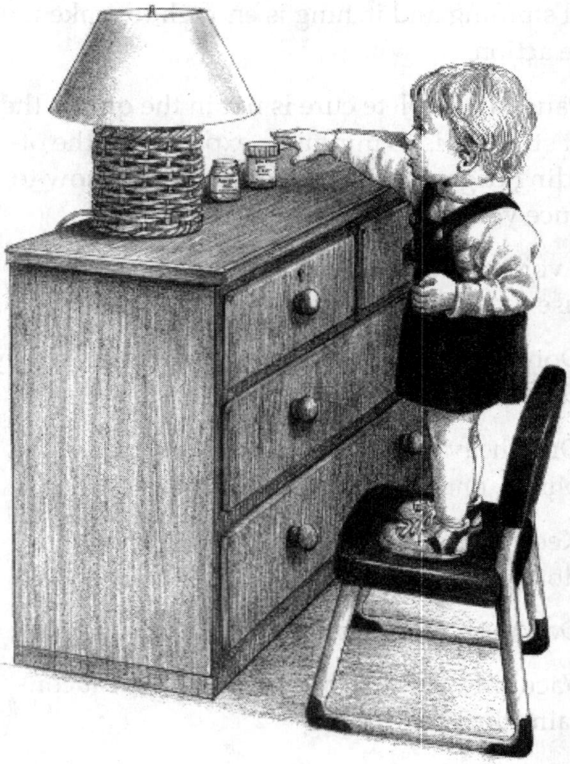

- Keep all household products and medicines out of children's reach, preferably in a locked cabinet.
- When you're using any of these products, never let them out of your sight, even if that means taking them with you when you answer the telephone or doorbell.
- Store medicines separately from household products.
- Keep medicines and household products in their original containers. Never transfer them to soft drink bottles, paper cups, or other containers.
- Leave original labels on all products and read the label before and after using. There are many look-alike bottles—such as various juices and cleaning liquids, grated cheese and cleansers, and candies and antihistamines. Adults, especially those with limited vision, can grab the wrong product just as easily as a child can.

- Pour liquids on the side opposite the label so the moisture doesn't blur the writing.
- Never give or take medicines in the dark.
- Avoid taking medicines in front of children as youngsters tend to imitate adults.
- Use child-resistant containers properly by closing them securely after each use. However, don't rely on "child-proof" caps to prevent your child from discovering a way to open a bottle of medicine or cleaning chemicals. They are merely "child-resistant," not "child-proof," and many youngsters can open them faster than adults can.
- Never refer to medicine as "candy" or to how good it tastes.
- Clean out your medicine cabinet at least twice a year. Dispose of medicines no longer used by flushing the contents down the toilet and rinsing out the container before throwing it away.
- Be more attentive at peak times. Most accidental poisonings occur between 4 and 6 P.M. when children are hungry and fussy and parents are tired and busy fixing dinner. Other peak times for an accidental poisoning to take place is when a parent or sibling is ill or the family is on a trip.
- Never store poisons in your pantry or food cabinet.
- Be alert when you have guests who may have medications in their purse or suitcase or when you visit someone else's home, which may not be poison-proofed.
- Never go to bed leaving dirty ashtrays or alcohol in glasses after a party. A child can awake early, get out of bed, and ingest these potentially toxic agents.
- Know the number of your closest Poison Control Center and keep it posted by every telephone in your home.

Children are not the only ones at risk for accidental poisoning. Those who take many prescription drugs, such as the elderly, may forget they have taken their medication and take another dose. Alcohol compounds the problem. It can lead to forgetfulness and taking too much medicine. Also, mixing alcohol with certain prescription drugs can create dangerously toxic effects.

In case of accidental poisoning, you need to know some basics so that at the very least, you don't make matters worse. The very first thing to do is contact the Poison Control Center and follow their instructions. Often, if the product ingested is caustic, such as lye, bleach, toilet bowl cleaner, or other corrosive household chemicals, you will be told not to induce vomiting, but to dilute the substance with water as rapidly as possible. Also, do not induce vomiting if you're unsure what was swallowed, or if it was an alkali or a petroleum product, such as gasoline or kerosene.

Some children may vomit when they have swallowed a poisonous substance. Others become sleepy or sluggish for no apparent reason. You may notice that the contents of a particular bottle have been reduced or that some of the substance remains around the child's mouth and teeth or has been spilled on the clothes. There may be burns around the lips or mouth from corrosive items or a breath odor from items such as alcohol or petroleum products.

Get medical advice even if you suspect, but don't know for sure, that your child has ingested a potentially hazardous product. Call your local Poison Control Center. It is staffed by registered nurses, pharmacists, and physicians. These professionals are familiar with how poisonous a particular substance is (known as its "toxicity") and can give you immediate information on what you should do to dilute or eliminate the poison, how to maintain the victim's breathing and circulation, and how to get medical aid. Their service is free and confidential.

ELECTRICITY

While most of us take electricity for granted, because it can't be seen or smelled, coming in contact with electricity can be dangerous and

How to Handle a Poisoning Emergency

It is vital, especially if you have small children, to have the Poison Control Center's telephone number posted on or near every phone in your home, and memorize it if you can. A call to the nearest Poison Control Center is the first step in saving a poisoning victim's life. Remember to:

- Keep calm.
- Tell the person taking your call the age of the victim, the name and amount of the medicine or other substance ingested (bring the container to the phone so you can give the exact name of the product and the amount you think was ingested), what if any first aid has been done thus far, and if the person has vomited.
- Have the name and address of your nearest hospital handy.
- Do not give fluids to an unconscious person or one having convulsions.
- Do not give syrup of ipecac to induce vomiting unless you are instructed to.

even deadly. Electrical shocks can knock you unconscious, cause deep tissue burns, and stop your breathing and heartbeat. Take the proper precautions with electricity, and you will reap the benefits without the dangers.

- Put safety plugs over all electrical outlets to prevent children from sticking screwdrivers, nails, pins, or other metal objects into them.
- Never use electrical appliances such as radios or hair dryers near a filled bathtub or sink. They could fall in and electrocute someone.
- Never touch anything electrical with wet hands or while standing in water.
- Don't run extension cords under the rug or carpet. The wires can quickly become frayed or broken from people walking on them, causing shocks and fires.
- Always turn off the circuit breaker before changing a lightbulb that has broken off from its base or before making any electrical repairs.
- Do not talk on the phone, take a bath, or use electric appliances during a lightning storm. The electrical charge can come in through the water pipes or telephone wires.

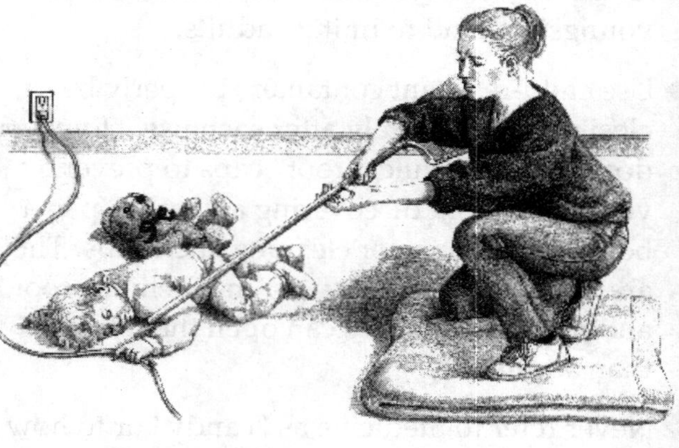

- Never touch someone who has been electrocuted without first shutting off the power source or moving them away from it with a nonmetal object, such as a wooden broom handle. The current could pass through the individual's body and shock you.

FALLS

Approximately 30 percent of those 65 and older fall each year. Accidental falls, especially around the home, kill more people over 65 than any other single type of injury, and they are the leading cause of accidental death for people over age 85. Those suffering from the residual effects of a stroke are especially susceptible to falling because of visual deficits, weakness, gait problems, and the effects of medication. In addition to breaking bones, falling can injure an older person's self-confidence, causing them to restrict their activities for fear of falling again.

Anyone can fall because of carelessness, stress, poor vision, or a loss of balance due to the side effects of drugs or alcohol. While the actual fall may result in nothing more than a bruise or slight cut, falling against a hot stove or hitting one's head against a hard object can cause a serious injury.

With awareness and preplanning, most of these falls can be avoided. Generally, you should take care to avoid high-risk situations: Don't jump right out of bed; the sudden change in blood pressure could make you feel dizzy. And NEVER use a chair as a step stool. Try to move more methodically; for example, take your time answering the phone; if you hurry, you could fall.

Here are some prevention tips:

- Install photocell nightlights in your hallways, bedrooms, bathrooms, and near the staircase so they light automatically when it is dark.

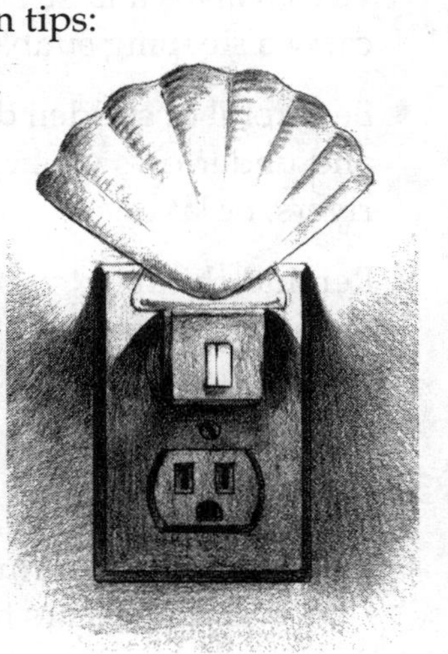

- If you need glasses for distance, be sure to wear them while walking around the house.
- Increase the wattage of lightbulbs lighting all staircases.
- Keep a flashlight on your nightstand so that late night trips are not attempted blind.
- Remove scatter rugs or be certain they are securely taped to the floor or have a nonskid backing. Air-dry bath mats so the rubber backing doesn't crack.
- Keep all staircases free from toys, shoes, or other clutter.
- Wear shoes and slippers with nonslip soles.
- Don't walk up or down stairs in stocking feet.
- Wipe up all kitchen spills immediately. A dab of butter, a grape, or a piece of lettuce can turn a kitchen floor into an ice rink, with potentially disastrous results.
- Relocate or tape down extension cords and telephone cords that might make someone trip.
- Be sure floor surfaces are not slippery. After washing them, block them off from traffic until they are totally dry.

Children and the elderly have the greatest risk of experiencing a fall and also of suffering a serious injury as a result. If you have young children or an older person in the house take these extra precautions:

- Install sturdy handrails on both sides of staircases.
- Install a safety gate at the top and bottom of stairs to prevent toddlers from climbing up and falling down the steps.
- Open windows from the top, not the bottom, to keep children from falling out; screens are not strong enough to hold even small children.
- If you suffer from osteoporosis or have an unsteady gait from multiple sclerosis, Parkinson disease, or any other disorder, use a walker or a cane for added support.
- Install grab bars in tubs, in showers, and near the toilet. You don't have to be old or pregnant to feel suddenly dizzy or weak.
- Use nonskid rubber mats or rubber stickers in bathtubs and shower stalls.
- Mark the bottom step with high-visibility tape, a different color paint, or some other highly visual marking.

WATER

In 1993 alone, 4,800 people in America died from drowning. Many of them knew how to swim, but either swam out too far, suffered a cramp, or just panicked and lost control. Drowning—especially in home pools—is the leading cause of death among toddlers in the United States. For every death, many more children will be rescued and survive but will live with serious brain damage. It only takes a few minutes for a child to drown. Young children are "head-heavy" for their bodies. They can drown in a bucket of water or the toilet because they can't lift their heads out.

Whether you have a pool at home or you like to swim at the community pool or beach, a few simple guidelines will help you safeguard your family from water hazards:

- Surround your pool or hot tub with a fence that cannot be climbed over or slipped through or under.
- Install locking gates on your pool and hot tub, and keep them locked. In one study, 70 percent of the pools where a drowning took place had broken or unlocked gates.
- Purchase a pool cover and pool alarm system.
- Learn cardiopulmonary resuscitation (CPR). Contact the American Red Cross, your community hospital, or a local adult-education program for information.
- Keep a telephone in the pool or spa area.
- Don't rely on swimming lessons to keep your child safe; you cannot "drown proof" a child.
- Never allow anyone of any age to swim alone; even expert swimmers develop cramps, get dizzy, or hit their heads.
- Don't rely on plastic arm floats or float toys to support your child; they may slip off or deflate.
- Teach your children and their guests proper water safety rules, including no running or pushing near a pool deck or on a diving board, no dunking other swimmers, and no yelling "help" unless you are actually in trouble.
- Never allow a child to remain in or near the bathtub, swimming pool, or any other body of water if you must leave—even for just a minute. Most toddler drownings occur when the caregiver is distracted by the telephone, chores, or socializing. A child can drown in only a few inches of water.
- Keep sandboxes covered tightly when not in use. Rainwater can collect inside and pose a danger of drowning to small children.
- Be sure to alert your baby-sitter to potential pool hazards.

When you're at the beach:

- Always swim parallel to the shoreline. If you get a sudden cramp or tire, you're not far from shore.
- Use caution with rafts and other flotation devices. Waves and strong currents can swiftly carry a sleeping sunbather far offshore.
- Be careful of sudden drop-offs, strong currents, and undertows when swimming in oceans, rivers, or lakes.
- Remind children to go into water feet first. Each year, diving into shallow water takes its toll in drownings and spinal cord injuries.
- Never swim during electrical storms.
- Never ride in a boat unless there is a life jacket for every passenger including children. Be sure everyone wears his or her jacket.
- Wear a life jacket when you water ski or jet ski. Even experienced skiers can fall and hit their heads.

FIRE

Approximately 6,000 Americans are killed each year by home fires. According to the National Safety Council, most of these deaths could be avoided if smoke detectors were properly installed and regularly maintained in the kitchen, stairwells, and near each bedroom. Check the batteries at least yearly to make sure they work.

The American Red Cross reports that 80 percent of all deaths due to fire take place when the family is sleeping. The cause is not the fire itself, but rather smoke inhalation and lack of oxygen. In addition, the fire may trigger the release of poisonous chemicals in upholstery, plastic material, and draperies.

No matter what the construction, no house is completely fireproof, but you can do a great deal to prevent home fires:

- If there are children in the home, lock up matches and cigarette lighters.

Hot Water Hazards

Hot water can cause painful and even life-threatening burns. Take these precautions:

- ◆ Lower the hot water temperature regulator to 120°F to prevent scalding in the tub or shower.
- ◆ Bathe children facing the front of the tub so they won't back into the hot metal of the water faucet. Child safety covers that protect the child from the spigot are also an option.
- ◆ Turn pot handles away from the edge of the stove to prevent someone from bumping into them and spilling the hot contents on themselves.

- ◆ Remove pot holders or dish towels that hang over the burners on the stove.
- ◆ Never smoke in bed.
- ◆ Never leave home or go to bed with your Christmas tree lights on.
- ◆ Never use a higher watt lightbulb than a lamp manufacturer suggests.
- ◆ Use salt or soda to put out a grease fire in your kitchen; never throw water on it.
- ◆ Have an established family escape route and have regular fire drills. If your house has more than one story, keep a fire safety ladder under each bed. Plan ahead where you'll all meet outside.
- ◆ Teach your family the American Red Cross rule if their clothes ever catch on fire: **Stop** running, **Drop** to the ground, and **Roll** over to put out the flames.
- ◆ Keep papers, curtains, and other flammable material away from hot radiators, portable heaters, and lighted fireplaces.
- ◆ Make sure that your child's sleepwear is flame resistant, and wash it according to manufacturer's instructions.
- ◆ Be very careful with portable kerosene heaters. Use them only when you are in the room; turn them off any time you leave the room.
- ◆ For homes with children, put up guards around space heaters, fireplaces, and wood-burning stoves.
- ◆ Don't overload circuits by putting too many plugs in an outlet.
- ◆ For lamps or small appliances, don't use extension cords that dangle and can be pulled. Children can pull the appliance down and injure themselves as well as start a fire.
- ◆ Don't let your children play with firecrackers or any type of explosives.
- ◆ Buy fire extinguishers, and learn how to use them. Place them where they are most likely to be needed, such as the kitchen. Check periodically to be sure they are in good working order.

CRIME AND ASSAULT PREVENTION

Preplanning and constant awareness reduce your chances of becoming a victim of crime or an assault. Unfortunately, it is a fact of life that we must take certain precautions to protect ourselves:

- ◆ Always lock the doors to your home and car.
- ◆ When you go on vacation, put lights on a timer. Stop the newspaper delivery, or have a trusted neighbor collect it for you. If you're away for a long time, arrange to have the grass cut, snow shoveled, and other chores done so it looks as though someone is home.
- ◆ Don't carry large amounts of cash, and only carry those credit cards you plan to use.
- ◆ Always be aware of your surroundings. Walk quickly and confidently.
- ◆ Scream if you're confronted by someone who frightens you. Don't feel embarrassed or let false pride threaten your safety.
- ◆ Don't wear flashy jewelry.
- ◆ Always park your car in well-lit areas.
- ◆ Have your key in hand when approaching your car. If someone is standing by your car,

Things to Teach Children

Some parents don't prepare their children to protect themselves against crime and possible assault because they don't want them to be afraid. However, the world is more violent than it was even twenty years ago. Children need to develop skills to maintain their safety.

- Encourage your child's school to show films about "The Friendly Stranger," so they know to avoid talking to strangers, even if they seem friendly.
- Make sure your child understands the difference between a "good" touch and a "bad" one.
- Encourage open communication. Make time for you and your youngster to talk. Be sure to listen.
- Teach your toddlers their last name, address, and phone number as soon as they are old enough to remember.
- Show your child how to call for emergency care. Explain the use of "911" if your community has this important service.
- Teach your children to turn and quickly run the other way if a car follows them.
- If you must have a gun in your home, keep it locked up, and put the key in a safe place. Teach your child gun safety.

return to the store or building and ask for an escort to your car.

- Drive with your windows up and the doors locked, even in the daytime.
- Never try to fight someone who has a knife or gun. It's better to lose your money, credit cards, and even family heirloom jewelry than your life.
- Take a class in personal protection. Check local community education programs.

SEX

Sex has always been a difficult subject for some to discuss because of the social and moral ramifications, but sex is also a health issue and, in some cases, a matter of life and death. Besides unplanned pregnancies and the age-old sexually transmitted diseases, unprotected sex can transmit AIDS—an incurable, fatal disease. Any discussion of staying well would be incomplete without discussing this touchy topic, because even though we don't often think of it as such, sex can be one of the most hazardous situations of all.

Sexually transmitted diseases. Anyone who is sexually active is potentially at risk for contracting a sexually transmitted disease (STD). These infections are far more serious than merely being an inconvenience or embarrassment. STDs can cause infertility, birth defects, and even death. The more sexual partners you have, the more at risk you become.

Avoiding STDs is a simple matter, but it isn't always easy. The best way to stay out of automobile accidents is to never get in a car, and the only 100 percent sure way to prevent STDs is to abstain from having sexual relations. However, having sex only with a noninfected, mutually monogamous partner also carries no risk, if you can be sure that he or she is actually not infected and is truly monogamous.

If neither of the situations is applicable or tolerable to you, it is vital to your health and your partners' health that you follow the rules of safe sex. At the very least, limit your number of sexual partners. Your chances of acquiring an STD go up with the number of partners you have. Use latex condoms with the spermicide nonoxynol-9 **every** time you have sex. Properly used condoms can protect both partners from a wide variety of STDs and can also prevent unwanted pregnancies.

It only takes one unprotected encounter to get pregnant and to transmit an STD, including HIV infection. Remember, condoms are not 100 percent effective; the only completely reliable method of avoiding STDs is to abstain from all sexual activity.

Do not assume you can tell if someone has an STD. Nice people from all economic levels and from all backgrounds can be carriers. Learn the signs and symptoms of STD infections. See your doctor immediately if you think you have any of them; you owe it to yourself and your partners to get tested. If you do have one, all of your partners need to be notified and possibly treated.

For free and confidential lists of clinics and private physicians who treat STDs, call the American Social Health Administration at 1-800-227-8922. HIV antibody testing is the only way to determine if you're infected with HIV. Most county public health units offer anonymous or confidential HIV testing. If you have any questions concerning AIDS or HIV, contact the National HIV and AIDS Hotline at 1-800-342-AIDS for free and confidential information.

Teenagers. As awkward and uncomfortable as it may be, talking frankly to teens about sex and STDs can be one of the most important preventive steps you can take for the health of your children. There are an estimated 12 million new STD infections each year in the United States. Teenagers are at the highest risk. One third of all new cases involve teens. They need to know that they can contract an STD and pass it on to others without ever feeling sick at all. Be sure they know about the virtues of abstinence, but don't just leave it at that—equip them to survive by teaching them the rules of safe sex.

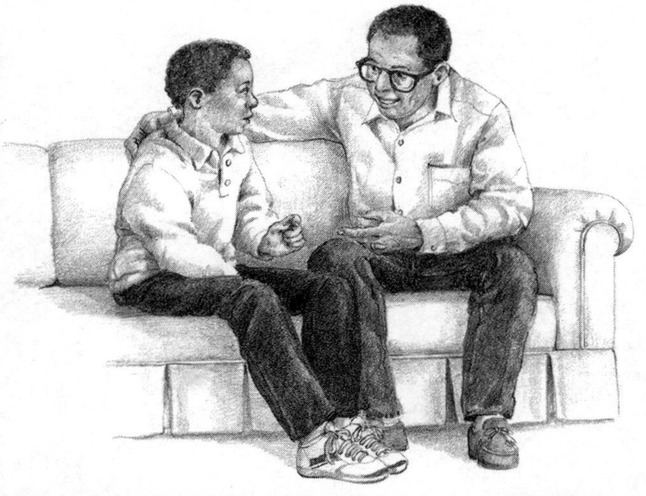

IN THE WORKPLACE

Repetitive motion disorders. Although carpal tunnel syndrome is the best known type of repetitive motion disorder, it is not the only one. Tendinitis and flexor tenosynovitis, or "trigger finger," are two additional forms of injury caused by overuse or improper positioning of muscles and tendons.

The use of computers has increased the number of carpal tunnel syndrome complaints. Carpal tunnel syndrome is caused when tissues swell around the median nerve as it passes through the canal just below the wrist. This swelling can occur through overuse of the wrist in a compressed position, as with computer operators, carpenters, secretaries, writers, surgeons, ditch diggers, knitters, and painters.

The best medicine for problems such as carpal tunnel syndrome is prevention. Set up your workstation correctly, and follow these guidelines to reduce your chances of suffering from these painful and debilitating disorders:

- If you work at a computer, take frequent breaks. Experts suggest a 15-minute rest for every two hours of repetitive movement.
- Alternate tasks. Type for an hour, then file. If you hammer or play the piano for long periods, alternate work or practice with another task not calling for similar hand motions.
- Sit in a chair that allows both feet to be flat on the floor with your thighs at right angles to your body.
- Use a desk that allows you to type with your wrists at right angles to the desk and not bent up or down.
- Look into orthopedic office aids such as pen and pencil grips, keyboard wrist rests, and ergonomically designed chairs and keyboards.
- Use your arms to open doors, rather than pushing with your hands.
- Be careful turning a key in the lock so you don't twist your wrist suddenly.
- If you sleep on your stomach, don't put a hand under the pillow and then rest your head on it.
- If it hurts to hold a heavy book, use a reading stand or a pillow to hold it.

- ◆ Avoid knitting, needlepoint, and other crafts that force your wrist in a compressed position.
- ◆ Become aware of the tension in your grip as you hold the steering wheel, especially if you're driving long distances. Music or books on tape may help you to relax.
- ◆ Card players should be aware of their grip when they hold playing cards. Too much tension can trigger carpal tunnel syndrome.
- ◆ Gripping a pen or pencil too hard also can cause an inflammation of the median nerve.

Lifting. Eight out of ten Americans will experience a back injury at some point in their lives. These painful injuries are seldom caused by a single event, but are triggered by improper, repetitive movements over a period of years. Work-related back injuries represent 15 to 30 percent of all worker's compensation injuries. Yet many of these injuries could be prevented by correcting poor posture, improving back-muscle flexibility, avoiding sudden twisting movements, and learning proper lifting techniques.

According to the Department of Labor, most on-the-job back injuries are triggered by incorrect lifting techniques. Don't bend over to lift a heavy object. Instead, use the "squat lift." Bend your knees and tuck the object to your chest. When you're ready to lift, tighten your stomach muscles and stand up, keeping your back straight. Most of the work should be done with your legs, not your back. For large or heavy items, get help or use a dolly or utility cart.

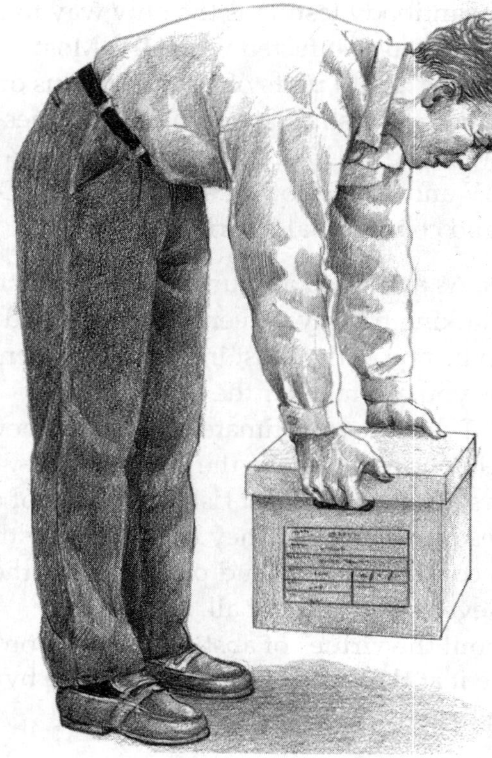

CARING FOR YOUR TEETH AND GUMS

The whine of the dentist's drill, the glaring white light in your eyes, the *U*-shaped plastic vacuum noisily sucking saliva out of your mouth—ugh! It's enough to make even a grown man shudder.

Of all the fears we harbor, visiting the dentist is one of the most universal, but there are ways to rid your semiannual appointment of little needles and big anxieties. In short, return to the basics. Think back to those first dental visits you had as a kid when the hygienist taught you how to take impeccable care of your teeth and gums. (Remember when she brought out that big plastic tooth and demonstrated the proper way to brush and floss?)

The plan is simple. Reduce your risk of developing cavities, gum disease, and other oral scourges by sticking to this fourfold strategy: Brush thoroughly and correctly after each meal; floss after each meal (or at the very least, once a day); use a fluoride toothpaste; and faithfully trudge to the dentist's office for a checkup and cleaning every six months.

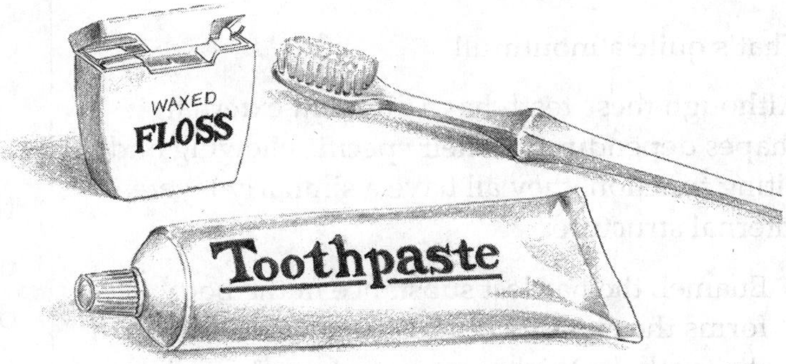

Also, remember that while the charming dental professionals in your life play a big role in keeping your mouth healthy and your smile brilliant, the bulk of the responsibility lies with you. Diligent home care can help you avoid tooth and gum disease and keep your pearly whites, well, pearly white.

YOUR TEETH AND GUMS

Before we look into what can go wrong and how to prevent it, let's find out what is standard equipment. Your teeth are very specialized structures that are well-designed for their task.

There are several types of teeth in your adult mouth:

- Eight to 12 molars (depending on whether you have your wisdom teeth or not)
- Eight bicuspids (which look like molars but are smaller)
- Four cuspids (also called canines)
- Four laterals (on either side of your upper and lower front teeth)
- Four centrals (the front teeth)

That's quite a mouthful!

Although these teeth have different external shapes depending on their specific chewing and biting function, they all have a similarly layered internal structure:

- Enamel, the hardest substance in the body, forms the exposed outer structure, or crown, of the tooth. Its thickness varies from 1.5 millimeters on the chewing surface to less than 0.5 millimeters on the sides.
- Beneath the crown's enamel lies dentin—the living, expanding tissue that makes up the bulk of your tooth.
- At the center of each tooth is a minute area of nerve tissue called pulp. As you age, the pulp shrinks and dentin tissue fills in the space left behind. (If the pulp dies, the dentin loses its source of nutrients, and a root canal is necessary to save the tooth from dying and falling out.)

Other structures that are important to know:

- Cementum—a thin layer below the gum line (Cementum, which is living tissue like dentin, functions as part of the anchor that keeps your tooth rooted to its position.)
- Gums, or gingiva—the pink tissue surrounding the root of the tooth
- Gingival, or periodontal, pocket—a small space between the tooth and the gum (*Periodontia* is a term to describe all of the tissues that surround and support the teeth, including the gums.)

The average, healthy periodontal pocket is about three millimeters deep or less. However, other factors, including receding gums, can affect this measurement. If the pocket grows deeper or wider, this situation can become grave, since it may lead to the tooth falling out. If you suffer from periodontal disease, your dentist may want to measure the gingival pocket in order to gauge the extent of the damage.

DENTAL DISEASE

The word *disease* may sound a bit scary, but we all know too well that things can go wrong with teeth. However, the good news is that since most dental afflictions begin with poor oral hygiene, they are quite preventable. To prepare yourself for oral self-defense, you must first know your enemies.

PLAQUE: YOUR TEETH'S WORST ENEMY

As unpleasant as it may sound, your mouth is a living swarm of bacteria and germs. Although a certain amount of bacteria is normal, excessive accumulations can destroy your teeth and periodontia (the teeth's support system).

The primary culprit is a sticky film called plaque. Plaque is a gelatinous substance that gives oral bacteria protection from the air (which can kill the germs). What's more, plaque pins the bacteria to your teeth, where they feast heartily on the leftover food particles in your mouth. They are especially fond of simple carbohydrates, such as refined sugar. Within a matter of hours, plaque bacteria can convert carbohydrates into enamel-decaying acids.

All forms of dental disease begin with plaque. For this reason, keeping this gummy substance under control is your first and most effective line of defense.

If plaque is left undisturbed on your teeth for an extended period (anywhere from two days to two weeks), it can start to harden into a substance called tartar (or calculus, in dentist's terms). Since tartar bonds even more tenaciously to your teeth than plaque does, it has the potential to do more damage. Given the opportunity, tartar spreads in all directions, even down below the gum line. At the same time, plaque continues to form on top of the hardened material. The result is an all-out bacterial feeding frenzy, and the toxic by-products of this frenzy destroy your teeth and periodontia.

Bad Breath

Many of us believe that onions, garlic, coffee, tea, and hot spices are the cause of bad breath, and that a simple mouthwash rinse can take care of the problem (at least until dinnertime). While it's true that mouthwash can temporarily alleviate bad breath, it is only a quick fix, not a cure. Also, what you are eating may not be the culprit: Periodontal disease, a dry mouth, and certain illnesses can all contribute to bad breath.

You should probably visit your dentist or doctor for an intractable, persistent case of bad breath. However, for a case of garden-variety halitosis, try the following:

- Drink plenty of water. When you become dehydrated, saliva—your mouth's natural cleanser—stops flowing. This allows bacteria and plaque to stick more persistently to your tongue, gums, and teeth (bacteria is often a cause of bad breath). Drinking water also helps to flush out loose food from between your teeth.
- To avoid smoker's breath, don't smoke.
- Stick with your regimen of diligent brushing and flossing. (We know—you've heard this one before.)
- Make like a bunny. Munching on a fresh sprig of parsley or mint clears the palate and the breath of food odors.
- Avoid the obvious offenders. While most food odors can be easily eliminated, some, like garlic and onions, tend to hang around a bit longer.

CAVITIES

When plaque accumulates in your mouth very rapidly, the acid-forming bacteria that colonize it start working immediately to break down your teeth's enamel. Holes in the enamel that have been eaten away by bacteria are called cavities (or caries), and these decayed pits in the tooth's surface must be drilled out and filled. There are three primary types of caries:

Pit-and-fissure caries form on the chewing surfaces of bicuspids and molars. Because of the uneven shape of these surfaces, they are the hardest to clean. Most people also have occasional dents and imperfections in these teeth, making them a target for bacterial decay.

Smooth-surface caries form on the smooth surfaces between your teeth. These caries are caused by prolonged exposure to acids (usually due to infrequent or improper cleaning).

Root caries, as their name implies, are found on the roots of your teeth. Decay in this area, too, is caused by prolonged exposure to plaque acids. Root caries are most evident in older people and those who have had extensive dental work or whose gums have eroded, exposing them to damaging acids.

PERIODONTAL DISEASE

Most of us have first-hand knowledge of cavities, but less well known—and more devastating—is what can happen when your gums succumb to disease. Periodontal (literally meaning around the tooth) disease can take several forms.

Gingivitis. Gingivitis is an inflammation of the gum tissue, or gingiva, caused by plaque and tartar. The deposits of plaque and calculus in the pocket irritate the surrounding gum tissue, causing it to swell and become tender.

Gingivitis sometimes goes undetected. The inflamed tissue can bleed easily, even with minor pressure from a toothbrush, but the condition does not usually cause pain or other noticeable symptoms. That's why it's so dangerous: Unchecked, it can lead to far more serious problems.

Periodontitis. Unchecked gingivitis can lead to a very serious periodontal disease called periodontitis (formerly known as pyorrhea). The deposits of plaque move deeper into the space between the teeth and gums, and the inflammation is often accompanied by gum recession and damage to the soft and hard tissues. When these underlying structures eventually succumb, tooth loss becomes a very real possibility.

In its advanced stages, periodontitis can invade the jawbone and ligaments. At this point, even the best oral hygiene won't be enough: If you want to save your teeth, you'll need to see a qualified dentist or, probably, a periodontist.

STRESS-RELATED DISORDERS

Stress affects the body in many ways. It has been linked to depression, high blood cholesterol levels, high blood pressure, and a number of other ills. What you may not be aware of, however, is that excessive stress can damage your teeth and jaws.

Two stress-related disorders that affect the mouth are temporomandibular joint syndrome (TMJ) and myofacial pain dysfunction (MPD). Although not technically diseases, these two disorders can be very unpleasant. TMJ causes pain in the joints and ligaments of the jaw. MPD is a similar affliction, although the term may refer to stress-related pain in any part of the face (not just the jaw). Both are (for unknown reasons) most likely to affect women in their 20s and 30s but can affect both sexes at any age.

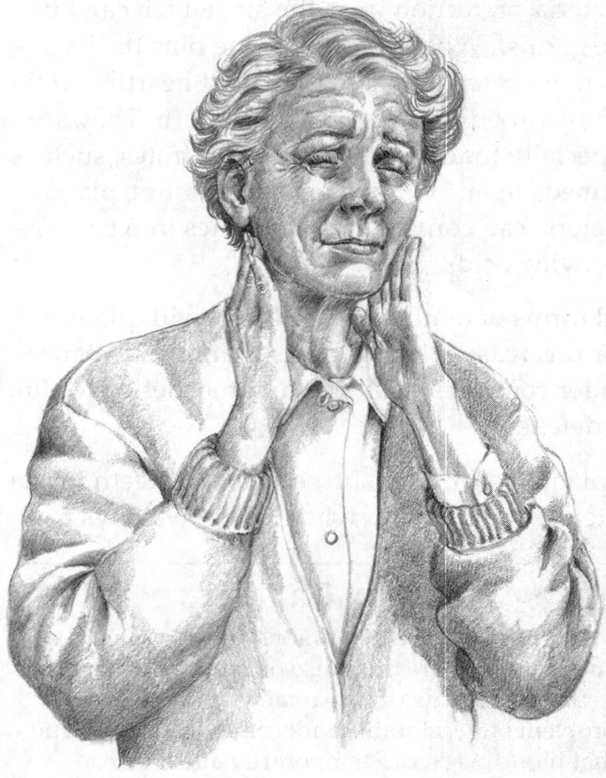

The following may be signs of TMJ or MPD:

- A clicking, cracking, or popping sensation when you open your mouth to yawn or laugh
- An inability to open your mouth wide
- Tension or tenderness in your cheek muscles (especially first thing in the morning)

If you experience any of these symptoms on a regular basis, you should probably consult your dentist, who may recommend one of the following therapies:

- Relaxation exercises (Since TMJ and MPD are related to tension, deliberate attempts at relaxation may help alleviate them. For more on stress and how to relieve it, see Chapter 6.)
- Gentle massage to ease the pain and help relax the affected muscles
- A custom polyurethane mouth guard made from an impression of your teeth (One of the prime causes of TMJ and MPD is nighttime teeth grinding or jaw clenching. A mouth guard worn over your lower set of teeth can

prevent them from grinding against the uppers. It also provides a cushioning effect, which may ease the stress on your tired jaw muscles and ligaments.)

- Avoiding excessive trauma to the painful areas (Stay away from hard and crunchy foods, try not to open your mouth too wide, and—if possible—postpone any unrelated dental surgery.)

ARE YOU AT INCREASED RISK?

Dental problems are often blamed on genetics: "I got my bad teeth from my mother." Certainly, heredity plays a roll in the composition and constitution of your teeth. In fact, many factors can contribute to the development of dental problems. As we know, poor oral hygiene is foremost among them, but there are others—both beyond and within your control. Here are some of the contributing factors:

- Malocclusion: Teeth that do not fit together properly or that grow in misaligned can be a contributing factor in both dental caries and periodontal disease. Correction of malocclusion early in life is the best way to prevent these problems.
- Chemical irritants: Some substances can weaken your teeth's own protective coating and make surrounding tissues more vulnerable to disease. Tobacco, both smoked and chewed, can have these effects, among other more devastating consequences.
- Hormone levels: Circulating hormones can cause changes in the structure of connective tissue. Pregnant women and women on certain oral contraceptives sometimes have spongier gums, making them more prone to cavities and gingivitis.
- Nonfluoridated water: People who live (or lived when they were children) in areas where the water is not fluoridated have an increased risk of developing dental disease. (For more on fluoridation, see pages 116–117.)

The Stuff That Fillings Are Made Of

For many years, there were only two types of fillings available—amalgam (a compound of zinc, copper, tin, silver, and mercury) and gold. However, advances in plastics technology have yielded some excellent alternatives to these old standbys.

The best material for fillings is indisputably gold. However, it can cost as much as ten times more to fill a tooth with gold than with amalgam or a plastic composite. Gold fillings can last up to 20 years—much longer than the others.

Although there have been inconclusive studies questioning the safety of amalgam fillings (because of their mercury content), most dentists still swear by them because of their relative durability, their ease of installation, and their low cost. The American Dental Association also remains committed to their position that the material is safe.

Perhaps because of the amalgam controversy, plastic composite fillings are gaining popularity. They also confer the advantage of being tooth-colored, rendering them practically invisible. Ongoing research promises to improve their future durability and ease of installation.

- Systemic disorders: Diabetes, disorders of the thyroid gland, and certain blood conditions can contribute to a person's risk of periodontal disease. Ask your doctor or dentist about your particular situation.

ORAL HYGIENE

Of all the health problems that can plague us, those involving our teeth are probably the most preventable. A few simple habits that most of us learned as children are pretty much all you need to maintain good oral hygiene.

However, just because we learned these habits as children doesn't mean we remember them today, and proper technique can make all the difference in the world. In this section, we'll elaborate on that elusive virtue called *oral hygiene*.

BACK TO BRUSHING BASICS

Brushing your teeth serves a number of purposes: It whisks away food particles, cleans and massages your gums, helps to eliminate decay-causing plaque, and freshens your breath. While not a panacea for all dental ills, brushing is an essential armament in the fight against decay, gingivitis, and periodontal disease.

Even though it's something most of us do every day, it doesn't hurt to get a refresher course on brushing, because using the proper brushing technique is just as important as vigilance.

- Choose a routine and stick to it. Establishing a proper and habitual method of brushing your teeth will go a long way toward preventing dental caries and gum disease.
- Always start in the same place in your mouth. This will help ensure that all parts of your mouth get cleaned every time. A good place to start is the hard-to-reach rear molars, which need the most time and attention.
- Press gently at a 45-degree angle. Scrub the front of the tooth and gum for a few seconds using a small circular motion. In the same manner, move slowly around your mouth until you get to the other side. Pay particular attention to your gum line, because this is where gingivitis takes hold.
- After you've worked your way to the other side of your mouth, rotate the brush so that it rests against the back of your tooth and gum, and use the same angle and same circular scrubbing motion as you return to the first tooth.
- Next, briskly brush along the top face, or chewing surface, of your teeth.
- Then repeat the entire process on your upper or lower set of teeth (depending on where you started).
- Lastly, don't neglect the roof of your mouth and your tongue. These surfaces also harbor harmful, plaque-causing bacteria.
- Rinse out your mouth.

This whole process should take at least three minutes, or you probably haven't done a thorough job. (Okay, all you speed demons—go back and start again!)

CHOOSING THE RIGHT BRUSH

Use a soft brush. Standard brushes with medium or hard bristles can, over time, wear away the gum line and create grooves and pocks in your teeth. As your gum line disappears, your risk of developing periodontal disease grows. Likewise, grooves and indentations in the teeth create more opportunities for plaque-causing bacteria to gather and eat away at the tooth enamel. A soft brush is sufficient for gentle—but still effective—cleaning.

Invest in high technology. A number of new, scientifically designed toothbrushes have emerged on the market, each with its own promise to remove plaque like no brush before it ever could. This is one area where innovation is more than just talk.

Comfort and ease of use are among the most valuable benefits conferred by the high-tech toothbrushes. Many come with tapered handles, finger grips, or flexible parts that make them easier to hold and manipulate in your mouth. These new toothbrushes may help you get to areas that were difficult to reach with the older, standard toothbrush shapes.

Another useful feature is variable-length bristles, which are cut into specific shapes. This can help the bristles penetrate the tight spaces between teeth and gums.

Trust the experts. If you'd like to try a new type of brush but can't make a choice, ask your dentist or hygienist for advice (they might even give you samples to try). If you're on your own, choose a brand that is approved by the American Dental Association (check the label).

Get plugged in. If, because of a disability, you are unable to use a manual toothbrush, an electric brush may be a good alternative. These products have become less expensive and more efficient in recent years.

FACTS ON FLOSSING

For many of us, a quick toothbrushing session in the morning and the evening serves as the meat and potatoes of our home dental care strategy. However, unless you've got a fetish for fillings, brushing by itself is not enough.

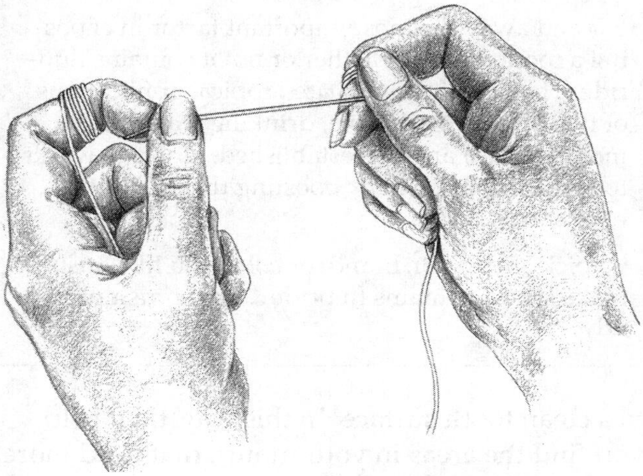

If you've ever been to the dentist, you've undoubtedly been told that flossing is the prime defense against periodontal disease. It also fights caries and decay. You should floss after each meal or, at the very least, once a day.

As with brushing, technique is important, so here are some flossing tips:

- Take an 18- to 24-inch length of floss, and wrap most of it around the index finger of one hand. Next, wrap all but about 4 inches around the index finger of the other hand.
- Gripping the floss between the thumb and bent forefinger, slowly work the floss between two teeth with a gentle sawing motion. Never snap or force the floss in. As with brushing, start in the same place each time you floss (the rear molars are a good place to begin).
- Gently scrape the floss around the tooth, going up into the gum line until you meet resistance. Work systematically in a *C* shape around each tooth.
- Using your fingers like spools, unwrap a clean section of floss from the hand with unused floss, and spin the used portion onto the other finger. Move on to the next space.
- Continue all the way around your mouth, using the same technique.

It's a good idea to rinse your mouth out every few teeth. Rinsing will help clear away the tartar and plaque you have dislodged. It will also show you if you are bleeding. (While a little blood is no cause for alarm, chronic or excessive bleeding may be a sign of gum disease.)

WHICH FLOSS SHOULD YOU USE?

Dental floss comes in a large variety of forms, flavors, and colors: There's waxed and unwaxed; thick and thin; mint-flavored and plain; white, clear, green, and blue. There are disposable floss holders and reusable floss threaders (sold in drugstores and supermarkets). There is even a tough Gore-Tex floss that is designed to slip into the tightest spaces without shredding or fraying.

Fortunately, there's no need to start an extensive research project on the most effective type of floss (the differences between brands and types are mostly for show). If you are just being initiated into the wonderful world of flossing, you might like to splurge on a few different kinds of dental floss to see which you like most. Here are a few hints to help you find the right floss:

- If your teeth are very close together, waxed, thin, or Gore-Tex floss may slide in between them more easily.
- Flavored flosses introduce a pleasant, distracting taste while you floss. (They're a great incentive for kids.)
- If you have wide spaces between your teeth, you might try using dental tape—a wider variety of floss.

◆ Floss holders and threaders may make flossing easier for you if you have extensive bridge work or partial dentures.

OTHER PREVENTIVE EQUIPMENT

A quest for better and easier weapons for the fight against dental decay and disease has produced mixed results. Better-designed toothbrushes do help some, but some other devices have provided more distraction than benefit.

Water irrigators are devices that force a concentrated jet of water through a tube and out of a nozzle designed to get to the hard-to-reach areas of your gums and teeth. Irrigators can be very useful if you have braces or any other dental work that resists a thorough flossing. However, if you are able to floss, irrigating is not an adequate replacement for that handy roll of string. It can serve as a useful adjunct to your regular brushing and flossing (the more ways you clean, the more likely you are to get everything). Carefully follow the manufacturer's directions, and consult your dentist if you have any questions.

Electric toothbrushes may help massage your gums, but cannot do anything more than a thorough manual brushing. They are not without their place: As stated earlier, they are a terrific boon to anyone who lacks the strength or the dexterity to brush their teeth with a manual brush.

New plastic and acrylic compounds used as sealants are making a big dent in parents' dental bills these days. Dentists have begun applying these durable, waterproof plastics to teeth (especially children's teeth) to keep out the plaque. The sealants are applied in a single office visit. They are especially effective on molars. These painless sealants can last for as long as five years, but may have to be redone every two or three years (depending on the amount of wear they suffer).

Disclosing tablets are an inexpensive, easy way to check up on your hygiene habits. These tablets contain harmless, colored vegetable dyes that adhere to plaque more readily than they adhere to a clean tooth surface. In this way, they help you find the areas in your mouth that need more attention.

Disclosing tablets are easy to use: After brushing your teeth, simply chew one up, swish it around your mouth, then spit it out. The stained areas are places that you missed or didn't clean thoroughly. Brush again to remove the stains, and remember to pay closer attention to those areas in the future. You can purchase disclosing tablets in your local drugstore, but don't overdo; they shouldn't be used more than once per week. Be sure to follow the manufacturer's directions carefully.

THE TRUTH ABOUT TOOTHPASTE

"Baking soda and peroxide." "Tartar control." "Especially for sensitive teeth." "All-natural ingredients." With so many types and flavors of toothpaste available, how should you make the choice?

The rule is to get back to basics: Sensitive-tooth formulations may make brushing a bit less painful. Tartar-control toothpastes may be slightly more effective for removing hardened plaque. (The baking soda–peroxide pastes don't do anything unique, aside from getting foamy.) But the truth is it's the mechanical action of brushing that does your teeth the most good.

Far and away the most important factor in choosing a toothpaste is whether or not it contains fluoride. The benefits of repeated topical applications of fluoride (in toothpaste, drinking water, and mouth rinses) are well established. Fluoride works to protect your teeth by boosting their ability to resist decay.

So pick any flavor, brand, or color you like. Just make sure it contains fluoride . . . and brush properly.

REMOVING STAINS

Stained teeth in themselves are not really a health hazard, but they can be an annoyance. Even worse, they can prompt you to do damaging things in an attempt to whiten them.

Some stains can be removed by your twice-yearly cleaning, while others may require more aggressive treatment. Still other stains may be almost impossible to remove. The best way to keep your teeth their whitest is to avoid staining them in the first place.

A variety of factors can contribute to or cause stained teeth. Some of the more common tooth stainers are cigarette smoke, chewing tobacco, and habitual coffee and tea drinking. Extensive decay and dead nerves may also cause some discoloration. Plaque left by improper or infrequent flossing and brushing is a magnet for foods that stain (remember, plaque is sticky stuff). And, of course, age—that notorious thief of beauty—robs your teeth of their original brilliant white color, leaving them slightly yellowed.

Exposure to certain drugs (such as the antibiotic tetracycline) either in utero or as a small child, can leave teeth a pearly gray. Excessive childhood ingestion of fluoride may also cause the enamel to appear mottled and uneven. These types of stains are often the most difficult to remove, although they may improve somewhat with the aid of a professional bleaching.

Here are some ideas to brighten your smile:

- Stick to your brushing and flossing regimen. (You knew that was coming, didn't you?) Once again, conscientious brushing and flossing wins—hands down—as the number-one preventer of dental problems, including staining.
- Avoid all forms of tobacco use, including pipes, cigars, chewing tobacco, and snuff.
- Cut down on your intake of coffee and tea. The less contact these fluids have with your teeth, the less opportunity they will have to leave stains.
- Disguise it. If you have a dark, highly visible amalgam filling (and a little disposable income), consider having it replaced with a tooth-colored plastic composite. A porcelain crown can also cover up a badly discolored or decayed tooth.
- Treat yourself to an extra cleaning or two. Keep your teeth whiter (and your hygienist happier) by scheduling visits just for professional cleanings. Extra cleanings may help prevent long-term staining.
- Get your teeth professionally bleached. Several excellent technologies have emerged for bleaching and whitening the teeth. Although some of these procedures must be performed in the dentist's office, a few can be done at home. Ask your dentist what he or she recommends.

The following are some definite tooth-whitening **don'ts**:

- Don't take aggressive measures on your own. You may end up compounding your problem. If your teeth are heavily stained or discolored, consult your dentist about professional or supervised treatments.
- Avoid home whitening kits. These kits are of dubious value, and some may even be dangerous. The American Dental Association has never put its seal of approval on any product currently marketed as tooth-bleaching. The bleaching ingredient used in most kits is carbamide peroxide, which is converted to hydrogen peroxide in your mouth. Hydrogen peroxide has the potential to damage soft tissues. If you're determined to do it yourself, consult your dentist beforehand.
- Never use any amount of chlorine bleach on your teeth. It is highly toxic.
- Don't overdo it with "whitening" toothpastes. Some stain-removing toothpastes are quite abrasive and can wear off enamel if used too often. To be cautious, don't use these products more than two or three times a week.

AN ANTICAVITY DIET

There is no perfect diet that will keep your teeth from all harm, but what you eat can have an effect on the health of your teeth and gums. Eating right has benefits on two fronts: By supplying your body with the right nutrients, a healthful diet strengthens your teeth from the inside; and by limiting the foods that promote bacterial growth, it protects your teeth from outside invaders.

BUILDING STRONG TEETH

Teeth are essentially a kind of bone. They are harder and more durable because they are on the outside, but the same nutrients that promote a strong skeleton promote strong teeth.

Calcium. The primary component of strong bone tissue is the mineral calcium. It gives the skeleton structure and hardness. It may seem that teeth, once they are fully grown, don't need any more calcium. Indeed, the most important time to ensure a proper amount of calcium in the diet is when teeth and bones are forming, but even after they are fully grown, teeth and bones still need to have an adequate supply. The body constantly takes calcium from bones and teeth and replaces it with new supplies. You should make sure that your body has plenty on hand.

Getting enough calcium in the diet can seem difficult for those who don't want to get too much fat. The best sources of calcium—dairy products—are often high in fat as well. However, there are alternatives: low-fat milk, low-fat and nonfat yogurt, some dark-green leafy vegetables, and calcium-fortified orange juice.

Vitamin D. Vitamin D works hand in hand with calcium. It doesn't add to the hardness of bones and teeth in itself, but it promotes the deposition of calcium in the skeleton. Without it, it wouldn't matter how much calcium your body had available, because the calcium would not be absorbed into bone tissue.

Vitamin D is added to almost all commercial milk, and many other foods are now fortified with it. Your body has the ability to make its own vitamin D also. The vitamin is produced in the

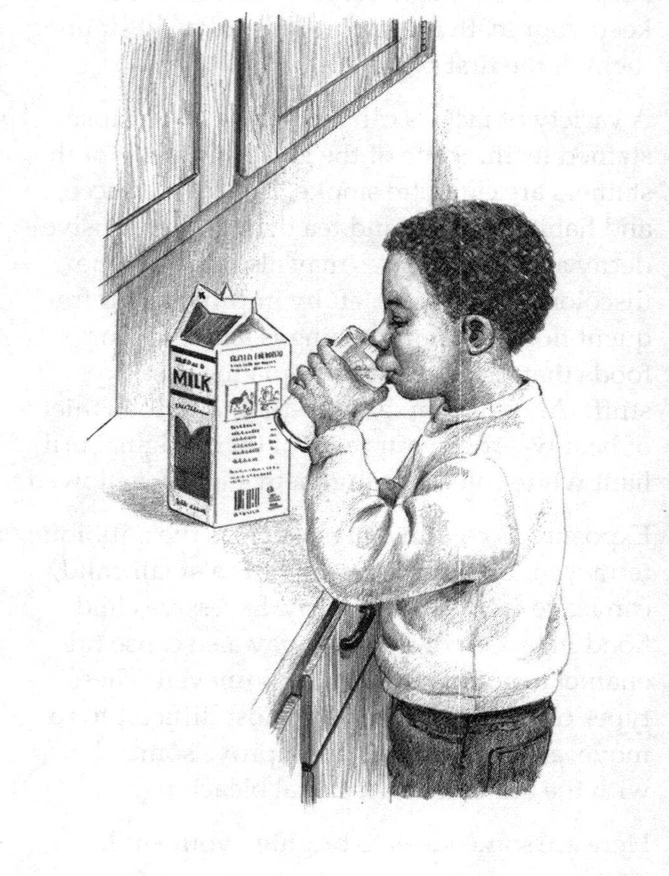

skin when your skin is exposed to the sun's ultraviolet radiation.

Vitamin C. Almost every ailment has been said to be "cured" by vitamin C, but here there is a real connection—connective tissue. Vitamin C is vital to the health of connective tissue such as your gums. In fact, one of the first symptoms of vitamin C deficiency, or scurvy, is weak, sore gums that bleed easily. Vitamin C can be found in citrus fruits and some vegetables such as broccoli and brussels sprouts.

Fluoride. The one nutrient that affects the health of your teeth the most is also one of the most controversial (see "Fluoride: Menace or Benefit?"). The mineral fluoride has been proved to make teeth harder and more resistant to decay. Study after study has shown that people living in areas where fluoride is added to the water have fewer cavities than those who do not. Although many of us do get our fluoride from fluoridated drinking water, some don't have that option in their communities. Ask your doctor or dentist if you are concerned.

PROBLEM FOODS

Because plaque formation is the start of virtually all types of dental disease, and plaque bacteria feed on leftover sugars, it stands to reason that cutting down on sugar—in all of its forms—will help prevent cavities. Easier said than done.

Sugar is one of the most insidious ingredients in the modern diet. If you look at almost any prepared food's ingredients, somewhere in that list will be sucrose or one of its close relatives (such as glucose, maltose, lactose, fructose, galactose, dextrose, corn syrup, molasses, brown sugar, raw sugar, and so on). Even honey, no matter how unrefined, contains simple sugars that serve as a banquet meal for plaque bacteria. The same goes for fructose (naturally occurring fruit sugar).

FLUORIDE: MENACE OR BENEFIT?

Artificially fluoridated drinking water was introduced in the United States in the 1940s, with the goal of enhancing our nation's dental health. Today, more than 60 percent of the population is supplied with it.

This supplemented water contains between 0.7 and 1.2 parts fluoride to 1 million parts water. At these levels, one quart of water contains about 1 milligram of fluoride (safe levels for adults lie somewhere between 1.5 milligrams to 10 milligrams per day, depending on body weight).

Although the World Health Organization and the American Dental Association contend that the amount of fluoride present in drinking water poses no health threat, other groups call attention to the fact that the chemical has been used as a rat poison and a pesticide. In addition, they ask, when you consider that fluoride is also present in many of the foods we eat (such as spinach and seafood), isn't our population at risk for fluoride overdose?

Before you make up your mind, consider the following: To get a lethal dose of one gram of fluoride, a child would have to drink 25 gallons of water in one day. And, unless you've got an extremely unusual kid, that's highly unlikely.

Complex carbohydrates can also provide food for bacteria in your mouth. In fact, some researchers suggest that starchy foods may be even more detrimental to your teeth than simple sugars. Starches are more sticky than sugar; the saliva that usually dissolves and washes away small amounts of sugar on the teeth might not be able to contend with the clumps of potato chips or crackers stuck in and around molars. Starchy foods that stick to your teeth and stay there for hours provide plenty of fuel for enamel-eroding microbes.

This doesn't mean that you should avoid starchy foods. On the contrary, they are the basis of a healthful diet (see Chapter 1). It only means that you must be more conscious of how these foods affect your teeth and more conscientious about cleaning them after you do enjoy those snack chips.

Although no other nutritional component besides sugar has been positively linked to tooth decay, the rest of your diet cannot be overlooked in your effort to maintain healthy teeth and gums. A diet that is full of sugars and overprocessed foods (or one devoid of vitamins, minerals, and crunchy fruits and vegetables) can eventually lead to decay, even in the mouths of the most avid brushers and flossers.

AT THE DENTIST

You cannot go it alone. No matter how well you care for your teeth at home, you will never be rid of the dreaded dentist's office. You still have to go for regular checkups and cleanings, and in the rare case of a dental emergency, you'll be glad the professionals are around.

THE CHECKUP

Has fear kept you away from the dentist for so long that your teeth hurt just thinking about it? If so, fight your fear with facts. A checkup is certainly nothing to worry about, and knowing what's going to happen should allay your fears. Here are a few things you can expect when you visit the dentist for your semi-annual cleaning and exam:

Cleaning. A professional cleaning involves more than a simple brushing and flossing. Your dentist has special instruments and techniques to clean your teeth more thoroughly than you can at home.

First, your dentist or dental hygienist removes the tartar, or calculus, that has built up on your teeth. This hardened plaque is removed with a sharp tool called a scaler. Some dentists now use a device that can remove the tartar with ultrasonic sound waves instead of a scaler, but both methods do the same thing.

After the tartar buildup has been removed, your teeth are polished with a special paste and a rotating rubber polisher. The polishing process not only brightens your teeth, but it also gives them a very smooth surface, making it difficult for bacteria and plaque to take hold.

In addition to these steps, children may also receive an extra treatment to make their teeth stronger and more cavity resistant. A fluoride

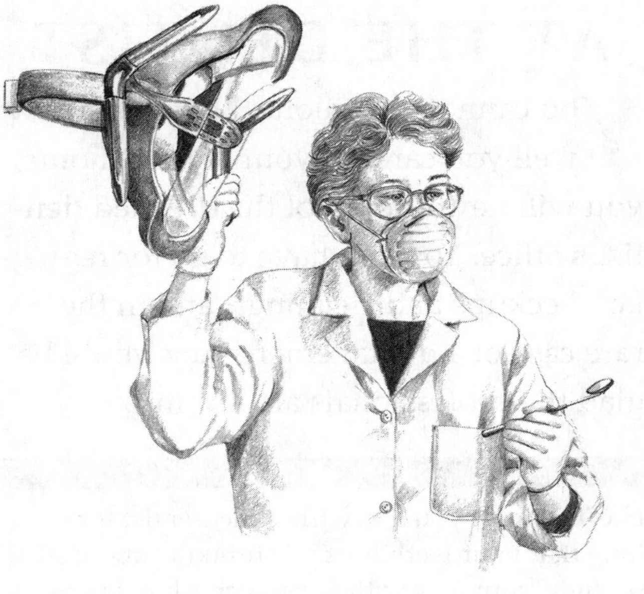

wash is a topical application of fluoride that can protect the tooth enamel.

Examination. After a thorough cleaning, the dentist checks on the health of your teeth and gums. This part of your visit includes:

- Examination of the soft tissue, during which the dentist checks the interior of your mouth for signs of any disease.
- Examination of the teeth with a small metal probe called an explorer to find any signs of decay.
- X rays to get a more accurate picture of any suspected decay, to examine teeth that have not yet emerged, or to assess the progress of periodontal disease. They can also locate any cysts or lesions on the jawbone. (X rays are usually considered optional unless it's your first visit to that particular dentist or regular examination reveals a problem that requires a more extensive evaluation.)

WHAT TO DO WHEN THINGS GO WRONG

Despite your flawless oral hygiene and your unbeatable genetic history, there may come a time when you are hit by a cataclysmic toothache or a roguish baseball to the upper left incisor.

Your first step should be to investigate the problem area and try to determine the source of the aggravation (in the case of the baseball, check out the extent of the damage). If you cannot attribute the pain to anything in particular (and especially if the site is extremely tender, bleeding, swollen, or lumpy), call your dentist at once. Also, if you notice any foul odor emanating from your mouth, it may be an indication of an infection or a decayed tooth requiring immediate attention.

The following are some suggestions for coping with pain and easing swelling until you can get to the dentist:

- Try oil of cloves. Oil of cloves is the numbing ingredient present in several over-the-counter toothache and tooth-pain remedies. Be sure to follow package directions carefully.

- Rinse your mouth with a solution of hydrogen peroxide and salt. Eight ounces of warm water mixed with one-half teaspoon each of table salt and fresh (not old) hydrogen peroxide may help soothe irritated tissues.
- Take an over-the-counter analgesic. Aspirin, acetaminophen (such as Tylenol), or ibuprofen (such as Advil or Motrin IB) may help keep your pain under control while you wait to receive professional treatment.
- Take good care of a burn. A burn inside your mouth can be extremely painful. Often, just keeping the affected area free of irritants (cigarette smoke, alcohol, hot drinks, and food) for a few hours will usually help. You can also apply ice cubes or ice chips directly to the site of the burn.

If you have burned your mouth with a chemical (such as aspirin or bleach), flush the area thoroughly with water and avoid allowing food, liquid, or your tongue to touch the area. If a chemical burn starts to bleed (or if it does not seem to be healing well), contact your dentist or physician.

A knocked-out tooth or a broken jaw are among the most serious of dental emergencies. A knocked-out tooth starts to die immediately. Get in touch with your dentist right away so that the whole tooth can be replanted. Meanwhile, place the tooth in sterile water if you can, and bring it with you to the dentist.

A broken jaw requires surgery. Go immediately to the nearest hospital emergency room. In the meantime, don't open your mouth, and do your best to immobilize the jaw.

TOOTH CARE IN UTERO

Your child's primary and secondary teeth begin to form before birth. There are certain precautions you can take while pregnant to protect those incubating jewels.

First off, make sure you get an adequate amount of calcium. (The RDA for calcium for pregnant women is 1,500 milligrams per day.) The pregnant woman's body will do almost anything to protect the developing fetus. If there is an inadequate supply of calcium on hand, the body will take calcium from the mother's bones and teeth to provide for the fetus, leaving the mother at risk for tooth problems and osteoporosis. If your obstetrician has recommended that you take a calcium supplement, do so diligently.

Second, avoid taking any form of the antibiotic tetracycline while you are pregnant or trying to conceive. Tetracycline can stain a child's primary and secondary teeth a pearly gray color.

Third, ask your dentist about taking fluoride tablets throughout your pregnancy, especially if you live in an area without fluoridated water. Some dentists believe that fluoride supplements can help your child build healthier, stronger teeth, right from the start.

YOUR CHILD'S TEETH

It is rare that a baby is born with any sign of teeth below its tiny gums. However, much to most parents' chagrin, the painful struggles with teething arrive all too quickly. Next comes the loss of these newly acquired baby (deciduous) teeth, followed by the grand finale—the arrival of the permanent teeth.

Although this emergence, loss, and re-emergence of teeth might seem a strange quirk of nature, understanding the processes behind the cycle will help you raise children with healthy teeth and gums. (The explanation might also serve as excellent ammunition for late-night fights over brushing and flossing.)

Both sets of teeth begin to form before birth. Four to eight months after birth (on average), the first tiny tooth starts to make its painful way through the gum, erupting amidst emphatic "oohs" and "ahs" from the baby's family.

Over the next 20 months, a new tooth will come in about once a month. At the end of this long cycle, the average child will end up with 20 primary teeth, which he will keep for another 30 to 36 months.

When a child is about six years of age, the first of her permanent molars erupts, and the baby teeth begin to fall out. As each tooth falls out, it is replaced by a shiny new permanent tooth. It will be another 10 years before the entire process is complete.

CARING FOR BABY'S TEETH

So, you may ask, if those first teeth are going to fall out anyway, do they really require much attention? The answer is a definitive *yes*.

First off, your child will have to live with those primary teeth for the next five years of his life. And, as we all know, children can be awfully cruel about things like discolored or decaying teeth.

Second, lifelong habits are established early. If you care about your children's long-term dental health, you need to start influencing them early.

Third, dental bills are expensive, even if you have great insurance. Just because baby teeth aren't permanent, doesn't mean they can't decay, and you can't tell a child to live the next two years with that toothache. What's more, you'll feel extraordinarily guilty as you stand by watching the dentist drill cavity after cavity out of your child's mouth.

So when do you start taking care of your baby's teeth? As soon as they erupt from the gum. The moment your baby's first tooth makes its momentous appearance, it will immediately come under siege by ravenously hungry plaque bacteria. As far as bacteria are concerned, the sugars found in breast milk, juice, and formula taste just as good as the sugars found in a candy bar.

Toy stores, drug stores, supermarkets, and baby specialty stores all sell tiny toothbrushes for babies. The best kind to start out with is a small rubber brush that fits on the end of your fingertip (if you can't find one, ask your dentist, who may keep some on hand). At this stage, you're probably better off not using toothpaste. (Conventional toothpastes are dangerous to swallow. The only safe kinds are the all-natural, calcium-carbonate pastes that do not contain added fluoride.)

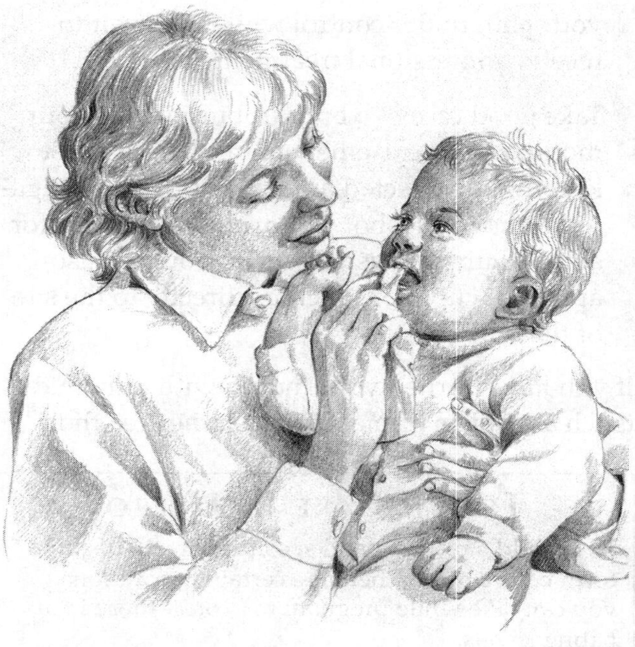

If you're not comfortable using a brush, you can start out by wiping the baby's teeth with a clean, soft cloth moistened with water.

Regardless of the method you choose, try to clean the teeth as often as you can, in particular, before naps and bedtime.

THUMB SUCKING AND PACIFIERS

Before the primary teeth come in, thumb sucking and pacifier use will probably have little or no effect on your child's future dental development. After the first teeth have erupted, however, their positions might be affected by the continuous presence of a thumb or a nonorthodontic pacifier. (Orthodontic pacifiers may be a little better due to their specially tapered shape.)

Many children who use a pacifier will lose interest in it at the age of about nine months—long before it can do any real damage. If you take the pacifier away at this time, many kids will forget about it altogether. Other children will stubbornly refuse to give up their pacifiers until much later. If you restrict the pacifier use to nap time and bedtime, you'll be able to keep the amount of damage it can do to a minimum. Most children become willing to give up this habit on their own by age three or four.

Thumb sucking often continues much longer than pacifier use—sometimes until age five or six. (After all, the thumb is always ready and accessible). And the damage it causes to the teeth can be far more extensive than that caused by a pacifier.

What should you do if your child is a persistent thumb sucker? First off, avoid turning the issue into a power struggle between you and your child. Chances are that if the child feels that it is you—not he—who has the big investment in discontinuing the habit, he will use it as a rebellion against you (two year olds excel in the rebellion department).

Unfortunately, many experts in the field of pediatric psychology say that you can't stop a child from thumb sucking until he perceives it as a problem (because it becomes fodder for teasing at school, for example). At that point, you can step in and devise a reward-based strategy for helping him stop.

For example, once your daughter tells you that she wants to stop sucking her thumb, you can make a big wall calendar together. For each day that your child succeeds in resisting the allure of her thumb, you can put a sticker on her calendar. You can also come up with a reward (dinner at her favorite restaurant or a toy) for each week or month that she successfully abstains.

Pediatricians differ in their opinions about using bitter liquids on the thumb as a deterrent. Some say that it reeks of cruelty; others say that it works only if the child feels that it will help her succeed. You'll need to make a decision that is right for you and your child.

If your child does not yet see thumb sucking as a problem (but you do), you might try telling her that she is welcome to suck her thumb as often as she wants, as long as she does it only when she is alone, in her own room. This sometimes will help interrupt the habit's association with activities, such as television watching, riding in the car, and so on. As with the use of a pacifier, sucking the thumb for a few hours a night, in bed, will help keep damage to a minimum.

Avoid Bottle Mouth Syndrome

Have you ever seen a child with bottle mouth? If you have, you probably remember it. The syndrome is characterized by gaping black holes in the front teeth—a result of long-term contact with a bottle nipple filled with formula, milk, or juice.

The biggest mistake you can make, in terms of your child's oral health, is to put him to bed with a bottle of milk or juice. These fluids are full of simple sugars (that's why babies love them). Long-term exposure can cause devastating decay.

Don't wait until a bedtime bottle is a habit your child tenaciously clings to (it's hard to talk a 14-month old out of anything, let alone his bottle). Your best strategy is simply to avoid the problem before it ever gets underway.

COPING WITH STRESS

Stress, as defined by Hans Selye, M.D., pioneer researcher in the field of stress, is "the nonspecific response of the body to any demand made upon it." It doesn't matter if the demand is pleasurable or frustrating, only that some modification or change is made.

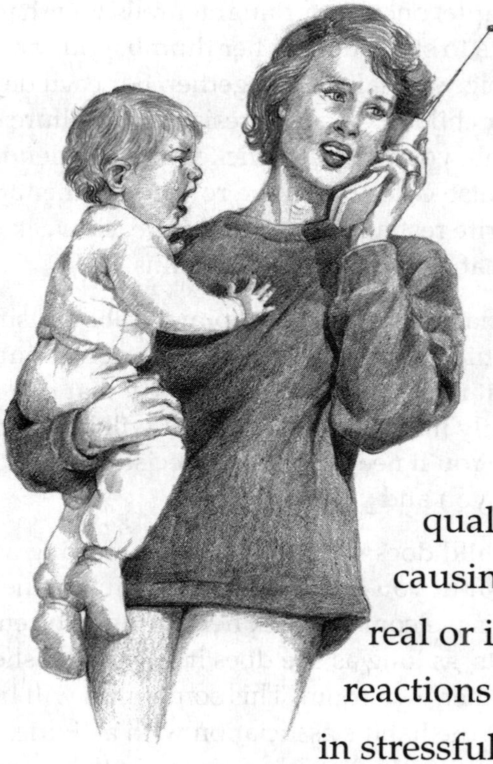

Stress, in and of itself, is not bad. Positive events such as winning an award, traveling, or completing a painting create stress, just as negative occurrences such as losing a job or approaching a deadline do. And a completely imagined fear or worry can trigger as much negative stress as an actual event.

What matters for your health is not the quality of the individual stressors—not the things causing the stress or whether they're good or bad, real or imagined—but your mental and physical reactions to them. In fact, it's what you do to yourself in stressful situations that makes stress dangerous.

Each of us reacts to stressors in our own way. What bothers one person may not seem the least bit troublesome to the next. What may create "distress" for each of us one day may hardly affect us at all the next. By learning to cope with stress and by changing those things creating distress, we can become healthier, happier, and better able to enjoy our lives.

THE DANGERS OF STRESS

Our bodies have been programmed genetically to react quickly to stressful situations. These reactions, called the "fight or flight" response, served our cave-dwelling progenitors well and offered them a chance for survival against wild animals, inhospitable environmental conditions, and warring neighbors. When faced with hostility, our ancestors' digestive systems shut down, and their heart rate, oxygen consumption, and blood pressure increased to enable them to go into action instantly, either fighting or escaping the enemy.

Although our caves are now condos or air-conditioned homes, our nervous systems remain the same. We're often at a constant state of readiness without the opportunity to swing into action, and that's the problem. With no outlet for this tense energy, it can turn on us. Like drops of water beating down on a slab of granite, the chemicals dumped into our bloodstream will eventually scar us physically and emotionally. After an extended period of time, stress—even good stress—can break through our resistance and weaken us.

CARDIOVASCULAR PROBLEMS

Blood pressure. Any kind of stress, either physical or emotional, makes the heart and blood vessels work harder, thereby raising blood pressure. Although this increase is only temporary during exercise and is beneficial to good health, during extended periods of stress, blood pressure can stay elevated constantly and can have serious long-term effects. Chronic high blood pressure is known as hypertension. In hypertension, the heart beats much faster than the normal rate of about 70 beats per minute. The heart has to work extremely hard to pump blood through the strained arteries. Hypertension often has no noticeable symptoms, making it all the more deadly as it quietly overtaxes the cardiovascular system.

Cholesterol levels. Extended stress can also trigger the production of specific hormones used by the body to fight or flee. When the stress continues without any action being taken, these agents elevate cholesterol levels in the blood. When cholesterol sticks to the walls of arteries, it makes them narrower, forcing the heart to work harder to pump blood through the smaller area.

IMMUNITY

The overwhelming majority of medical professionals today now acknowledge that the mind and body are interconnected. What we think does affect our physical body. Studies at major medical institutions reveal that Norman Vincent Peale was right when he wrote the *Power of Positive Thinking*. Research indicates that learning to reduce stress in our lives through various means can enhance our immune system.

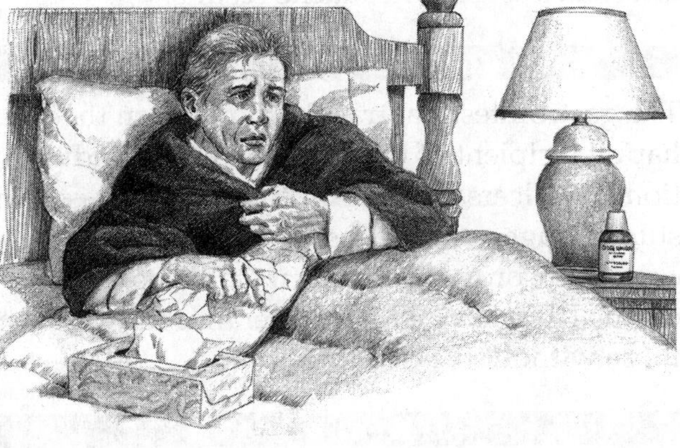

A strong immune system helps to protect us from cold and flu viruses that are always in our environment. You don't get colds from getting wet feet or sitting in drafts. You "catch" a cold when a virus is introduced into your system. Quite often, you inhale virus particles or transfer them into your respiratory tract with dirty hands. But not every time a virus enters your system does it produce a cold. Your immune system can usually fight off common viruses. However, when your immune system is weakened by stress, you have less resistance to the cold or flu and more of the little invaders will get through and make you sick.

What's more, your immune system has a roll in diseases other than simple infections. To some extent, your immune system is involved in defending against the development of cancerous growths—certainly a good reason to want it working at its best. Also, autoimmune diseases, in which the immune system attacks healthy body tissue, have been associated with or exacerbated by stress.

HEADACHES

More than 45 million Americans suffer from regular headaches, the majority of which are triggered by muscle tension. In fact, stress was named most often by those suffering from recurring headaches as the primary contributing cause.

Stress causes the adrenal glands to release a hormone called norepinephrine, which transmits nerve impulses and constricts blood vessels. When the vessels and muscles in your head are affected, a tension headache results.

GASTROINTESTINAL SYMPTOMS

The gastrointestinal tract has long been the unhappy recipient of the effects of stress. Indigestion and ulcers can be exacerbated by stress. And studies suggest that those suffering from a chronic disorder known as irritable bowel syndrome (IBS) have a lower tolerance to stress than those without the disorder.

MENTAL HEALTH

Substance abuse. People suffering from stress often turn to alcohol or other chemical substances to help them relax. However, alcohol and many drugs such as barbiturates and some tranquilizers can actually compound the problem. Alcohol and recreational drugs can trigger additional stress by interfering with normal thought processes. People may drive too fast, become physically or verbally abusive, or otherwise behave inappropriately while under the influence of drugs or alcohol. Later, many moan, "I'm so sorry. I wasn't thinking. I was drunk," or "I was stoned out of my mind. I didn't know what I was doing." This type of antisocial behavior resulting from substance abuse adds to stress.

Depression. As stress builds, a person can often become angry at the boss who is increasing the workload and withholding praise, at the spouse who doesn't seem understanding, at the kids who can't seem to be controlled, at the world for being so frustrating and unfriendly. Unable to fight everyone and everything, the person suffering from stress can turn it inward, onto him or herself. Feeling totally unable to cope can lead to depression and have devastating effects on physical and mental health.

Lowering of self-esteem. Stress can lower a person's self-esteem in many areas—work, sexual relationships, child rearing, and friendships, just to mention a few. If you don't feel good about yourself, others won't either. At work, stress might cause you to feel distracted so you miss deadlines or turn out mediocre work. When the boss complains, you might feel a loss of self-esteem, which in turn, creates additional stress, and the next project suffers even more.

Sexual dysfunction. Experts agree that stress is one of the major causes of sexual dysfunction, especially a man's inability to have or maintain an erection. Once stress triggers this problem, additional stress is created by performance anxiety, which increases the likelihood of more failures in the future.

It can become a vicious cycle. Men suffering from stress may have occasional bouts of impotence. Their self-esteem plummets. "I'm no good as a lover," they may think and avoid making love. The spouse feels stress from what she perceives as rejection. "I'm not attractive enough for him," she thinks.

Measuring Your Stress Level

In 1967, two psychiatrists at the University of Washington Medical School, Drs. Thomas H. Holmes and Richard H. Rahe, devised a rating scale of stressful life events. According to their study, a person's vulnerability to illness can be predicted fairly accurately by the number of points scored. Circle all the events you have experienced in the past year. Then total your score.

Event	Points
1) Death of a spouse	100
2) Divorce	73
3) Marital separation	65
4) Jail term	63
5) Death of a close family member	63
6) Personal injury or severe illness	53
7) Marriage	50
8) Fired at work	47
9) Marital reconciliation	45
10) Retirement	45
11) Change in health of family member	44
12) Pregnancy	40
13) Sex difficulties	39
14) Gain of a new family member	39
15) Business readjustment	39
16) Change in financial state	38
17) Death of a close friend	37
18) Change in work or school major	36
19) More arguments with spouse	35
20) Home mortgage over $50,000*	31
21) Loan foreclosures or unpaid bills	30
22) Change in work/school responsibilities	29

Event	Points
23) Son or daughter leaving home	29
24) Trouble with in-laws	29
25) Outstanding personal achievement	28
26) Spouse begins or stops work	26
27) Begin or end school	26
28) Revision of personal habits	24
29) Trouble with boss or school instructors	23
30) Change in work or social hours	20
31) Change in residence	20
32) Change in schools	20
33) Change in recreation	19
34) Change in church activities	18
35) Change in school activities	18
36) Mortgage or loan less than $50,000*	17
37) Change in sleeping habits	16
38) Change in number of family gatherings	15
39) Change in eating habits	15
40) Vacation	13
41) Christmas	12
42) Minor violation of the law	11
Total:	—

*This figure has been revised from the original scale to represent present mortgage rates more accurately.

Scoring

If you score:	You have a:
150–199	Mild chance of incurring some form of illness in the next year
200–299	Moderate risk of incurring some form of illness in the next year
300+	Very likely risk of serious physical or emotional illness

Remember, the scoring of this scale does not represent an exact prediction of a future event, but simply an increased likelihood based on observations and research in the general population. That does not mean that you should dismiss the significance of a high score. If you find your score soaring, you might want to think about delaying some stressful life changes until things settle down, or look into ways to handle stress better (see page 128).

Thomas Holmes and Richard Rahe. "The Social Readjustment Rating Scale," *J Psychosom Res* 11:212–218, 1967.

Women suffering from continued stress may develop hormonal imbalances, which can lead to menstrual problems such as irregular periods or heavy bleeding or a loss of sex drive.

Eating disorders. Stress is often the trigger for eating disorders including anorexia, bulimia, and obesity. Going off to college, getting married or divorced, starting a new job, or having a baby are a few common stress situations that can lead to an eating disorder.

Anorexia is a illness in which the person—usually a woman—has a distorted body image. Although her weight may be normal or considerably below what it should be for her height and build, she is obsessed with the conviction that she is fat. People with anorexia may suffer from abdominal bloating, downy hair on their face and arms, brittle lackluster hair, irregular heartbeat, and constant chills. Over 15 percent of those suffering from anorexia will die from starvation or conditions triggered by the eating disorder.

Those suffering from bulimia stuff themselves with a large amount of food, then take laxatives, enemas, or emetics to rid themselves of the unwanted calories. People with bulimia often suffer from dental problems due to the stomach acid in the vomitus, and irregular heartbeats due to upsetting the delicate chemical balance of their bodies. They may have liver and kidney damage as well as internal bleeding. In some cases, the constant irritation from stomach acid can ruptue the esophagus. Many people with bulimia suffer from constant infections due to their weakened immune systems. Bulimia sufferers are often those under stress to maintain a specific weight, such as ballet dancers, high school and college wrestlers, gymnasts, and models.

Obesity is an eating disorder suffered by almost 25 percent of Americans. "Obesity" is defined as at least 20 percent over the weight that is considered standard for a person's sex, height, and build. Many people become obese because they eat under stress. The more stress they feel, the more they eat. The more weight they gain, the more stress they experience. Often a health professional's help is needed to break this self-destructive cycle.

ACCIDENT PRONENESS

It's impossible to focus on two things at once. When stress overwhelms us, we concentrate so completely on our problems and the way we feel that we lose track of what else is going on in the world. That's why the person under stress walks in front of moving traffic, grabs bug spray rather than vegetable spray, spills hot coffee, or climbs up on a cane-bottom chair, rather than getting out a ladder or step stool.

ALLERGIES

Most specialists in environmental medicine agree that certain allergies may be associated with stress. That doesn't mean that it's all in your head. The condition is real. It just means that stress can lower your tolerence to some allergens.

Asthma, hay fever, sinusitis, hives, irritable bowel syndrome, and headaches are just a few of the many medical conditions that may be caused by allergies and exacerbated by stress. In many cases, such as asthma, there is additional stress once the allergic reaction takes hold. The person has trouble breathing and naturally becomes frightened, and the stress from the fear makes the condition even worse.

People suffering from various types of allergies can often reduce the severity of their symptoms by learning stress-reduction techniques.

IDENTIFYING STRESSORS

There are many factors that create stress in our lives. It would be extremely simple to eliminate them if everyone reacted to the same stressor at the same time and in the same way. As we are all individuals, however, each person must learn what triggers stress in his or her life. Recognizing those situations and influences that cause stress is the first crucial step in coping with it.

FAMILY

Why is it that those closest to us create the most stress in our lives? It is for precisely that reason: Because they are closest to us, they know our trigger points, and we care what they think.

Many women, for example, find their jobs to be supportive and rewarding yet feel stress piling up as soon as they walk in the door to their home. The kids are fussing and fighting, her husband calls to say that he'll be late and that what she's fixing for dinner is exactly what he had for lunch, and her mother has left a message on the answering machine asking her to pick up a prescription at the drugstore.

Women who try to be all things to all people will almost certainly find that being superwoman is impossible. Two parts of the superwoman costume are stress and guilt. Regardless of what hat she is wearing at a particular moment, superwoman frets about what she isn't doing.

Men don't have it much easier, however. Today's male has no guidelines or role models by which to judge his behavior. Mixed messages from the media, women, and other men create overwhelming stress. Despite changing roles, many men still feel in the position of the provider—and, unfortunately, the failure if they can't make ends meet. Family tensions and time constraints created by a working spouse often create additional stress, forcing the "breadwinner" to be thankful for the extra income on the one hand, while on the other, he wonders if he's a failure for not being able to be the sole supporter for his family.

As family patterns change, as they must when someone dies, marries, divorces, becomes chronically ill, or leaves to go off to school or work, the

EARLY SIGNS OF STRESS

1) Do you often feel distracted, unable to focus on the task at hand?

2) Do you have difficulty falling asleep at night, or once asleep, do you keep waking up?

3) Do you find yourself "having a short fuse," losing your temper easily, or becoming over-critical?

4) Do you overeat at meals and between meals?

5) Does your stomach hurt after you've eaten?

6) Do you often have diarrhea shortly after eating?

7) If you drink alcohol, do you drink more now than before?

8) Are you having any problems related to the reproductive system, such as impotence in men or menstrual difficulties in women?

9) If you smoke, are you smoking more now than before?

10) Do you demonstrate excess motor activity such as tapping your fingers, jiggling your foot as you sit, clenching your teeth, or juggling coins or keys in your pockets?

11) Do you have new and noticeable tics, such as wrinkling your nose, blinking, clearing your throat, or biting your lip?

12) Does your mouth often feel dry?

13) Has your skin broken out in rashes or pimples? Cold sores or eczema?

14) Have you begun to experience asthma attacks?

15) Do you suffer from frequent headaches?

16) Do you often feel your heart beating loudly or skipping a beat?

17) Do you have to urinate frequently?

18) Are your hands and feet often cold and clammy?

19) Do you often complain of feeling "bone tired"?

20) Do you have frequent back and neck aches?

21) Do you have difficulty in making decisions?

All of these symptoms may indicate other disorders, but they also are common signs of stress. If you've said "yes" to more than two, you may be suffering from excessive stress. However, if you suspect something else may be the cause, check with your physician.

family members may experience overwhelming stress as they accept and act out different roles.

WORK AND SCHOOL

For some men and women, work is where they earn their paycheck, nothing more. The job may be boringly repetitive or a dead end with no chance of advancement. Others may feel they have no control over what they do, let alone how or when they must do it. Still others may report to supervisors whom they do not respect or who have no leadership or communication skills. For these workers, their place of employment may become a source of frustration, stress, and often, self-doubt.

Children with learning disorders, attention deficit disorders, hyperactivity, obsessive compulsive disorder, Tourette syndrome, or other neurologic problems that infringe on learning and social skills may also experience great stress at school. For those whose conditions are undiagnosed or misdiagnosed, the frustration is even greater as they may begin to believe that their teachers and peers consider them "stupid."

NEW SITUATIONS

New situations are stressful for most of us because we often are unsure just how to react and don't want to embarrass ourselves. Public speaking ranks high as one of the most stressful situations even for those who are experienced at it. Even the late actress Helen Hayes admitted that she suffered from extreme stage fright before every performance.

Walking into a room at a party with many strangers can trigger anxiety as will interviewing for a job. Single men and women find meeting a blind date extremely stressful.

CHRONIC ILLNESS

Chronic illness creates tremendous stress on everyone involved—both the sick person and his or her friends and family. Chronic illness changes interpersonal relationships. Those who have been in control now find themselves dependent on others. Those who depended on the one who is now ill find themselves in a new and often time-consuming role. In addition, the illness itself creates stress on the patient's physical and emotional well-being.

WORRYING

Chronic worry is an exhausting and extremely stressful lesson in futility. The worrier becomes so obsessed by the worries that fill his or her mind that nothing else can be accomplished.

ENVIRONMENTAL FACTORS

There are numerous environmental influences that can create stress for an individual. Some of them include noise pollution, poor air quality, over-crowding, lack of sunlight, and even chemical agents in the water or air.

STRATEGIES FOR DEALING WITH STRESS

Fortunately, there are many demonstrated ways to control the negative stress in our lives once we've recognized it. Experiment with a variety of the techniques described until you find the combination that works best for you in your particular situation.

EXERCISE

As if you didn't already have enough reasons to get moving: Exercise can really burn off the pent-up tension that stress creates. With regular exercise, you can channel that negative, self-destructive energy into something positive for your mind and body. There is a form of exercise that is just right for everyone. It may not be the one your best friend selects, but it's one you enjoy, which means it's far more likely you'll continue doing it.

Take time to determine how you like to exercise—whether you prefer to exercise in a group situation or if you prefer doing it alone. Is morning your best time or would you like to exercise through the lunch hour or after work? Determining your favorite exercise is important because the more that the type and time of exercise fits your individual needs, the more consistent you'll be in doing it.

You may think that trying to fit exercise into an already over-committed schedule would create even more stress in your life, but it won't. Once you begin to make time to exercise, you'll find yourself more relaxed, better able to handle existing stressors, and looking forward to your regular exercise period.

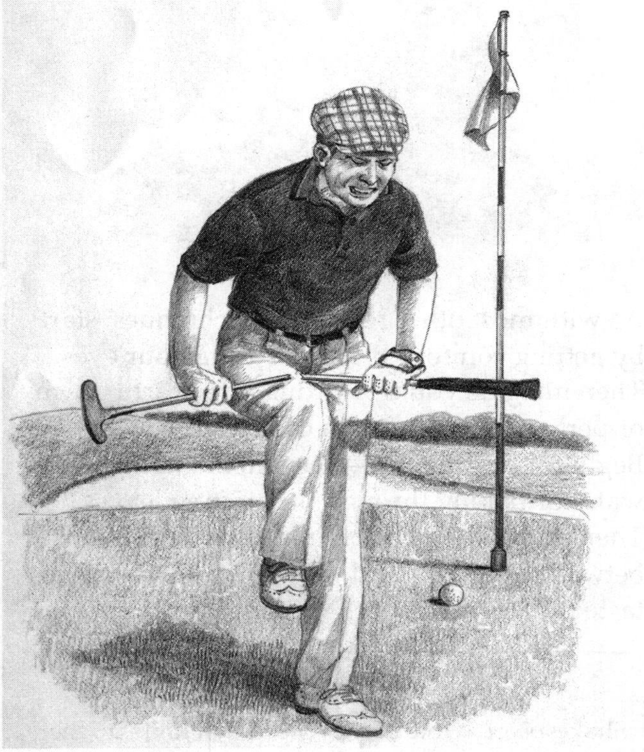

If you're competitive by nature, however, stay away from sports where you push yourself hard to win. That takes exercise out of the "fun" category and puts it into one marked "stressful." You're trying to reduce your stress level, not add to it. (For more information on starting an exercise program, see Chapter 3.)

RELAXATION TECHNIQUES

These are some of the best means of reducing stress; they are scientifically proven, medically accepted, and easily learned. Most of them take very little time to practice, and only one of them, biofeedback, requires any type of equipment. These relaxation techniques help you to block out stress and focus on serenity, thereby lowering your blood pressure, slowing down your heartbeat, and reducing wear and tear on your joints, muscles, and organs.

Progressive relaxation. As a form of stress reduction, this technique has been around since the 1930s. The basis of this type of relaxation is the isolation and elimination of the sensation of being stressed. Many of us walk around with frowns, tensed jaws or neck muscles, and clenched fists without even knowing it. Progressive relaxation brings this tension into our circle of awareness.

There are actually two forms of progressive relaxation. The first is active relaxation, in which you consciously tighten a particular muscle group before relaxing it. The second method is passive relaxation, in which you concentrate on a particular muscle group and become aware of its existing tension; then you consciously relax it by imagining the tension unwinding and the weight of the muscles sinking limply. Experiment with both methods. Both are effective and easy to learn.

The National Institute of Mental Health lists ten ways to help yourself deal with stress. They include:

1) **Trying physical activity**
2) **Sharing your stress by talking to others**
3) **Knowing your limits**
4) **Taking care of yourself**
5) **Making time for fun**
6) **Volunteering**
7) **Listing and checking off your tasks**
8) **Cooperating rather than fighting**
9) **Creating a quiet scene**
10) **Avoiding self-medication**

Here is the active form of relaxation. Get comfortable and loosen any tight clothing. Find a place and a time that you will not be disturbed. Then, sitting or lying comfortably with your legs uncrossed, slowly begin the exercise:

- Close your eyes and breathe deeply through your nose.
- Tense your face and head—furrow your brow; squeeze your eyes closed; grit your teeth; and tense your neck.
- Hold the tension for five to seven seconds, but don't hold your breath. Continue to breathe through your nose.
- Release all the tension at once. Feel all the muscles of your face, head, and neck go limp and relax.
- Take a few deep breaths before moving on to the next muscle group.
- Repeat the tension and release method with each of the other body groups: the arms, the chest and abdomen, and the legs. Don't forget to breathe normally.
- When you are finished with all groups, feel the warmth and heaviness of your entire body and the tingling in your feet and hands. Imagine the relaxation moving up and down through your body like a wave.
- Finally, when you are ready, open your eyes.

Meditation. Unfortunately, meditation is erroneously dismissed by many people as some strange "new age" hocus pocus. It isn't, of course. Meditation has been used for centuries by Native Americans, yogis, religious leaders throughout the world, and performers in sports and entertainment. Through meditation, you learn to clear your mind of extraneous thought and focus inward by favoring a mantra—a single word such as *peace, love,* or *God*. Some people focus on a flickering flame of a candle, while others stare at a leaf, flower, or other object of nature. Meditation—a mental time-out from the stressful world—allows you to enter a state similar to that of hypnosis, filling your physical and mental being with a sense of tranquility and peace.

Mental imagery. In this technique, you reduce stress by remembering or imagining a place or situation that is extremely calm and relaxing. It's almost like telling yourself a story in which the only character is you, the setting is the most idyllic spot you can think of, and the plot is practically nonexistent.

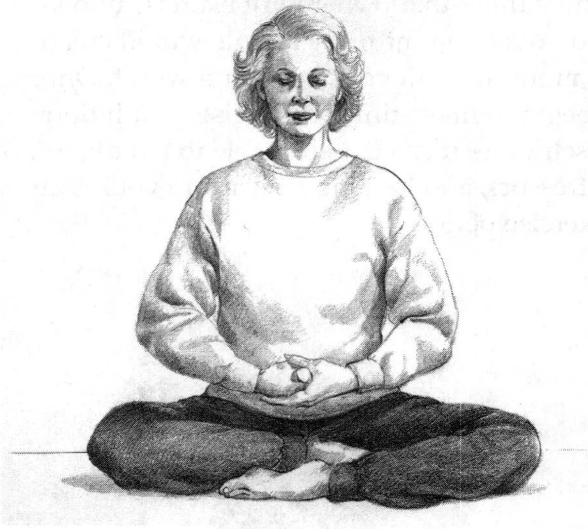

As with most other relaxation techniques, start by getting comfortable and closing your eyes. Then imagine yourself sitting on a warm beach or perhaps the porch of a cabin in the woods. Begin to see the scene—the sun flickering on the water or poking through the shifting leaves. Then add each of the other senses: Feel the sand between your toes and the breeze on your face; taste the salt air from the ocean; hear the waves

Sleep Away Stress?

Shakespeare wrote of the "Sleep that knits up the ravell'd sleave of care..." According to *American Demographics,* a recent survey revealed that adults who sleep seven or eight hours a night are less likely to feel stress every day than those who sleep less.

The 1994 Prevention Index reported that 43 percent of people who sleep six hours or less feel great stress daily, compared to 14 percent of those who sleep seven to eight hours each night.

or rustling leaves; smell the dark damp dirt of the forest floor. Get comfortable in this new setting, and take the time to enjoy it after you have conjured it up. When you are ready to leave, slowly open your eyes and get up refreshed.

Biofeedback. Biofeedback most vividly demonstrates the importance of the mind and body connection, showing that we can learn to control various body stresses by using our minds. To learn the technique you will need to work with a psychologist, psychiatrist, or other health professional trained in biofeedback. Through sensors attached to your head or fingers, you are connected to a special computerlike machine that translates your heartbeat, muscle tension, skin temperature, blood pressure, and other signs of tension into audio or video signals.

With practice, you can learn to slow or regulate your heartbeat as you watch or hear your effectiveness in achieving a state of relaxation on the biofeedback machine. You can have the same success in lowering blood pressure, reducing muscle tension, and adjusting your breathing in order to reduce stress. Once you feel confident doing it on your own, you can continue using biofeedback in conjunction with some of the other relaxing techniques, as well.

Self-hypnosis. Once considered a mere parlor trick or carnival act, hypnosis is now considered a useful way to reduce stress. As with biofeedback, it's helpful to work with a trained health professional before using this relaxation technique on your own. Once mastered, however, you will find that it can be applied in many potentially stressful situations: in the dentist's chair, before giving a speech, or while waiting for a job interview to start.

Although learning self-hypnosis takes practice, it is relatively simple. It's merely a way of focusing our mind's attention. Most of us already experience self-hypnosis when we are so focused on a television show that we don't see someone entering the room or when we arrive at a destination and don't remember driving there.

Using Self-Hypnosis to Reduce Stress

1) Sit in a comfortable chair and loosen your collar and waistband.
2) Focus your attention on a spot across the room.
3) Take a deep breath, hold it, then let it out. Repeat two more times.
4) Feel your eyes growing heavy and allow them to close.
5) Keep focusing on your breathing.
6) Picture a sturdy staircase in your mind. Take hold of the bannister and slowly walk down its 20 steps, counting as you go.
7) Feel yourself going more deeply into the hypnotic state with every step you count down.
8) When you get to the bottom step, you should feel very relaxed. Let yourself go to a safe place where you feel very secure and very relaxed.
9) Stay in your safe place until you wish to return.
10) When you want to come out of the hypnotic state, count slowly to three, becoming more alert with each number. At three, open your eyes.

This technique works very well for many people. Don't be easily discouraged, as it can take some practice and some getting used to. Certainly, don't be afraid of it; remember, you are in total control at all times and can leave the hypnotic state at any time you choose.

HOBBIES

A hobby is a pursuit, other than one's occupation, done for relaxation or pleasure. The operative words, of course, are "relaxation" and "pleasure." As long as you don't take them too seriously, hobbies are good ways to reduce stress. They alter the pattern of your day and allow you more sense of control in what you're doing.

Some hobbies, such as fishing, bird watching, or gardening, actually slow our breathing and get us in touch with the rhythm of nature. Playing a musical instrument, writing, dancing, knitting, and making pottery all put us in touch with our creative side. We focus on these efforts and forget about some of the tensions and dissatisfactions in our lives. The arts play an important part in bringing peace and beauty into our lives.

Sports are a healthy way to reduce stress *if* you can enjoy them without being overly competitive. Slamming the tennis ball down your opponent's throat or throwing your putter in the pond are not good ways to rid yourself of tension.

MASSAGE

The "laying on of hands" has been used for relaxation and therapeutic purposes since ancient times in Greece and Rome. Although there are many different styles of massage therapy, they all involve some degree of kneading, rubbing, or otherwise stroking the skin. Most of us quickly learn the type of stroke we prefer, whether we relax better with background music or silence, and what type of oil or cream is most soothing.

Before allowing a massage therapist into your home, be sure to ask for references. Some states required massage therapists to be licensed before working on clients.

Many individuals prefer to get their massage from the waters in a Jacuzzi or whirlpool tub. Others just relax in a bubble bath, letting the water and the scent of the bath salts, oil, or bubbles relax them.

LAUGHTER

The late Norman Cousins is often credited with the recent acceptance by health professionals of the healing power of laughter. A good laugh is the body's natural tranquilizer: It triggers the release of endorphins, which help the body reduce stress; laughing makes you breathe more deeply, therefore bringing more air into your lungs; and it also helps to reduce blood pressure and muscle tension and to improve blood circulation. Laughter is what Norman Cousins called "inner jogging."

VOLUNTEERISM

Volunteerism is an American tradition. Ralph Waldo Emerson said, "It is the most beautiful of compensations of this life that no man can try to help another without helping himself."

When we reach out to help others, we turn our attention away from ourselves and our problems. Many volunteers report actually feeling a "helper's high," similar to the sensation of well-being they get through exercise, along with a sense of tranquility and heightened self-confidence. This is one of the reasons that many schools and businesses require their students and employees to volunteer in their community.

In addition, studies reveal that middle managers who have been laid-off are more likely to find new employment when they do volunteer work. It may be that they make more contacts through their volunteer efforts or that they feel good about themselves and therefore make a better impression during interviews. In any case, volunteerism is a good way to reduce stress.

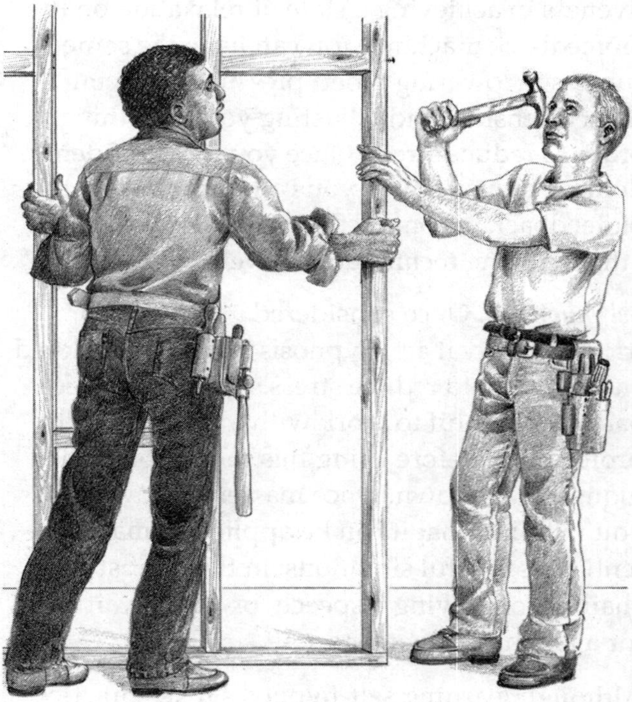

Consider the following:

- Prepare food or serve at the neighborhood soup kitchen.
- Give a day of your weekend to Habitat for Humanity and help build needed housing.

- ◆ Help out at a homeless shelter.
- ◆ Play Santa Claus at the childrens' hospital.
- ◆ Deliver groceries to shut-ins.

There are so many volunteer opportunities available through church and civic organizations. Find one that you are suited for, and help yourself and others at the same time.

HEADING OFF STRESS

So far, our focus has been on coping with stress by learning to get rid of it. However, in some situations, even the most experienced of relaxers can't shake off the stress of their environments. Seeing that prevention is our general goal, perhaps there are ways of removing stress from our lives entirely—or at least trying.

ALTERING CIRCUMSTANCES

One way to prevent stress is to avoid all stressful situations or, at least, minimize their occurrence. Many events need not be the crunch time that they appear to be, and some common sense and forward thinking can head off some stressful situations before you ever have to deal with them.

Time management. Some people think proper time management means doing two or more things at once or racing madly from place to place trying to get everything accomplished. Unfortunately, all they usually manage to achieve is extra stress as they fight with the frustration of never getting caught up.

True time management means establishing priorities and preplanning, so that you can become more effective in what you do without feeling anxious about what isn't getting done. Few of us will ever attain every goal we've set. What we need to learn is how to handle what's most important to us and to allow ourselves to experience joy in what we have accomplished.

Most of our time pressures are self-imposed. They are often the result of our procrastination and drifting without establishing priorities. It's like beginning a trip without determining where you want to go or how you'll get there and without even looking at a map. However, once you sit down and list what you hope to achieve, you've begun a plan and thought about your priorities. That puts you in charge of your life. Stress can be triggered by a sense that things are out of control. You gain control by first determining your priorities, then creating and carrying out your plan.

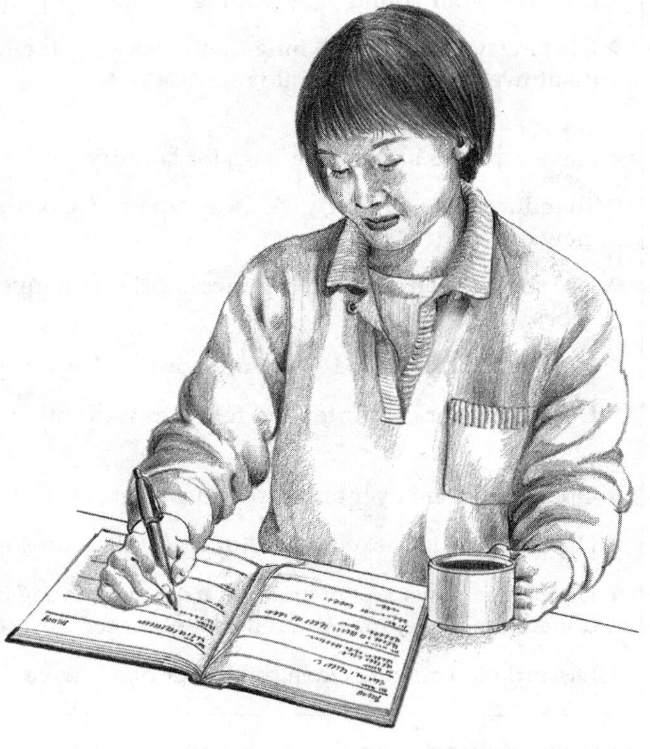

Clearing your mind. Albert Einstein once said that he never cluttered his mind with anything that he could write down. The multimillion-dollar industry of pocket and desk calendars and computerized date and schedule reminders demonstrates that he was certainly on the right track. Some people, however, get so caught up in rewriting their "to do" list and copying entries

How to Reduce Mess Stress

You may have become so used to your clutter that you don't even see it. Take a photograph of every room in your home (and your office) and you'll suddenly become aware of the mess that causes you unnecessary stress.

General tips

- Establish priorities.
- "Things" tend to have natural resting places; try to work within them.
- Don't try to do things perfectly.
- Have a place for things so you know where they *should* be.
- Don't buy things you really don't need.
- Divide cleaning tasks into small, manageable pieces.

Kitchen clutter

- Store any small appliance you don't use at least weekly.
- Other than ones you use frequently, store cookbooks on bookshelves.
- Clean off your counters by putting spices in cupboards or on a shelf on the wall.
- Give away pans, dishes, mugs, and glasses you never use and utensils that have rusted, and throw away torn dishtowels or turn them into rags.

Bedroom clutter

- Have separate hampers or bags for laundry and dry cleaning.
- To reduce closet clutter, give away a pair of shoes, a suit, a purse, or a sweater every time you purchase a new one.
- Use some of the closet storage accessories that give you better visibility and more space for your clothes and shoes.
- Have a "tidy box" and a "dump it drawer" where you can throw junk, and go through it monthly.
- Use a duvet or comforter and few, if any, throw-pillows.

Living room

- Open your mail over an oversized wastebasket.
- Have a specific basket or box for your bills, envelopes, stamps, calculator, and pen.
- Don't save newspapers more than a week or magazines more than a month. Recycle the newspapers and donate the magazines to a retirement center, hospital, school, or doctor's office.
- Discard old catalogs when the newer ones arrive.

from one reminder book to the next, that they create even more time pressures and stress.

The easiest way to clear your mind is to have one calendar or diary in which you record everything. There are hundreds of choices, so you'll need to take time to find the one that "fits" you best. In this book, write down phone numbers, addresses, appointments, gift preferences and sizes, books you want to read, birthdays, and any other notations that now fill your mind. Once listed, you're freed from the stress of trying to remember everything and can instead turn your thoughts to more productive and satisfying considerations.

Communication skills: Although most of us have been talking since we were slightly more than a year old, many people still are not good communicators. Faulty communication skills often trigger stress in both the speaker and the listener because no message or the wrong message was received.

Reduce your stress from miscommunication by checking with your listener after saying something, rather than waiting to discover that they didn't understand. Active listening is as important to effective communication as talking. Improve your listening skills by giving others your full attention when they are speaking, and offer feedback from time to time, either verbally or through body language, to be sure what you heard is what the speaker actually meant to say. Communication skills can be improved with practice. Don't get discouraged.

COGNITIVE COPING SKILLS

For most of us, the complete avoidance of stressful situations is not possible. This brings us to a second way to head off stress: Stop it before a situation gets to you.

Even though all of us have to deal with stressful situations from time to time, we don't necessarily have to come away from all of them stressed. Remember, it's not the events themselves that cause stress; it's the way we react to those events. Quite often, we get anxious about events that don't have to be stressful. We just make them stressful by the way we think about them. See if any of the following techniques for changing your outlook might help you avoid the automatic stress response.

Correcting distorted thinking. Believe it or not, many of us walk around judging the world by standards and assumptions that are just plain wrong. We don't even realize that the conclusions we draw are based on these false assumptions. However, many of these forms of distorted thinking create stressful situations for us out of thin air.

It takes a keen eye to spot the distorted thinking that we bring to situations, and there are many different forms. For example, there is the all-or-nothing fallacy that makes us put everything into one of two polar opposite categories with no middle ground. Perhaps you've caught yourself dwelling on the fact that you didn't get that big raise, so now you think you're going to be fired. Big raise or fired—are those really the only two choices? What if profits were down, and your supervisor, who really does like you and your work, just can't fit that raise in the budget? There are always shades of gray.

Other examples of distorted thinking are:

- Blaming: For everything that goes wrong, there is someone responsible who should be blamed.
- Disqualifying: When people compliment me, they are not serious; they really mean quite the opposite.
- Overgeneralization: Having seen one example of something, I know all I need to know about all those things.
- Shoulds: There are certain ways that the world should be and people should act.
- Labeling: Everyone and everything fits into easy stereotypical categories.
- Magnification: Everything is really important and could turn into a tragedy at any moment.

There are many others. Try to recognize the fallacies that you hold to be true. Seeing how you trick yourself into creating worrisome and anxious feelings and thoughts can help you stop the self-created stress. The next time you find yourself steaming over a situation, looking for someone to blame, or feeling guilty and unworthy, take a second look at the assumptions that got you there. Make sure that distorted thinking isn't really the problem.

Using creative imagination. Sometimes an impending event has you so worried that you can't stop thinking about it. *Thinking* about it is not a problem; *worrying* about it, however, creates stress. Thinking in the proper manner can actually help you overcome the anxiety that you feel about upcoming situations. You can use the proper thinking we're talking about with a technique called creative imagination.

We use our imaginations to create scenarios all the time. Why not put that powerful ability to work for you? Imagine the potentially stressful scene in its entirety and in detail, and see how harmless it really is. Imagine the whole thing coming off perfectly: You are relaxed and sharp; others are impressed and charmed; you feel proud and completely satisfied.

The technique is simple, but for it to work best, you've got to put a little into it. Here are some important tips:

- Be sure that your picture of what will happen is as complete and as real as you can make it.
- To enhance the reality, include in your scene at least one example of each of the five senses (sight, sound, touch, taste, and smell).
- Think about the scene in the present tense as if you were living it right now.
- Picture all the desired results actually happening (the audience applauding, the boss smiling and shaking your hand).
- Finally, let yourself really feel your own emotional reaction. You might even notice a smile coming across your face as you feel the satisfaction of a perfect performance.

Using creative imagination can change more than just your outlook. It can change the reality of the situation as well. Practice makes perfect and using creative imagination to conjure up situations you must face is really just a form of prac-

Preparing for Stress-Free Sleep

While insomnia, restless sleep, and early waking are all signs of stress, proper preparation can help to reduce stress, thereby paving the way for a restful night of sleep.

- Do not rely on artificial aids such as sleeping pills or alcohol to help you sleep.
- Have nothing to eat or drink after your evening meal, which should end at least three hours before bedtime. The only exception to this is a glass of milk (which contains L-tryptophan, a natural sedative)
- Use your bed only for lovemaking and sleep. Read and do paperwork in another room. If you associate your bed with work, you are more likely to worry about it there.
- Have a regular bedtime schedule and follow it.
- Relax before bedtime. Listen to relaxing music, meditate, or take a warm bath. Skip the late news if it tends to bother you.
- Take a stroll after work or after dinner. Do not engage in strenuous exercise just before bedtime.
- Improve your bedroom environment with drapes or blackout shades to keep it dark; set the thermostat to 60 to 65°F; and remember that mattresses *do* wear out. If yours feels lumpy, slants to one side, or is too soft, you may need to replace it.
- Stop worrying. Set aside a specific period after work to write down all your worries and anxieties. Spend five minutes by the clock worrying about everything on your list. Then put the list aside until the next day. If the troubling thought pops into your head once you're in bed, remind yourself that it's on the list and you'll worry about it tomorrow.
- Use visual imagery to picture a relaxing scene, such as vacationing at the beach. Feel the warm sun on your face, hear the calming sound of the surf, relax and let yourself go . . . to sleep.
- Don't toss and turn. If you don't fall asleep in 10 to 15 minutes, get up and read or listen to music. Then, when you begin to feel drowsy, go back to bed.

tice. So next time you're faced with a potentially stressful event, don't dwell on it, practice it.

Self-acceptance: No one is perfect and those who demand it of themselves create unnecessary stress. Don't call yourself stupid when you make a mistake; call yourself human. Many of us are far kinder to others than we are to ourselves.

Self-talk is the mechanism by which we encourage and chide ourselves. Many of us continually bombard ourselves with negative self-talk messages and then wonder why we don't accept or like ourselves. Listen to what you say to yourself. Is it encouraging? Or are you running yourself down and predicting doom around every corner?

Negative self-talk can make us ruin our own best efforts and create stress. You can turn this around, though. Self-talk doesn't come from anyone else; it comes from you. Take control of the messages you send to yourself. Vow today to make those messages positive.

- Make a list of all the things you do well or like about yourself and repeat them often to yourself.
- Stay away from others who make you feel bad about yourself.
- When you hear yourself returning to a negative thought, concentrate on it, count to three, and yell "Stop!" to banish it from your mind.

Remember, you have control over what goes on in your head. Eleanor Roosevelt once said, "No one can make you feel inferior without your consent." Don't give that power to anyone, including that little self-talk voice.

PROFESSIONAL HELP

Although you often can learn to reduce stress by using the techniques that are described above, sometimes you can't do it on your own or solely with the help of friends or family. Enlisting the help of a professional, someone trained to listen and to coach those who are feeling the pain of unrelieved stress, is an option that you should not overlook.

HOW CAN IT HELP?

Others help us deal with stress by gently guiding us along the path we would take if we weren't under so much pressure. A high stress level makes it difficult to think straight. Others cut through the stress fog by helping to light the way and by letting us know we are not alone.

When we feel that we are no longer passive, but can take some type of action against our stress, feelings of helplessness dissipate. Our immune system strengthens; we develop more self-confidence; and we begin to feel back in control once more.

FINDING APPROPRIATE HELP

The different types of professional guidance available are daunting. Choosing one that makes you feel comfortable is vital to the therapy's success. Here are just a few of the options:

Support groups are attended by over 15 million people in 500,000 group meetings a week. Groups are effective for two essential reasons: 1) you learn to tell the truth about yourself and see that truth in the context of other people's lives; and 2) you learn to listen to other people without judging them. Your local newspaper usually lists various support groups and the time and place of their meetings.

One-on-one therapy makes some people more comfortable than the group approach. In this more intimate setting, they can work on their problems related to stress with a medical or other healthcare professional. Still others prefer to confide in a social worker, a religious leader, or other therapist trained to listen and to help you determine solutions (see "A Therapists' Who's Who," page 138).

A Therapists' Who's Who

There are many kinds of therapists out there who can help you cope with problems. The trick is finding the one kind that will do you the most good. Here is a list of some of the professionals that you can turn to.

An *Alcohol/Drug Abuse Counselor* often has a degree in either social work, psychology, or psychiatry and works in a variety of settings, including drug treatment centers and family service agencies. Training and experience are primarily in substance abuse.

An *Employee Assistance Professional* is a mental health professional provided by an employer to offer confidential services to employees and, often, to their families. These counselors can be occupational physicians, nurses, psychologists, social workers, or trained union members. They provide assessment, brief counseling, and when appropriate, referral to community resources. Some are Certified Employee Assistance Professionals (CEAP).

A *Marriage Counselor* or *Family Therapist* has a degree in social work, psychology, or psychiatry with postgraduate study and training in marital and family problems.

A *Pastoral Counselor* is a minister, priest, or rabbi who has a bachelor's degree or master's degree in divinity (religion) and additional training in psychology or counseling. They can identify mental health problems and make appropriate referrals. Certified Pastoral Counselors have an advanced degree in mental health and may provide counseling.

A *Psychiatric Nurse* holds a degree in nursing, either as a registered nurse (R.N.), a bachelor's degree in nursing (B.S.N.), or a master's degree in nursing (M.S.N.). In addition, they have specialized training in the care and treatment of psychiatric patients.

A *Psychiatrist* is a medical doctor (M.D.) or doctor of osteopathy (D.O.) who has had a three- or four-year residency in a psychiatric facility and is board certified in psychiatry. A psychiatrist is the only mental health professional who can prescribe medication or medical treatments.

A *Psychoanalyst* is a psychiatrist, clinical psychologist, or social worker who has had specialized training in psychoanalysis and has gone through psychoanalysis.

A *Psychologist* has received either a doctorate in psychology, education, or counselling (Ph.D., Psy.D., or Ed.D.). This professional must also complete a one-year internship in a psychiatric hospital or mental health center and have specific training to do psychotherapy.

A *Social Worker* has earned at least a bachelor's degree (B.S.), master's degree (M.S.W.), or doctorate (D.S.W.) in social work. Graduate training involves course work dealing with individual and family assessment and psychotherapy.

KEEPING TABS ON YOUR HEALTH

Some people take better care of their cars than they do their bodies. They religiously change their oil every 3,000 miles and always make sure they see a mechanic for a tune-up once a year. They'd never dream of using anything but premium gasoline.

Ask one of these automobile aficionados why they're so careful, and they're apt to answer that routine maintenance helps keep a car in tip-top condition and alerts them to problems before they become too serious. Ask the same person about the last time they took themselves in to the doctor for a checkup, and you're likely to receive a blank stare.

Just as you would check the oil in your car, so should you regularly check into the state of your own health. You don't want the first sign that you've run out of oil to be when your engine suddenly seizes up.

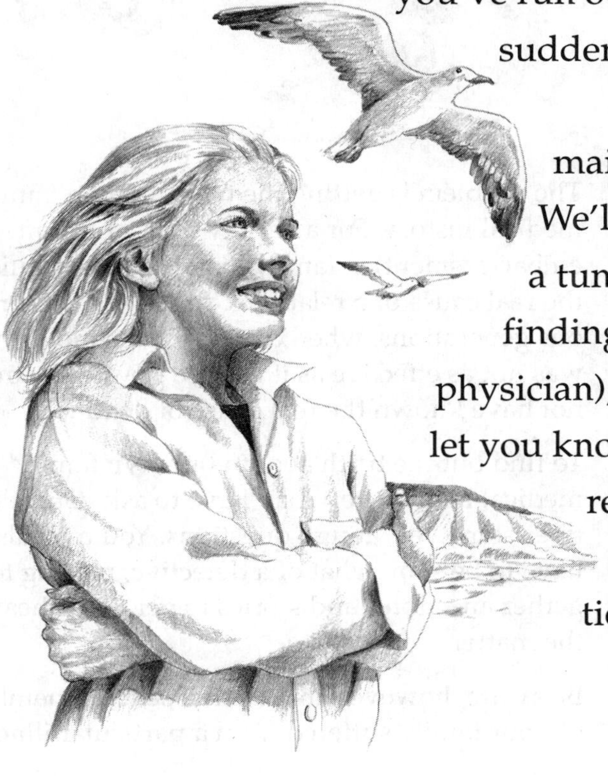

Consider this chapter a routine maintenance manual for your body. We'll tell you how often you need to get a tune-up (or a checkup), give you tips on finding a competent mechanic (or a physician), tell you which knocks and squeaks let you know it's time to take yourself to the repair shop, and teach you how to check your timing (do self-examinations for common conditions).

ASSESSING YOUR OWN HEALTH

Wouldn't it be nice if there were one universal home diagnostic test kit that could determine how healthy you are, warn you about potential problems, and offer suggestions on how to head off problems before they ever come to the surface?

Unfortunately, an infinite number of variables intertwine to form the mosaic of an individual's health and well-being. Some of these factors are handed down through generations of a family. Some of them might result from drugs a mother took when she was pregnant or a father's workplace exposure to toxic chemicals. Still others relate to the way an individual has lived his or her life.

Evaluating the state of your health, then, is a complex issue, rife with approximations, theories, and guesses. The following sections describe the interplay of several important factors that you should be aware of because they can influence your health.

YOUR FAMILY'S MEDICAL HISTORY

Genealogy used to be an exercise in simple curiosity—tracing your family tree to learn where your clan came from and how they lived. Increasingly, the search for identity and family has taken on the goal of revealing a medical legacy. Instead of mere curiosity about who the father of Aunt Flo's children was, the goal becomes finding out how old your uncle was when he died, and—perhaps more importantly—whether he died of any illnesses that might have been passed along to you and yours.

What does your family history say about your health? Research is increasingly linking diseases and conditions—from lactose intolerance to depression to premature heart disease—to inherited traits. If your father and all of his brothers developed coronary blockages in their 40s, chances are, your risk is higher than that of the general population. Knowing this gives you the power to take preventive measures early in life, possibly heading off an early heart attack.

Likewise, researchers have discovered that a woman with two immediate relatives with breast cancer is far more likely to develop the disease than a woman without breast cancer in her family. Knowing this, she might opt to get an early start on a program of annual mammograms (see page 150).

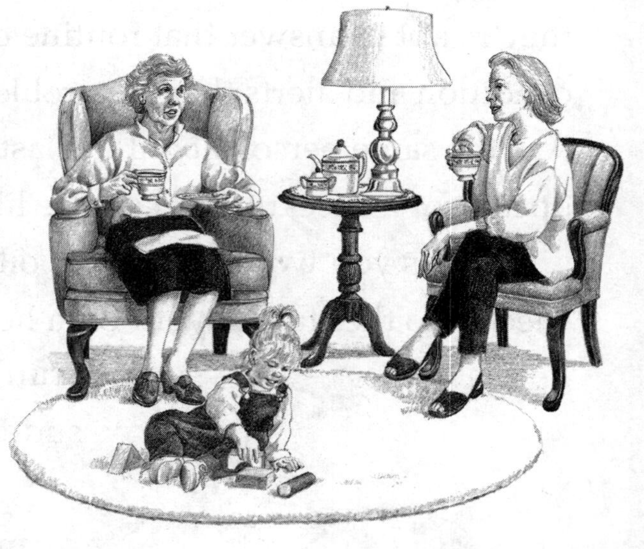

The problem is getting the truth about a family's medical history. For a variety of reasons (often embarrassment), a family may hide or disguise the real cause of a relative's death. Also, in previous generations, when diagnostic technology was not as effective as it is now, physicians may not have known the real cause of death.

To find out the truth about your own family's medical history, you may have to ask your relatives some very tough questions. You may also have to be somewhat of a detective, piecing together anecdotes and stories to get to the heart of the matter.

Be aware, however, that even if several members of your family suffered from a particular illness or health condition, you are not automatically condemned to the same fate. First of all, families pass on habits to each other, as well as genes. Many risk factors for disease are environmental—meaning that they are affected by chemicals in the environment, diet, activity, stress levels, and so on. People in the same family may suffer from the same diseases because they live their lives in similar ways.

Also, you may not have been born with the same genes that caused an illness in a relative. Your genes come equally from both of your parents. For this reason, your personal characteristics (eye color, hair color, tendency to develop a particular illness, and so on) are a merger of your parents' individual characteristics. Some genes—such as the gene for brown eyes—are dominant, meaning that it only takes one gene from one parent to produce the trait in the offspring. Other genes—such as the gene for blue or green eyes—are recessive, meaning that one must be passed on from each parent to produce the trait in the offspring.

Some diseases, such as Tay-Sachs and sickle-cell disease, tend to run in particular ethnic groups. However, if an individual marries outside of that ethnic group, the chances are lower that both parents will carry the gene for an inherited disease. For example, if a woman of Jewish descent has children with a non-Jewish man, the chances that her children will develop Tay-Sachs are much lower than if she had married a Jewish man. Hence, even though a disease may run in your family, your particular genetic makeup may spare you from developing it.

Also, some genetic tendencies skip a generation or are linked to the sex of the offspring. For example, the gene for baldness seems to be handed down from the maternal grandfather.

The bottom line is that while you should pay close attention to your family's medical history, the interpretation of what that history means to you may not always be clear. A genetic counselor may be able to clarify your risk factors. The important thing is to be aware of the legacy that has been handed you by your ancestors.

Recessive Traits Common to Ethnic Groups

The most prevalent recessive gene afflictions are those that run in ethnic groups. Here are three of the more well known:

Cystic fibrosis causes the lungs and respiratory system to fill with mucus. It may also contribute to the development of lung disease. The disorder is caused by a recessive gene most commonly found in white people of Northern European descent.

Sickle-cell disease occurs in about 1 out of every 625 African Americans. This disorder causes a crescent-shaped deformity of the red blood cells (normal red blood cells are circular). The crescent-shaped cells have a tendency to get caught in and clog narrow blood vessels. This action cuts off oxygen to tissues and causes localized pain.

Tay-Sachs disease occurs most often in Jews of Eastern European descent. Starting shortly after birth, a child with Tay-Sachs begins to show signs of retardation and blindness. Often, seizures and death follow within a few years.

If you belong to one of the above ethnic groups, it would be wise to discuss your risks with a genetic counselor before you decide to have children (or while you are pregnant). Many of these and other inherited diseases can be detected by prenatal screening tests.

YOUR LIFESTYLE

You are free to live your life in the style you choose. You can eat what you want, drink what you like, live where you want to live, work wherever they'll hire you. (After all, the pursuit of happiness is the American way.) However, although your lifestyle choices may not affect anyone else, you may (consciously or unconsciously) be writing the conclusion to your own life.

Many life-threatening diseases—including heart disease, emphysema, stroke, and certain forms of cancer—are linked to lifestyle factors. In other words, these illnesses are partly caused by poor eating habits, drug abuse, a lack of physical activity, and so on.

These diseases are largely preventable but seldom reversible. Only you—not your doctor or any miracle drug—have the power to reduce your risk of developing them. If you really want to keep tabs on your health, start by taking stock of your lifestyle. Are any of the following habits part of your routine?

Smoking. Perhaps the most insidious and damaging lifestyle choice you can make is to smoke cigarettes. Smoking is the most preventable cause of illness and death in the United States.

Aside from commonly known health repercussions of smoking (lung cancer, emphysema, and other respiratory diseases), cigarette smoking or second-hand smoke has also been implicated in skin cancer, ulcers, bronchitis, sudden infant death syndrome, ear infections, and strokes.

Smoking also affects your health in more indirect ways. For example, heavy smokers often have a hard time breathing deeply. For this reason, they may engage in less physical activity. A sedentary lifestyle can lead to other problems, including osteoporosis, obesity, low energy, and an impaired immune system.

Of the 4,000 or so chemicals in tobacco smoke, 200 are known to be poisonous to human beings. Carbon monoxide, tar, and nicotine are the three most dangerous. Carbon monoxide decreases the amount of oxygen that your red blood cells can carry. Tar coats and clogs up the lungs and carries known carcinogens. Nicotine—the addictive agent in cigarette smoke—affects the cardiovascular and nervous systems. (For more on smoking, see Chapter 4.)

Alcohol abuse. The most popular and accepted drug in America is alcohol. Its abuse can affect almost every system in the body. As a result, heavy drinkers often begin a gradual downward cycle, in which their bodies begin to degenerate slowly.

The liver, of course, is most vulnerable to the effects of alcohol. Cirrhosis—or chronic inflammation—of the liver occurs in about 20 percent of all heavy drinkers. Heavy drinking is also thought to contribute to high blood pressure, which is a leading risk factor for strokes. Other possible physical manifestations of alcohol abuse include trembling hands, chronic gastrointestinal problems, and easy bruising.

Heavy drinking and alcoholism can also take a toll on your emotional health and your relationships. Many people, when drunk, become physically or verbally abusive and are not in control of their actions.

Alcoholism is an illness. In fact, like heart disease or diabetes, alcoholism tends to run in families. For this reason, if your mother, father, grandparents, or aunts and uncles suffered from alcoholism, it would be wise for you to be very prudent about your own drinking.

How much drinking is considered "heavy"? Since everyone has a different tolerance to the effects of alcohol, there is no real answer to this question. However, if you drink daily—and especially if you drink more than two drinks per day—it is likely that you are overdoing it. (For more on alcohol, see Chapter 4.)

YOUR MEDICAL HISTORY

Another factor that may influence your overall health is your personal medical history. Certain health conditions, such as a high blood cholesterol level or high blood pressure, can be important predictors of problems you may face in the future. In addition, some medical treatments, such as chemotherapy and radiation treatments, can impair your immune system and put you at increased risk for developing other, seemingly unrelated health problems.

Be sure to provide each new physician you visit with a complete medical history. Include all major illnesses, hospitalizations, and all of the prescription and nonprescription drugs you take. Don't forget to discuss lifestyle habits, such as diet, exercise, and stress.

Also, if you have any questions about how your past medical history might affect you in the future, ask your doctor. He or she may be able to give you an idea of whether previous conditions might recur or cause other problems in the years to come.

Risky sexual behavior. It's gotten enough publicity that you're probably aware of it, but it never hurts to restate the obvious: Having unprotected sex with an individual who carries a sexually transmitted disease (such as AIDS or hepatitis B) can be fatal.

What is unprotected sex? Traditional sexual intercourse without a latex condom, anal intercourse without a latex condom, oral contact with the sexual organs or anus without a latex condom or dental dam, or any activity that brings an individual in contact with an open sore or lesion (such as a venereal wart or cold sore).

How do you know if you're with an infected individual? Frankly, you don't. Viruses are not selective, and anyone who has had sex can be infected. In other words, moral convictions and personal habits aside, the only way to know if you have been exposed to a communicable virus is to get tested. Early detection will allow you to get early treatment, a factor associated with longer survival rates. Also, early detection will help you protect those you love.

Your activity level. Regular exercise confers many health benefits:

- Building lean body mass (which helps prevent obesity)
- Preserving bone density (which helps stave off osteoporosis)
- Improving the ratio of "bad" low-density lipoprotein cholesterol (LDL) to "good" high-density lipoprotein cholesterol (HDL) in the blood (which can help prevent heart disease)
- Reducing blood pressure
- Reducing resting heart rate
- Increasing energy and vigor
- Improving sleep
- Alleviating mild stress or depression

How much exercise do you need to stay healthy? The current recommendations include at least 20 minutes (but preferably 30 minutes) of moderate aerobic exercise three times a week, along with two strength-training workouts that target the body's major muscle groups. If you do less exercise than that, your physical fitness may be below optimal levels. (For more on fitness and exercise, see Chapter 3.)

Your diet. The American Dietetic Association recommends that you get no more than 30 percent of your daily calories from fat, about 55 percent from carbohydrates, and 15 to 20 percent from protein. Here are some other recommendations:

- Eat at least five servings of fruits and vegetables per day.
- Eat 6 to 11 servings of breads, cereal, and other grain products per day.
- Eat two to four servings of lean protein (for example, lean meat or legumes) per day.
- Eat at least two servings of low-fat dairy products per day.
- Eat minimally processed, high-fiber grain products.
- Moderate your intake of salt, sugar, and processed foods.

A diet that meets these requirements can help prevent cancer, gastrointestinal illnesses, and a host of other health problems. Conversely, a high-fat, low-fiber, high-sugar diet can set you up for unnecessary health problems down the road. (For more on food and nutrition, see Chapter 1.)

YOUR HEALTH REPORT CARD

Now that you have an idea of the most important factors that can influence an individual's overall health, here is an opportunity to rate your own. The following quiz is not meant to be a substitute for a doctor's assessment. However, it may serve as a useful starting point for a discussion with your physician. In addition, your score may prompt you to make some sensible improvements to your lifestyle.

Answer the following questions:

1) Is there a history of heart disease, cancer, stroke, or other inherited illnesses in your family?

2) Do you smoke cigarettes?

3) Do you drink more than two alcoholic beverages daily?

4) Do you use illegal drugs?

5) Have you engaged in unprotected sexual intercourse?

6) Do you drive under the influence of alcohol or drugs?

7) Do you always wear your seat belt?

8) Do you engage in a program of regular exercise?

9) Does your diet meet The American Dietetic Association's recommendations?

10) Are you within five pounds of your recommended weight for your height and age?

For questions 1–6, give yourself 10 points for each "no" answer. For questions 7–10, give yourself 10 points for every "yes." Add up your score, and grade yourself on a traditional scale:

90–100 = A

80–90 = B

70–80 = C

60–70 = D

below 60 = F (a failing grade)

Remember, honesty is the best policy. If you cheat, you're only cheating yourself.

Once you know where you stand you can reassess how your lifestyle is affecting your health. If your score is not where you would like it to be, what changes can you make to improve it? Which categories need the most work? If, for example, your diet is not the best, check out the information in Chapter 1 again to see if any of the suggestions there can help you make improvements. Chapter 2 can help you maintain a healthy weight. Chapter 4 has suggestions on where to go for help with quitting smoking.

SELF-EXAMINATIONS

Although doctors are usually very thorough and keep scrupulous records, no one has the daily access to your health status that you yourself do. When it comes to monitoring for early warning signs, you are, by far, the best person for the job.

SKIN CANCER

Skin that has been evenly browned by the sun may look healthy. However, as you've no doubt heard, sun exposure—even the amount that it takes to give your cheeks just a hint of ruddy glow—can damage your skin. It may even cause skin cancer.

Skin cancer is the most common form of cancer, with some 700,000 new cases occurring each year in the United States. It is also largely preventable. The best defense is protective clothing and sunscreen with a sun protection factor (SPF) of 15 or higher.

The effects of sun damage are cumulative. Often, the effects go unnoticed and untreated from year to year. The worst damage is usually caused by exposure to the sun during the first ten years of a person's life.

Early detection and treatment of skin cancer greatly improve a patient's prognosis. Fortunately, unlike other cancers, skin cancers are usually visible to the naked eye, even in their early stages. If you are in a high-risk group, dermatologists recommend that you conduct a thorough self-examination for skin cancer regularly. Follow the procedure outlined below. You will need a full-length mirror, a handheld mirror, and good lighting.

- Disrobe and examine all parts of your body for moles, birthmarks, discolorations, and new or unusual-looking lesions.

  Use the handheld mirror to examine your buttocks, back, neck, and face. Lift your hair out of the way to get a clear view of your ears and hairline. If you cannot clearly see a part of your body, ask your spouse or a close friend to help you. Don't neglect parts of your body that never see the sun. Cancers can develop in those areas, too.

- Make mental or handwritten notes of the size, location, and appearance of your most significant moles and birthmarks. Keep these notes on hand to review during your next examination. Be sure to write down any changes you see developing over time.

- Pay special attention to dark, pigmented, or irregularly shaped lesions.

When evaluating a mole or other lesion, remember the A, B, C, and D of skin-cancer warning signs:

- *A* stands for asymmetry.
- *B* is for border irregularity (frilly or poorly defined edges).
- *C* is for color variation (especially black, tan, brown, white, or red).
- *D* is for diameter larger than 6 millimeters (the size of a pencil eraser).

If you notice anything suspicious during your monthly examination, see your doctor or a dermatologist as soon as possible.

TESTICULAR CANCER

The hormones that bring on the physical changes of puberty bring with them another, more worrisome possibility: testicular cancer. Fortunately, testicular cancer is relatively rare (fewer than 6,500 new cases occur each year in the United States) and is usually curable if it is detected early.

To be safe, you should examine your testicles monthly. Regular examinations will help you get familiar with your body's natural architecture, so that you'll more easily recognize any unusual symptoms.

In the shower, roll each testicle between the forefinger and thumb, carefully checking all areas for hard lumps or bumps. Make note of any pain you experience. Later, in a mirror, look for evidence of discoloration, changes in skin texture, or open sores. If you notice anything suspicious, see your physician as soon as possible.

BREAST CANCER

Breast cancers are more treatable when they are detected in early stages. For this reason, the American Cancer Society recommends that all women conduct monthly breast self-examinations.

If you are still menstruating, the week after your period has ended is the ideal time for a self-examination, but regardless of when in the cycle you choose, do it the same

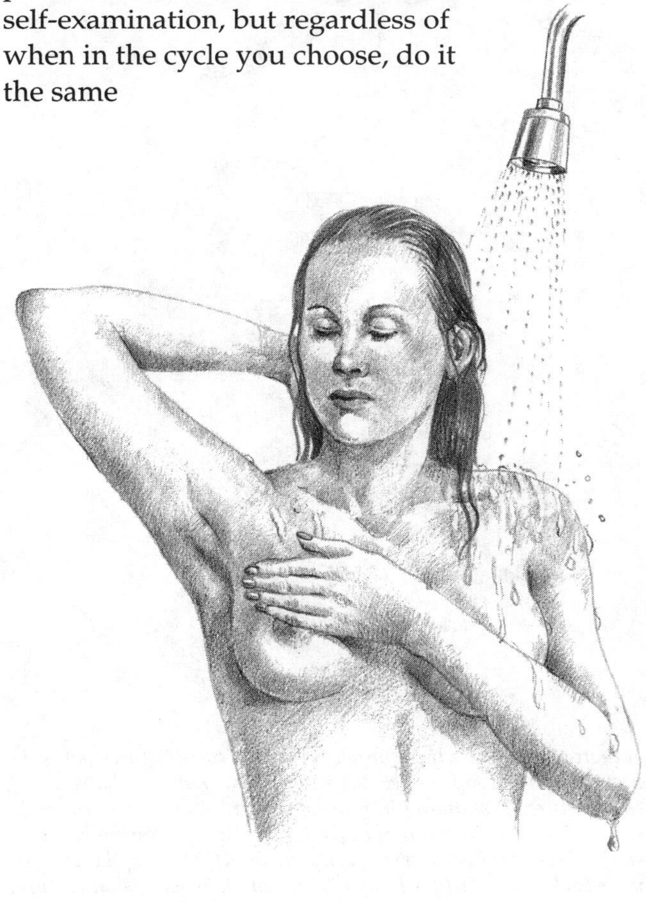

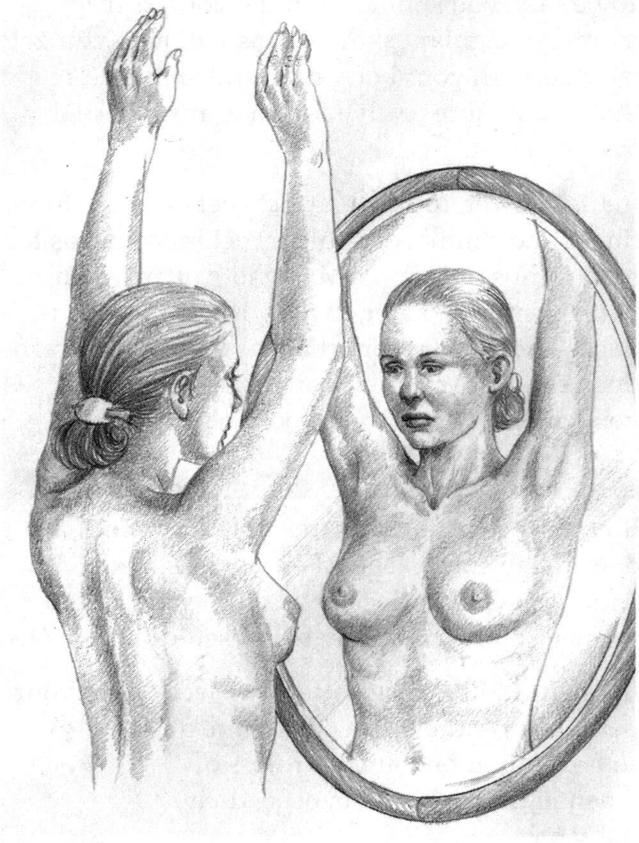

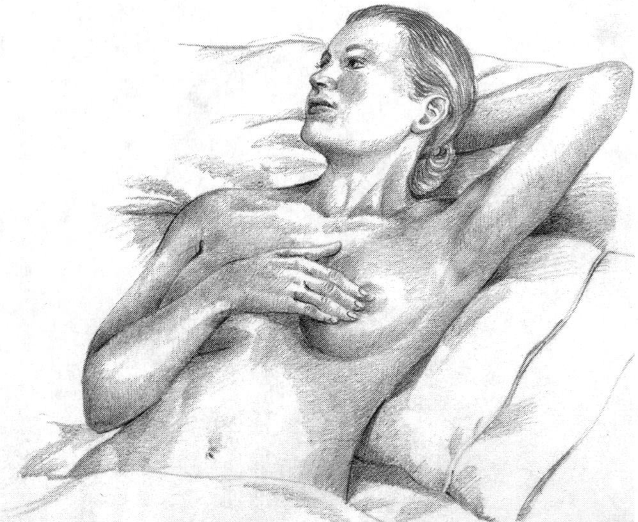

A thorough breast self-examination should include three parts: 1) Standing in the shower, feel for any lumps, knots, or changes in skin texture; 2) standing in front of a mirror with your arms at your sides, look for changes in contour or any puckering of the skin (repeat with your arms over your head); 3) lying flat on your back, again feel for lumps, knots, or changes in skin texture.

time each month. The same goes for postmenopausal women: Do it the same time each month. Conducting regular breast self-examinations will help you become familiar with the normal landscape of your breasts. In this way, any unusual lumps or growths that surface will be more obvious.

A thorough breast self-examination should have at least two parts.

In the shower:

1) Use your left hand to examine your right breast, and vice-versa.

2) Start by pressing your fingers firmly against each area of your breast, working your way around in a circular pattern from the outside of the breast inward toward the nipple.

3) Carefully feel for lumps, knots, or changes in skin texture.

4) Do not skip the area underneath your arms. This is breast tissue, too.

In front of a mirror:

1) Stand, topless, with your hands at your sides and note the natural contour of your breasts.

2) Raise your arms above your head and look for changes in the size, shape, and contour of your breasts. Also, note any dimpling, puckering, or changes in skin texture.

3) Squeeze each nipple gently and look for non-milky discharge (if you have given birth or nursed a baby within the last year, some clear or milky discharge is probably normal).

Some experts also suggest examining your breasts while lying flat on your back with one arm raised over your head; it gives you one more angle and helps ensure a thorough examination. You should report any suspicious symptoms to your physician immediately. Remember, your regular breast self-examinations are an adjunct to—not a replacement for—your regular visits to the doctor.

THE IMPORTANCE OF REGULAR CHECKUPS

While the self-examinations described in this chapter can play an important role in helping you keep tabs on your health, they cannot serve as a substitute for periodic evaluations conducted by an experienced physician.

The frequency and type of checkups you should have depends on your age, your sex, and the state of your health. If your physician believes you to be at high risk for developing a particular illness (because of your family or personal medical history), he or she may recommend that you come in for more frequent visits than you would if you did not have those risk factors. Likewise, if you already suffer from a specific health condition, your doctor will probably want to see you at frequent, regular intervals.

CHOOSING A PRIMARY-CARE PHYSICIAN

You already know that it's not wise to wait until you're ill to see a physician. It's best to start shopping for a primary-care physician (family physician, general practitioner, or internist) while you are in good health.

Thousands of physicians graduate from medical school each year. However, only a small percentage go on to become primary-care physicians. Why? Because being a generalist is not quite as glamorous (or as high paying) as being a specialist. After all, an average family doctor sees about 100 run-of-the-mill colds before ever encountering an unusual or exotic virus.

It also takes a special temperament to treat patients of all ages, sexes, and backgrounds. Because a family doctor cares for such a wide variety of patients, he or she must be familiar with an equally wide range of health problems. As a result, a generalist is part pediatrician, part internist, part allergist, part pathologist, and part counselor.

He or she is also the health care professional most likely to give you advice on staying healthy (as opposed to a specialist, who may be consulted only when you are ill).

Where should you begin your search for a primary-care physician? Not in the Yellow Pages. Instead, ask your trusted friends and relatives about their doctors. Are they happy with them? Whom have they had a bad experience with? Referrals are a valuable source of information. If you belong to a health maintenance organization (HMO) or a preferred provider organization (PPO), your health plan may limit your choice of doctor. Check to see if your plan has a list of available doctors.

When you have a list of four or five local physicians who come highly recommended, you can call your local or state medical board to be sure that each physician is properly licensed. You can further screen candidates by calling their offices and asking the following questions:

- Does the office accept your insurance?
- Does the doctor see patients in your age range?
- Does the doctor encourage regular checkups?
- What hospitals is the doctor affiliated with?
- Does the doctor deliver babies or provide prenatal care (if appropriate)?
- What is the fee schedule for office visits?
- Will the doctor refill prescriptions over the phone?
- Who will cover for the doctor in the event that he or she is not available or in an emergency?
- Does the doctor make emergency house calls?
- What hours is the office open?
- What is the average waiting time to see the doctor?

Keeping Track of Your Medical Records

The average person moves more than seven times in the course of his or her life. More mobile folks may move 15 or 20 times.

Just as you leave a paper trail for your mail to follow when you move, so should you make sure that your medical records accompany you to your final destination. Ask your physicians, dentists, and specialists to give you a copy of your records, or you can provide them with a signed release form, asking them to pass on your records to your new health care providers.

Here are some items you'd be wise to keep track of:

- Any recent X rays
- Hospital records
- Prescription records
- Immunization records for all family members
- Dental records

Prudence suggests making back-up copies of all of these items and storing the copies in a secure, fireproof location.

The best, most reliable test of a physician's (or any health care professional's) suitability for you is your own gut instinct. After all, if you don't feel comfortable with your practitioner, you are not apt to work well together in your health care partnership and not apt to receive satisfactory health care from him or her.

CHOOSING A GYNECOLOGIST

The relationship between a woman and her gynecologist is often more intimate than the relationship between a patient and a general practitioner. A woman needs to discuss very personal topics with this health care provider, including her sexual practices and birth-control choices.

Also, recent studies have shown that many women use their gynecologists as their primary-care physicians; this type of arrangement may be beneficial, depending on how well the gynecologist can deal with nongynecologic problems. Most primary care physicians are well-equipped to deal with women's health issues, but research reveals that women who see only a general practitioner sometimes miss out on the very important vaginal examinations and Pap smears.

For all of these reasons, the choice of a gynecologist should not be taken lightly. As with choosing a general practitioner, referrals from friends and family are a good place to start. And don't be afraid to go with your gut instinct.

THE CUSTOMER IS ALWAYS RIGHT

A physician works for the patient—not the other way around. Most physicians want to work with you as a partner, but it is still your responsibility to make sure that any candidates for the position are licensed, competent professionals.

Aside from checking his or her credentials, how else can you avoid receiving services from someone who does not promote your best interests?

- First off, don't make the mistake of giving your personal power away to any physician. Ask questions about the treatment you are receiving, and insist on thorough answers.
- If you feel that a physician is on the wrong track, speak up. If your physician is unreceptive, get a second opinion. Never allow yourself to be bullied by a doctor. After all, it's your body, and you don't have to consent to any treatment or procedure that you feel unsure of.
- Read current health magazines and books—especially those written about topics relevant to your health needs. Take note of current treatments, and question your doctor if his or her methods differ from the norm.
- Compare notes with friends who have experienced conditions similar to your own. Ask what treatment they received—for example, what medications they were given, in what dosages, and for what length of time. Ask how much they pay for a doctor's visit or a lab test.
- Don't be afraid to change doctors. If your doctor will not provide the services you need, find another.

- If you think your doctor may be incompetent or dishonest, report him or her to your local medical review board. These boards are empowered to investigate allegations of misconduct.

PRENATAL TESTING

Pregnancy and childbirth are exciting and often nerve-wracking experiences. Throughout the long nine months, prospective parents are likely to be preoccupied with worries about the baby's health.

Prenatal tests can help allay some of those fears. Aside from confirming that the fetus is healthy, the results of these tests can also prepare prospective parents for the likelihood of an inherited illness or a birth defect. Early detection of health problems may also pave the way for life-saving treatments, some of which are even performed before birth. Listed here are some common prenatal tests.

Maternal serum alpha-fetoprotein (MSAFP) screening. MSAFP screening is a blood test that measures the amount of a certain substance called alpha-fetoprotein in a pregnant woman's blood. The results of this test give the physician an idea of the likelihood that the fetus suffers from a defect, such as spina bifida or Down syndrome.

Although the MSAFP screening poses no danger to either mother or child, parents should be aware that this is a screening, not a diagnostic test. Therefore, even an abnormal result does not confirm or deny the presence of a problem. It only suggests that further tests should be conducted.

Amniocentesis. Amniocentesis is a genetic analysis performed on the uterine amniotic fluid. Using a long, thin needle inserted through the abdominal wall, a physician extracts a small sample of the fluid from the sac that surrounds the fetus. Cells from the sample are later reproduced and analyzed.

Unlike the MSAFP screening, amniocentesis is a diagnostic test—meaning it can be used to confirm conclusively the presence or absence of a specific genetic defect, such as spina bifida or Down syndrome. It can also definitively disclose the sex of the fetus.

Because amniocentesis carries with it a very slight risk of infection, amniotic fluid leakage, bleeding, and miscarriage, it is only performed when there is a specific reason to do so. Such indications can include a mother over 35 years of age or an abnormal MSAFP screening result.

Inherited Disorders: An Unfortunate Game of Roulette

When a prenatal test reveals that a fetus has a deformity or a serious illness, the first question that often comes to mind is "Why?" A child may be born with an affliction because both parents are carriers of a recessive gene for the trait and unknowingly passed these genes along to their offspring.

However, being a carrier of a gene for an inheritable illness does not necessarily condemn your child to developing the illness. Even if both parents carry one recessive gene for a particular disorder, the chances of the child inheriting the affliction is only 25 percent (one in four). If only one parent is a carrier of a disorder caused by a recessive gene, the child cannot inherit the problem, but still has a 50 percent chance of becoming a carrier.

Since carrying a gene causes no symptoms in the carrier, people are often unaware that they run the risk of passing a disorder on to their children. If you know of any inherited diseases that run in your family or your spouse's family, genetic testing and counseling may give you a clearer picture of the risks you face as a prospective parent.

Ultrasonography. Fetal ultrasonography (sometimes called simply *ultrasound*) is the only noninvasive method of examining a fetus while it is still inside the mother's womb. It carries little risk of damage to the fetus and can be a useful way to confirm that a pregnancy is progressing as it should.

Ultrasonography uses the echo of sound waves to create a black-and-white picture on a televisionlike screen. The ultrasound picture can show the fetus' anatomy (even the beating of its tiny heart). This technology can help a physician determine the exact age of a fetus (which can help set the timing of other tests), confirm the fetus' position in the womb, and rule out ectopic (tubal) pregnancies. Ultrasound can also be helpful in diagnosing certain birth defects.

Chorionic villus sampling (CVS). CVS is an alternative to amniocentesis. Because it is a little riskier than the other procedure, CVS is usually only performed if earlier detection of a defect is necessary (amniocentesis cannot usually be performed until about the 16th week of pregnancy). The test analyzes a tiny piece of tissue taken from the chorionic villi (small projections on the surface of the fetal membrane). Like amniocentesis, CVS can conclusively determine the fetus' sex. It is also used for genetic analyses.

CHECKUPS THROUGH CHILDHOOD

Most children will first visit their pediatrician's office at the age of about two weeks. This is usually the first time the doctor will see a child after he or she has been discharged from the hospital.

From there, a common checkup schedule is 1 month (or six weeks, depending on the physician), 2 months, 4 months, 6 months, 9 months, 12 months, 15 months, 18 months, 24 months, and annually thereafter.

In the earlier visits, a pediatrician or family physician will check an infant's length, weight, and head circumference. Immunizations may be administered (see pages 152–154 for information on childhood immunization), or blood tests taken. Usually, a doctor will ask the parents questions about the baby's behavior in an effort to determine whether the child's development is proceeding at a normal pace.

The checkup—especially in infancy—is a perfect opportunity to ask the physician questions about nutrition, feeding schedules, diaper rash, sleep patterns, discipline, and anything else of concern to the parent. Later (after the third year), the physician may check the child's vision, hearing, gait, spinal development, and school readiness.

CHECKUPS IN YOUNG ADULTHOOD

Fortunately, adolescence through age 30 is often a healthy period for most individuals. For those who have no obvious health problems, the following is a conventional schedule for checkups and well visits:

- A general physical examination every five years
- A serum cholesterol test every five years; more often for people with a family history of cardiovascular diseases

CHECKUPS AT A GLANCE

AGE	PHYSICAL EXAM	VISION CHECK	CHOLESTEROL SCREENING	RECTAL EXAM	DENTAL EXAM	PELVIC EXAM	MAMMOGRAPHY
Childhood	Annually after 2 years	Annually	Every 5 years	Annually	Every 6 months after 3 years	None unless problems arise	None
Adolescence to 30 years	Every 5 years	Every 1 to 3 years†	Every 5 years	Every 5 years	Every 6 months	Every 1 to 3 years§	None
30 to 40 years	Every 1 to 3 years‡	Every 1 to 3 years†	Every 5 years*	Every 5 years*	Annually	Every 1 to 3 years§	None*
40 to 50 years	Every 1 to 3 years‡	Every 1 to 3 years†	Every 5 years*	Annually	Annually	Every 1 to 3 years§	None*
Over 50 years	Annually	Annually†	Every 5 years*	Annually, plus sigmoidoscopy every 10 years	Annually	Every 1 to 3 years§	Every 1 to 2 years*

*unless personal or family medical history dictates more frequent testing
†more often if you wear glasses, have diabetes, or have a family history of glaucoma or high blood pressure
‡closer to every 3 years for men; closer to annually for women
§depending on sexual practices (for example, closer to annually for women with a history of sexually transmitted disease or multiple partners)

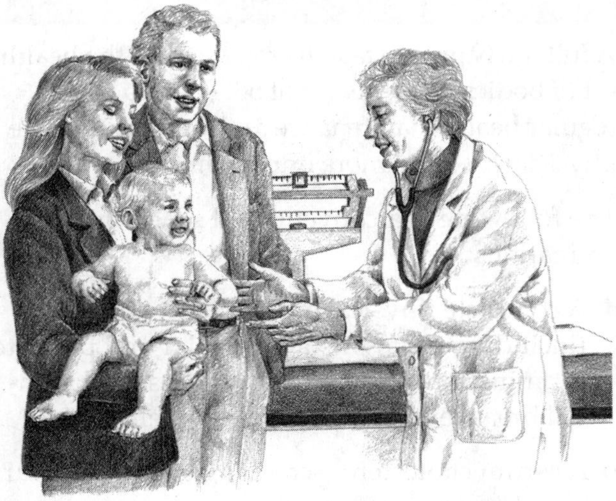

- An annual pelvic examination and Pap smear for sexually active women
- A vision exam every one to three years (more often for those who are at higher risk for eye problems, including those who wear glasses, suffer from diabetes, or have a family history of glaucoma or high blood pressure)

CHECKUPS THROUGH MIDDLE AGE

Health becomes a bigger issue for most of us between the ages of 30 and 50. The little aches and pains that were easily overlooked in our 20s become more difficult to ignore. We don't have quite as much energy as we used to. Our stamina begins to fail, ever so slightly. We become aware that our dietary indiscretions—once quickly atoned for—are now more likely to stick around and haunt us.

All these little realizations serve to drive home the message that we cannot take our health for granted. From this point onward, quality of life depends on proper self-care, regular preventive checkups, and appropriate medical care when necessary.

At this point, visits to the doctor become more frequent and a little more involved. A conventional schedule of health maintenance might proceed as follows:

- A complete physical examination every three to five years (including professional testicular and prostate examinations for men and professional manual breast examinations for women)
- A serum cholesterol test at least every five years (more often if a previous test came out on the high side)
- For women, an annual pelvic examination and cervical Pap smear (After the age of 40, women who have a family history of breast cancer or some other risk factor may want to discuss with their physician the benefits and risks of regular mammography.)

What to Expect from Your Regular Checkup

Your plain old, run-of-the-mill checkup serves several important functions: It is designed to check the progress of any existing conditions you may suffer from, and to determine if anything unexpected has developed. It also presents an opportunity for you to ask your doctor questions (about mild symptoms, changes in your body's functions, and so on) and get feedback on ways to improve the overall state of your health.

When you go in for your check-up, expect the following tests:

- Vision
- Hearing (only performed occasionally)
- Blood pressure
- Weight
- Temperature
- Heart, lungs, and breathing (performed with the aid of a stethoscope)
- Ears, eyes, nose, and throat (performed with a small scope)
- A blood test for serum cholesterol or other factors (under certain circumstances)
- A urinalysis (under certain circumstances)
- A breast examination (for women)
- A manual testicular and prostate examination (for adult men)
- An examination designed to evaluate the state of any specific conditions you may suffer from or suspect

When to Call the Doctor

Besides the obvious emergencies and the periodic checkups, there are other times when you should see the doctor. You should consult a doctor for any unusual symptoms, but be especially wary of the following:

- Unexplained lumps or swelling
- Frequent nosebleeds
- Blackouts
- Dizzy spells
- Frequent earaches
- Severe depression
- Persistently hoarse voice
- Difficulty swallowing
- Frequent or painful urination
- Recurring colds, sweating, or fever
- Blood-streaked urine or stools
- Chronic cough
- Swollen ankles
- Enlarged lymph nodes
- Loss of motor function (stumbling)
- Severe insomnia or fatigue
- Persistent thirst
- Convulsions
- Chest pressure
- Unexplained weight loss or gain
- Unrelieved constipation or diarrhea

Adapted from *365 Health Hints.* © 1993 Don R. Powell, Ph.D.

- An eye examination every one to three years (more often for those who wear glasses, suffer from diabetes, or have a family history of glaucoma or high blood pressure)
- After 40, an annual rectal exam, followed by a flexible sigmoidoscopy (an internal examination performed with the aid of a tiny camera) if a manual examination or examination of a stool sample turns up any suspicious results

CHECKUPS AFTER AGE 50

A full life begins to take its toll on even the healthiest of bodies after the age of 50. For this reason, regular health maintenance and well visits to the physician become more important than ever.

The following is a conventional schedule of examinations:

- A complete physical examination annually (including professional testicular and prostate examinations for men and professional manual breast examinations for women)
- A serum cholesterol screening every five years
- An annual gynecologic exam and mammogram for all women
- A cervical Pap smear annually, or every three years for postmenopausal women whose previous ones were normal
- An annual eye exam, especially for those who continue to drive after the age of 65
- A manual rectal examination and stool sample for occult blood once per year, plus a flexible sigmoidoscopy every ten years (or if indicated by the less invasive tests)

IMMUNIZATIONS: A SHOT FOR ALL REASONS

To immunize means, quite simply, to render your body immune to a foreign invader, such as a virus. Immunizations help your system defend itself against specific diseases and infections.

Immunization is a way to teach your body to recognize a certain invader. So the next time it detects that invader, your immune system can get a head start on preparing to fight that particular organism.

PEDIATRIC VACCINATION SCHEDULES

Before the invention of vaccines, millions of children succumbed to crippling or fatal illnesses before they ever reached adulthood. Fortunately for children today, technology has advanced to the point where many of the diseases that our grandparents feared have been all but eradicated (at least in this country).

There is a catch, however: Maintaining control over the life-threatening diseases of the past requires every citizen's full cooperation. If even one child is not vaccinated and contracts a disease, he or she can give it to fetuses or to newborns who have not yet received the vaccination. It is for this reason that most cities and states require all children to be up to date with their immunizations before entering a public school (with a few religious and medical exemptions).

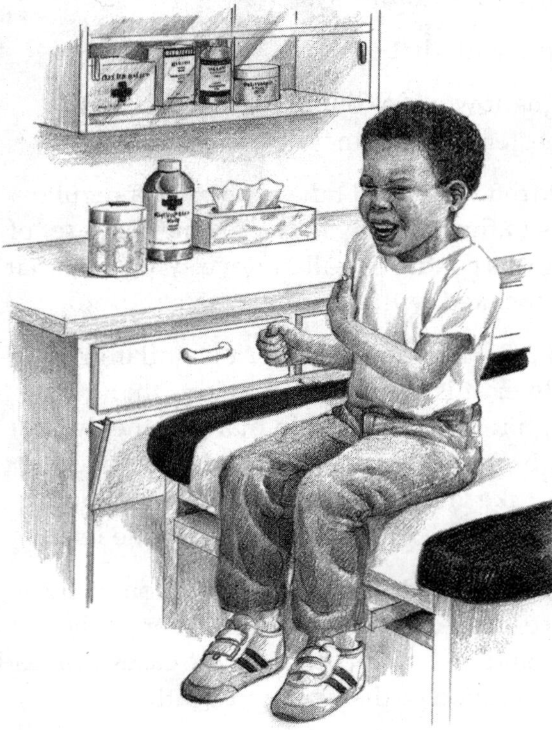

To make the process of immunizing children as nontraumatic as possible (remember how you hated getting shots as a child?), many vaccines are now given simultaneously. Thus, American children receive an MMR (measles-mumps-rubella), a DTP (diphtheria-tetanus-pertussis), and so on. Single-agent vaccines include the OPV (oral polio vaccine) and the HiB (*Hemophilus influenzae,* type B). A new vaccine against chicken pox (varicella zoster virus) has just become available, too. Children also receive a test for tuberculosis, in which they are exposed to a tiny amount of the bacteria to see how their bodies react.

In the absence of any health conditions that would preclude the administration of vaccines

THE CONTROVERSY OVER PERTUSSIS VACCINES

While few people argue about the benefits of vaccines in general, the vaccine for whooping cough (pertussis) has been the topic of continuing debate. The concern is over the whole-cell vaccine used for the first three pertussis boosters, which is made from the inactivated particles of the virus *Bordatella pertussis*. This vaccine has been linked to side effects ranging from fever and high-pitched crying to brain damage and death.

Proponents of the whole-cell vaccine say that the immunization has never been conclusively proved to cause the more serious side effects. And regardless, they say, any dangers posed by the vaccine are much less of a threat than the threat of contracting a bad case of whooping cough.

The 1991 approval of a new synthetic pertussis vaccine has made the situation even more complicated. This vaccine, which is widely used in Japan and Europe, is not associated with the same side effects as the whole-cell vaccine. However, it is also not as effective at protecting children against whooping cough. (It is effective when it is used in children who have already received three doses of the whole-cell vaccine, according to the Food and Drug Administration.)

Since children are required to have full immunizations before entering school, many parents find themselves facing a dilemma: Should they take the risk of immunizing their child? And, if not, how will their child enter school?

If you have any fears about your child receiving the whole-cell pertussis vaccine, arrange a time to discuss the matter with your child's physician.

(such as an impaired immune system), pediatric immunizations are usually given according to the following schedule:

DTP: Given at age 2 months, 4 months, 6 months, 12 to 18 months, and 4 to 6 years

OPV: Given at age 2 months, 4 months, 6 to 18 months, and 4 to 6 years

Tine test for tuberculosis: Given around the first birthday

MMR: Given at age 12 to15 months; second dose at either 4 to 6 years OR 11 to 12 years

HiB: Given at age 2 months, 4 months, 6 months, and 12 to 15 months

Hepatitis B: Given at birth to 2 months, 2 to 4 months, and 6 to 18 months

Varricella zoster vaccine: Given at 12 to 18 months and 11 to 12 years

Payment Assistance

If you cannot afford to pay for your children's required immunizations, you may be eligible to receive help from federal, state, or local programs that subsidize the cost of the vaccines or administer them free of charge. (Eligibility for and availability of subsidized programs will vary in every community.) Contact your state or local health agency to ask about programs in your area.

VACCINES FOR ADULTS

Vaccinations aren't just for children. Adults can also receive protection against illnesses:

The flu. It may not seem a formidable threat, but the flu (the common name for influenza) can be a serious illness. It kills thousands of Americans every year. It poses a special danger to the elderly and immunocompromised individuals.

The flu is really any one of millions of different viruses. Fortunately, scientists at the Centers for Disease Control and Prevention in Atlanta are always busily at work formulating new vaccines against the latest mutation of the flu bug.

Who should get a flu shot? In general, anyone who is concerned about getting the flu (and who can afford to pay for it). However, some populations should take the flu threat more seriously:

- People over the age of 65
- People whose immune systems are impaired by AIDS or another chronic illness
- People who reside in chronic-care facilities, such as nursing homes
- All health care workers and public-service employees (police officers, firefighters, child-care workers, and so on)
- Those who suffer from chronic lung problems, such as asthma or cystic fibrosis
- Smokers
- People who are taking medications that suppress their immune systems
- People with diabetes
- Pregnant women (but only after the first trimester of pregnancy)
- Children who must take aspirin on a regular basis (a flu shot may help prevent the onset of a serious condition called Reye syndrome that is associated with aspirin use in children)

Hepatitis B. Hepatitis B is a serious inflammation of the liver. It is far more contagious than HIV, although it is transmitted in many of the same ways (through semen, blood, and other bodily fluids). Like HIV, it can also be passed through the placenta of a pregnant woman to the fetus.

Symptoms of acute hepatitis B infection include jaundice, dark urine, pale stools, fever, loss of energy, and loss of appetite. Severe cases can lead to degeneration of the liver and death.

The immunization is now routinely given to children and is also recommended for those at the highest risk of contracting hepatitis B:

- Health care workers
- Patients receiving kidney dialysis

- Tourists visiting Asia (where the disease is common)
- Intravenous drug users
- Individuals who engage in unprotected sexual intercourse with multiple partners (or with one infected individual)

Immunization against hepatitis B is done by injection. The effects of the vaccine usually last for several years.

Pneumonia. Pneumonia, which is also called pneumonitis, is an umbrella term for an entire category of illnesses causing an inflammation of the lungs. It can be caused by bacteria, viruses, or chemical irritants. Its severity can range from a simple upper-respiratory infection to a life-threatening illness.

About 1.5 percent of Americans get pneumonia every year, and many die from it. (Because pneumonia is often a secondary infection caused by another illness, it is difficult to ascertain whether the cause of death was the primary illness or the pneumonia.) Fortunately, a pneumonia vaccine does exist.

The elderly are particularly susceptible to lung infections. The vaccine is recommended for everyone at age 65 (sooner if the individual is at an increased risk). People with chronic heart or lung disease, diabetes, Hodgkin disease, or any other disorder that impairs the immune system are at increased risk and should be immunized. The effectiveness of pneumonia immunization depends on the overall health of the patient receiving it.

CURRENT HEALTH INFORMATION

It seems that "revolutionary" medical breakthroughs, "incredible" scientific discoveries, and "miraculous" technologic wizardry abound of late. Barely a day goes by without a report of a spectacular new cure for a formerly incurable illness.

To make matters even more confusing, it seems that each new study contradicts the last: One day, drinking alcohol is detrimental to your health; the next day, it is reported to help prevent heart disease. It is becoming harder and harder to interpret the news.

EVALUATING THE NEWS

How can an average individual sort out the useful information from the bogus reports? First off, take everything you hear with a grain of salt. (Absolute truth exists only in fairy tales.) Here are some tips:

- Use your common sense. Things that seem too good to be true (like thigh cream) usually are.
- Ask your doctor. Your physician is an invaluable source of health information. (After all, he or she has been reading and digesting medical studies for years.) If a new study has piqued your curiosity, ask your doctor to help you put the findings in context.
- Look for a confirming report. Information that is reported by at least two independent sources is more likely to have merit.
- Consider the source. The *Journal of the American Medical Association* is a much more reliable source for medical news than the *National Enquirer*. (Perhaps this tip falls under the "use your common sense" heading.)

HELPFUL ORGANIZATIONS

There are thousands of consumer and professional organizations dedicated to health promotion and education. Some of these groups are privately funded, while others operate on a not-for-profit basis. Still others are affiliated with (or are divisions of) government agencies.

Even if a group has a profit motive (such as a large pharmaceutical company does), it may still provide useful health information to consumers. However, be aware that these companies often have an unspoken agenda (for you to buy their products).

Here are some organizations you can turn to in your search for sound health information:

American Academy of Dermatology
930 North Meacham Road, P.O. Box 4014
Schaumburg, IL 60168-4014
(708) 330-0230

American Cancer Society
1599 Clifton Road NE
Atlanta, GA 30329-4251
(800) ACS-2345

American College of Obstetricians and Gynecologists
409 12th Street SW
Washington, DC 20024-2188
(202) 484-3321

American Diabetes Association
1660 Duke Street
Alexandria, VA 22314
(800) 232-3472

American Heart Association
7320 Greenville Avenue
Dallas, TX 75231
(214) 373-6300
(800) 242-8721

American Lung Association
1740 Broadway
New York, NY 10019
(212) 315-8700

Gay Men's Health Crisis
129 West 20th Street
New York, NY 10011
Hotline: (212) 807-6655

Juvenile Diabetes Foundation International
432 Park Avenue South
16th Floor
New York, NY 10016
(212) 889-7575

March of Dimes Birth Defects Foundation
1275 Mamaroneck Avenue
White Plains, NY 10605
(914) 428-7100

National Alliance of Breast Cancer Organizations (NABCO)
1180 Avenue of the Americas
New York, NY 10036
(212) 719-0154

National Easter Seals Society (Cerebral Palsy)
230 West Monroe Street
Suite 1800
Chicago, IL 60606-4802
(312) 726-6200

National Multiple Sclerosis Society
733 3rd Avenue
New York, NY 10017
(212) 986-3240

National Women's Health Network
514 10th Street NW
Suite 400
Washington, DC 20004
(202) 347-1140

Project Inform (AIDS information)
1965 Market Street, Room 220
San Francisco, CA 94103
(800) 822-7422

The U.S. Food and Drug Administration (FDA)
Consumer Affairs Department
5600 Fishers Lane—HFE 88
Rockville, MD 20857
(301) 443-3170

PART II: SYMPTOMS, ILLNESSES, TESTS & SURGERIES

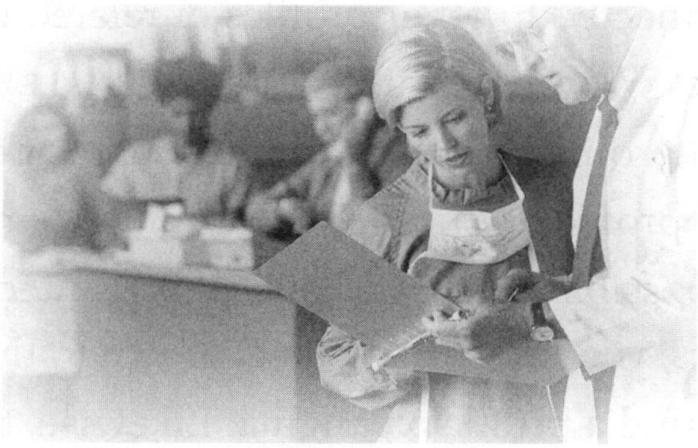

We all get sick at one time or another, and when you or a family member is ill, you need to get the facts. Whether you have something as simple as a child with a cold or as serious as a loved one facing the specter of cancer, you can turn to the following pages for hard information. Here is a place you can go to get quick answers to your questions and to help you ask the right ones at the doctor's office.

Part I outlined those aspects of health that you can control. Part II is your entry into the world of professional health care. There are three sections—1) Symptoms, 2) Illnesses, and 3) Tests & Surgeries—each containing concise information from the experts at Northwestern University Medical School.

The profiles are arranged alphabetically in each section, and they are all connected to other profiles of related interest by cross-references. Words that are printed in SMALL CAPITAL LETTERS have their own profile elsewhere in the book. For example, if you are reading the profile on chest pain, you might find ANGINA mentioned under possible causes; because it is printed in SMALL CAPITAL LETTERS, you know that you can turn to the Illnesses section and find a profile on angina. Likewise, the profile on angina might mention ANGIOPLASTY as a possible treatment; because it is printed in SMALL CAPITAL LETTERS, you know you can turn to the Tests & Surgeries section and find a profile on the procedure. The names of the prescription drugs listed in Part III of the book are also printed in SMALL CAPITAL LETTERS, so you know when you can turn to that part to learn more about the medications mentioned.

Whether you need to know about an operation or you just want to learn what could be causing those sniffles, all the information is at your fingertips. And knowing the facts is one of the first steps toward getting quality health care.

ABDOMINAL PAIN

The causes of abdominal pain are many, and the complaint is one of the most frequent reasons patients seek medical attention or advice.

Most causes of abdominal pain are not dangerous and need little, if any, investigation. Some features, however, that point to more serious causes include abdominal pain

- That is constant and prolonged (over two hours)
- Associated with persistent VOMITING
- Associated with a high FEVER (over 101°F)
- That is sudden and awakens the patient
- Made worse by movement, coughing, or sneezing

CAUSES

The causes of abdominal pain range from the very common (GASTROENTERITIS, IRRITABLE BOWEL SYNDROME, and indigestion) to the less frequent (appendicitis, GALLSTONES, ULCER, PANCREATITIS, and DIVERTICULAR DISEASE) and uncommon (aortic ANEURYSM, and INTESTINAL OBSTRUCTION).

APPROACH

The patient's MEDICAL HISTORY provides the clue to the cause of abdominal pain in many instances. Pain made better or worse by meals may point to ULCER or PANCREATITIS. Pain made better with bowel movements suggests IRRITABLE BOWEL SYNDROME or narrowing of the large intestine. Pain associated with VOMITING may suggest an INTESTINAL OBSTRUCTION. Women are prone to gynecologic causes of abdominal pain, and a menstrual history may be helpful.

The location of the pain and the way it radiates are important features. For example, the pain of ULCER is typically pinpointed just below the end of the breast bone; pain emanating from PANCREATITIS or GALLSTONES frequently starts above the belly button and travels straight into the back.

Laboratory tests may include evaluation of the BLOOD COUNT or other BLOOD TESTS. If the MEDICAL HISTORY or PHYSICAL EXAMINATION indicates serious problems, X rays (RADIOGRAPHY) of the stomach and intestine, COMPUTED TOMOGRAPHY, ULTRASOUND, or ENDOSCOPY may be in order.

TREATMENT OPTIONS

If the pain is severe, prolonged, or associated with the dangerous symptoms noted above, it is best to avoid solid food. The patient may take clear liquids, if tolerated, and should seek medical attention.

ABDOMINAL SWELLING

Many people feel some abdominal swelling, or distension, after a meal. Even though they may keenly sense the distension, the symptom in this situation is without serious medical cause or consequence.

Although usually benign, many illnesses can be signaled by abdominal swelling. If the abdominal swelling is prolonged and visibly obvious to others, this symptom could represent serious medical problems.

CAUSES

The intestine itself lacks typical pain receptors and when the wall of the intestine is minimally stimulated or stretched, patients may experience the subjective symptom of distension without any objective evidence of it. This is very common in patients with IRRITABLE BOWEL SYNDROME whose intestinal nerve receptors may have a lower threshold for sensing intestinal action.

Fluid accumulation within the abdomen can also cause abdominal swelling. Fluid accumulation can result from various causes such as

- CONGESTIVE HEART FAILURE
- Cirrhosis of the liver
- Nephrotic syndrome of the kidney including KIDNEY FAILURE
- Intra-abdominal cancer (especially OVARIAN CANCER in women)

INTESTINAL OBSTRUCTION from many causes may also result in this symptom, but is typically accompanied by ABDOMINAL PAIN and VOMITING.

APPROACH

The PHYSICAL EXAMINATION will frequently detect if any serious cause is present for abdominal swelling. At times, ULTRASOUND probing or COMPUTED TOMOGRAPHY of the abdomen may be done to rule out the more potentially dangerous causes of abdominal swelling.

TREATMENT OPTIONS

Minor dietary modifications such as restricting dairy products and reducing fat content may benefit some patients with benign abdominal swelling (see IRRITABLE BOWEL SYNDROME).

More serious underlying conditions such as various forms of cancer or cirrhosis of the liver must be addressed directly.

ANKLE SWELLING

The term *swollen ankles* includes any visibly apparent increase in size or puffiness in the lower legs. It is a sign of excess fluid pooling in the lower legs, called *edema*.

Ankle swelling is an example of a symptom that affects one area of the body but indicates possible systemic problems.

CAUSES

The most common cause of ankle swelling is VARICOSE VEINS. Less commonly, ankle swelling can be caused by an injury such as a sprain or bone damage.

Less common but more serious causes include

- Thrombophlebitis
- CONGESTIVE HEART FAILURE
- Nephrotic syndrome—damage to the filtering function of the kidneys (see KIDNEY FAILURE)
- Liver damage that causes decreased protein production and fluid retention

APPROACH

Clues from an individual's MEDICAL HISTORY include any known heart, kidney, or liver disease or any symptoms related to those organs, especially if swelling is associated with BREATHING DIFFICULTY. Without shortness of breath and with fluid retention limited to the leg, VARICOSE VEINS would be the most common explanation.

A PHYSICAL EXAMINATION might focus on the neck veins and signs of fluid retention in other parts of the body with close attention to any bone tenderness.

Diagnostic tests might include blood flow studies of the leg to look for blood clots (ULTRASOUND), X rays of the bones (RADIOGRAPHY) if an injury is suspected, or BLOOD TESTS to assess kidney and liver function. Tests of cardiac function include echocardiography (ULTRASOUND).

TREATMENT OPTIONS

Treatment of the underlying condition should, in general, alleviate ankle swelling; however, general measures to treat the symptom include

- Elevation of the leg above the level of the heart
- Elastic stockings that prevent blood and fluid from pooling in the lower leg
- Rarely, diuretics such as HYDROCHLOROTHIAZIDE or FUROSEMIDE to control severe edema

ANXIETY

Although not easy to define, anxiety is a very real symptom. It can appear by itself, or it can accompany other physical and psychological problems.

Anxiety is a very common symptom that occurs in a variety of forms. Some people feel nervous, worried, or fearful. Others feel a wide range of body sensations, including

- Restlessness
- TREMBLING
- Muscle tension
- Muscle aches and pains
- HEADACHES
- Nausea
- ABDOMINAL PAIN
- DIARRHEA
- Sweating (see SWEATING, EXCESSIVE)
- Palpitations
- CHEST PAINS
- BREATHING DIFFICULTY
- DIZZINESS
- FATIGUE
- Irritability
- SLEEPING PROBLEMS

Anxiety can be present constantly or it can come and go, sometimes in distinct episodes known as panic attacks.

CAUSES

A variety of internal and external factors produce anxiety. Life stress is the most common cause of mild to moderate anxiety. Exposure to, or withdrawal from, certain substances—caffeine, alcohol, tobacco, amphetamines, sedatives, marijuana, thyroid hormone, decongestants, theophylline, other asthma medications, and weight-reduction medication—can also provoke anxiety.

Anxiety may be associated with a specific psychiatric diagnosis such as

- DEPRESSION
- Panic disorder
- Phobias
- Post-traumatic stress disorder
- Generalized anxiety disorder

Anxiety can also accompany a wide range of medical conditions such as

- HYPERTHYROIDISM
- Heart rhythm disturbances (ARRHYTHMIAS)
- ANGINA pectoris
- Low blood sugar

APPROACH

A physician usually starts by asking about specific physical and psychological symptoms and about exposures to caffeine, alcohol, tobacco, recreational drugs, and medications that could potentially contribute to symptoms. Sources of stress and the individual's methods of coping with them are also of interest. A general PHYSICAL EXAMINATION is useful, focusing on BLOOD PRESSURE TESTING, the thyroid gland, the heart, the lungs, and the nerve reflexes.

No tests are absolutely essential, but if symptoms and the results of the PHYSICAL EXAMINATION are suggestive, the doctor might want to do a BLOOD TEST for thyroid function, ELECTROCARDIOGRAPHY, or any of a wide range of tests for specific conditions.

TREATMENT OPTIONS

Treatment depends on the underlying cause of the anxiety. If a specific medical or psychiatric diagnosis is made, it should be treated accordingly.

Reducing or eliminating exposure to caffeine, alcohol, tobacco, recreational drugs, or medications that can worsen anxiety is helpful. Finding constructive ways of coping with stress is also important. Some strategies include

- Eating appropriate foods
- Exercising regularly
- Reading
- Meditation

Specific medications that are sometimes used for anxiety disorders include

- DIAZEPAM and related sedatives
- Antidepressants such as FLUOXETINE, AMITRIPTYLINE, or nefazodone
- Beta-blockers such as PROPRANOLOL
- Antihistamines such as HYDROXYZINE
- The anxiolytic buspirone

APPETITE, LOSS OF

The medical term for loss of appetite is *anorexia*. Many situations and medical problems can contribute to the loss of appetite.

The symptom of anorexia by itself has limited diagnostic significance. The degree of anorexia, however, does provide a useful index of the severity of many diseases.

CAUSES

Loss of appetite is quite common to a large number of debilitating diseases, but if it is the only symptom, it has very limited diagnostic value. Many people with chronic diseases such as MULTIPLE SCLEROSIS, CROHN DISEASE, RHEUMATOID ARTHRITIS, and AIDS can lose their appetite. Stress, ANXIETY, and DEPRESSION are certainly frequent contributors to a loss of appetite. If the anorexia persists and is *not* accompanied by WEIGHT LOSS, it is less likely to be related to an illness.

Anorexia can be the first sign of infectious HEPATITIS, even preceding yellowing of the skin. Cancers of various types, including STOMACH CANCER and PANCREATIC CANCER, can cause loss of appetite and progressive WEIGHT LOSS.

Anorexia nervosa is a psychophysiologic condition usually occurring in women and girls; it is characterized by refusal of food, fear of becoming obese, distorted sense of body image, and MENSTRUAL IRREGULARITIES.

APPROACH

Loss of appetite deserves investigation if it is protracted and is accompanied by WEIGHT LOSS. Stress, ANXIETY, and DEPRESSION are very common causes and their presence may be explanation enough for the symptom. A general PHYSICAL EXAMINATION will provide a clue whether or not it is appropriate to pursue diagnostic testing. BLOOD TESTS, including a BLOOD COUNT, test of thyroid function, and screening chemistries provide a good picture regarding general health and can be an effective screen for any serious illness responsible for the anorexia.

TREATMENT OPTIONS

Treatment should be directed specifically at the underlying cause of the loss of appetite. Pharmacologic appetite stimulants, as a general rule, are not very effective and carry some risk, although agents such as megestrol acetate are useful in some patients with chronic debilitating illnesses such as AIDS and cancer.

BACKACHE

Although many episodes may come on after lifting or straining, back pain may also occur without an inciting cause. The vast majority of back pain episodes improve or resolve within about six weeks.

Backache is a common symptom that may affect as many of 20 percent of all Americans at any one time. The lifetime chance that one may have an episode of back pain at some time is 90 percent.

CAUSES

The vast majority of backaches occur because of overuse problems. Heavy lifting or repetitive twisting and turning activities may contribute to backache.

Inflammatory conditions such as RHEUMATOID ARTHRITIS, systemic LUPUS ERYTHEMATOSUS, and others may cause backache. Backache is also a primary symptom of ankylosing spondylitis—a condition that occurs in a very small population segment, mostly in men.

OSTEOPOROSIS may cause a localized compression fracture in the spine, causing pain.

Tumors and infections of the spine, all of which can cause back pain, are very rare.

Kidney infection can also cause back pain.

In rare instances sudden severe back pain may be caused by the rupture of an aortic ANEURYSM.

APPROACH

The course of the backache is an important feature; for example, if it started with an injury or overuse episode other causes can be ruled out. The PHYSICAL EXAMINATION will be directed toward the muscles, range of motion, and response to stresses on the spine. The doctor will also be interested in any sensation or reflex changes in the lower extremities.

More involved diagnostic studies, such as RADIOGRAPHY, COMPUTED TOMOGRAPHY, and MAGNETIC RESONANCE IMAGING are useful in only a small number of cases.

TREATMENT OPTIONS

The initial treatment for backache is usually common sense and can be self-directed. Rest and over-the-counter analgesics such as ASPIRIN, acetaminophen, or IBUPROFEN are usually all that is required. Persistent pain may benefit from treatment with prescription medicines and some exercises or physical therapy. In rare cases, LUMBAR DISK REMOVAL surgery may be needed for a persistently problematic HERNIATED DISK.

BOWEL CONTROL, LOSS OF

Fecal incontinence is rarely seen in younger populations; it is noted most often in older groups.

An isolated episode of fecal incontinence is not an uncommon experience and should not be a source of major concern. Recurrent episodes of fecal incontinence, however, are abnormal and require medical evaluation.

Bowel control involves five aspects; they are

- The ability to sense stool filling the rectum
- The ability to distinguish the nature of rectal contents (gas, liquid, or solid)
- The ability of the rectum and large bowel to store feces for variable periods of time
- The ability of valves (rectal sphincters) to open and close in a controlled fashion
- The ability of the pelvic muscles to maintain the rectum at a sharp angle in the abdomen, retarding the passage of stool by mechanical means

Disruption of any of these mechanisms can cause fecal incontinence.

CAUSES

The isolated instance of fecal incontinence is usually related to intestinal hurry induced by sensitivity to food, by stress, or by an acute episode of DIARRHEA. In the case of prolonged or recurrent fecal incontinence, the causes may be multiple and relate to several general categories, including

- Functional impairment or decreased mental capacity including any severe chronic debilitating illness resulting in a bed-ridden state such as ALZHEIMER DISEASE
- Decreased capacity of the rectum as a result of a tumor (COLORECTAL CANCER), surgical resection of part of the intestine, or aging
- Decreased rectal sensation because of DIABETES or stool impaction (see INTESTINAL OBSTRUCTION)
- Damaged rectal sphincters or damage to the nerves that control their function such as unrecognized trauma from vaginal delivery in women, spinal cord problems, or laxity of pelvic muscles with aging

APPROACH

Isolated episodes of fecal incontinence, although obviously distressing to the patient, may need no extensive evaluation. A PHYSICAL EXAMINATION would involve a digital examination of the rectal sphincter and a test of the sensation around the rectum to assess for stool impaction (see INTESTINAL OBSTRUCTION), local inflammation, or nerve damage.

Repeated episodes of fecal incontinence would be evaluated by several measures including

- Sigmoidoscopy or colonoscopy (see ENDOSCOPY) to assess the capacity of the rectum and reveal any obstruction or inflammation
- A barium X ray (RADIOGRAPHY) of the colon
- In complicated cases, tests of rectal sphincter and nerve function or tests of anorectal motility, which involve placing a small balloon in the rectum

At times, X-ray studies (RADIOGRAPHY) of rectal function called *defecography* or *proctography* may be done by placing small amounts of barium within the rectum and recording the process of defecation.

TREATMENT OPTIONS

If fecal incontinence is related to stool impaction (see INTESTINAL OBSTRUCTION), the impaction needs to be evacuated with cleansing enemas and the physician may implement a treatment program for chronic CONSTIPATION. In other circumstances, a variety of therapeutic options may be employed depending on the underlying cause of fecal incontinence.

Other options that may help with a fecal incontinence problem include

- Bowel training programs
- Biofeedback techniques
- Pharmacologic agents (such as psyllium to increase the bulk of the stool)
- Surgical procedures

Except for incontinence related to obvious prolapse of the rectum, in which the rectum drops out through the anus, surgery should be employed only after nonsurgical methods have failed.

BREAST PAIN OR LUMPS

Cancer is what most women think of when they find a lump or have breast pain. However, most often something else is the cause. It is still very important, however, to pursue such breast symptoms if persistent.

Women of all ages can have breast pain or lumps. About one in ten women will get BREAST CANCER at sometime in their life, usually between the ages of 50 and 70. Ninety percent of women, therefore, will never get BREAST CANCER. It is important to remember that many other things besides cancer can cause breast symptoms, and most are not serious.

CAUSES

Breast pain and tenderness can be caused by

- FIBROCYSTIC BREAST DISEASE
- Benign tumors
- BREAST CANCER
- Infection such as mastitis or an abscess
- Tenderness from hormones related to pregnancy, estrogen replacement therapy, birth control pills, or premenstrual syndrome

APPROACH

The MEDICAL HISTORY and PHYSICAL EXAMINATION will focus on caffeine intake, risk factors for BREAST CANCER, signs of infection such as FEVER, CELLULITIS near the nipple, and any recent medication intake. The examination will help distinguish a cyst from a more suspicious lump. A follow-up examination in one month or at a different time in a woman's cycle may help.

Persistent or suspicious lumps generally need to undergo BIOPSY. Mammogram (RADIOGRAPHY) and ULTRASOUND may be helpful, but about ten percent of BREAST CANCER is not seen by mammography so BIOPSY remains necessary.

TREATMENT OPTIONS

Decreasing caffeine and increasing vitamin E intake to 400 to 800 IU per day seems to help many women with FIBROCYSTIC BREAST DISEASE pain.

BREATH, BAD SMELLING

Bad breath is rarely a sign of serious illness and can usually be helped by improving dental hygiene and by avoiding spicy, aromatic foods.

Many patients sense that they have bad breath, or halitosis, but in reality do not. Breath that is offensive to others is a more reliable symptom than halitosis that is reported only by the patient.

CAUSES

Oral bacteria contribute substantially to halitosis. The normal activities of eating and drinking stimulate saliva, which cleanses the mouth and reduces bacterial count. Salivation and normal mouth cleansing are reduced during sleep, contributing to breath odor noted in the morning. Other causes include

- Diseases of the mouth, gums, and teeth
- Aromatic foods, such as onions and garlic
- Dairy products and large amounts of sugar, which provide a good substrate for oral bacteria
- Chronic infections of the sinuses (a rare cause)
- Problems related to delayed emptying of the stomach (peptic ULCER or INTESTINAL OBSTRUCTION)
- Gastroesophageal reflux (heartburn)

APPROACH

If the problem is corroborated by others and is persistent, dental and mouth examination by a dentist is a logical first step. If no problem is noted on examination of the mouth, a physician may ask about symptoms that could represent heartburn, peptic ULCER, or chronic sinus infection. Rarely, barium X rays (RADIOGRAPHY) of the esophagus or stomach, or even ENDOSCOPY of the stomach may be recommended.

TREATMENT OPTIONS

Dental hygiene with frequent brushing, flossing, and occasional use of antiseptic mouthwash is a logical first step in treating halitosis. Occasional use of breath spray is acceptable. The chewing of sugar-free gum or use of sugar-free candy or breath mints stimulates salivary flow and decreases oral bacteria counts. Review of dietary habits and elimination or reduction of dairy products (especially milk and cheese) and spicy or aromatic foods may also be beneficial.

BREATHING DIFFICULTY

Most people with breathing difficulties adopt an increasingly inactive lifestyle, which can, in many cases, aggravate their condition.

In the normal state, breathing is not a conscious activity, except during exercise. A number of medical conditions alter this state, so that breathing is noticeable with minimal or no activity. Such conscious or labored breathing is often described as air hunger or shortness of breath. The medical term is *dyspnea*.

CAUSES

The most obvious and most common causes of breathing difficulties are lung conditions such as

- ASTHMA
- Chronic bronchitis (BRONCHITIS, CHRONIC)
- EMPHYSEMA
- PNEUMONIA

When lung conditions are the cause, other respiratory symptoms such as wheeze, COUGH, sputum production, and chest pain may be present.

A number of nonlung conditions cause dyspnea as well, but they are usually accompanied by other symptoms. For example

- CONGESTIVE HEART FAILURE results in episodes of shortness of breath that cause SLEEP PROBLEMS and ANKLE SWELLING.
- Severe ANEMIA is often accompanied by pale-colored nail beds and conjunctiva (the lining of the eyelids).
- Neuromuscular weakness may cause generalized weakness or specific coordination problems such as difficulty rising from a chair or SWALLOWING DIFFICULTIES.
- ANXIETY and hyperventilation are suspected in patients with certain personality traits and no other evidence of disease.

It should be noted that most dyspneic patients minimize their sense of breathlessness by adopting an increasingly sedentary lifestyle. This lack of any regular physical exercise results in general deconditioning and possibly overweight or OBESITY, all of which can further aggravate the sense of shortness of breath.

APPROACH

The approach to the dyspneic patient begins with a careful MEDICAL HISTORY and PHYSICAL EXAMINATION. More extensive testing is often needed to confirm the cause of dyspnea, including

- Chest X ray (RADIOGRAPHY)
- PULMONARY FUNCTION TESTING
- Arterial blood gas analysis (BLOOD TESTS)
- Complete BLOOD COUNT

If the diagnosis is not apparent after these tests, further information may be gathered with a formal exercise test, which is useful to distinguish lung from nonlung causes of breathlessness and echocardiography (ULTRASOUND) to assess cardiac function.

TREATMENT OPTIONS

Dyspnea is most effectively treated by addressing the underlying medical condition. For example

- In patients with lung disease, such as EMPHYSEMA, treatment should be aimed at improving lung function.
- In patients with CONGESTIVE HEART FAILURE, drugs such as DIGOXIN, FUROSEMIDE, or ENALAPRIL should be prescribed to improve heart function, thus decreasing breathing problems.
- In patients with ANEMIA, the red BLOOD COUNT should be restored by nutritional supplementation after the underlying cause of the ANEMIA is determined.

BRUISING, UNEXPLAINED

Unexplained bruising of the skin can be insignificant, or it can be a sign of a blood or bone marrow disorder. Therefore, a sudden onset of unexplained bruising should be evaluated.

A bruise is nothing more than blood under the skin. If blood leaks out of a blood vessel due to any cause, a bruise forms. It may be red, yellow, orange, or blue. Blue usually indicates a deeper bruise; the color is caused by the blood pigment, hemoglobin, reflected through skin tissue.

CAUSES

The most common cause of a bruise is blunt trauma to the skin, causing an opening in one of the skin blood vessels. Even after an insect bite, the injured skin vessel may leak into the skin and cause a bruise. People who have accumulated a lot of sunlight over a lifetime tend to have fragile skin blood vessels. They will notice very easy bruising in sunlight-exposed areas, such as the forearms. In these individuals, often bruises form just from normal pressure on the skin, without any injury or trauma.

A severe vitamin C deficiency can cause easy bruising. The classic sign of this deficiency, called *scurvy*, is a little bruise with a corkscrew-shaped hair rising from the bruise. Scurvy is very rare today.

When injured, the blood vessels should clot. If a problem exists with the elements in the blood that clot the vessels, the result may be thin blood that does not clot well and readily seeps out of the skin blood vessels, causing a bruise with even minor trauma. Possible causes include

- LEUKEMIA
- A defect in one of the clotting elements of the blood, particularly the platelets (thrombocytopenia)
- A problem with the bone marrow (which makes blood elements and cells) such as that caused by chemotherapy, alcohol, or insecticides.

If a person takes a lot of ASPIRIN or another nonsteroidal anti-inflammatory drug such as IBUPROFEN, the platelets in his or her blood do not clot properly and easy bruising may occur. In addition, patients who take systemic corticosteroid medications such as PREDNISONE often have easy bruising of the skin and overall thin skin.

The sudden onset of small red bruises on the lower legs and feet or forearms and wrists in conjunction with FEVER and general illness must be taken very seriously because it may mean an acute life-threatening infection such as Rocky Mountain spotted fever or spinal meningitis. Viral illness, drug allergies, and connective tissue diseases such as systemic LUPUS ERYTHEMATOSUS are other serious conditions in which the skin blood vessels become inflamed and leak blood, causing small bruises.

APPROACH

Often, a MEDICAL HISTORY combined with a PHYSICAL EXAMINATION can indicate the cause of the bruising problem. For example, sun-induced bruising is very common in middle-aged and elderly people, particularly those with fair complexions. The appearance of bruises on sun exposed areas of the body usually makes this diagnosis self-evident. The physician may inquire about any medications the patient is taking such as ASPIRIN, IBUPROFEN, or PREDNISONE.

The sudden onset of generalized bruising or bruising after an activity in which such bruising usually does not occur (such as water skiing, light exercise, rowing, jumping, and so on) dictates a careful examination by a physician. In addition, laboratory tests to evaluate the clotting elements in the blood and to make sure that the bone marrow is producing the right amounts of blood cells and platelets (see BLOOD TESTS; BLOOD COUNT) should be done.

The sudden onset of small bruises over the arms, hands, lower legs, and feet in association with FEVER and generalized illness must be considered a serious infection or vasculitis until proved otherwise. BLOOD TESTS (white BLOOD COUNT, bacterial CULTURE) may taken to evaluate whether the patient has an infection. To determine the possibility of vasculitis, the physician will ask about any recent illnesses and medications. To diagnose vasculitis, BLOOD TESTS and a BIOPSY of the skin are often necessary.

TREATMENT OPTIONS

When bruising stems from a serious condition such as LEUKEMIA, bone marrow disorders, systemic infection, or vasculitis, the treatment depends upon the cause. For simple, benign causes of bruising (use of ASPIRIN, IBUPROFEN, corticosteroids, or other medications), the treatment is stopping the medication if possible. Sometimes use of these medications is necessary, and the patient must learn to live with some easy bruising of the skin. For easy bruising due to the accumulation of sunlight and perhaps other types of light over a lifetime, the only effective treatment is keeping the skin covered.

BURPING

Burping is rarely a sign of any serious medical problem.

Burping is the voluntary expelling of trapped air from the stomach into the esophagus.

CAUSES

Most burping is related to conscious or unrecognized air swallowing. The swallowed air builds to a certain pressure within the stomach, causing relaxation of the valve between the stomach and esophagus (called the *lower esophageal sphincter*). Air is then expelled into the esophagus and mouth. Burping certainly can occur after ingesting large amounts of food or carbonated beverages and may be related to acid reflux (heartburn), but in rare instances, it can be caused by significant gastrointestinal disease.

APPROACH

Typically, no special tests or examinations need to be done. A physician may elicit a history of heartburn which may be a rare cause of burping. Frequently, it is difficult for patients to realize that they are swallowing air and causing the burp simply because the problem has been present for a long time and has become an unconscious habit.

TREATMENT OPTIONS

Reassurance without specific therapy is usually all that is needed. Appropriate preventive maneuvers include

- Avoiding large quantities of carbonated beverages
- Avoiding chewing gum
- Eating slowly
- Chewing food thoroughly

CHEST PAIN

Sudden severe chest discomfort is a potentially ominous symptom; it should be considered an emergency that requires rapid evaluation by a medical professional. Milder, recurrent, episodic chest discomfort, however, can be evaluated more leisurely in the setting of an office visit.

Although many people associate this symptom with heart attack, chest discomfort is not always a sign of life-threatening illness. Many conditions—some very mild—can cause pain in the chest.

CAUSES

Common causes of chest pain include

- Muscle or ligament strain in the chest wall
- Gastrointestinal problems such as inflammation of the esophagus, peptic ulcer disease (see ULCER), upper colon problems, and heartburn
- Psychological problems such as ANXIETY, DEPRESSION, or panic attacks
- Heart and lung problems such as pleurisy, pericarditis, and ANGINA (the most common cardiac cause)

HEART ATTACK (called *myocardial infarction*), tears in the aorta sometimes associated with ANEURYSM, and PULMONARY EMBOLISM are among the life-threatening causes.

APPROACH

Severe sudden chest pain needs to be evaluated rapidly with a careful MEDICAL HISTORY, PHYSICAL EXAMINATION, ELECTROCARDIOGRAPHY, and often a chest X ray (RADIOGRAPHY) to ascertain whether the symptom is being caused by a life-threatening condition. Characteristics of the pain can be important clues. Some questions might include

- What brings on the pain—effort, cold wind, swallowing, changes in position?
- What makes the pain go away—antacids, rest, changes in position?
- What is associated with the pain—BREATHING DIFFICULTY, nausea?
- What is the nature of the pain—burning, pressure, or sharp pain?

Tests that may be useful include

- ELECTROCARDIOGRAPHY
- BLOOD PRESSURE TESTING
- X ray (RADIOGRAPHY) of the chest and stomach
- Treadmill tests (CARDIAC STRESS TEST)
- Exploration of the psychosocial stressors and other clues to ANXIETY or DEPRESSION

CONFUSION

Confusion can be difficult to define and even harder to recognize as a symptom, but it can be a manifestation of significant disease.

Confusion is a disordered thought process that can be caused by a variety of diseases affecting the brain. It can be a difficult symptom to understand because it is very subjective and can have many manifestations. Confusion can be a disorientation regarding

- Time
- Place
- Situation
- People

Failure to recognize or understand any of these appropriately could be evidence of medically significant confusion.

Depending on the cause of the confusion, the symptoms can be mild and fleeting or they can be quite severe and prolonged. The severity may also vary or progress over time. In some instances, people can experience periods of extremely confused behavior immediately preceded and followed by absolutely normal behavior.

The fact that periods of confusion are sometimes transient and resolve on their own should not lead the patient to ignore the symptom. Confusion can be a sign of significant disease and should be evaluated by a health professional.

CAUSES

Confusion is produced when the brain's normal functioning is altered. There are several possible ways this can happen. One possibility is any of the diseases that affect the brain directly. Causes that fall under this category include

- Degenerative diseases of the brain such as ALZHEIMER DISEASE and PARKINSON DISEASE
- Some brain tumors
- Some infections of the brain such as meningitis, encephalitis, and syphilis
- Some types of seizures seen in the disease epilepsy

Other possible causes of confusion not directly related to the brain include

- Low or very high blood sugar levels that can occur in people with diabetes when tight control is not maintained
- Systemic diseases such as severe liver disease or kidney disease
- The side effects or overdose of certain medications such as tranquilizers, sedatives (LORAZEPAM and TRIAZOLAM), and narcotics (CODEINE and MORPHINE)

APPROACH

Because of the many potential causes of confusion, there is no set approach to determining the cause. Information about the period of confusion is usually the most helpful. Significant factors sought in the MEDICAL HISTORY are

- How and when the confusion first began or became noticeable
- Whether it has been constant, progressive, or intermittent
- Any past illness
- Any medication use including prescription, over-the-counter, and illicit drug use

Tests that may be performed include

- A general PHYSICAL EXAMINATION
- A neurologic examination
- Blood testing (see BLOOD TESTS)
- Urine testing (URINALYSIS)
- COMPUTED TOMOGRAPHY of the head and neck area
- MAGNETIC RESONANCE IMAGING of the head and neck area
- ELECTROENCEPHALOGRAPHY, if a brain disease is suspected

TREATMENT OPTIONS

A trial period in which medications that could be contributing to the confusion are stopped may be one possible course of action. Optimizing the treatment of other conditions may also help.

COUGH

Coughing is a common symptom that rarely signifies a serious problem, but a cough that continues for months or years invariably disrupts life, resulting in fatigue, sleep problems, and isolation.

In general, cough protects the lung by forcefully eliminating harmful elements from the tracheobronchial tree. It is a vital mechanism to clear foreign material (as when food "goes down the wrong pipe"), pus (as in PNEUMONIA), and excess mucus (as in ASTHMA and chronic bronchitis [BRONCHITIS, CHRONIC]). On the other hand, cough that does not produce mucus—a dry cough—may not be of obvious benefit.

All of us experience cough during upper respiratory tract infections such as the COMMON COLD. Cough in this setting may last for several weeks, but it invariably goes away on its own. Cough that is present for more than a month is distinctly unusual, and suggests another medical condition.

CAUSES

The most common causes of cough include

- Cigarette smoking (chronic smoker's cough)
- Air pollution
- Postnasal drip (see NOSE, STUFFY OR RUNNY)
- ASTHMA
- Gastroesophageal reflux (heartburn)
- EMPHYSEMA
- Chronic bronchitis (BRONCHITIS, CHRONIC)
- Cystic fibrosis
- Upper respiratory tract infections such as the COMMON COLD or INFLUENZA
- Head and neck cancer, such as LARYNGEAL CANCER
- LUNG CANCER
- Bronchiectasis (abnormal dilation of the bronchial tree leading to collection of mucus)
- CONGESTIVE HEART FAILURE
- ANXIETY
- Pulmonary fibrosis or scarring
- PNEUMONIA
- Tuberculosis
- Some medications such as ACE inhibitors (ENALAPRIL or CAPTOPRIL) commonly used in HYPERTENSION

APPROACH

The single most important factor in patients with chronic cough is whether or not they smoke. In smokers, the complete cessation of smoking effectively eliminates cough about 50 percent of the time.

Next, it is significant whether cough is productive of mucus or whether it is dry. Productive cough is seen in conditions such as chronic bronchitis (BRONCHITIS, CHRONIC) and bronchiectasis, whereas chronic dry cough or minimally productive cough may be seen in chronic postnasal drip, ASTHMA, heartburn, or drug-induced cough.

Routine tests to establish the cause of cough include

- Chest or sinus X rays (RADIOGRAPHY)
- PULMONARY FUNCTION TESTING
- A provocative test when ASTHMA is suspected (but not proved by routine PULMONARY FUNCTION TESTING)
- Monitoring of esophageal acidity or radiographic studies (RADIOGRAPHY) when heartburn is suspected

TREATMENT OPTIONS

The most effective treatment of cough is to treat the underlying condition. For example

- For cough associated with the COMMON COLD, expectorants are useful to loosen thick and difficult to clear sputum.
- For dry cough, cough suppressants may be tried; increasing water intake decreases the sense of throat tickle in many cases.
- For cough associated with smoking, complete cessation of smoking is the only effective treatment.
- For chronic productive cough related to chronic bronchitis (BRONCHITIS, CHRONIC) and EMPHYSEMA, smoking cessation combined with bronchodilator medications such as THEOPHYLLINE or ALBUTEROL improves cough.
- For productive cough, cough suppressants and antihistamines are best avoided for fear that these medications will interfere with mucus clearance.
- For a dry or minimally productive cough in nonsmokers with a normal chest X ray (RADIOGRAPHY), speech therapy techniques and specific breathing techniques are extremely helpful to decrease unnecessary throat clearing and cough. Such techniques are preferable to cough suppressant medications, which are generally quite disappointing for these patients.

DIARRHEA

Diarrhea is a very common symptom and is usually not a serious sign of illness; it usually resolves after a few days.

Although most patients know what it is intuitively and think it superfluous to define diarrhea, it is important to define this very common symptom objectively. Diarrhea is the passage of large volumes of unformed or liquid stool. Some patients feel that frequent trips to the toilet equate to diarrhea, but physicians define diarrhea as a volume of stool greater than 200 grams (approximately six ounces) in a 24-hour period. Some patients may have the urge to defecate frequently, but unless the stool is unformed and the volume large enough, it does not constitute diarrhea.

CAUSES

Diarrhea is most frequently a self-limited illness of three or four days and is usually caused by an infection. The most common infection is caused by a virus such as rotavirus or Norwalk agent virus, but bacteria such as *Salmonella*, *Shigella*, *Campylobacter*, and toxigenic *Escherichia coli* (the cause of "traveler's diarrhea") are also culprits.

Dietary causes of diarrhea are also very common but tend to last 24 hours or less and include overindulgence in rich food, lactose intolerance, and food poisoning. Overuse of artificially sweetened foods, candies, or soft drinks may also induce diarrhea.

Various medications (prescription and over the counter) such as antacids and antibiotics are also very common causes of diarrhea.

Diarrhea that lasts more than three or four weeks brings in the possibility of a large variety of diseases, including chronic PANCREATITIS, sprue (a rare sensitivity to wheat protein), and bacterial overgrowth that cause diarrhea by interfering with intestinal absorption of nutrients.

Recurrent diarrhea can also be a sign of IRRITABLE BOWEL SYNDROME.

APPROACH

Most diarrhea is self-limited and runs its course in several days and does not need extensive evaluation. However, investigation by a physician is warranted if the patient experiences

- Diarrhea that lasts more than four weeks
- High FEVER (higher than 101°F)
- ABDOMINAL PAIN

- Diarrhea that awakens one from a good sleep
- RECTAL BLEEDING

Evaluation includes a PHYSICAL EXAMINATION and possibly a stool sample to determine if a serious bacterial infection has occurred. The physician focuses on whether the patient is suffering from DEHYDRATION and whether the abdomen is tender or distended (see ABDOMINAL PAIN; ABDOMINAL SWELLING).

The patient's recent history may provide important clues. Viral diarrhea, for example, may start in infants or young children and be spread through the family. Travel (even travel to modern and industrialized areas) may expose the patient to new bacteria or viruses, and certain foods may induce diarrhea.

TREATMENT OPTIONS

Because most diarrhea will run its course in several days, direct treatment is often not needed. There is no effective medication for the most common cause of diarrhea—viral infection—and it remains quite controversial whether antibiotics make any major difference even in bacterial infections that lead to diarrhea.

The most important option to prevent complications is to insure adequate hydration. This can be achieved by limiting solid food and maintaining a diet of clear liquids (soft drinks, broth, juices, and water) supplemented by some source of sodium such as crackers. Liquid supplements are also commercially available but are not always needed, especially if the patient can maintain hydration through the liberal use of clear liquids (two quarts or more in a 24 hour period).

Over-the-counter medications to slow diarrhea such as LOPERAMIDE can be used with discretion, but it must be remembered that these agents provide only some symptomatic relief and do not cure diarrhea. These agents should be avoided if there is substantial ABDOMINAL PAIN, FEVER, or RECTAL BLEEDING. Agents such as pectin that act as absorbers of water are probably safe, but their benefits are questionable.

Patients can resume their normal diets once the volume of diarrhea has decreased and their appetite returns. In some patients, use of dairy products may produce a temporary relapse because the diarrheal illness has temporarily depleted the intestine of the enzyme, lactase, that helps digest milk.

DIZZINESS

People use the word dizziness to describe a number of different feelings. These feelings can range from brief light-headedness to a near fainting spell. Dizziness is not usually serious, but on rare ocassion, it can be caused by problems that should not be ignored.

Doctors find it useful to divide dizziness into four categories:

- *Light-headedness* is a mild sensation that represents about one third of all people who see the doctor for dizziness.
- *Vertigo* is a more intense spinning sensation; it represents another third of cases.
- *Dysequilibrium* involves unsteadiness, balance problems, or stumbling; it represents about one fifth of cases.
- *Presyncope* is an episode of near FAINTING OR FAINTNESS; it represents only a few percent of cases.

CAUSES

As a general rule, light-headedness is associated with ANXIETY, DEPRESSION, panic attacks, or stress-related problems.

Vertigo is usually caused by an inner ear problem or a problem in a related portion of the brain. The body uses minute changes in position in the inner ear as a balancing device, hence these structures are suspect in cases of vertigo.

Dysequilibrium or unsteadiness can be caused by a number of problems with the body's sensory systems. These include problems with the nerves in the legs that help tell the brain the exact position of the ground. Vision problems (for example, CATARACTS) can also cause unsteadiness as can problems with the balance centers of the brain and inner ear.

Presyncope, or near-fainting spells, are usually caused by low blood pressure. Most commonly, low blood pressure is related to problems with the tone of the blood vessels and the nervous system reflexes responsible for maintaining adequate blood pressure when standing up. Less often, presyncope is related to heart rhythm irregularities (ARRHYTHMIAS). Actual FAINTING OR FAINTNESS and its causes are discussed elsewhere.

APPROACH

Other symptoms associated with dizziness can be a clue to the underlying cause.

- Changes in hearing or a ringing in the ears (EAR, RINGING OR BUZZING) when combined with vertigo-like dizziness suggests the inner ear or the nerves in that area might be involved.

- VOMITING and HEADACHE combined with dizziness can be signs of serious problems with the nervous system.
- Dizziness associated with certain types of head movements may be clues to inner ear problems or problems with the circulation to the brain.
- Dizziness associated with arm or leg weakness; NUMBNESS in the arm, leg, or face; difficulty talking; VISION DISTURBANCES; or clumsiness may all be clues to a circulation problem in the brain such as a transient ischemic attack (see STROKE).

Besides asking questions about related symptoms such as the ones mentioned above, the doctor may perform standing BLOOD PRESSURE TESTS and some BLOOD TESTS and may also listen to the heartbeat.

To examine the nervous system, the doctor may want to observe walking and certain head motions. A hearing test may also be needed. Depending on the initial results, more involved tests of the nervous system may be required, including MAGNETIC RESONANCE IMAGING, COMPUTED TOMOGRAPHY, and ELECTROENCEPHALOGRAPHY.

TREATMENT OPTIONS

Treatment of dizziness involves treating the underlying cause. The two most common types of vertigolike dizziness are benign positional vertigo and labyrinthitis (an inflammation of the inner ear). These problems are usually treated with the drug meclizine. Problems associated with low blood pressure can be treated with certain drugs to raise the blood pressure, such as fludrocortisone, or drugs to treat the ARRHYTHMIA causing the problem, such as PROCAINAMIDE, ATENOLOL, and DIGOXIN. For patients with dysequilibrium, sometimes correcting vision problems is the answer.

If the problem is persistent and has no apparent cause, certain exercises are sometimes useful in suppressing the feeling of vertigo. Using assisted walking devices such as canes or walkers can also be helpful. Stress reduction techniques and treatment for ANXIETY or DEPRESSION help many patients with light-headedness.

Rarely, surgery could be required for some of the inner ear and brain stem problems that cause dizziness.

EAR, RINGING OR BUZZING

A ringing or buzzing in the ear is a symptom frequently associated with hearing loss. All patients who experience it should have a hearing test done.

Tinnitus is the name for a noise that is heard in one or both ears without any obvious external stimulus. It may be described as a ringing, buzzing, or even hissing. The pitch and intensity varies among individuals. Tinnitus can be present without any obvious cause, but is usually a symptom of another illness. Therefore, all patients with tinnitus should be evaluated by a physician.

CAUSES

It is thought that the source of tinnitus is the hair cells that conduct hearing. The damaged hair cells in the inner ear send an abnormal signal to the brain that is interpreted as tinnitus.

Tinnitus is frequently caused by medications, including over-the-counter drugs. The most common medications that can cause tinnitus are ASPIRIN, IBUPROFEN, and medications for RHEUMATOID ARTHRITIS such as hydroxychloroquine.

There are a variety of ear-related problems that can cause tinnitus. Frequently, processes involving the middle ear can cause ringing. These include fluid or infections in the middle ear, eustachian tube dysfunction (inability to clear or pop one's ear), or disorders of the middle ear bones.

Tinnitus can also be caused by inner ear disorders. One of the more common ones is Meniere disease. This disease usually has a triad of symptoms including tinnitus, fluctuating hearing loss, and vertigo (DIZZINESS). There are some systemic illnesses that may affect the inner ear, too. These include inflammatory or infectious illness such as labyrinthitis.

Unfortunately, tinnitus can be associated with more severe illnesses. There are patients whose tinnitus can be heard by an observer. Usually this type of tinnitus is pulsatile in nature, being heard with every heartbeat. This can be a sign of vascular tumor affecting the ear and is frequently accompanied by a hearing loss. Tinnitus that affects only one ear that also has a hearing loss can be a sign of a problem involving the hearing nerve or the brain stem. There are tumors known as acoustic neuromas that can cause this scenario. Fortunately, these tumors are uncommon and benign.

If the tinnitus is associated with weakness, VISION DISTURBANCES, and incoordination, the possibility of a transient ischemic attack should be considered (see STROKE).

Trauma that causes a concussion or damage to the ear drum can also provoke tinnitus.

APPROACH

The evaluation of this symptom would start with a MEDICAL HISTORY focusing especially on recent medication use, past illnesses, and possibly any acoustically traumatic events. Other associated symptoms, such as DIZZINESS or hearing loss, may help narrow the possibilities. A hearing test and an examination of the ear in question with an otoscope (a device for looking in the ear canal) are also usually performed. A general PHYSICAL EXAMINATION, particularly a neurologic examination of the head, is helpful.

More extensive tests may be necessary depending on the suspected diagnosis. MAGNETIC RESONANCE IMAGING of the head may be done to locate structural problems in the ear or tumors that affect hearing. A BLOOD COUNT to rule out ANEMIA and blood flow studies (ULTRASOUND) to test the circulation to the brain may also be appropriate.

TREATMENT OPTIONS

There are several medications that may be of some benefit. They include several antidepressant medications such as AMITRIPTYLINE, anti-anxiety medications such as DIAZEPAM, diuretics such as HYDROCHLOROTHIAZIDE, and steroids such as PREDNISONE.

For people with moderate to severe hearing loss, a hearing aid can sometimes help. The increased sound delivered to the ear through the hearing aid can help make the tinnitus less noticeable.

There are also devices that can produce white noise that can help mask the tinnitus. Such a device can either be worn in the ear, or a larger one can be placed in the environment. The results with these devices have not been encouraging.

Many patients join support groups usually sponsored through the American Tinnitus Association. This association provides continuing education to the affected individuals through seminars and newsletters. In some severe cases, patients are referred for psychiatric counseling. There are many individuals who have stressors in life that can make the tinnitus worse, and counseling may be an option for those people. Biofeedback has also been used with some success.

EARACHE

Earache is a common complaint that prompts many visits to doctors' offices and emergency departments.

Although commonly thought of as a problem that affects children, earaches can and do occur in people of all ages. In an effort to identify the cause of and best treatment for this symptom, careful evaluation of the ear and its surrounding anatomy is essential.

CAUSES

Common causes of earache include

- Middle ear infections
- Ear canal infections (swimmer's ear)
- Swelling of the lymph glands in the area
- External ear infections
- Disturbances of the joint of the jaw (TEMPOROMANDIBULAR DISORDER)

Less common causes of ear pain include

- Infections of the mastoid bone behind the ear (mastoiditis)
- Foreign bodies in the external ear canal
- Tonsillitis
- Herpes zoster infections (SHINGLES) of the nerve pathway around the ear
- Pressure-related injury (called *barotrauma*) to the eardrum
- Wax impactions

APPROACH

The history of the symptom including the onset, duration, character, specific location, and the intensity of the earache is very important in identifying the cause of the symptom.

Intense pain in the ear followed by rapid resolution and purulent discharge from the ear suggests a middle ear infection with subsequent perforation of the eardrum. Viral infections of the middle ear usually accompany or immediately follow an upper respiratory tract infection such as the COMMON COLD or INFLUENZA.

Earache associated with chewing suggests TEMPOROMANDIBULAR DISORDER or an infection of the external areas of the ear.

Pain behind the ear in an individual who has experienced recurrent ear infections for a long time suggests infection of the mastoid bone (mastoiditis). This type of radiating pain can also be a sign that the pain is being referred from another area such as infected tonsils (tonsillitis). A vague or intense pain around the ear can herald the eruption of a herpes zoster rash (SHINGLES).

People who swim regularly can develop an infection of the external ear canal, so a history of recent swimming can be a diagnostic clue. Recent airline travel may also be a clue; airline travel is associated with pressure injuries. An acute onset of pain and a diminished sense of hearing after swimming, showering, or attempting to clean one's ears could be evidence of an earwax blockage in the external canal.

Most of the above conditions can be quickly diagnosed by a physician who listens to the relevant MEDICAL HISTORY and inspects the ear. During an examination of the ear, the physician will probably look in the ear canal with a special device called an *otoscope* and may feel the surrounding structures for clues as to the exact location of the pain.

Occasionally, a specialist in ear, nose, and throat medicine (an otolaryngologist) may be needed to perform more thorough or complex diagnostic evaluations.

TREATMENT OPTIONS

Treatment of earache involves treating the underlying cause:

- Bacterial infections of the middle and external ear necessitate antibiotic therapy with AMOXICILLIN, trimethoprim, or sulfamethoxazole.
- Viral infections may require antiviral therapy (acyclovir for herpes zoster infection) and therapy, such as decongestant medication, aimed at relieving specific aspects of the symptom.
- The presence of foreign matter in the ear canal or wax impactions require removal of the offending material.

EYE PAIN

Eye pain ranges from minor irritation to achiness to stinging. Although it usually heralds a problem with the eye itself, it can also be associated with conditions elsewhere.

Eye pain can be characterized in three ways. A patient may complain of

- A foreign body sensation—irritation, scratchiness, a sandy sensation, or a stinging feeling, like something is in the eye
- Aching or deep discomfort, like a toothache or dull pressure
- ITCHING of the eye

CAUSES

A foreign body sensation nearly always feels like something is indeed in the eye. More often than not there is no true foreign body. However, if one has been out in the wind, working under a car, grinding metal, or otherwise at risk for a foreign body, it is possible.

This type of discomfort can also be the first symptom of an eye infection. Conjunctivitis and corneal ulcers may be heralded by this symptom. Contact lens wearers at risk for infections involving the front tissue of the eye should immediately remove the contact lens from the affected eye.

Chronic dry eye or corneal abrasion are examples of noninfectious causes of foreign body sensation.

Aching discomfort is often a symptom of deeper inflammation of the eye. However, this symptom may occur in patients who need glasses, but choose not to wear them. It can occur in patients prone to crossed or wall eyes.

It can also be caused from head or neck problems away from the eye such as

- Tooth decay
- Abnormal jaw function (see TEMPOROMANDIBULAR DISORDER)
- Sinus disease
- RHEUMATOID ARTHRITIS of the neck.

Pain that occurs away from the true source is called *referred pain*. Infections or inflammations within the eye or the eye socket (such as blepharitis) and sudden elevations in the inner fluid pressure of the eye (GLAUCOMA) can cause this type of discomfort.

ITCHING is usually associated with allergy. This can be a drug allergy, a reaction to make-up, hay fever, or a reaction to some other environmental stimulus.

APPROACH

Persistent pain, especially in the presence of redness or VISION DISTURBANCES, should prompt a call to the ophthalmologist. The eye doctor will ask several questions, such as

- What was happening when the pain began?
- Was the onset of pain sudden or gradual and how long has it gone on?
- Has it ever occurred before?
- Is the pain constant or intermittent?
- Is it severe or mild and is the intensity changing?
- Are there associated eye problems such as redness, light sensitivity, VISION DISTURBANCES, or eye discharge?
- Was the eye injured in any way?
- Are there any significant past medical or eye problems?

A foreign body sensation must be carefully evaluated by a doctor. The affected eye needs to be inspected for the presence of a foreign particle; this includes flipping the upper lid to look for a hidden foreign body.

TREATMENT OPTIONS

Avoiding the allergen or causal substance will prevent the release of the chemicals in the eye responsible for the symptoms. Cold compresses made by soaking a wash cloth in cold tap water should be held over the closed eyes for a few minutes several times each day for symptomatic relief.

Unless the symptom is quite mild, a physician and possibly an ophthalmologist should be consulted. An eye examination may be necessary to determine the best course of action. While ASPIRIN or acetaminophen may help reduce pain from any cause, the best solution is to uncover the source of the problem and address it.

FAINTING OR FAINTNESS

The feeling of almost passing out is a common experience. About one third of healthy young people report having had at least one episode of fainting.

Fainting or faintness (known medically as *syncope*) is not usually the sign of a major problem. Most people will feel faintness from simply standing up too quickly after squatting or lying down. Less often, fainting or faintness is a sign of a serious disease.

CAUSES

Fainting is generally caused by the body's inability to maintain adequate blood pressure in the brain, thus depriving the brain of oxygen and leading to a loss of consciousness. This inadequate blood pressure can be caused by something as simple as standing for extended periods.

Less common causes include

- Seizures
- Heart rhythm abnormalities (ARRHYTHMIAS) or pumping problems
- Low blood sugar levels
- Low blood oxygen levels
- Specific physical situations that interfere with brain circulation (for example, coughing)

In approximately one fourth of all cases, no exact cause is ever determined despite reasonable efforts.

APPROACH

Clues that may indicate the underlying cause of fainting or faintness include

- The position of the individual at the time of the episode (for example, getting up from bed)
- The activity the individual was engaged in (for example, straining physical work)
- The general situation (for example, standing in a hot, stuffy, crowded room)
- Any specific provocation (for example, the sight of blood or a large needle)

A further investigation into an episode of fainting would also include consideration of any associated symptoms such as

- Weakness in the arm
- BREATHING DIFFICULTY
- Nausea
- CHEST PAIN
- Seizures

A MEDICAL HISTORY of underlying heart disease and the use of medications that commonly affect blood pressure or heart rhythm may also help with the diagnosis. Certain drugs used to treat hypertension that may be pertinent include

- HYDROCHLOROTHIAZIDE
- CAPTOPRIL
- ATENOLOL
- NIFEDIPINE

Psychotropic drugs may also be of interest. These include

- AMITRIPTYLINE
- CHLORPROMAZINE

A PHYSICAL EXAMINATION would focus on BLOOD PRESSURE TESTING while lying down and then while standing for at least two minutes. The physician may also check the arteries in the neck, the heart, and neurologic function depending on what he or she suspects the underlying cause to be.

Additional tests are usually not necessary, but may include

- ELECTROCARDIOGRAPHY
- Various BLOOD TESTS
- Tilt-table testing

TREATMENT OPTIONS

Most fainting spells are isolated events, but they do warrant the review of a physician. Recurrent episodes are treated based on the underlying cause. For example, fainting caused by inadequate blood pressure when standing may be treated with elastic stockings that keep blood from pooling in the legs, a high-salt diet to increase blood pressure, or drugs such as fludrocortisone.

FATIGUE

As many as one quarter of the people seeing their primary care physician have fatigue of sufficient severity that it significantly compromises their ability to meet their daily responsibilities and to enjoy life.

Fatigue is discomfort or loss of efficiency experienced after physical or mental activity. It is distinct from weakness, which is a loss of power or strength, and from sleepiness, which is a difficulty or inability to stay awake.

When fatigue lasts for more than a few months, it is classified as chronic. Chronic fatigue is an exceedingly common symptom. It is one of the top ten reasons adults seek medical attention.

CAUSES

A wide range of illnesses and circumstances can cause chronic fatigue, including

- Psychological conditions such as DEPRESSION, ANXIETY, bereavement, and stress
- Excessive use of caffeine, alcohol, sedatives, or illicit drugs
- Some prescription drugs such as ATENOLOL and methyldopa used to treat HYPERTENSION
- Disorders that interfere with sleep such as irregular nighttime breathing, called *sleep apnea* or restless leg syndrome, called *nocturnal myoclonus* (see SLEEP PROBLEMS)
- Illnesses that affect the major body systems or organs such as the heart, lungs, kidneys, liver, blood, and nervous system
- Chronic infections, particularly viral HEPATITIS and certain forms of tuberculosis

The chronic fatigue syndrome is a well-publicized, rare cause of unremitting fatigue. It is 50 to 100 times less common than any other cause of chronic fatigue. In a significant minority of patients, a cause of the fatigue is never identified despite an extensive medical and psychological evaluation.

APPROACH

In some cases, the illness inducing the fatigue is readily apparent, but if not, the investigation into the symptom usually begins with a discussion of possible related symptoms. For example, if the fatigue is accompanied by BREATHING DIFFICULTY during exertion, heart and lung problems may be suspected; sleepiness, loud snoring, and HEADACHE may indicate a sleep disorder.

Given that psychological disorders are exceedingly common causes of fatigue, an inquiry into an individual's mood, intellectual functioning, and stress level is important. Referral to a mental health professional may be helpful.

A complete MEDICAL HISTORY may uncover clues from the health of other family members or from recent use of prescription or nonprescription drugs. Although the results of a PHYSICAL EXAMINATION are usually normal, in some cases, it can reveal an underlying illness.

More sophisticated diagnostic tests are usually reserved until a specific cause is suspected. However, if no illness or cause can be suspected from the MEDICAL HISTORY and PHYSICAL EXAMINATION, further investigation may include BLOOD TESTS to assess the patient's

- BLOOD COUNT
- Liver function
- Kidney function
- Pancreas function
- Thyroid function

TREATMENT OPTIONS

Therapy is, of course, aimed at treating the underlying disease. However, even when a specific cause is never identified, symptoms can usually be minimized by therapies that are designed to

- Enhance sleep
- Improve physical fitness
- Maintain mental health

FEVER

Fever that persists for days, is very high (104°F or higher), or is associated with other worrisome symptoms needs medical evaluation.

Fever is usually a sign of infection and is usually self-limited. Low-grade fever (that is, a fever less than 100.5°F) is commonplace with upper respiratory infections such as the COMMON COLD. Higher temperatures (101°F to 104°F) are seen with flu-like illness (INFLUENZA). The associated symptoms are the main determining factor in deciding about further diagnostic tests or specific treatment.

CAUSES

Viral illnesses are a common cause of fever. Examples include

- COMMON COLD
- INFLUENZA
- HEPATITIS
- Viral meningitis
- AIDS
- Mononucleosis

Bacterial illnesses that can cause a fever include

- PNEUMONIA
- Bacterial meningitis
- Otitis (ear infection)
- Sinusitis
- Urinary tract infection (BLADDER INFECTION)
- PELVIC INFLAMMATORY DISEASE
- Appendicitis
- Lyme disease
- Toxic shock syndrome
- Tuberculosis
- BLOOD POISONING
- Endocarditis

Fever can be a symptom of some forms of cancer, including

- HODGKIN DISEASE
- LEUKEMIA
- Lymphoma (LYMPHOMA, NON-HODGKIN)

Autoimmune diseases that can cause fever include

- LUPUS ERYTHEMATOSUS
- Sarcoidosis
- CROHN DISEASE
- SCLERODERMA

Parasitic diseases such as malaria and amebiasis also cause fever.

APPROACH

A MEDICAL HISTORY and PHYSICAL EXAMINATION will usually provide sufficient clues to make a diagnosis. CULTURES of the blood, urine, sputum, or spinal fluid (see LUMBAR PUNCTURE) may be necessary in some cases.

The most useful clues leading to a diagnosis include

- Any RASH or bruising (BRUISING, UNEXPLAINED) on the skin or mucous membranes of the mouth
- COUGH or BREATHING DIFFICULTY
- HEADACHE
- Nausea, VOMITING, or DIARRHEA
- Swollen glands
- Any localized pain
- Night sweats (SWEATING, EXCESSIVE)
- Bladder or pelvic symptoms such as pain during urination (URINATION, PAINFUL), urethral or VAGINAL DISCHARGE; painful testes (TESTICLES, PAINFUL OR SWOLLEN)

TREATMENT OPTIONS

For self-limited viral infections, treatments may include

- Acetaminophen or IBUPROFEN (ASPIRIN is to be avoided in children and young adults)
- Antibiotics for specific bacterial or parasitic infections
- Adequate fluids to replace the additional losses from perspiration

For any persistent fever, a diagnosis should be sought so that specific treatment can be given for the underlying cause.

HALLUCINATIONS

Hallucinations can be symptoms of serious disease, but more often, they have a simple cause.

Hallucinations are false sensory perceptions. They can involve vision, hearing, or occasionally touch and feeling. In some instances, the hallucinating individual is aware that the perceptions are not real, but in other cases, the hallucinations are perceived as being real. When hallucinations occur as part of mental illness, there are usually other behavioral and thought disturbances that accompany them, and the hallucinations are typically voices.

CAUSES

Drugs and psychiatric illness are the most common causes of hallucinations. Drugs including alcohol, prescription drugs, and especially illicit psychedelic drugs (LSD, psilocybin, and mescaline) can produce all types of hallucinations.

Less commonly, the symptom can be produced by brain diseases such as

- STROKE
- Transient ischemic attack
- Tumor
- Seizures such as those in epilepsy

APPROACH

Evaluation of the patient with hallucinations includes

- A MEDICAL HISTORY, in which the onset and nature of the hallucinations are determined, as are any other problems that preceded or appear to be related to their onset, such as drug and alcohol use
- A PHYSICAL EXAMINATION, which usually focuses on mental and neurologic function as well as any evidence of systemic illness
- Laboratory tests, the nature and extent of which are determined by the initial clinical examination and commonly include BLOOD TESTS and URINALYSIS
- Psychiatric evaluation for patients who appear to have no physical cause for their hallucinations

TREATMENT OPTIONS

Treatment is determined by the cause. Drugs such as HALOPERIDOL, risperidone, and THIORIDAZINE can be very effective in psychiatric causes and can also counteract hallucinations produced by other drugs.

HEADACHE

At one time or another almost 100 percent of the population will experience a headache.

There are many different types of headaches, but they can roughly be divided into two categories: 1) those that are not dangerous or not associated with a dangerous disease or condition; and 2) those that require immediate medical attention. Fortunately the vast majority of headaches are trivial and fall into the former category.

CAUSES

Benign headaches have a variety of causes, and although they can be very unpleasant, they are usually self-limiting to some degree. The most common causes are

- Muscle tension
- Eye strain
- Mild viral infection such as the COMMON COLD or INFLUENZA
- Stress, ANXIETY, or mild DEPRESSION
- Dental pain such as a toothache
- MIGRAINE HEADACHE
- Caffeine withdrawal
- HYPERTENSION
- Side effects of some medications such as FLUOXETINE, NITROGLYCERIN, antihypertensive drugs such as NIFEDIPINE, and bronchodilator drugs such as THEOPHYLLINE
- Minor trauma to the head

Less common are headaches that are caused by very serious problems:

- The "thunder clap" headache—the sudden onset of intense head pain—could be caused by a ruptured ANEURYSM.
- Headache associated with FEVER, malaise (general feeling of being unwell), CONFUSION, and NECK PAIN could be caused by meningitis (inflammation of the membrane surrounding the brain and spinal cord).
- Headache after a head cold associated with FEVER, malaise, and purulent nasal discharge could be caused by acute sinusitis.
- Headache associated with low-grade FEVER, malaise, muscle pain, and a loss of appetite (APPETITE, LOSS OF) in patients older than 50 could be caused by an inflammation of the arteries called *temporal arteritis*.
- Headache associated with nausea and VOMITING, weakness on one side of the body, NUMBNESS,

seizures, speech difficulty, SWALLOWING DIFFICULTIES, VISION DISTURBANCES, HALLUCINATIONS, or personality changes could be caused by a brain tumor or a clot in the brain (hematoma).

APPROACH

The physician will probably begin with a detailed medical history focusing on medication use, previous illness, and family medical history. The nature of and symptoms associated with the headache are also crucial. Important aspects include

- How long they have been occurring
- Whether they have changed over time
- Their frequency
- Their duration
- Whether they have a distinct location
- Whether they are preceded by specific symptoms such as vision disturbances or nausea (see MIGRAINE HEADACHE)
- Their character
- What makes them worse or better

A complete PHYSICAL EXAMINATION is usually performed, with special attention paid to the cranial nerves, which give function and sensation to the head, and the blood vessels in the head and neck. BLOOD TESTS and an eye examination (VISUAL ACUITY) may provide more clues. More complex diagnostic tests may include

- MAGNETIC RESONANCE IMAGING of the head and neck
- Angiography (a form of RADIOGRAPHY used to image blood vessels)
- ELECTROENCEPHALOGRAPHY

TREATMENT OPTIONS

Treatment, of course, depends on the underlying cause of the headaches. Most benign headaches respond to pain killers, either over-the-counter varieties (such as ASPIRIN, acetaminophen, and IBUPROFEN) or prescription (for example, mild narcotics such as CODEINE). Stress headaches can sometimes be treated by removing the stressor or by learning stress reduction techniques. MIGRAINE HEADACHES can sometimes be prevented with medical treatment.

ITCHING

Itching is common and most often due to a benign condition.

Itching is a symptom that is related to a mild pain but is perceived differently. Scratching probably helps relieve itching by overstimulating the area to the point where the nerve impulses from the skin to the brain are no longer perceived. People tend to itch and scratch more in the evenings and around bedtime when other external stimuli are lessened and the itching is more noticeable.

CAUSES

There are many internal and external causes of this symptom, including

- Any common skin disease, such as PSORIASIS or DERMATITIS
- A topical agent that irritates the skin or to which a person is allergic such as poison ivy resin, a perfume, a type of clothing, or a cosmetic
- A product that a person has used for many years without a problem, which suddenly becomes a source of itching
- Dry skin, very common in the middle-aged and elderly, which can result from the use of hot water, frequent bathing, and the generous use of soaps and detergents
- A complex of conditions consisting of easily irritable skin, hay fever, ASTHMA, and frank periods of skin DERMATITIS
- A number of diseases of the internal organs such as chronic KIDNEY FAILURE or primary biliary cirrhosis
- A high red blood cell count (see BLOOD COUNT), due either to genetics or to chronic lung diseases, which causes itching especially when one is getting out of a hot shower
- Reaction to certain medications such as HYDROCHLOROTHIAZIDE
- An underlying malignancy, especially lymphoma (see LYMPHOMA, NON-HODGKIN), although this is rare

APPROACH

A MEDICAL HISTORY of childhood or other skin diseases, ASTHMA or hay fever, and systemic diseases is taken. A list of current medications is needed along with a critical evaluation of the need for these medications and whether the onset of the itching corresponded to the onset of the use of one or more of the current medications. The types of personal soaps, fragrances, moisturizing creams, fabric softeners, laundry powders, and bathing habits may give clues to the cause of itching. The frequent habit of bathing with harsh soaps and hot water suggests that dry skin is the culprit.

PHYSICAL EXAMINATION of the skin is necessary, and skin conditions such as DERMATITIS are directly viewed. When skin dries out, it may invoke a patchy DERMATITIS (redness with scale). A localized scaly red patch on the feet, soles, groin, or flank may suggest a fungal infection that may itch. In this case, the scale must be scraped and examined for fungi.

When no obvious cause for the itching can be ascertained and when the itching is persistent, the physician is obligated to search for an underlying cause. This evaluation will include a chest X ray (RADIOGRAPHY), evaluation of the BLOOD COUNT, and examination of certain biochemical elements associated with blood, kidney, and liver disease (see BLOOD TESTS). When lymphoma (LYMPHOMA, NON-HODGKIN) limited to the skin is considered, a skin BIOPSY must be obtained for microscopic examination. If a drug is being used and can be discontinued, it should be to see if the itching improves or abates.

TREATMENT OPTIONS

- Avoiding frequent bathing, hot water, and harsh soaps
- Using topical agents that bring moisture back to the skin
- Soaking in a tub without soap and then applying these topical agents immediately after soaking
- The use of antihistamines such as DIPHENHYDRAMINE or HYDROXYZINE
- Avoiding wool or polyester fabrics and potentially irritating topical preparations such as fragrances, harsh body soaps, cosmetics, and astringents
- Treating any underlying skin disease or systemic disease
- Specific therapy for itching due to certain internal diseases (Patients with severe kidney disease may need to have their itching treated with ultraviolet light treatments.)

MEMORY PROBLEMS

Nearly everyone notices changes in memory as they get older, but not all components of memory are affected by the aging process.

Mild changes in memory function do occur as people age, but these changes should not substantially interfere with performance. Some changes are signs of other problems.

From a practical point of view, what people notice as they age is particular difficulty remembering names, the need for additional repetitions to learn new items, and some degree of randomness to the memory errors they make (that is, items are not consistently forgotten). When the memory system is affected by actual disease, there is a more consistent inability to recall items and repetition of material is less and less effective in improving memory performance. Progressive decline in memory eventually affects old knowledge—usually minimally affected by the aging process—and performance is affected in most, if not all, daily activities.

CAUSES

There are many factors that affect memory processes. Even in healthy people, the decreased attentiveness that can accompany a lack of sleep or moderate illness may be enough to cause apparent difficulties in memory performance. However, performance usually returns to normal when the offending factor resolves.

Drug intoxicants can cause varying degrees of memory problems. Prescription drugs that can cause subtle deficits in attention or metabolic processes involved in memory include

- Sedatives such as LORAZEPAM and TRIAZOLAM
- Psychoactive drugs such as antidepressants or major tranquilizers
- Diuretics such as HYDROCHLOROTHIAZIDE and FUROSEMIDE
- Steroid hormones such as PREDNISONE

Chemical intoxicants other than medications can affect memory and attention functions. These substances include

- Alcohol
- Volatile agents or gases such as toluene and carbon monoxide
- Illicit drugs
- Heavy metals such as lead, arsenic, and mercury

Systemic disorders affecting the body in general can interfere with memory. These disorders include

- Cardiovascular disorders such as CONGESTIVE HEART FAILURE

- Pulmonary disorders such as EMPHYSEMA
- Renal (kidney) disorders such as KIDNEY FAILURE
- Hepatic (liver) disorders such as cirrhosis
- Endocrine (glandular) disorders such as CUSHING SYNDROME, HYPOTHYROIDISM, and HYPERTHYROIDISM
- Certain cancers such as small-cell LUNG CANCER
- Deficiencies of vitamin B_{12} or thiamin
- Infections that cause FEVER, particularly in the elderly

Environmental agents or situations can cause disorientation and apparent memory problems. These include

- Hospitalization
- Isolation
- Absence of day and night cues

Finally, brain disorders can directly affect memory areas. These disorders include

- Degenerative disorders such as ALZHEIMER DISEASE and PARKINSON DISEASE
- Vascular diseases of the brain such as ATHEROSCLEROSIS, ANEURYSM, and STROKE
- Trauma such as concussion
- Brain infections such as meningitis, encephalitis, and syphilis
- Brain tumors
- Severe epilepsy

APPROACH

Diagnosis of memory disorders almost always begins with a detailed MEDICAL HISTORY and a PHYSICAL EXAMINATION, including a complete neurologic and mental status assessment. Mental status examination is a detailed review of various cognitive functions to check performance of attention, memory, language, visual-spatial function, abstract reasoning, insight, behavior, and judgement.

BLOOD TESTS can be useful to check for metabolic disturbances, systemic infections, and nutrient deficiencies.

Further tests, performed only when unusual features have been detected on earlier examination, can include

- ELECTROENCEPHALOGRAPHY
- COMPUTED TOMOGRAPHY
- MAGNETIC RESONANCE IMAGING
- LUMBAR PUNCTURE

MENSTRUAL IRREGULARITIES

Some variation in regularity and length of menses is normal, but persistent changes may be related to an underlying problem. Common menstrual irregularities include

- Mid-cycle spotting
- Missed period
- Heavier or lighter menstrual flow

(See VAGINAL BLEEDING for related problems.)

Menstruation is not always a perfectly predictable process and many irregularities in the cycle are not cause for concern.

CAUSES

Of course, pregnancy may be the cause of a missed period, but stress, both emotional and physical, can also cause a missed or delayed period. Birth control pills often help regulate menses but any variation in type of pill, time of day one takes the pill, or missed pills may throw off the cycle.

Other common causes of menstrual irregularity are

- FIBROID TUMORS
- Systemic bleeding disorders such as decreased number of platelets or other clotting protein disorders
- ENDOMETRIOSIS
- Thyroid imbalance (HYPERTHYROIDISM or HYPOTHYROIDISM)

APPROACH

The common diagnostic approach includes

- A MEDICAL HISTORY, focusing especially on past menstrual history and any clues to systemic illness (hormone imbalances, bleeding disorders)
- PHYSICAL EXAMINATION, including pelvic examination and PAP SMEAR
- Pregnancy test, either by BLOOD TEST or URINALYSIS
- BLOOD TESTS to check the level of thyroid hormone
- Other diagnostic tests (see VAGINAL BLEEDING)

TREATMENT OPTIONS

- Different preparations of birth control pills are frequently tried.
- Special causes of VAGINAL BLEEDING may require other therapies.
- Progressively bothersome FIBROID TUMORS may require surgical FIBROID TUMOR REMOVAL.

NECK PAIN

Neck pain occurs in a large percentage of the population, most often due to an overuse episode.

Most people experience some neck pain or ache for a limited period of time after an overuse episode or injury. Neck pain after an automobile crash or a severe fall or injury should be evaluated to exclude a BONE FRACTURE or ligament injury.

CAUSES

The most common cause of neck ache or neck pain is overuse of the neck muscle; this may be due to a positioning problem (as in working on the computer) or because of repetitive motions. Injuries involving falls or automobile crashes are also common; these should be carefully evaluated and may require some amount of time to resolve.

Rarely, meningitis and inflammatory conditions such as RHEUMATOID ARTHRITIS can be the cause of neck pain. Pain from the heart may also radiate into the neck (see ANGINA).

APPROACH

A MEDICAL HISTORY will be taken, including how the neck pain started. If the injury was traumatic, the way in which the neck was stressed may be helpful in deciding which part of the neck (disk, ligaments, muscles) may have been injured. Radiating pains into the arms or shoulders may be associated with nerve root problems; the doctor will also ask about any sensation or muscle strength changes.

The PHYSICAL EXAMINATION will be focused on the neck; range of motion testing, as well as direct examination of the muscles, may point toward the diagnosis. Upper extremity strength and sensation testing for those patients with radiating pain complaints may point out a specific level where the nerve roots are irritated. X rays (RADIOGRAPHY) are especially useful in cases where the neck pain has a traumatic cause, in order to eliminate the chance that a BONE FRACTURE is present.

TREATMENT OPTIONS

Most neck pain will respond to

- Rest and over-the-counter analgesics such as IBUPROFEN or acetaminophen
- A change in sleeping position to let the neck rest in the neutral position
- Prescription medicines such as etodolac and exercises or physical therapy

NOSE, STUFFY OR RUNNY

Stuffy or runny nose results when the lining of the mucous membranes in the nasal passages become inflamed (stuffy) and produce excess mucus (runny). Although a stuffy or runny nose is not usually a serious sign of illness, any nasal congestion lasting longer than a week should be investigated by a physician.

Perhaps the most commonly experienced symptom, stuffy nose can be a result of everything from minor irritations to major illnesses.

CAUSES

Stuffy or runny nose can be the result of

- Allergies, usually to pollen, dust, or molds
- Infections, either viral (the COMMON COLD or INFLUENZA), bacterial, or fungal
- Anatomic abnormalities, such as a deviated septum
- Nasal polyps or enlarged adenoids
- Systemic disease such as granulomatosis—a rare disorder affecting the sinuses, lungs, and kidneys
- Tumors, either benign or malignant

APPROACH

The investigation into the cause of a stuffy nose usually begins with a PHYSICAL EXAMINATION, in which the nose may be inspected visually. More extensive evaluation along these lines might include ENDOSCOPY of the nasal passages. To examine the internal structures, plain X rays (RADIOGRAPHY) may be useful, but COMPUTED TOMOGRAPHY is often the choice.

If specific causes are suspected, more targeted diagnostic testing may be performed, including

- ALLERGY TESTING
- Nasal air-flow measurements
- BIOPSY of suspicious areas

TREATMENT OPTIONS

Obstructions can sometimes be treated surgically, sometimes with lasers or cryosurgery. Septoplasty is a procedure to correct a deviated septum. Adenoidectomy is a procedure to remove enlarged adenoids.

Treatments aimed at alleviating the symptom include

- Topical steroid nasal sprays
- Decongestants such as pseudoephedrine
- Antihistamines such as chlorpheniramine
- Allergy shots

NUMBNESS

Numbness itself is difficult to treat without knowledge of the underlying cause.

Numbness is a sensory disturbance that consists of loss of sensation, the occurrence of abnormal sensations, or pain. When a sensory disturbance takes the form of an abnormal spontaneous sensation, such as burning, tingling, or "pins and needles," it is called a *paresthesia*. A *dysesthesia* is a disturbance in which an unpleasant and painful sensation is produced by a stimulus that is usually painless.

CAUSES

There are many causes of numbness. The location of the symptoms, the mode of onset, and the accompanying symptoms help to determine what part of the nervous system is causing the numbness. In general, sensory impairment can happen as a result of brain, spinal cord, or peripheral nerve involvement.

Some characteristics that suggest a serious cause of numbness are

- A sudden onset
- Involvement on one side of the body only
- Association with other symptoms such as VISION DISTUBANCES, slurred speech, weakness, and disequilibrium (see DIZZINESS)

Common types of sensory loss and their causes include

- Sciatica, characterized by shooting pain and sensory loss in the back of the leg, most often caused by a HERNIATED DISK or RHEUMATIOID ARTHRITIS of the lower back
- Peripheral neuropathy, characterized by an insidious onset of numbness and tingling of both feet, caused by damage to the ends of long nerves that such diseases as DIABETES and ALCOHOLISM can do
- Benign forms of sensory loss, in which a person may, for example, hyperventilate and experience tingling of all the extremities and of the mouth, caused by ANXIETY
- The combination of numbness of one part of the body and slurred speech possibly caused by a STROKE
- Sensory loss involving only a part of a limb and associated with sharp pain, suggesting a pinched nerve

APPROACH

Testing for numbness includes

- A complete MEDICAL HISTORY to assess possible drug-related or injury-related problems
- A PHYSICAL EXAMINATION, including a full neurologic examination, to determine what parts of the body are involved, how the numbness started, how it has progressed, and if there are any associated symptoms such as weakness, VISION DISTURBANCES, DIZZINESS, or difficulties with walking or any other specific tasks
- Depending on the patient's MEDICAL HISTORY and PHYSICAL EXAMINATION results, electromyography and nerve conduction studies to evaluate the peripheral nerves and help determine whether numbness is caused by a "pinched nerve" or a peripheral neuropathy
- BLOOD TESTS to find out if a peripheral neuropathy is the cause of numbness, to exclude DIABETES, vitamin deficiencies, and other possible causes related to systemic illness
- MAGNETIC RESONANCE IMAGING or COMPUTED TOMOGRAPHY of the brain and spinal cord, if abnormalities in these structures are believed to be the origin of the numbness

TREATMENT OPTIONS

The treatment of a sensory disturbance is directed at the underlying cause.

RASH

Rashes are very common and have a variety of causes ranging from infections to irritants to serious internal problems.

Rashes appear in various forms: small clear fluid-filled bumps (vesicles), red raised bumps (papules), flat red spots (macules), and raised red bumps with pus inside that may drain (pustules).

CAUSES

- Infections such as SHINGLES, Lyme disease, syphilis, ringworm, and scabies; childhood infections such as measles, rubella, and chicken pox; rare infections such as Rocky Mountain spotted fever and toxic shock syndrome
- Allergic or autoimmune diseases such as systemic LUPUS ERYTHEMATOSUS, hives (allergic drug reactions, some types of DERMATITIS), and sarcoidosis
- PSORIASIS
- Forms of SKIN CANCER (rare)

APPROACH

The MEDICAL HISTORY can be helpful in identifying irritants such as detergents, oils, and heavy metals like nickel or mercury found in leather products. Clues to a more systemic illness include mouth ulcers and swollen joints or lymph glands. Any new drug ingestion, including over-the-counter or health food store products, or viral infection should be reported to the doctor. Family history of PSORIASIS or DERMATITIS may be suggestive—ITCHING may be a useful clue.

The PHYSICAL EXAMINATION may include looking at the entire body's skin, the lymph nodes, and the abdomen. Characterizing the rash by location and type of rash helps to limit the possibilities of causes.

FEVER is an important clue. Scrapings, CULTURE, or even BIOPSY may be needed as well as certain BLOOD TESTS. ALLERGY TESTING for contact DERMATITIS may occasionally be necessary.

TREATMENT OPTIONS

Antihistamines such as DIPHENHYDRAMINE may be used for ITCHING. Steroid creams such as TRIAMCINOLONE, anti-fungal drugs such as griseofulvin and FLUCONAZOLE, or even systemic treatment with antibiotics or PREDNISONE may be needed depending on the underlying disease.

RECTAL BLEEDING

Most frequently, even if recurrent, rectal bleeding is not dangerous or life threatening.

Rectal bleeding is the passage of visible red blood through the rectum, usually with a bowel movement. It is a very common occurrence. It is seen primarily on the toilet paper or streaking the stool; on rare occasion, it is large in volume with clots. Most often the amount of blood passed is quite small and not immediately dangerous, although it should ultimately be discussed with a health care professional.

CAUSES

The most common causes of rectal bleeding are HEMORRHOIDS and anal fissures. HEMORRHOIDS are present in nearly all of us and are cushions of vascular tissue that line the rectal opening. Since HEMORRHOIDS are rich in blood vessels, they can bleed easily. Anal fissures are small cuts or scrapes in the anus that occur with straining during bowel movements. Anal fissures will frequently cause pain with defecation or burning after a bowel movement and at times can squirt blood into the toilet. Other causes of rectal bleeding occur less often but are more serious, including COLON POLYPS, COLORECTAL CANCER, and vascular malformations.

APPROACH

It is always appropriate to consult with a health professional about rectal bleeding. The physician will examine the rectum digitally. If the bleeding is recurrent or the source is not obvious, the physician may use anoscopy, sigmoidoscopy, or colonoscopy (all forms of ENDOSCOPY).

TREATMENT OPTIONS

Bleeding from HEMORRHOIDS or anal fissures can be alleviated by

- Stool softeners or fiber in the diet
- Sitting in a warm bath or tub
- Cleansing the anus with mild soap and water after bowel movements
- Tissues medicated with nonallergenic lotions
- Multiple local surgical techniques (HEMORRHOID BANDING, HEMORRHOID REMOVAL, application of cautery or heat, topical injection), especially in severe or repeatedly bothersome cases

SKIN CHANGES

Moles are sometimes present at birth, but they more often appear during childhood and adolescence. Skin changes are likely during pregnancy as well.

Moles are cells related to pigment-producing cells called *melanocytes* and can have a tan, brown, or black color. When a mole changes, this may be cause for some concern. A mole that bleeds, becomes elevated, becomes larger, changes color, or changes shape should be evaluated by a professional.

CAUSES

Benign causes of moles becoming darker or appearing larger occur

- During pregnancy
- While taking hormones such as oral contraceptives or estrogen replacement therapy
- With increased exposure to sunlight
- After injury to the mole and during the natural healing process

However, the main significant concern is when a mole changes because the cells within the mole become cancerous (SKIN CANCER). Melanoma is a pigmented SKIN CANCER that is of great concern, and this is the most dangerous cause of skin changes.

APPROACH

Melanoma can be cured when it is caught early and the pigmented tumor has not invaded the skin too deeply (see MALIGNANT MELANOMA REMOVAL). Therefore, the most conservative approach is to have any changing mole evaluated as soon as possible.

The doctor will evaluate the mole visually, perhaps with the aid of an optivisor or dermatoscope, which helps bring out the detailed features of the mole. During the evaluation, the clinician will make credit and debit columns out of the features of the mole.

On the credit side, he or she would like to see a symmetric mole that is

- Flat and nonpalpable
- Even, homogeneous color
- Regular, clear border
- No notching of the perimeter or fingers of pigment extending from the border

All of these features are on the side of the mole being benign. Some moles may have one or more hairs growing from them, and this also is usually considered a benign feature.

On the debit side, an asymmetric mole with an irregular border and containing variegated hues of tan, yellow, brown, red, and black would have features that signal atypical cells and perhaps a melanoma.

TREATMENT OPTIONS

Benign moles, or nevi, do not need to be treated. Moreover, if the patient desires to have the mole removed for cosmetic purposes, the clinician needs to inform the patient that he or she will be trading the mole for a scar.

One approach is to remove the mole by performing a shave BIOPSY. This type of wound does not require sutures, but the patient is inconvenienced by the necessity of tending to the wound on a daily basis for 10 to 16 days. There is also a recurrence rate of about 5 to 7 percent.

Alternatively, the mole can be excised with an elliptical incision and the margins of the ellipse sutured closed. The patient can have the sutures removed in 7 to 14 days, depending upon the site.

If there is a high index of suspicion that the lesion may be a melanoma (SKIN CANCER), the physician will excise the lesion (MALIGNANT MELANOMA REMOVAL) in order to provide enough material for the pathologist to determine the depth of the melanoma. This is important because the thickness and depth of the melanoma have implications for prognosis and treatment options.

If the index of suspicion for melanoma is low but there are features of the mole that are atypical or of concern, the physician may elect to remove it or at least obtain a BIOPSY of the specimen for viewing under the microscope by a trained dermatopathologist.

SLEEP PROBLEMS

Although 20 to 40 percent of the general population complain of insomnia occasionally, only about 15 percent feel they have a serious problem.

The most common sleep disorder is insomnia. Insomnia is the perception that sleep is not adequate. Insomnia may involve difficulty getting to sleep or difficulty remaining asleep. A closely related problem is sleepiness during the day, which can occur if nighttime sleep is not adequate.

CAUSES

Insomnia may be caused by many different conditions. Sometimes an acute stress in the life of the patient may cause insomnia. This acute insomnia may resolve when the life stress has abated, but this temporary insomnia may also become chronic if the patient develops poor sleep habits or hygiene.

Insomnia may also be associated with psychiatric disorders such as ANXIETY and DEPRESSION.

Certain medical conditions may be experienced as insomnia including

- Sleep apnea
- Nocturnal leg movements
- Urinary problems
- IRRITABLE BOWEL SYNDROME

Excessive daytime sleepiness may be caused by many conditions. The most serious medical condition associated with daytime sleepiness is the sleep apnea syndrome, in which the patient stops breathing for short periods of time at frequent intervals during the night. Narcolepsy, in which the patient requires an abnormal amount of sleep, also causes daytime sleeping as can leg movements occurring frequently during the night that continually wake the individual from a sound sleep.

APPROACH

The most important aspect of diagnosing the cause of insomnia involves a careful MEDICAL HISTORY, which can reveal important information about the duration of the problem, possible precipitating stresses, and poor sleep habits. Occasionally, it is necessary to do an overnight sleep study in a sleep laboratory to make sure that there are no breathing problems such as sleep apnea or leg movements that are disturbing sleep.

Evaluating excessive daytime somnolence also involves taking a careful MEDICAL HISTORY. Patients who are in their teens and 20s are more likely to have narcolepsy as a cause of their sleepiness, whereas breathing difficulties are more common in middle-aged men who snore. The overnight sleep study, and occasionally a daytime nap study, which measures just how sleepy the patient is, are very helpful in evaluating this problem.

TREATMENT OPTIONS

The treatment of insomnia depends on the cause. If a specific psychiatric or medical cause is found, treatment of this underlying problem frequently helps the insomnia. If no specific cause for insomnia is found, treatments that can be beneficial include

- Progressive relaxation
- Stress-reduction techniques
- Biofeedback

Sleeping medications such as temazepam may be useful in certain patients, but are usually prescribed for a limited time period.

The treatment of daytime somnolence also depends on the cause of the problem. Narcolepsy is treated with stimulant medications such as methylphenidate.

Sleep apnea responds best to a nasal mask (continuous positive airway pressure) that is worn at night and prevents the respiratory events from occurring. Sleep apnea responds less well to surgery on the palate.

Various medications may be used to treat leg movements at night, such as

- Dopaminergic medications (LEVODOPA)
- Benzodiazepines (CLONAZEPAM)
- Narcotics (CODEINE)

STOOL, ABNORMAL APPEARANCE

Only a few abnormalities in stool appearance, such as blackened stool or red blood with stools, may be cause for concern; other problems are usually not significant.

Many things influence the color and consistency of stool. Variations in size and color most frequently relate to changes in the diet and transit through the digestive tract. It is not unusual to see vegetable material (corn kernels, tomato skin) in stool. Bile from the liver and gallbladder interacts with dietary substances to give stool its color, which may normally vary from brown to green or even yellow. The amount of fiber in the diet dramatically influences the volume and consistency of stool.

CAUSES

Only several abnormalities in stool appearance should give rise to some concern. Stools that are pitch black and looser in consistency may represent bleeding in the stomach or upper intestinal system. Bacteria degrading small amounts of blood will cause the stool to turn black. In addition, the use of iron, bismuth subsalicylate, and occasionally beets or spinach may also cause stool to turn black.

The shape of stools is quite variable and rarely an indicator of underlying disease. Although physicians have worried that narrowing of stools may represent the development of cancer, it is rare that this symptom is of any dangerous significance.

Stools frequently float in the toilet and this is not a marker of illness but relates to the volume of air trapped within the stool. Stools that are greasy or have visible oil droplets may represent problems with adequate intestinal digestion or absorption of food.

Visible red blood with stools should raise some concern and, although most frequently relate to minor RECTAL BLEEDING from HEMORRHOIDS, deserve discussion with a health professional.

APPROACH

A dietary and MEDICAL HISTORY are usually the beginning of an inquiry into this symptom. The physician will digitally examine the rectum to be sure that no abnormalities are present. OCCULT BLOOD TESTING can detect any tiny amounts of blood hidden in the stool. At times, sigmoidoscopy (a form of ENDOSCOPY) may be performed through the rectum. If there is concern that there is internal bleeding or that digestive organs are not functioning properly, barium X rays (RADIOGRAPHY) of the stomach, small intestine, or colon may be done.

SWALLOWING DIFFICULTIES

The esophagus is a long muscular tube that runs from the throat into the stomach. It has no function in digesting food but serves as a conduit for food to pass into the stomach. Although gravity does most of the work, the esophagus has a muscular coat that aids in propelling food forward. The patient may experience food getting caught in the back of the throat, behind the breast bone, or in the "pit" of the stomach. Swallowing may also be painful.

Swallowing difficulties may result from problems within the esophagus itself or the muscles in the throat that initiate swallowing.

CAUSES

Swallowing difficulties should be attended to, as their causes can be serious. Causes include

- Narrowing of the esophagus due to scarring from acid reflux (peptic stricture)
- Development of a tumor
- Muscular weakness of the esophagus due to neurologic illness (myasthenia gravis) or STROKE
- Excessive muscular contraction of the esophagus
- Lower esophageal sphincter's lack of contraction
- Acid reflux and infections of the esophagus

APPROACH

Most swallowing problems require careful investigation. Barium X rays (RADIOGRAPHY) of the esophagus or gastrointestinal ENDOSCOPY are frequently the initial studies. More sophisticated tests of swallowing function, such as motility testing and video fluoroscopy (RADIOGRAPHY) of the throat and larynx, performed while a patient swallows a small amount of barium paste, may also be required.

TREATMENT OPTIONS

Treatment should be specifically directed toward the underlying cause of the problem. Empiric treatment with acid-blocking drugs (CIMETIDINE) or motility agents (METOCLOPRAMIDE) before diagnostic testing is rarely done and only when gastroesophageal reflux is the cause. Retraining of swallowing by a speech pathologist may be helpful in those patients with a neurologic illness.

SWEATING, EXCESSIVE

Although inconvenient to the patient, excessive sweating usually does not indicate a medical problem.

Excessive sweating, particularly of the palms, soles, and underarms, is a common problem. Excessive sweating, called *essential hyperhidrosis*, is rarely an indicator of a medical problem, but there are very rare causes of excessive sweating that stem from a significant underlying disorder.

CAUSES

Excessive sweating can be caused by

- Rare neurologic diseases in which there is a genetic imbalance in the autonomic nervous system
- A disturbance in the hypothalamus of the brain
- A metabolic condition, such as DIABETES, HYPERTHYROIDISM, OBESITY, or pregnancy
- Spinal cord disorders
- Chronic infection, such as tuberculosis or malaria
- Medications, such as INSULIN
- Genetic skin disorders
- Lymphoma (LYMPHOMA, NON-HODGKIN)

APPROACH

An underlying neurologic disease can usually be detected during a careful MEDICAL HISTORY and a PHYSICAL EXAMINATION including neurologic examination. Most of the time, an extensive search for the cause of the excessive sweating is not done. However, if other clues are suggestive of possible metabolic disorders, BLOOD TESTS to assess factors such as thyroid function may be performed.

TREATMENT OPTIONS

Treatment can be difficult. The topical application of aluminum chloride, either alone or under clear plastic cling wrap, to the area of excessive sweating can control (not cure) the problem. The use of medicated powders such as Zeasorb applied to the skin after a bath or shower and after drying well may be helpful. If excessive sweating of the feet is associated with severe odor, the additional application of an antibiotic solution such as CLINDAMYCIN or ERYTHROMYCIN to decrease the bacterial flora of the skin may help.

Another approach to excessive sweating of the palms, soles, or underarms is iontophoresis. This procedure involves placing the skin in a solution with a mild electric current.

TESTICLE, PAINFUL OR SWOLLEN

At times, men may develop a severe pain or a swelling in the scrotum. Not every one of the causes of testicular pain and swelling have serious repercussions, but every scrotal swelling should be evaluated by a physician.

Regular testicular self-examination should be a part of every man's hygiene routine, and abnormalities should be reported to a physician.

CAUSES

Acute pain in the scrotum may occur as a result of

- Viral infections such as mumps in young men
- Bacterial infections such as epididymitis
- Torsion or twisting of the testicle that compromises the blood supply to the testicle

Nontender swellings of the scrotum may represent

- Benign cysts in the epididymis
- A collection of fluid around the testicle (hydrocele)
- Malignant tumors of the testicle (TESTICULAR CANCER)

APPROACH

The most important clues to scrotal pain and swelling are found in the patient's MEDICAL HISTORY. Information about the onset of the symptoms, the duration of the mass or swelling, and the degree of tenderness in various positions is very helpful. The PHYSICAL EXAMINATION by the doctor can often reveal the source of the problem. When necessary, an ULTRASOUND of the scrotum may be very useful to image the mass.

TREATMENT OPTIONS

In general, many scrotal swellings or other benign conditions need not be treated unless they cause symptoms because of their large size. Viral inflammation of the testicles, such as that in mumps, often resolves spontaneously. Bacterial infections respond well to antibiotics.

Testicular torsion represents a surgical emergency because of possible damage to the testicle from impaired blood supply; in this case, a simple surgical procedure to untwist the testicle is performed immediately.

Solid masses in the scrotum may represent a malignancy (TESTICULAR CANCER) and require surgical exploration and removal.

THROAT, SORE

A sore throat is a relatively common symptom that ranges from a slight tickle to scratchiness to real pain.

The first noticeable sign of a sore throat is usually pain when swallowing, but it can also be a persistent pain or rawness, too. A sore throat is often not an isolated symptom; it is usually associated with other symptoms of an infection.

CAUSES

Causes of a sore throat include

- Viral infection such as the COMMON COLD, mononucleosis, or INFLUENZA
- Bacterial infections such as strep throat and tonsillitis (less common than viral infections)
- Tumors such as LARYNGEAL CANCER (rare)

APPROACH

The most useful clues from an individual's MEDICAL HISTORY include whether the sore throat is associated with a COUGH or other signs of an infection such as FEVER and swollen glands. The location of any purulent discharge in the throat or on the tonsils can be an additional clue.

Throat CULTURES, rapid strep screens, and other tests, including X rays (RADIOGRAPHY) on occasion, may be necessary to determine the exact cause and the appropriate treatment.

TREATMENT OPTIONS

Most sore throats can be treated symptomatically; that is, without ever determining the underlying cause. Depending on the severity of the pain any of the following may be used:

- Saltwater gargles
- ASPIRIN in adults and acetaminophen in younger patients
- Local anesthetics such as xylocaine

If laboratory tests reveal a bacterial infection or if the likelihood is high enough from other evidence, a trial of antibiotics such as PENICILLIN, AMOXICILLIN, or ERYTHROMYCIN can be useful. Even in bacterial infections, however, antibiotics may not shorten the duration of the sore throat. If a sore throat persists for more than a few weeks, a more thorough evaluation will be necessary.

TONGUE PAIN

Tongue pain is a symptom that must never be ignored. Unless there is a history of recent trauma (such as biting or burning the tongue) the complaint requires a medical or dental examination.

Tongue pain is an unusual symptom but often an important one. It is not the same as generalized mouth pain; it is usually more specific.

CAUSES

The most obvious cause of tongue pain would be trauma. Biting one's tongue or eating scalding hot food can leave acute as well as residual pain.

Infections of the tongue are another possible explanation. Bacterial, fungal, and viral infections can lead to generalized tongue pain. These are usually accompanied by other symptoms associated with infection, such as swelling and redness.

Sore tongue is a symptom seen in several vitamin deficiency syndromes. Sore tongue associated with ANEMIA and neurologic weakness may be a sign of vitamin B_{12} deficiency. Folate deficiency can also lead to a red, sore tongue with ANEMIA and weakness.

Among the more serious conditions heralded by a sore tongue are ORAL CANCER and DIABETES.

APPROACH

A PHYSICAL EXAMINATION would involve visual examination and palpation (directly feeling the area) of the tongue. A MEDICAL HISTORY might focus on eating habits, alcohol use, tobacco use, and surgical history to explore the possibility of a vitamin deficiency. Diagnostic tests include

- CULTURE to test for and identify infection
- X ray (RADIOGRAPHY) to examine structures
- BIOPSY to evaluate any suspicious lesions

TREATMENT OPTIONS

The underlying condition is the focus of treatment. Some treatment strategies include

- Vitamin supplementation for deficiencies
- Antibiotics such as AMOXICILLIN for any bacterial infection
- Antifungals such as ketoconazole or nystatin for fungal infection
- Denture adjustment for traumatic injury or irritation
- Surgery, chemotherapy, or radiation for ORAL CANCER

TREMBLING

Although most tremors are either barely noticeable or a mere nuisance, some can become disabling.

Trembling is an involuntary, rhythmic, visible shaking or quivering of all or part of the body. Most commonly affected are the hands, head, and voice; less commonly affected are the legs and trunk. Typically, tremors occur only during waking hours and cease during sleep.

CAUSES

By far the most common cause of tremor is essential tremor, also called *benign tremor* or *familial tremor* (because some patients can inherit it) or *senile tremor* (when a benign tremor begins in old age).

Other causes are

- PARKINSON DISEASE
- Diseases that involve the cerebellum (the back part of the brain that is largely responsible for coordination), such as inherited diseases, degenerative diseases, MULTIPLE SCLEROSIS, STROKES, tumors, and ALCOHOLISM
- Alcohol withdrawal after several days (or more) of heavy drinking
- A forearm tremor that occurs during prolonged writing
- Diseases that produce weakness such as MULTIPLE SCLEROSIS or STROKES
- Chorea, which is frequently confused with tremor, especially in the initial stages when there are involuntary, arrhythmic, rapid jerks
- Other causes not associated with disease states, such as ANXIETY, stress, and FATIGUE
- Stimulant beverages, such as coffee, tea, and sodas and other caffeine-containing foods
- Nicotine in cigarettes and nicotine patches

Tremor may also be a side effect of some medicines, such as

- Drugs used in the treatment of lung conditions such as ASTHMA or EMPHYSEMA (THEOPHYLLINE or ALBUTEROL inhalers)
- Valproic acid and sodium valproate compound used in the treatment of epilepsy
- LITHIUM, a medication used in the treatment of manic illness

- Antipsychotics and antidepressants such as FLUOXETINE, sertraline, and PAROXETINE
- Too much thyroid hormone, either as part of a disease state (HYPERTHYROIDISM) or if administered in excess to patients undergoing treatment for HYPOTHYROIDISM

APPROACH

A MEDICAL HISTORY would focus on

- Drug use
- Alcohol use
- Family history

These points can be very useful. The results of a PHYSICAL EXAMINATION, particularly a neurologic examination, and the characteristics of the tremor—whether it occurs only while at rest or only during purposeful movement—usually provide adequate information to make a diagnosis.

TREATMENT OPTIONS

For essential tremor, PROPRANOLOL, a drug otherwise used in the treatment of heart disease and HYPERTENSION, is the treatment of choice, although the patient's response is often incomplete.

Other drugs to treat essential tremor include primidone and ALPRAZOLAM (a sedative drug related to DIAZEPAM).

URINATION, FREQUENT

A person's bladder habits can change over time without having a discernable medical cause, but sudden changes in bladder function or habit warrant medical evaluation.

Frequent urination is commonly defined as the need to urinate more often than every two hours. It is a disturbing symptom and can affect lifestyle and cause SLEEP PROBLEMS.

CAUSES

Frequent urination may result from

- BLADDER INFECTION or bladder tumor
- Enlarged prostate (PROSTATE, ENLARGED)
- Neurologic disease or aging

Urinary frequency may also occur in the absence of a specific identifiable cause and may be related to subtle changes in a person's response to bladder sensations.

APPROACH

The diagnostic approach to urinary frequency involves a careful MEDICAL HISTORY of symptoms and habits. A PHYSICAL EXAMINATION may focus on prostate problems in men.

The adequacy of bladder emptying may be assessed by an ULTRASOUND examination of the bladder or by catheterization to determine how much urine is left in the bladder after voiding. In some cases, a urodynamic study, which measures responses of the bladder to filling and the behavior of the bladder during urination, may be performed.

URINALYSIS is performed in all patients to rule out infection, and in some cases urine CYTOLOGY or cystoscopy (a form of ENDOSCOPY) may be performed to rule out the presence of a bladder tumor.

TREATMENT OPTIONS

Treatment depends on the cause:

- In men with a large obstructing prostate (PROSTATE, ENLARGED), medical therapy may be used to alleviate symptoms or surgical therapy may be recommended to remove the prostatic obstruction.
- In patients with neurologic disease or age-related changes in bladder function, medication may be used to reduce the irritative symptoms.
- In patients with BLADDER INFECTION, antibiotic therapy can usually clear the infection.
- In patients with BLADDER STONES or a tumor, surgical removal may be an option.

URINATION, PAINFUL

Dysuria is the medical term for painful urination. Although sometimes caused by irritation, painful urination is usually a sign of an infection. These infections are rarely serious, but a physician should be consulted if the condition persists, especially if it is associated with FEVER or BACKACHE.

Painful urination is most frequently caused by infections that are rarely serious and usually subside with antibiotic treatment.

CAUSES

The most common cause of painful urination is a bacterial infection of the lower urinary tract, the urethra, or the bladder (BLADDER INFECTION). It is important to treat this infection promptly to prevent it from ascending the urinary tract to the kidneys, which can be more serious. Other causes of painful urination include

- Sexually transmitted diseases
- Prostatitis
- Yeast infections
- Atrophic VAGINITIS
- KIDNEY STONES

APPROACH

In order to diagnose the cause of painful urination, a careful MEDICAL HISTORY needs to be taken about the symptom and any associated symptoms, such as

- A change in urine appearance (URINE, ABNORMAL APPEARANCE)
- A change in bladder habits (URINATION, FREQUENT)
- FEVER
- BACKACHE
- Penile or VAGINAL DISCHARGE

The PHYSICAL EXAMINATION includes palpation of the bladder as well as pounding on the back to determine if there is any tenderness over the kidneys. Additionally, a URINALYSIS will be performed. Other procedures may include a pelvic examination or urethral swabs for CULTURE.

TREATMENT OPTIONS

Treatment of the underlying cause should alleviate the symptom. Most causes of persistent painful urination are from infections (see BLADDER INFECTION), which are treated with antibiotics. KIDNEY STONES can be resolved by medical or surgical means (see ULTRASONIC LITHOTRIPSY).

URINE, ABNORMAL APPEARANCE

Although a sudden change in the appearance of one's urine can be an alarming symptom, it is not usually an ominous one.

Abnormal appearance of the urine most commonly results from the presence of blood in the urine or the presence of infection. Blood in the urine may turn the urine pink or red depending on the concentration of blood. Cloudy urine, sometimes emitting a foul odor, may indicate infection.

CAUSES

Some of the possible conditions that could cause urine to change appearance include

- BLADDER STONES
- KIDNEY STONES
- Severe BLADDER INFECTION
- Bladder tumors
- Kidney tumors
- Other diseases of the lower urinary tract such as atrophic VAGINITIS affecting the opening for urine
- Certain diseases affecting the function of the kidneys such as glomerulonephritis
- Infection such as malaria
- Crystals in the urine that are benign

APPROACH

The MEDICAL HISTORY of the patient, including onset and duration of the symptom, gives important clues for diagnosis. The single most important test is the URINALYSIS, in which the doctor performs a microscopic examination of the urine to determine whether blood or pus cells are present.

Depending on the findings on URINALYSIS, tests may be performed to look for a source of bleeding in the kidneys or bladder such as an intravenous pyelogram (a form of RADIOGRAPHY) of the kidney or cystoscopy (a form of ENDOSCOPY) of the bladder.

If infection is suspected, a urine CULTURE may be performed.

TREATMENT OPTIONS

Treatment for blood in the urine depends on finding the cause and then treating it appropriately. For tumors, surgery may be required. KIDNEY STONES and BLADDER STONES can be removed with certain procedures (see ULTRASONIC LITHOTRIPSY). Infections are usually cleared with antibiotics.

VAGINAL BLEEDING

A woman should keep a good record of her menstrual history to aid in the evaluation of vaginal bleeding.

Although some vaginal bleeding is usually not an ominous sign, excessive bleeding can be a medical emergency. If the bleeding soaks through a regular sanitary napkin within 30 minutes, a physician should be notified. Also, if bleeding is associated with DIZZINESS or FAINTING OR FAINTNESS, immediate evaluation is necessary. Postmenopausal women should always have unexpected bleeding evaluated.

CAUSES

In postmenopausal women, vaginal bleeding may be attributable to

- Atrophic VAGINITIS
- Uterine prolapse
- Endometrial polyps
- UTERINE CANCER
- Vaginal cancer
- CERVICAL CANCER
- Systemic bleeding disorders

In premenopausal women, the above causes are possible, but it may also be attributable to

- MENSTRUAL IRREGULARITIES
- Complications of pregnancy (often unsuspected)
- ENDOMETRIOSIS
- PELVIC INFLAMMATORY DISEASE
- VAGINITIS
- Endometrial hyperplasia
- HYPERTHYROIDISM or HYPOTHYROIDISM
- OVARIAN CYST
- OVARIAN CANCER
- Rare endocrine disorders such as CUSHING SYNDROME

APPROACH

A MEDICAL HISTORY, including a complete menstrual history, and a pelvic examination are probably the first steps in evaluating vaginal bleeding. A BLOOD COUNT to check for ANEMIA and BLOOD TESTS to test for thyroid function, pregnancy (if it is at all possible), and other problems may also be performed.

Further tests could include

- Hysteroscopy (a form of ENDOSCOPY)
- A BIOPSY of the uterine lining (endometrium)
- DILATION AND CURETTAGE for cases in which biopsy is not easily obtainable

VAGINAL DISCHARGE

A small amount of discharge, especially in the middle days between periods, is normal and related to ovulation.

Normal vaginal discharge can sometimes lead women to try products like sprays and douches that may create a problem. If any blood is present, it should be evaluated (see VAGINAL BLEEDING).

CAUSES

- VAGINITIS from lack of estrogen or from infection with yeast or *Trichomonas* or *Chlamydia* bacteria not normally present in large numbers
- Irritation from products such as douches, sprays, or contraceptive foam
- PELVIC INFLAMMATORY DISEASE
- Foreign bodies including intrauterine devices (IUDs), cervical caps, tampons, or diaphragms
- Cervical, uterine, or vaginal polyps or cancer (see CERVICAL CANCER; UTERINE CANCER)
- OVARIAN CYSTS
- Urethral infection (BLADDER INFECTION)

APPROACH

A MEDICAL HISTORY would focus on the use of any materials inserted into the vagina, presence of a FEVER, sexual contacts, and changes in contraceptive pills or devices. Recent antibiotic use commonly alters the bacterial balance of the vagina and may lead to infection.

PHYSICAL EXAMINATION, especially pelvic and abdominal examination, is useful in determining a diagnosis. Laboratory tests could include CULTURES, microscopic examination of secretions, and a PAP SMEAR. If intrauterine, tubal, or ovarian problems are suspected, BIOPSY and ULTRASOUND may be used.

TREATMENT OPTIONS

Antifungal creams such as clotrimazole and antibiotics such as METRONIDAZOLE—or more specific prescriptions—may be recommended, depending on the underlying cause.

VISION DISTURBANCES

Early treatment of vision disturbances may reduce the chance of progressive or permanent sight loss.

Vision can be defined in many ways. Aside from the ability to read the newspaper or street signs, vision can be the ability to perceive color, to see at night, or to see out of the corner of the eye. A disturbance in vision can mean any disruption in the above or the perception of light flashes or sparks and the appearance of floaters in the eyes.

CAUSES

Different types of visual disturbances have different causes. For example, flashes of light suggest something may be tugging at or tearing the retina.

Floaters are noted when some opacity is floating in the interior of the eye. This could simply be some spot of localized degeneration, but it could also be blood or inflammatory material.

A reduction in central vision may simply mean that spectacles need updating to reflect a change that has occurred within the focusing elements of the eye. Nearsightedness usually progresses until age 30 and may not begin until the mid-20s. At around age 40, the ability to focus up close decreases to the point of causing symptoms. Reading glasses may be needed shortly after the initial observation of change.

Some systemic diseases, such as DIABETES with high blood sugar, can induce a nearsighted shift. A reduction in night vision may occur after laser treatment for eye disease related to DIABETES.

Retinitis pigmentosa causes a chronic, progressive, and permanent loss of night vision. Visual obscuration from CATARACT also may reduce visual function at night. CATARACT is a reversible cause of central vision loss, while macular degeneration causes permanent reduction in central visual function.

The sudden loss of side vision may occur in retinal detachment or in blockage of blood vessels within the retina. A STROKE involving the visual pathways could also cause this symptom. Episodic loss of vision may be due to bits of material within the arteries temporarily blocking blood flow in the retina.

MIGRAINE HEADACHE may initially be experienced as a blurring of side vision. This usually passes within 20 minutes. The gradual perception of a side vision abnormality could be related to GLAUCOMA or a tumor within the eye. It could also be caused by CATARACT.

Loss of color vision is usually caused by an abnormality in the function of the optic nerve that transmits the visual message to the brain. Inflammation, poor circulation to the nerve, or a drop in the speed at which the signal can be sent, may make colors appear washed out. Inherited color vision problems do not occur suddenly and are usually present from birth.

Any eyedrop, drug, or eye disease that causes the pupils to decrease in size will limit the amount of light that enters the eye, thereby decreasing night vision. Pilocarpine, a common GLAUCOMA drop, reduces pupil size.

APPROACH

Visual problems that clear with a blink or that clear when the glasses are used are generally not of a serious nature. However, a change in visual function that is not simply remedied at home should prompt a call to the doctor. A MEDICAL HISTORY is necessary, including information about

- The onset of the symptom (sudden or gradual)
- The duration of the symptom (still present or over)
- The number of episodes
- The timing of the most recent episode
- Whether both eyes were involved
- Any associated symptoms such as HEADACHE, eye redness or EYE PAIN, weakness, or NUMBNESS

The examination will include a measurement of VISUAL ACUITY. It is important to bring the best pair of spectacles to the examination. Side vision testing may also be done. The ability of the pupils to react to light will be checked. Careful examination with the microscope, including a measurement of eye pressure, is necessary. The pupils will likely be dilated, so sunglasses and perhaps a friend or relative to drive are often necessary. Dilation is needed to get the best possible view of the inside of the eye including the retina and optic nerve.

TREATMENT OPTIONS

Treatment will depend on the cause of the problem. Treatment may be as simple as a new pair of glasses or use of tear-supplement drops. The key to treatment is prompt evaluation. Early treatment may reduce the chance of progressive or permanent sight loss.

VOMITING

Vomiting is a very common and typically transient or self-limited symptom. Its occasional occurrence should not cause alarm. More serious instances that may demand medical attention include

- Persistent vomiting (lasting more than two days)
- Vomiting associated with severe ABDOMINAL PAIN
- Vomiting associated with severe HEADACHES
- Vomiting of undigested food that was eaten many hours earlier
- Vomiting of foul- or feculent-smelling material
- Vomiting associated with a significant amount of blood

Although some cases of vomiting demand medical attention, most are due to overindulgence in food or drink or to simple food poisoning and resolve in a matter of hours.

CAUSES

The most common causes of vomiting, which are typically self-limited and resolve in a matter of hours, are most often related to

- Dietary indiscretion
- Overindulgence in food or drink, especially too much alcohol
- Simple food poisoning

Other causes of vomiting include

- GASTROENTERITIS, which is due to a viral infection and is typically associated with a low-grade FEVER, generalized muscle aches and pains, and some DIARRHEA, and resolves in a few days
- Stomach or INTESTINAL OBSTRUCTION, PANCREATITIS, and gallbladder disease (see GALLSTONES; CHOLECYSTITIS AND CHOLANGITIS)
- Neurologic illness that ranges from MIGRAINE HEADACHES to problems within the brain that elevate spinal fluid pressure (rare)
- Pregnancy, especially in the early stage ("morning sickness")

APPROACH

Evaluation is needed only for those rare cases of persistent, prolonged, or recurrent vomiting. A description of the specific circumstances may point to the need for more diagnostic evaluation.

The PHYSICAL EXAMINATION will focus on signs of dehydration BLOOD PRESSURE TESTING and pulse while lying down and standing up, degree of moisture in the skin and mouth) and abnormalities of the abdomen and rectum. At times, a neurologic examination or evaluation of the eyes and retina will be done.

Laboratory tests will be ordered only if the preliminary examination is abnormal. These may include BLOOD COUNT, serum electrolytes, and serum amylase (see BLOOD TESTS).

Further tests may include

- X rays (RADIOGRAPHY) of the abdomen if INTESTINAL OBSTRUCTION is suspected
- COMPUTED TOMOGRAPHY or MAGNETIC RESONANCE IMAGING of the brain if neurologic disease is suspected
- Barium X rays (RADIOGRAPHY) of the intestine and ULTRASOUNDS or COMPUTED TOMOGRAPHY of the abdomen in unclear cases

TREATMENT OPTIONS

Most episodes of vomiting resolve within a short period of time and are not caused by a persistent medical problem. Food intake should be limited to clear liquids, such as soft drinks, juices, and broth, until the problem resolves and the patient feels up to eating regular food. Physicians may prescribe antinausea medications, including

- CHLORPROMAZINE
- PROCHLORPERAZINE
- Promethazine
- Thiethylperazine
- METOCLOPRAMIDE
- Trimethobenzamide

WEIGHT GAIN

In most cases, progressive weight gain is due to increased caloric intake accompanied by decreased physical activity.

Concern about weight is ubiquitous. But for all the worry, there is no absolute value of weight that is desirable. Tables that list "ideal" body weights, adjusted for body build, age, sex, and height, are readily available but not always useful for individuals.

Although many people find it difficult to accept, almost all instances of increased body weight relate to increased caloric intake, decreased caloric expenditure because of decreased physical activity, or a combination of both factors. Problems stemming from a slow metabolism rarely explain weight gain.

Rapid fluctuation in weight (on the order of one to two pounds per day) is almost always due to fluid retention and is quite commonly noted premenstrually in women.

CAUSES

Increased caloric intake, coupled with decreased activity, accounts for the overwhelming majority of cases of progressive weight gain. Illnesses that result in rapid weight gain from fluid and salt accumulation within the body include

- CONGESTIVE HEART FAILURE
- Cirrhosis of the liver
- Nephrotic syndrome of the kidney (see KIDNEY FAILURE)

These diseases are frequently associated with other symptoms, including

- Abdominal distension and ABDOMINAL SWELLING
- Swelling of the legs (ANKLE SWELLING)
- BREATHING DIFFICULTY

An underactive thyroid gland (HYPOTHYROIDISM) on occasion may result in weight gain.

APPROACH

The patient's weight is adjusted for body build, height, sex, and age to determine whether the weight gain is normal or excessive. The weight should be taken in the same manner each time, preferably without clothes or shoes. A dietary history should be reviewed to estimate caloric intake on a daily basis. Some sense of energy expenditure can be ascertained by reviewing job responsibilities, hobbies, and exercise habits.

Abnormal fluid retention can be detected from the PHYSICAL EXAMINATION by examining the heart, neck, lungs, abdomen, and legs. If abnormalities are suspected because of findings from the PHYSICAL EXAMINATION, the following are more extensive tests that may be performed:

- The heart may be assessed with ELECTROCARDIOGRAPHY or chest X ray (RADIOGRAPHY).
- The liver may be assessed with blood liver function tests (see BLOOD TESTS) or ULTRASOUND examination of the liver itself.
- The kidneys may be assessed with URINALYSIS.
- The thyroid gland may be assessed with blood thyroid function tests (see BLOOD TESTS).

TREATMENT OPTIONS

Weight gain due to increased oral intake can be treated by dietary restrictions in fat and total calories as well as a graded exercise program. Quick fixes such as crash diets almost never work in the long term. Programs that result in permanent lifestyle adjustments are the only ones with the potential for long-term success.

Fluid overload states can be treated with salt restriction and diuretics such as HYDROCHLOROTHIAZIDE.

Appetite suppressant pills, although touted by lay advertisers, are usually ineffective in the long term.

WEIGHT LOSS

Small fluctuations in weight are not unusual, but progressive weight loss without an obvious explanation merits some concern.

Unexpected weight loss—that is, weight loss not related to dieting or increased exercise—can represent serious illness. Weight loss should be interpreted within the context of a patient's usual weight. Physicians begin to worry seriously about an underlying illness when weight loss reaches approximately ten percent of the individual's stable weight.

CAUSES

Decreased intake of food is obviously the most common cause of weight loss; dietary changes, such as a reduction in total fat intake, can easily explain weight loss. If the dietary changes are associated with a poor appetite (see APPETITE, LOSS OF), substantial weight loss may point to DEPRESSION, PANCREATIC CANCER, STOMACH CANCER, some other undiscovered malignancy, or AIDS.

At times, patients lose weight despite maintaining or even increasing their dietary intake. In this instance, an overactive thyroid gland (HYPERTHYROIDISM) or DIABETES needs consideration. Diseases of the small intestine or pancreas that interfere with complete digestion and absorption of food may lead to weight loss, although changes in bowel habits or even DIARRHEA are usually present as well.

Anorexia nervosa may be a cause of weight loss in young women (see APPETITE, LOSS OF).

APPROACH

General nutritional information, MEDICAL HISTORY, PHYSICAL EXAMINATION, and baseline laboratory tests—BLOOD COUNT, screening chemistries (see BLOOD TESTS), and OCCULT BLOOD TESTING—will determine the need for additional testing. Testing would be directed toward abnormalities noted on the general evaluation.

TREATMENT OPTIONS

Many oral nutritional supplements are commercially available and can be used without harm in an effort to gain weight. The first step, however, is to determine whether weight loss is a sign of a medical problem and whether weight gain is necessary for the patient.

ILLNESSES

AIDS

In the United States, there are between 1 and 1.5 million people infected with the human immunodeficiency virus (HIV); there are as many as 20 million people infected worldwide. AIDS—which stands for *acquired immunodeficiency syndrome*—affects all races and ethnic groups as well as people of all ages.

Few infections are associated with as much panic and misinformation as infection with the human immunodeficiency virus—the virus that causes AIDS—but without a cure, education and prevention are the best weapons with which to fight it.

CAUSES

AIDS is caused by infection with HIV. There are two types of HIV: type 1 and type 2. HIV type 1 is the only virus that causes AIDS in the United States. However, infection with HIV type 2 occurs in Africa.

The groups at highest risk for HIV infection are

- Gay and bisexual men
- Injection drug users
- Hemophiliacs
- Children born to mothers with HIV
- Sexually active heterosexuals

Transmission of HIV by blood transfusion is extremely rare in the United States.

SYMPTOMS

After exposure to HIV, some patients develop an *acute retroviral syndrome* characterized by FEVER, RASH, and swollen lymph nodes. This is often indistinguishable from other viral illnesses.

The patient is generally without symptoms, though, for several years until the immune system deteriorates. At that time, symptoms suggestive of HIV infection include

- WEIGHT LOSS greater than ten percent of total body weight
- DIARRHEA for longer than one month
- FEVER for longer than one month
- COUGH for longer than one month
- Skin RASH
- Recurrent SHINGLES
- Oral thrush (yeast infection in mouth)
- Swollen glands all over the body

Unfortunately, these symptoms are not specific to HIV infection and can mimic other infections or cancer.

DIAGNOSIS

HIV infection can be detected by a BLOOD TEST. If the first screening test is positive, a second is performed for confirmation. More sophisticated testing can be performed in research studies or at many university medical centers.

A positive result on an HIV test is not, however, a diagnosis of AIDS. An HIV-infected person is considered to have AIDS only when they develop any one of a number of diseases that occur in individuals with abnormalities in their immune system. In addition, when the patient's T-cell count (a measure of the immune system's function) falls below 200 (the normal range is 750 to 1,250), the patient is considered to have AIDS.

COMPLICATIONS

The complications related to infection with HIV are the result of infections that develop due to deteriorating immune function. These include

- PNEUMONIA
- Tuberculosis
- Meningitis

Patients with HIV infection also have an increased risk of developing cancer.

Patients with HIV should contact their health care provider if they develop

- A high FEVER
- Severe or persistent HEADACHE
- VOMITING
- BREATHING DIFFICULTY
- Persistent DIARRHEA
- VISION DISTURBANCES
- Significant WEIGHT LOSS

The complexity of this syndrome prohibits a more detailed explanation of the complications. All patients with HIV disease should be closely monitored by a physician with experience treating AIDS patients.

TREATMENT

SELF TREATMENT:

While there is no cure for AIDS, there are many things that patients can do to help prolong their life. Common sense dictates that patients with HIV infection should eat well-balanced meals, exercise regularly, and get plenty of sleep. Tobacco and illicit drug use should be stopped. Alcohol is acceptable in moderation, unless it interacts with a medication the patient is taking. There is no benefit to megadoses of vitamins, but a daily multivitamin is acceptable.

MEDICAL TREATMENT:

There are many drugs that can be used to treat patients with HIV. The antiviral medications that are commonly used are zidovudine (AZT), didanosine (ddI), zalcitabine (ddC), and stavudine (d4T). There are several other experimental medications that are undergoing clinical evaluations. Additional therapy for HIV and its associated complications is beyond the scope of this book and should be discussed with a health care provider.

SURGICAL TREATMENT:

None, except for cases in which there is a surgical treatment for a secondary condition, such as an enlarged spleen or cancer.

PREVENTION

The best way to avoid HIV is by prevention. This means that condoms should be worn during intercourse and needles should not be shared. There is no evidence that HIV is transmitted via casual contact.

There are many medications that can prevent infections in patients already infected with HIV. A sulfamethoxazole and trimethoprim combination can be used to prevent PNEUMONIA; ISONIAZID can be used to prevent tuberculosis; and FLUCONAZOLE is effective in preventing fungal infections.

Once again, the preventive measures for patients with AIDS are in constant evolution and should be discussed with a health care provider.

ALCOHOLISM

About five percent of the population abuse alcohol and an additional eight percent are dependant on alcohol at some time in their lives. Men are affected about three times as often as women.

Alcohol *abuse* is defined as a pattern of repeated drinking that interferes with a person's work, family, or social life or that exposes a person to physical dangers (driving or operating machinery while drunk, for example) or legal problems (such as drunk-driving arrests).

Alcohol *dependence* is more severe and includes the above problems as well as physical tolerance to the effects of alcohol (being able to drink large amounts without getting drunk), physical symptoms of withdrawal when the person stops drinking, difficulty quitting drinking, or rearranging activities to keep drinking.

CAUSES

People who have close relatives with these conditions are three or four times more likely to develop alcohol problems than they would be otherwise. Sometimes people drink in response to another inadequately treated psychological disorder, such as DEPRESSION or schizophrenia. Most people with alcohol abuse or dependence, though, probably do not have any of these associated conditions.

SYMPTOMS

Symptoms of alcohol intoxication are well known and include

- Impaired attention or MEMORY PROBLEMS
- Incoordination
- Slurred speech
- Unsteady walking
- Possibly stupor or coma

Alcohol withdrawal can cause

- Hand TREMBLING
- ANXIETY
- Restlessness
- SLEEP PROBLEMS
- Nausea
- Rapid heartbeat
- Sweating (see SWEATING, EXCESSIVE)
- Seizures
- HALLUCINATIONS and delirium

DIAGNOSIS

There is no specific level of alcohol intake that qualifies a person for an alcohol-related disorder. The diagnosis of alcohol abuse or dependence is made according to the impact of drinking on a person's work, family, and social life and on the basis of physical symptoms.

Four questions, known as the CAGE questionnaire, are a good screening test for alcoholism. These questions are

- Have you ever felt you should **C**ut down on your drinking?
- Have people **A**nnoyed you criticizing your drinking?
- Have you felt **G**uilty about your drinking?
- Have you ever had a drink first thing in the morning (an **E**ye-opener) to steady your nerves or get rid of a hangover?

Two "yes" answers indicate the chance of having an alcohol-related disorder is high; three or four "yes" answers indicate alcohol dependence.

COMPLICATIONS

In addition to the acute symptoms of intoxication and withdrawal, chronic alcohol abuse produces many physical complications, including

- HEPATITIS
- Cirrhosis of the liver
- Liver failure
- Jaundice
- Leg and ABDOMINAL SWELLING
- Damage to the nerves of the feet and hands
- Malnutrition, including vitamin deficiencies
- Brain damage, including MEMORY PROBLEMS
- Breast development and shrinking testicles in men
- IMPOTENCE
- Stomach irritation and ULCERS
- PANCREATITIS
- Dilated veins in the esophagus
- HEMORRHOIDS
- Stomach or intestinal bleeding
- High blood pressure (HYPERTENSION)
- Irregular heartbeat (ARRHYTHMIAS)
- CONGESTIVE HEART FAILURE
- Death

Alcohol abuse can also bring on symptoms of psychological disorders such as DEPRESSION and ANXIETY. Even moderate alcohol use during pregnancy can cause birth defects.

Alcohol abuse disrupts work, family, and social relationships. It can lead to legal difficulties and physical injuries. Alcohol use is involved in half of all fatal car accidents, one third of all suicides, and two-thirds of all murders.

TREATMENT

SELF TREATMENT:

Alcohol-related disorders can be difficult to control without help. Most who have an alcohol-related disorder find it easier to avoid drinking completely than to drink a little. It is important for many alcoholics to avoid situations that are likely to involve drinking.

MEDICAL TREATMENT:

A variety of inpatient and outpatient treatment programs exist; the main focus of these programs is on the psychological aspects of quitting drinking. Alcoholics Anonymous, the most widely known alcohol abuse recovery program, provides a supportive context for learning about the damaging effects of alcohol, contact with others who are struggling with the same problem, and practical techniques for avoiding drinking and restoring one's life.

Medical detoxification is usually accomplished with gradually tapering doses of sedatives such as CHLORDIAZEPOXIDE or LORAZEPAM. Some people find it easier to avoid drinking if they take DISULFIRAM, a medicine which makes people sick if they drink alcohol.

SURGICAL TREATMENT:

None.

PREVENTION

Because alcohol use is widespread in our culture, alcohol abuse can be difficult to recognize. Being aware of the symptoms of alcohol abuse and dependence can lead one to seek treatment early and avoid the potentially devastating consequences.

ALZHEIMER DISEASE

Alzheimer disease is a degenerative disorder of the brain that causes the progressive loss of intellectual abilities. The disease usually affects memory (see MEMORY PROBLEMS) and at least one other cognitive domain such as language, attention, visual-perceptual skills, reasoning, judgement, or behavior.

Alzheimer disease is the most common cause of dementia, accounting for up to 80 percent of all cases.

CAUSES

The underlying cause of Alzheimer disease is unknown, but there have been recent advances in understanding the disorder. It appears that the disease is probably several diseases that cause similar changes in the metabolism of the brain.

Heredity may play a role; several genetic markers have been linked to the disease.

Although aluminum poisoning was once thought to be a factor, recent studies have not supported that theory.

SYMPTOMS

The initial symptoms of the disease are usually subtle and may not be recognized at all by the affected person. Often the family of the person are the first to notice increasingly frequent MEMORY PROBLEMS. Often the individual will

- Display a lack of interest in work or social activities
- Neglect or have difficulty with routine tasks
- Become withdrawn

Signs of more advanced disease include

- CONFUSION
- Need for assistance eating or dressing
- INCONTINENCE

DIAGNOSIS

Diagnosis of memory disorders almost always begins with a detailed MEDICAL HISTORY and a PHYSICAL EXAMINATION, including a complete neurologic and mental status assessment. Mental status examination is a detailed review of various cognitive functions to check performance of attention, memory, language, visual-spatial function, abstract reasoning, insight, behavior, and judgement.

BLOOD TESTS and a BLOOD COUNT can be useful to check for metabolic disturbances, systemic infections, and nutrient deficiencies.

Further tests can include
- ELECTROENCEPHALOGRAPHY
- COMPUTED TOMOGRAPHY
- MAGNETIC RESONANCE IMAGING
- LUMBAR PUNCTURE

Sometimes, cognitive and PHYSICAL EXAMINATIONS are repeated over the course of several months to determine if the disease is progressing.

The diagnosis of Alzheimer disease is made by finding the characteristic pattern of symptoms in the absence of any other causes after a reasonable search.

COMPLICATIONS

DEPRESSION is often associated with the disease, and overall life expectancy decreases on account of a number of factors. Inability to care for oneself and reduced mental function can precipitate problems ranging from vitamin deficiencies to automobile accidents.

TREATMENT

SELF TREATMENT:

None.

MEDICAL TREATMENT:

At this time, there are no good treatments available; no medication has been shown even to slow the disease significantly. The only drug approved for use in Alzheimer disease is tacrine, but its effects are modest, at best. Other medications used to treat associated disorders are
- Antidepressants such as sertraline
- Mild sedatives such as low doses of HALOPERIDOL used sparingly
- Antianxiety drugs such as LORAZEPAM

SURGICAL TREATMENT:

None.

PREVENTION

There seems to be a protective effect in education; studies show that the risk of developing dementia is two to five times more likely in those with little or no education.

ANEMIA

Anemia is a condition in which the blood has a reduced number of red blood cells. These cells are responsible for carrying oxygen from the lungs to all body tissues, so a lessened number of them leads to less efficient oxygen distribution.

The course of anemia can be reversed with medical treatment, but severe untreated cases can be dangerous.

CAUSES

The multiple causes of anemia can be divided into two main categories: decreased production of red blood cells in the bone marrow and increased destruction or loss of red blood cells. Decreased production is seen in

- Deficiencies of vitamin B_{12}, folate, or iron
- Bone marrow disorders such as LEUKEMIA
- Chronic inflammatory disorders such as RHEUMATOID ARTHRITIS
- Thalassemia

Increased destruction is seen in

- Hereditary diseases such as sickle-cell disease
- Infections
- Use of drugs such as methyldopa
- Autoimmune disorders (LUPUS ERYTHEMATOSUS)
- Blood loss

SYMPTOMS

- FATIGUE
- BREATHING DIFFICULTY
- Pallor
- Fast heart rate
- CHEST PAIN
- DIZZINESS
- Blood in stool (RECTAL BLEEDING) or in vomit
- Excessive menstruation (MENSTRUAL IRREGULARITIES)
- Jaundice
- Dark-colored urine (URINE, ABNORMAL APPEARANCE)

DIAGNOSIS

Anemia is diagnosed with tests such as

- Complete BLOOD COUNT
- BLOOD TESTS for vitamin B_{12}, folate, and iron to check for deficiencies

- BLOOD TESTS for hemoglobin electrophoresis to check for hereditary diseases
- BLOOD TESTS to check for red cell destruction and evidence of chronic diseases
- Stool and urine samples to check for the presence of blood (OCCULT BLOOD TESTING; URINALYSIS)

If no diagnosis can be made, a bone marrow BIOPSY may be performed.

COMPLICATIONS

In cases of severe or rapidly developing anemia, body organs may be damaged from a lack of oxygen. This can result in STROKE, HEART ATTACK, KIDNEY FAILURE, liver failure, and in severe cases, death.

TREATMENT

SELF TREATMENT:

Iron supplements are recommended for women with heavy menstrual periods. A diet consisting of vegetables, fruits, and meats should provide enough of the necessary nutrients to prevent anemia.

MEDICAL TREATMENT:

Medical therapy is dependent on the underlying cause. Usually, treatment of the underlying cause or of the chronic disease will reverse the anemia. In cases of severe anemia, blood transfusions can be given. Iron can be given in cases of chronic blood loss, and erythropoietin is helpful in patients with KIDNEY FAILURE.

SURGICAL TREATMENT:

Surgical intervention may be needed to treat sources of blood loss such as COLON POLYPS or tumors.

PREVENTION

- A well-balanced diet with adequate iron and vitamins is helpful.
- Exposure to solvents such as benzene and insecticides, which can damage the bone marrow, should be avoided.

ANEURYSM

An aneurysm is a weak spot in the wall of a blood vessel. Common locations for an aneurysm include the small blood vessels, such as those in the brain, and the largest blood vessels, such as the aorta as it travels from the heart, through the chest, and into the abdomen.

Aneurysms in and of themselves are not a serious danger, but the very real potential for rupture and clot formation at the site is life-threatening.

An aneurysm is a balloonlike swelling of a blood vessel. Because of this abnormal shape and wall strength, rupture and clot formation in the area of the defect are a serious danger.

CAUSES

Most aneurysms of the aorta are caused by ATHEROSCLEROSIS. Less often, infections or hereditary diseases can also contribute to aneurysm formation. Aneurysm formation in the blood vessels in the brain also appears to have some hereditary factor, but it can be associated with other diseases, as well.

High blood pressure (HYPERTENSION) increases the stress on the weak spot of the blood vessel wall causing the aneurysm to increase in size like a balloon and the risk of rupture to increase.

SYMPTOMS

Aneurysms are usually without symptoms until a catastrophe occurs. Occasionally, an aneurysm in the brain will cause HEADACHES before it ruptures.

In the aorta, an aneurysm can also go completely unnoticed until disaster strikes, but in rare cases, it can cause

- CHEST PAIN or discomfort
- Hoarseness
- SWALLOWING DIFFICULTIES
- Persistent COUGH

For an aortic aneurysm in the abdomen, a throbbing so-called *pulsatile mass* may be an indicator.

Usually, when an aortic aneurysm ruptures, there is sudden severe pain, severe drop in blood pressure, and even loss of consciousness. Even with emergency surgery, aortic aneurysms are associated with a very high mortality.

DIAGNOSIS

An aortic aneurysm in the abdomen can usually be diagnosed in a PHYSICAL EXAMINATION by feeling the abdominal pulsatile mass.

An aneurysm in the chest can be suspected by marked differences in BLOOD PRESSURE TESTS and pulse between the right and left arm. Chest X ray (RADIOGRAPHY) can also be useful in the diagnosis of an aortic aneurysm in the chest.

Aneurysms in the brain can be detected by

- COMPUTED TOMOGRAPHY
- MAGNETIC RESONANCE IMAGING
- Angiography (a form of RADIOGRAPHY)

Angiography may be needed to detect or confirm the presence of an aneurysm in all three locations. ULTRASOUND may also be useful.

COMPLICATIONS

The two major complications associated with aneurysm are rupture, in which the walls of the blood vessel actually break at the site of the aneurysm, and clot formation, in which the widened space of the aneurysm provides a place where blood can start to coagulate. Depending on the size of the vessel, rupture can lead to serious internal bleeding or damage to surrounding tissue. A clot, particularly in an aortic aneurysm, can break off and travel farther down the blood stream causing GANGRENE in the leg or internal abdominal organs.

WARNING SIGNS:

Sudden rupture in the brain leads to

- Extremely severe HEADACHE
- NECK PAIN
- Neurologic weakness

Rupture in the abdomen or chest results in

- Severe pain often in the back near the rupture site
- Extremely low blood pressure
- Loss of consciousness
- Shock

TREATMENT

SELF TREATMENT:

Limitations in exercise may be necessary to decrease the chance of temporarily elevated blood pressure that could cause rupture.

MEDICAL TREATMENT:

Medical therapies include beta-blockers, such as PROPRANOLOL, to lower blood pressure and stress on the blood vessel wall. Nimodipine is sometimes prescribed for a ruptured aneurysm in the brain.

SURGICAL TREATMENT:

Surgical therapy may be necessary when an aneurysm is identified but has not yet ruptured. The timing of surgery for aortic aneurysm is a controversial area, but it is based on the speed at which the aneurysm is expanding and its size at the time of detection. Aneurysms can be managed surgically by removal and repair with Dacron or other techniques to reinforce the walls of the vessel (see ANEURYSM REMOVAL).

Recently, special prosthetic devices called *stents* delivered to the area of weakness by a catheter threaded through the blood vessels have been used with increasing frequency. This technique is a less invasive alternative to open surgical repair.

PREVENTION

Prevention of aneurysm formation and progression includes controlling the risk factors for ATHEROSCLEROSIS and HYPERTENSION. Strategies include

- Avoiding smoking
- Following a low-fat, low-cholesterol diet
- Limiting intake of sodium
- Participating in regular exercise (if so advised by a physician)
- Diligently taking all prescribed blood pressure medication

ANGINA

Angina is a discomfort or pain usually in the center of the chest caused by a lack of blood flow to the heart muscle. Although not life-threatening in itself, it can progress to more serious heart problems.

The heart muscle gets its blood from the coronary arteries; when this blood flow is momentarily interrupted or limited, the heart muscle doesn't get the food and fuel it needs, and the CHEST PAIN of angina is the result.

CAUSES

The most common cause of angina is ATHEROSCLEROSIS. Much less common causes include spasms of the coronary arteries or disease of the smallest branches of these vessels. Spasms can be triggered by

- Nicotine in cigarettes
- Cold air
- Emotional stress
- Cocaine and other stimulant drugs

The risk factors for ATHEROSCLEROSIS include

- HYPERTENSION
- Smoking
- High blood cholesterol level (HYPERLIPIDEMIA)
- DIABETES
- Male sex (Men are more susceptible than women.)
- Family history of the disease

SYMPTOMS

Angina is most commonly described as a pressure, squeezing, or heavy sensation in the center of the chest. Less often, it can be an achy feeling or burning. The discomfort is sometimes experienced in other locations, including the left or right side of the chest, the upper abdomen, the neck, the jaw, and the arms. The discomfort is usually precipitated by some type of physical effort and is relieved with rest. An angina attack commonly lasts approximately one to two minutes.

DIAGNOSIS

The diagnosis of angina is usually made from the characteristic symptoms and the individual's MEDICAL HISTORY and risk factors for ATHEROSCLEROSIS. ELECTROCARDIOGRAPHY performed *during* the pain usually shows some abnormalities but can be totally normal in between episodes. A CARDIAC STRESS TEST can usually help sort out atypical symptoms. A CARDIAC CATHETERIZATION or angiogram (RADIOGRAPHY) may be necessary.

COMPLICATIONS

Angina can progress to unstable angina or directly to a myocardial infarction (HEART ATTACK).

WARNING SIGNS:

- Longer episodes of pain
- More frequent episodes
- Episodes precipitated more easily
- Episodes less responsive to medications

TREATMENT

SELF TREATMENT:

(See Prevention below.)

MEDICAL TREATMENT:

NITROGLYCERIN is the most commonly used drug to treat or prevent episodes of angina. Calcium channel blockers, such as DILTIAZEM and NIFEDIPINE, and beta-blockers, such as ATENOLOL and METOPROLOL, are also used to prevent episodes.

ASPIRIN and drugs to reduce blood cholesterol levels, such as CHOLESTYRAMINE and LOVASTATIN, are also helpful in treating underlying coronary artery ATHEROSCLEROSIS.

SURGICAL TREATMENT:

Procedures to clear blockages and improve blood flow in the coronary arteries include

- CORONARY ARTERY BYPASS GRAFT SURGERY
- Percutaneous transluminal coronary ANGIOPLASTY

PREVENTION

- Avoidance of smoking
- Low-fat, low-cholesterol diet
- Control of HYPERTENSION by low-sodium diet and diligent use of prescribed medication
- Regular exercise as recommended by a physician
- Estrogen replacement therapy for postmenopausal women (probably)
- Adequate vitamin E intake (possibly)

ARRHYTHMIA

Almost everyone will experience a heart rhythm abnormality—whether it be a skipped beat or a minor palpitation—and most of these occurrences are not serious. However, persistent rhythm problems can be dangerous.

A normal heart rhythm is regular and beats between approximately 50 and 100 times per minute during periods of rest—faster during periods of exertion. A heart rhythm that is abnormal is an arrhythmia. When the heart rhythm is too slow, it's called *bradycardia,* and when the rhythm is too fast, it's called *tachycardia*. Rhythm abnormalities can be either intermittent (called *paroxysmal*) or persistent.

CAUSES

The heart's rhythm is controlled by electrical impulses originating from areas in the heart called *nodes*. Disruptions in the normal rhythm can be caused by

- Scar tissue in the electrical system of the heart or in other parts of the heart muscle
- Degenerative changes in heart tissue
- Side effects of certain drugs—for example, ERYTHROMYCIN combined with TERFENADINE, or caffeine or cocaine
- Coronary artery disease (ATHEROSCLEROSIS and other problems)
- MYOCARDITIS
- Excessive thyroid hormone
- Potassium and magnesium deficiency

SYMPTOMS

Many people with rhythm abnormalities do not have any symptoms. When someone does have symptoms, palpitations are probably one of the most common feelings. More serious rhythm abnormalities cause

- FAINTING OR FAINTNESS
- DIZZINESS
- Light-headedness
- BREATHING DIFFICULTY

The most severe rhythm disturbances can lead to sudden cardiac death.

DIAGNOSIS

Many rhythm abnormalities can be detected by a careful PHYSICAL EXAMINATION, especially of the pulse and neck veins.

The most definite diagnosis is by ELECTROCARDIOGRAPHY, which can be performed in many ways: Holter monitors are portable recorders usually worn for a 24-hour period. Longer-event monitors and even subcutaneous implants to monitor the heart rhythm are being used in selected cases to capture and record an intermittent arrhythmia.

Electrophysiologic studies using pacing catheters are commonly used today both to detect and even treat rhythm abnormalities.

COMPLICATIONS

The most serious rhythm abnormalities can lead to unconsciousness, FAINTING OR FAINTNESS, and if prolonged, sudden cardiac death. Rhythm disturbances may also lead to the formation of emboli (see PULMONARY EMBOLISM and STROKE).

TREATMENT

SELF TREATMENT:

A physician may teach a patient certain "vagal maneuvers" in order to turn off an intermittent arrhythmia. This technique can trigger the nervous system to terminate certain types of rhythm abnormalities. These maneuvers include straining, gagging, or putting one's face in a bowl full of ice water. These should be attempted, however, only when one's physician has directed to do so.

Stress reduction many also help certain types of rhythm disturbances. Emotional stress can both precipitate rhythm disturbances and make someone more distressed by otherwise innocent rhythm disturbances.

MEDICAL TREATMENT:

Drug therapy may be necessary in extremely bothersome rhythm disturbances, such as palpitations that persistently keep someone from sleeping, or in otherwise harmless rhythm disturbances that are distressing despite reassurance. Drugs are usually reserved for serious rhythm abnormalities that have led to symptoms of FAINTING OR FAINTNESS or warning signs of sudden cardiac death.

Commonly used drugs include

- PROCAINAMIDE
- Amiodarone
- VERAPAMIL
- PROPRANOLOL
- DIGOXIN

Because some of these drugs can actually aggravate rhythm problems, drug therapy is generally reserved for the most serious disturbances. Anticoagulation drugs such as WARFARIN can also be used to cut down the chance of emboli in certain types of rhythm abnormalities, such as ATRIAL FIBRILLATION.

SURGICAL TREATMENT:

Electronic PACEMAKER INSERTION is commonly used to treat heart rhythms that are too slow and are causing distressing symptoms.

Some cases of tachycardia can be treated with a special catheter technique in which part of the faulty electrical system is destroyed. Some tachycardias that can lead to sudden cardiac death have a high rate of recurrence; in survivors, recurrences have been successfully treated with specialized pacemaker-like devices called implantable defibrillators.

Occasionally, open heart surgery is necessary to control some types of serious tachycardia.

PREVENTION

A generally heart-healthy lifestyle that may decrease the chance of rhythm disturbances includes

- Regular exercise
- Not smoking
- Avoiding excessive amounts of alcohol and caffeine
- Avoiding illegal drug use (especially cocaine)

ASTHMA

Although asthma can be quite severe and problematic for some sufferers, most do not have debilitating disease, and symptoms are controllable.

Asthma is a chronic inflammation disorder of the bronchial tubes that causes excess mucus formation, muscular constriction, and variable degrees of reversible airflow obstruction, resulting in incomplete emptying of the lung and lung over-inflation. Unlike chronic bronchitis (BRONCHITIS, CHRONIC) though, asthma appears to be episodic in nature, and it can often be set off by various triggers such as allergens, cold air, and exercise.

CAUSES

The exact cause of asthma is not completely understood. It seems to have a genetic component because people with a family history of the disease have a greater risk of eventually developing it.

Other factors that may precipitate asthma in susceptible individuals include

- Childhood exposure to allergens such as warm-blooded animals and dust
- Exposure to tobacco smoke
- Certain respiratory infections
- Occupational exposure to plastics and some inorganic chemicals

SYMPTOMS

In the classic case of asthma, the patient experiences recurrent episodes of

- Wheezing
- BREATHING DIFFICULTY
- COUGH
- Chest tightness, particularly at night and in the early morning

Not every case is the classic case, and various combinations of these symptoms are possible in individual cases. Some patients, for example, experience COUGH alone; others experience BREATHING DIFFICULTY only during exercise or only at certain times of the year.

DIAGNOSIS

Asthma can usually be diagnosed from the symptoms and the MEDICAL HISTORY. A PHYSICAL EXAMINATION provides support for the diagnosis.

Other tests include measurements of lung function using a spirometer or peak flow meter (see PULMONARY FUNCTION TESTING). People with asthma have lower peak flow readings than healthy people, especially after exercise.

Another common test for asthma is the methacholine challenge. It is a test of bronchial wall inflammation in the presence of the chemical methacholine. In people with asthma, methacholine causes a drop in lung function, which can be reversed with medication.

COMPLICATIONS

All patients with asthma are at risk of developing a severe asthma attack that can lead to respiratory failure—a disorder called *status asthmaticus*. Attacks in status asthmaticus can come on suddenly or, more commonly, the symptoms develop over a number of days until the patient ends up in the emergency room with respiratory distress. Regardless of the circumstance, status asthmaticus is a life-threatening disorder that can require mechanical ventilation in an intensive care unit.

Overinflated lungs may rupture, allowing air to escape into the chest cavity and compressing the lung tissue because the air can get in, but it can't get back out—a potentially life-threatening condition called *pneumothorax* that may require immediate treatment.

Because medication is used on a long-term basis in asthma, cumulative side effects can cause problems. Long-term steroid use can lead to

- WEIGHT GAIN
- Muscle loss
- Bone thinning (OSTEOPOROSIS)
- CATARACT
- High blood pressure (HYPERTENSION)
- CUSHING SYNDROME

TREATMENT

SELF TREATMENT:

Avoiding asthma triggers, such as smoke or specific pollutants, and caring for general health, such as ensuring proper nutrition, are appropriate measures. Contact with pets may need to be limited.

MEDICAL TREATMENT:

For patients with infrequent symptoms, inhaled medications such as ALBUTEROL or METAPROTERENOL provide adequate control.

For patients with more severe symptoms (episodes one to two times per week), specific treatment of bronchial wall inflammations is recommended. Inhaled anti-inflammatory medications such as steroids (beclomethasone), nedocromil sodium, or cromolyn sodium are effective. The nonsteroidal medication is preferred for children because steroids can retard growth. THEOPHYLLINE, a bronchodilator, may have useful anti-inflammatory effects as well.

SURGICAL TREATMENT:

None.

PREVENTION

Primary prevention—preventing the development of asthma—includes altering the environment of those at risk for the disease, such as infants of asthmatic parents. Decreasing exposure to allergens, such as dust mites and warm-blooded pets, and to environmental tobacco smoke can help. Vaccinations for children can prevent respiratory infections that may precipitate asthma.

Secondary prevention—preventing attacks in those who already have asthma—includes avoiding triggers, including some food additives, some drugs (beta-blockers) used to treat HYPERTENSION and GLAUCOMA, and anti-inflammatory agents such as ASPIRIN and IBUPROFEN. Vaccinations and frequent hand washing can limit respiratory tract infections.

ATHEROSCLEROSIS

Atherosclerosis is a condition that can lead to some of the biggest killers, including heart attacks and stroke.

In atherosclerosis, also commonly called hardening of the arteries, fat and sometimes calcium deposits build up on the inner wall of blood vessels. Although the condition can affect blood vessels anywhere in the body, the vessels in which atherosclerosis causes the most noticeable problems include the coronary arteries, which feed the heart muscle, the carotid and vertebral arteries, which feed the brain, and the iliac and femoral arteries, which feed the legs.

CAUSES

Although the exact cause of atherosclerotic build-up in the blood vessels is not known, certain risk factors for atherosclerosis have been identified, including

- High blood pressure (HYPERTENSION)
- Smoking
- High blood cholesterol level (HYPERLIPIDEMIA)
- DIABETES
- Being male
- Family history of the disease

SYMPTOMS

For long periods of time while deposits build up on the walls of blood vessels, atherosclerosis can be quite silent, causing no noticeable symptoms at all. Ultimately, though, the progressive occlusion of the blood vessels by fat and calcium deposits can lead to symptoms. Gradually progressive symptoms can stem from the slowly diminishing blood flow to the area, or sudden serious symptoms can appear when there is a sudden total blockage, or occlusion, of the blood vessel.

When a localized deposit of cholesterol and fats (called atherosclerotic *plaque*) ruptures and causes a blood clot to form, the blood vessel can become completely blocked and the flow of blood stopped. The specific symptoms of such an occurrence depend on the location of the affected blood vessels

- If the arteries to the brain are affected, then the common symptoms include those of a transient ischemic attack—brief episodes of weakness in an arm or leg, difficulty speaking, or loss of vision in one eye—or STROKE.
- If the coronary arteries are affected, then symptoms related to ANGINA or HEART ATTACK can result.

- If the blood vessels to the bowels are affected (mesenteric ischemia), severe ABDOMINAL PAIN after meals can be a manifestation (especially in older people).
- If the vessels of the legs are affected, a reproducible, consistent ache that occurs most commonly in the back of the calf when walking and that is relieved with rest (a symptom known as *claudication*) is the most common manifestation.

DIAGNOSIS

Atherosclerosis can be diagnosed on the basis of typical symptoms. Sometimes a PHYSICAL EXAMINATION reveals a decreased circulation; examination of the pulses or listening for a turbulent flow (called *bruits*) are also clues.

Diagnostic tests include

- CARDIAC STRESS TEST to evaluate signs of atherosclerosis to the heart
- Carotid artery blood-flow studies (including ULTRASOUND) for evidence of decreased flow or blockages to the brain and legs
- Angiography (CARDIAC CATHETERIZATION and RADIOGRAPHY) of the affected area to show signs of narrowing caused by atherosclerosis

COMPLICATIONS

The complications of atherosclerosis are related to the area in which the circulation is affected. The most serious ones are

- STROKE—if the blood vessels in the brain are affected
- HEART ATTACK—if the coronary arteries are affected
- GANGRENE—if the blood vessels of an extremity are affected

TREATMENT

SELF TREATMENT:

- Avoidance of smoking
- A low-fat, low-cholesterol diet
- Regular exercise

MEDICAL TREATMENT:

Because blockages are a dangerous consequence of atherosclerosis, drug therapy is aimed at promoting good blood flow. To this end, calcium-channel blockers, such as DILTIAZEM and NIFEDIPINE, are sometimes prescribed. NITROGLYCERIN is commonly used to treat or prevent episodes of ANGINA caused by atherosclerosis. Beta-blockers, such as ATENOLOL and METOPROLOL, are also used to help compensate for a lack of blood flow.

ASPIRIN, WARFARIN, and ticlopidine are sometimes used to decrease the chance of blood clots forming on a ruptured atherosclerotic plaque.

In recent years aggressive attempts to lower blood cholesterol levels have been shown to slow and even reverse progressive plaque buildup in the blood vessels to the brain, heart, and legs. Drugs such as SIMVASTATIN, LOVASTATIN, CHOLESTYRAMINE, and niacin have been the most frequently used for this purpose.

SURGICAL TREATMENT:

Surgical procedures designed to treat more advanced cases of atherosclerosis include

- CORONARY ARTERY BYPASS GRAFT SURGERY
- Percutaneous transluminal ANGIOPLASTY
- CAROTID ENDARTECTOMY
- Peripheral vascular surgery (using veins to bypass blockages in the legs)

PREVENTION

- Avoidance of smoking
- Low-fat, low-cholesterol diet
- Control of HYPERTENSION
- Regular exercise
- Estrogen replacement therapy for postmenopausal women (probably)
- Adequate vitamin E intake (possibly)

ATRIAL FIBRILLATION

Atrial fibrillation is an irregular heartbeat caused by rapid chaotic discharge of the upper chambers of the heart (called the *atria*). These erratic signals travel through the heart's electrical system to the bottom chambers (called the *ventricles*), leading to a rapid and irregular pulse.

The frequency of atrial fibrillation increases with age; as many as a few percent of people over 65 experience the condition.

CAUSES

Atrial fibrillation is most commonly related to some underlying heart disease, such as

- Hypertensive heart disease related to long-standing high blood pressure (see HYPERTENSION)
- HEART VALVE DISEASE
- Ischemic heart disease (such as prior HEART ATTACK)

Other causes include HYPERTHYROIDISM and excessive alcohol consumption that can cause heart rhythm and heart muscle problems.

SYMPTOMS

Atrial fibrillation in many cases can be completely without symptoms for years at a time. When it does cause symptoms, it may be noted as palpitation or an awareness of one's own heartbeat. Unfortunately, one of the complications of atrial fibrillation is sometimes the first sign to be noticed.

DIAGNOSIS

A PHYSICAL EXAMINATION that reveals a randomly irregular pulse may signal the presence of atrial fibrillation. The diagnosis is usually confirmed by ELECTROCARDIOGRAPHY.

COMPLICATIONS

The complications of atrial fibrillation include formation of blood clots in the atria that can travel to various parts of the body including the brain (leading to a STROKE or a transient ischemic attack), the abdominal organs (for example, the bowels), or the extremities (causing a suddenly cold and painful pulseless arm or leg and possibly GANGRENE). This complication is called an *embolism*.

Because atrial fibrillation is a less efficient form of heart function, it may also lead to a worsening of CONGESTIVE HEART FAILURE or ANGINA.

TREATMENT

SELF TREATMENT:

Lifestyle changes that decrease the underlying causes of atrial fibrillation (HYPERTENSION, ALCOHOLISM, or coronary artery disease) are the most helpful. Measures include

- Low-salt diet
- Moderate exercise
- Avoidance of alcohol
- Avoidance of other risk factors for ATHEROSCLEROSIS

MEDICAL TREATMENT:

Pharmaceutical treatment can help control the heart rate with DIGOXIN, VERAPAMIL, and beta-blockers such as PROPRANOLOL. Attempts to convert the heart rhythm to a more normal rhythm (called a *sinus* rhythm) may include the use of the drugs quinidine, PROCAINAMIDE, or amiodarone.

Drugs can also be useful in the control of potential embolic complications. The drugs WARFARIN and ASPIRIN reduce the blood's clotting ability, thus decreasing the chance of blood-clot formation in the atria and the risk of embolism.

Another medical therapy is electrical cardioversion, which involves using electrical paddles in a monitored setting to convert the atrial fibrillation to a normal sinus rhythm.

SURGICAL TREATMENT:

Surgical therapies are rarely used to treat atrial fibrillation, but some persistent and severe atrial rhythm abnormalities that do not respond to drug treatment may warrant surgery. Certain electrical oblation techniques involving catheters passed through blood vessels to the heart or open heart surgery to change the electrical pathways within the heart can be used to treat these rare severe cases.

PREVENTION

- Avoidance of excessive alcohol consumption
- Appropriate treatment of strep throat infection to decrease the chance of rheumatic heart disease and HEART VALVE DISEASE
- Measures to decrease the risk of ATHEROSCLEROSIS
- Weight control and adherence to a low-salt diet

BLADDER INFECTION

Bladder infections are almost always bacterial infections. In women, these infections can recur sporadically, and although they are often uncomfortable and inconvenient, they are rarely dangerous.

In men, bladder infections are often a signal of some underlying urologic problem.

Women are much more susceptible to bladder infections than are men simply because women's urethras are much shorter than men's, thus leaving less distance for infecting bacteria to travel up to the bladder.

CAUSES

Bladder infections are usually caused by bacteria migrating up the urethra to the bladder. Often bacteria from other parts of the body are involved; bacteria that normally live in the digestive tract, for example, are frequently implicated in bladder infections because of the close proximity of the anus and the urethra, especially in women. Recurrent infections in women may sometimes be associated with sexual intercourse (see Prevention below).

In men, a bladder infection is usually caused by an infection of the prostate gland that has spread to the bladder or by bacteria trapped in the bladder by an enlarged prostate (PROSTATE, ENLARGED).

SYMPTOMS

The symptoms of a bladder infection include

- Frequent and often urgent need to urinate (URINATION, FREQUENT)
- Burning sensation upon urination (URINATION, PAINFUL)
- Lower back pain (occasionally)
- FEVER (occasionally)
- Rarely, blood in the urine (usually seen in women only)

DIAGNOSIS

Bladder infection can usually be suspected from the symptoms, but the definitive diagnosis of bladder infection relies primarily on two basic tests

- URINALYSIS
- Urine CULTURE

COMPLICATIONS

Left untreated, bladder infection can lead to kidney infection, which can, in turn, progress to BLOOD POISONING, KIDNEY STONES, and kidney damage.

TREATMENT

SELF TREATMENT:

Drinking plenty of fluids can help.

MEDICAL TREATMENT:

The main weapons used to fight bladder infection are antibiotics such as

- TRIMETHOPRIM
- AMPICILLIN
- Sulfamethoxazole
- OFLOXACIN

For men whose infection is associated with an underlying urologic problem such as an enlarged prostate (PROSTATE, ENLARGED), the underlying condition is also treated.

SURGICAL TREATMENT:

None.

PREVENTION

- Drinking plenty of fluids and not delaying urination help to flush the bladder regularly.
- Front-to-back wiping with toilet tissue can prevent contamination of the urethra by bacteria from the anal area.
- For women who experience recurrent bladder infections associated with sexual intercourse, urinating immediately after intercourse may prevent some infections.

BLADDER STONES

Bladder stones are conglomerates of minerals that form in the urinary bladder for various reasons. The stones can vary considerably in size and shape, but many can cause severe discomfort.

The urine produced by the kidneys and stored in the urinary bladder contains various inorganic minerals that can, under certain circumstances, precipitate and form stones.

CAUSES

Although the exact cause of stones is quite often never determined, most commonly, stones form when the bladder does not empty completely, allowing time for minerals in the urine to coalesce. This condition can be brought on by an obstruction or by an anatomic abnormality that allows the urine to pool.

BLADDER INFECTIONS can change the chemical nature of the urine, contributing to stone formation. Less often, the stones can be a result of KIDNEY STONES that have passed down the ureter and lodged in the bladder.

There may be a hereditary tendency to develop bladder stones; people with a family history of bladder stones appear to have an increased chance of developing them.

SYMPTOMS

The symptoms are relatively obvious and include

- Sharp pain in the bladder region (lower ABDOMINAL PAIN) that can come in waves
- Sudden, painful interruption of flow during urination

The pain of bladder stones is sometimes associated with

- Profuse sweating (SWEATING, EXCESSIVE)
- VOMITING and nausea
- Blood in the urine (URINE, ABNORMAL APPEARANCE)

DIAGNOSIS

Besides the tell-tale symptoms, diagnosis can include

- X ray (RADIOGRAPHY) of the bladder
- ULTRASOUND of the bladder

COMPLICATIONS

- Bladder stones can set the stage for a BLADDER INFECTION.
- Prolonged obstruction of the urinary tract can lead to kidney damage.

TREATMENT

SELF TREATMENT:

(See Prevention below.)

MEDICAL TREATMENT:

(See Prevention below.)

SURGICAL TREATMENT:

If the stones are not passed, they are removed surgically with either an open surgical technique or with a cystoscope—a flexible tube that passes up through the urethra. The latter procedure is less expensive and requires no incision, but might not be appropriate for all kinds of stones.

PREVENTION

Adequate fluid intake ensures proper hydration and may discourage stone formation.

Drugs such as HYDROCHLOROTHIAZIDE and ALLOPURINOL may be used to prevent additional stone formation depending on the type of stone and the likelihood of recurrence. This preventive therapy is not appropriate for all patients.

BLOOD POISONING

Blood poisoning is a nonmedical term used to describe patients that have a serious bacterial infection that is causing widespread reaction in the body.

The technical term for blood poisoning is *septicemia*, or *sepsis*. The danger of septicemia can be caused by the rampant infection itself or by toxins being released by the bacteria and spread through the blood. By definition the whole body is affected because the blood distributes the bacteria and toxins throughout the body.

CAUSES

An infection in any one portion of the body that gets out of control and spreads throughout the body is the cause of blood poisoning. Examples of conditions that can lead to septicemia include

- Ruptured appendix in appendicitis
- Ruptured gallbladder (see CHOLECYSTITIS AND CHOLANGITIS)
- Kidney infection
- PELVIC INFLAMMATORY DISEASE
- GANGRENE
- Tooth abscess

Immunosuppressive drugs such as PREDNISONE and diseases such as DIABETES and LEUKEMIA that interfere with the body's immune system can also precipitate septicemia.

SYMPTOMS

Any one symptom is not sufficient to label a patient as having blood poisoning. However, the increasing number and constellation of them does. These symptoms include

- Shaking chills
- High FEVER
- Fast heart rate
- CONFUSION or other symptoms of mental impairment such as MEMORY PROBLEMS
- Low blood pressure
- General malaise (a feeling of being unwell)

DIAGNOSIS

Diagnosis is based on the symptoms. Additional tests that may be helpful include white blood cell count (see BLOOD COUNT) and blood CULTURES looking for bacteria.

In severely ill patients with low blood pressure additional measurements may be made with a catheter threaded up to the right side of the heart (see CARDIAC CATHETERIZATION). The additional cardiovascular measurements may further confirm a picture of sepsis and aid in the proper treatment.

COMPLICATIONS

Very low blood pressure can progress to shock, with multiple organ failure and even death. Organs that can fail during sepsis are the kidneys and lungs and, less often, the liver. Also, any underlying heart disease would be aggravated during the period of low blood pressure because of the extreme stress sepsis puts on the heart.

TREATMENT

SELF TREATMENT:

A person with symptoms of septicemia requires prompt medical attention; however, general measures include reducing the FEVER with acetaminophen and maintaining adequate hydration by drinking enough fluids.

MEDICAL TREATMENT:

Generally, broad-spectrum antibiotics such as gentamicin and large volumes of intravenous fluids are the initial treatments for sepsis. Temporary measures to assist with any organ failure may be necessary, including drugs such as FUROSEMIDE to maintain urine flow, oxygen to assist the lungs, and drugs such as dopamine to help the heart.

Occasionally, if sepsis progresses to total KIDNEY FAILURE or respiratory failure, mechanical devices such as dialysis or mechanical ventilation may be required on a temporary basis.

SURGICAL TREATMENT:

Surgical drainage may be required of the original source of the infection such as a ruptured appendix, a ruptured gallbladder, or an abscess located elsewhere in the body.

PREVENTION

Prompt attention to bacterial infections can generally prevent them from progressing to blood poisoning. For certain high-risk individuals, vaccinations are appropriate such as pneumococcal vaccine for older adults or patients with significant heart or lung disease or DIABETES.

BOIL

A boil, also called a *carbuncle*, is an infection of the follicle of a hair. Accordingly, they occur only in areas of the skin that have hair follicles. Areas of the skin that are subject to friction and perspiration are common sites of boils, including the neck, face, underarms, skin folds, and buttocks.

As the boil progresses, the infected hair follicle becomes a firm, deep-seated, inflammatory bump (or nodule). It can be warm and tender and usually is red. It may eventually drain pus, especially if manipulated.

Boils are usually more unsightly than dangerous, but they can precipitate dangerous complications, especially if treated improperly.

CAUSES

Boils are caused by infection of the hair follicle by the bacteria *Staphylococcus aureus*.

SYMPTOMS

A boil is a firm, warm, tender, deep-seated, red nodule in a hair-bearing region of the skin. The nodule may drain pus or feel like it has liquid inside of it. If the nodule drains the pus, the tenderness usually improves rapidly, and the nodule may resolve itself over several days.

DIAGNOSIS

A physician can usually recognize a boil, or carbuncle. The diagnosis may be confirmed by sampling the pus and performing a gram stain and CULTURE to identify *Staphylococcus aureus*. Sometimes a BIOPSY is performed on the lesion to confirm that it is, in fact, just a boil.

COMPLICATIONS

- The infection of the hair follicle may spread to involve surrounding soft tissue and even bone.
- A chronic deeper infection involving fibrotic firm connective tissue may occur; this is called a *furuncle* and can be difficult to eradicate.
- A diffuse infection of the skin around the hair follicle may occur. This is called CELLULITIS.
- Sometimes the bacteria in the infected hair follicle can spread to the blood stream (sepsis, or BLOOD POISONING) and cause a systemic infection involving other organs.

TREATMENT

SELF TREATMENT:

- Moist warm compresses should be applied to the boil to encourage it to drain spontaneously.
- The patient should make every effort to avoid manipulating the boil or squeezing it.
- After the boil ruptures and releases its contents, the area can be soaked with aluminum acetate solution for one hour two to four times a day.
- An over-the-counter ointment containing polymyxin B sulfate and bacitracin (such as Polysporin) applied between soaks can be helpful.
- The lesion should be washed with an antibacterial soap (such as Hibiclens) daily, and the patient should wash his or her hands very well with the same soap after changing dressings.

MEDICAL TREATMENT:

Systemic antibiotics against *Staphylococcus aureus*, such as PENICILLIN or DICLOXACILLIN, are usually the first medical treatments indicated. For patients who are allergic to PENICILLIN, CLINDAMYCIN and ERYTHROMYCIN are good alternative antibiotics. Unresponsive or recurrent boils can be treated with another antibiotic, RIFAMPIN.

All of the above Self treatment measures should be instituted by the physician if the patient has not yet started them.

SURGICAL TREATMENT:

Boils can be lanced and drained by a physician, but warm moist compresses accomplish the same thing and allow the lesion to drain spontaneously with minimal trauma to the tissues.

PREVENTION

- Washing and changing clothes, towels, and bed linens frequently
- Use of antibacterial soap in areas of previous boil eruption
- Meticulous hygiene and daily bathing

BONE FRACTURE

A bone fracture is a partial or complete break through a part of the skeleton; this can occur in large bones like the femur (thigh bone) as well as in small bones like the phalanges (finger bones).

Bone fractures are relatively common injuries and can occur at any age.

CAUSES

Most bone fractures are caused by traumatic injury. Occasionally, fractures can occur because of repetitive stress (stress fractures), but this is rare by comparison.

OSTEOPOROSIS and other diseases affecting the strength and structure of bone can make an individual more susceptible to this type of injury.

SYMPTOMS

The most common symptom of a bone fracture is pain over the broken portion. In cases where the fracture is displaced (moved out of its normal alignment) a deformity of the bone or joint can sometimes be seen.

DIAGNOSIS

Most bone fractures are definitively identified by X rays (RADIOGRAPHY) of the affected area. Fractures in very small bones, hairline fractures, or stress fractures may occasionally require a specialized test called a bone scan to confirm the diagnosis (see NUCLEAR MEDICINE).

COMPLICATIONS

The main complication of a bone fracture is a failure to heal, which can lead to an unstable area in the bone or instability of the adjacent joint. If the bone heals in a malunion (that is, out of alignment), there may be an angular or rotational deformity, which can cause some loss of range of motion at adjacent joints.

TREATMENT

SELF TREATMENT:

Fractures are difficult to manage, and evaluation by a physician is always recommended. First aid measures are appropriate such as

- Immobilizing the injured area
- Controlling any bleeding
- Applying ice if there is no bleeding

However, these measures are not to replace medical treatment, which should be sought immediately.

MEDICAL TREATMENT:

Nonsurgical treatment of fractures requires a period of immobilization in a splint or cast until the bone is healed. Pain medication such as an ACETAMINOPHEN AND CODEINE COMBINATION may be prescribed if needed.

SURGICAL TREATMENT:

Open reduction and internal fixation of the fracture, in which the bone is reshaped and mechanically held together by a pin or some other device, can be necessary in serious fractures.

PREVENTION

Fractures of bones generally occur as accidental trauma. General safety measures, such as the use of automobile seat belts and protective sports gear, may help prevent some fractures.

Many occupational injuries are related to alcohol abuse (see ALCOHOLISM) and are, therefore, also avoidable.

BREAST CANCER

Breast cancer is a cancer that originates in the breast tissue of women and men. It can spread to the lymph nodes under the arm before diagnosis. With advanced disease, metastasis can be seen in many body organs, including bone, brain, lung, liver, and skin.

About one in ten women will get breast cancer at sometime in their life, usually between the ages of 50 and 70.

CAUSES

Risk factors for developing breast cancer include
- Early onset of menses or late menopause
- First pregnancy after age 30
- Family history of the disease
- Radiation exposure

Possible risk factors include
- High-fat diet
- Excessive alcohol intake
- Estrogen replacement therapy
- Oral contraceptive use

SYMPTOMS

Breast cancer is usually manifest as a painless lump anywhere in the breast or under the arm (see BREAST PAIN OR LUMPS). Occasionally, its symptoms can be more subtle, such as
- An inverted nipple
- Bloody discharge from the nipple
- Changes in the skin overlying the breast making it resemble the skin of an orange

DIAGNOSIS

Any BREAST PAIN OR LUMPS felt on PHYSICAL EXAMINATION by a woman or her physician, and any lumps found on mammography (RADIOGRAPHY) should be considered for BIOPSY. Lumps seen on mammography but not palpable on examination can be located by ULTRASOUND or mammogram for BIOPSY.

If a diagnosis of breast cancer is established, staging tests include
- Liver function tests (see BLOOD TESTS)
- Alkaline phosphatase test to check for bone disease (see BLOOD TESTS)
- Chest X ray (RADIOGRAPHY)
- Bone scan (NUCLEAR MEDICINE)

COMPLICATIONS

Complications of breast cancer are related to areas of metastasis:

- Metastasis to bone can cause pain, BONE FRACTURES, or elevated calcium levels in the blood.
- Metastasis to the brain or spinal cord can cause seizures, HEADACHES, weakness, NUMBNESS, or CONFUSION.
- Metastasis to the lungs can cause BREATHING DIFFICULTY, CHEST PAIN, or swelling of the face and neck.

TREATMENT

SELF TREATMENT:

- A well-balanced diet should be maintained.
- Once a diagnosis of breast cancer is made, all estrogen medication should be stopped, including birth control pills.

MEDICAL TREATMENT:

Many women will require additional drug therapy after surgery to prevent breast cancer from returning. Either tamoxifen (a hormonal pill) or chemotherapy (intravenous medication) may be recommended, depending on the type of tumor. More advanced breast cancer is also treated with chemotherapy or hormonal therapy.

SURGICAL TREATMENT:

Two alternative initial treatments for breast cancer are

- Lumpectomy with lymph node dissection followed by radiation therapy to the breast
- Mastectomy (MASTECTOMY, PARTIAL; or MASTECTOMY, MODIFIED RADICAL)

PREVENTION

Early detection of breast cancer by regular breast self-examination and regular mammography (RADIOGRAPHY) screening is important. A low-fat diet and moderate alcohol intake may be important. Some researchers theorize that exercise for preadolescent girls may be helpful as it delays the age of onset of menstruation.

BRONCHITIS, CHRONIC

Chronic bronchitis is a condition of the lung characterized by excess mucus in the bronchial tubes and a COUGH present on most days. In patients with chronic bronchitis, there is an increase in the number and size of mucus-secreting glands in the bronchial tubes.

Because the condition is so closely associated with smoking, people with chronic bronchitis often have EMPHYSEMA as well.

Chronic bronchitis is distinguished from acute bronchitis by its duration and cause. The acute condition is an inflammation of the bronchial tubes caused by an infection; the chronic condition causes ongoing symptoms even without infection.

CAUSES

The most important cause of chronic bronchitis is smoking. The greater the extent and duration of smoking, the greater the likelihood of developing bronchitis. Other causes include occupational exposures to chemicals and exposure to air pollutants. There are cases that have no apparent cause. Infections generally do not cause chronic bronchitis but can aggravate the condition.

SYMPTOMS

The hallmarks of chronic bronchitis are

- Persistent COUGH
- Excess mucus
- BREATHING DIFFICULTY
- Wheezing (occasionally)
- ANKLE SWELLING in cases of heart strain

Respiratory symptoms tend to wax and wane, resulting in "good days" and "bad days." The coughing and mucus production are often worse first thing in the morning.

DIAGNOSIS

The diagnosis of chronic bronchitis is made from the characteristic symptoms and characteristic MEDICAL HISTORY that includes a long history of smoking. PHYSICAL EXAMINATION often reveals wheezes and a prolonged expiratory phase during breathing similar to but not as pronounced as that seen in ASTHMA and EMPHYSEMA. Other tests include

- PULMONARY FUNCTION TESTING
- Chest X rays (RADIOGRAPHY)
- Testing of blood oxygen and carbon dioxide levels (see BLOOD TESTS)

COMPLICATIONS

Patients with chronic bronchitis tend to minimize their symptoms by adopting a sedentary lifestyle, resulting in general deconditioning and WEIGHT GAIN—both of which can aggravate BREATHING DIFFICULTY.

Because the condition can lead to decreased levels of oxygen in the blood and a subsequent constriction of pulmonary blood vessels, chronic bronchitis can lead to heart strain and symptoms of CONGESTIVE HEART FAILURE.

Infections are particularly dangerous in chronic bronchitis and can lead to life-threatening PNEUMONIA.

TREATMENT

SELF TREATMENT:

- Quitting smoking
- Embarking on a sensible exercise program
- Washing hands frequently to decrease the risk of infection

MEDICAL TREATMENT:

- Oxygen for patients whose blood level is too low
- Inhaled bronchodilators such as ALBUTEROL and ipratropium bromide and oral bronchodilators such as THEOPHYLLINE to improve airflow
- Corticosteroids (PREDNISONE) to reduce swelling and inflammation in the bronchial tubes
- Antibiotics to address infections promptly
- Guaifenesin to loosen mucus

INFLUENZA vaccine given in the fall can protect against the usual outbreak of INFLUENZA seen in the winter months. Pneumococcal vaccine offers protection against one of the most common causes of PNEUMONIA.

SURGICAL TREATMENT:

None.

PREVENTION

Avoidance of smoking and exposure to smoke and pollutants is the most important preventive step.

BURSITIS

Bursitis can usually be attributed to some overuse or injury, but not all cases have an obvious cause.

Bursitis is an inflammatory condition of the small fluid filled sacs (called *bursas*) overlying prominent parts of the skeleton. A bursa normally consists of a thin sac with lining cells that decrease the gliding friction of tendons or other soft tissues as they move and rub against each other. In bursitis, the inflamed lining cells increase the fluid production and cause swelling and tension.

Patients who have bursitis in an area may have recurrent episodes, as the lining cells become more susceptible to pressure or friction.

CAUSES

Bursitis is frequently caused by minor trauma or overuse in the area of the bursa or by adjacent tendons. Repeated physical activities, such as swinging a tennis racket or sweeping can cause bursitis.

There are also medical conditions, such as gout, that cause inflammatory changes in joints and tendons throughout the body that can involve the bursas.

SYMPTOMS

Patients may notice pain and swelling in the area, and painful motion as they use a particular joint. The overlying skin may become red, or feel warm. Bursitis can cause swelling of the bursa to such a degree that the overlying skin may appear swollen, too. Bursitis is most commonly seen in the shoulders, elbows, wrist, lateral area of the hip, knees, and ankles.

DIAGNOSIS

Diagnosis of bursitis is generally made clinically by combining the patient's recent activity history with the findings of a PHYSICAL EXAMINATION; the findings are usually similar to those noted by the patients themselves.

Occasionally, fluid can be removed for testing, primarily when there is concern that the bursa might be infected. X rays (RADIOGRAPHY) may be helpful in evaluating the painful joint, but the film will not show the bursa itself.

COMPLICATIONS

The main complication of bursitis is an infection of the bursa. The bursa is frequently just under the skin, and it is possible that skin bacteria could cause an infection.

TREATMENT

SELF TREATMENT:

- Decreasing the activity involving the joint gives the inflammation time to go down.
- Over-the-counter anti-inflammatory and analgesic medication such as IBUPROFEN can reduce pain and inflammation.

MEDICAL TREATMENT:

- Splinting may help the joint rest by limiting its motion.
- Anti-inflammatory and analgesic medication such as IBUPROFEN and NAPROXEN can reduce pain and inflammation.

SURGICAL TREATMENT:

In severe or recurrent cases, bursal drainage (in which the fluid is drawn out of the swollen bursa) and bursectomy (in which the affected bursa is removed) are options.

PREVENTION

Many times, bursitis is caused by repetitive overuse or minimal traumas associated with sports or work. Early recognition of overuse problems and treatment with rest and anti-inflammatory medications may resolve the problem before serious problems arise.

CARDIOMYOPATHY

When a disease of the heart muscle affects its ability to pump blood normally, the term *cardiomyopathy* is used.

There are three basic categories of cardiomyopathy based on the cause and the mechanical difficulty with the heart muscle: 1) the heart balloons out in size (dilated); 2) the heart thickens excessively (hypertrophic); or 3) the heart loses its ability to relax between heartbeats and refill for the next contraction (restrictive).

CAUSES

A wide variety of causes have been identified, although many cases do not have any apparent cause. Common causes include

- Advanced HYPERTENSION or coronary artery disease (ATHEROSCLEROSIS)
- Familial hypertrophic cardiomyopathies
- Chronic excessive alcohol intake (ALCOHOLISM)
- Vitamin deficiencies (for example, thiamin)
- Viral infections causing MYOCARDITIS
- Pregnancy-related cardiomyopathy

OBESITY and DIABETES may also contribute to the problem. In some cases, medications such as thyroid hormone may contribute to the problem and need to be regulated.

SYMPTOMS

Many times, some decrease in heart muscle performance is without symptoms. In more advanced stages, signs of CONGESTIVE HEART FAILURE (BREATHING DIFFICULTY, ANKLE SWELLING) or symptoms from complications may be the first clue.

DIAGNOSIS

A MEDICAL HISTORY and PHYSICAL EXAMINATION compatible with CONGESTIVE HEART FAILURE would be the initial step in diagnosis. A chest X ray (RADIOGRAPHY) and ELECTROCARDIOGRAPHY provide additional information. The absence of other causes of CONGESTIVE HEART FAILURE, such as HYPERTENSION, ATHEROSCLEROSIS, HEART VALVE DISEASE, or pericardial or congenital heart disease, increases the likelihood of a primary heart muscle problem. An echocardiogram (ULTRASOUND) or NUCLEAR MEDICINE study can confirm a cardiomyopathy. In some cases, CARDIAC CATHETERIZATION, angiography (RADIOGRAPHY), and BIOPSY may be needed.

COMPLICATIONS

Cardiomyopathy may lead to ARRHYTHMIAS (ventricular tachycardia, heart block), causing FAINTING OR FAINTNESS or even cardiac arrest. When young people in athletic events die unexpectedly, this is often the cause. Dilated heart muscles may allow blood clots to form along the inner walls of the heart, and these may break off and travel to the brain or limbs, causing a STROKE or GANGRENE.

TREATMENT

SELF TREATMENT:

(See Prevention below.)

MEDICAL TREATMENT:

- Control of hypertension with medication such as HYDROCHLOROTHIAZIDE
- Treatment of CONGESTIVE HEART FAILURE with medications such as DIGOXIN, FUROSEMIDE, and ACE inhibitors (ENALAPRIL)
- In selected cases of MYOCARDITIS, immunosuppressive treatment with medication such as PREDNISONE
- The suspension, at least on a trial basis, of medications that may aggravate CONGESTIVE HEART FAILURE, such as steroids, beta-blockers (ATENOLOL, PROPRANOLOL), DISOPYRAMIDE, and VERAPAMIL

SURGICAL TREATMENT:

- Heart transplant or related surgery may be warranted in advanced refractory cases where the prognosis is otherwise poor.
- Occasionally, CORONARY ARTERY BYPASS GRAFT SURGERY may help in very carefully selected patients.

PREVENTION

- Control of HYPERTENSION
- Treatment of ATHEROSCLEROSIS
- Avoidance of excessive alcohol intake
- Maintenance of a healthy weight
- Other strategies to prevent ATHEROSCLEROSIS (not smoking, low-fat diet, regular exercise)

CARPAL TUNNEL SYNDROME

Carpal tunnel syndrome is a grouping of symptoms involving the median nerve in the wrist and hand. Symptoms include NUMBNESS, tingling, weakness, and pain in the palm side of the wrist and hand, which are innervated by the median nerve. Symptoms in the fingers are most frequently noted in the thumb-side fingers (thumb, index finger, and middle finger).

Carpal tunnel syndrome can affect anyone, but the most commonly affected group is women in their 30s and 40s.

CAUSES

Carpal tunnel syndrome is caused by a decrease in the local blood supply to the median nerve as it moves through a tunnel-like area in the wrist. The nerve shares the tunnel with the flexor tendons of the wrist (the tendons of muscles that flex the wrist and fingers), and may be under pressure if the tendons swell from overuse.

Swelling of the soft tissues caused by increased fluid volume (particularly in pregnancy) may also increase the pressure in the carpal tunnel and decrease the blood supply to the nerve.

SYMPTOMS

The symptoms of carpal tunnel syndrome include

- NUMBNESS and tingling on the thumb side of the hand, including the thumb, index finger, and middle finger
- Weakness of thumb-side grip strength
- Pain in the hand and wrist that may worsen with repetitive motions or increase when the wrist is flexed

DIAGNOSIS

The diagnosis of carpal tunnel syndrome includes noting the symptoms and finding NUMBNESS or weakness on PHYSICAL EXAMINATION. These findings may be determined by sensory testing and by objective measurements of grip and finger strength. Several tests may briefly increase the pressure on the median nerve and provoke the symptoms.

Definitive evidence of nerve compression with slowing of the nerve signals of the median nerve can be demonstrated with electrical testing (electromyography) in which electrodes are attached to the forearm.

COMPLICATIONS

Episodic NUMBNESS and tingling complaints can resolve with time; prolonged and continuous loss of sensory abilities and motor strength may suggest more severe compression of the nerve, which can lead to permanent nerve damage and chronic symptoms.

TREATMENT

SELF TREATMENT:

Avoidance of repetitive activities that cause symptoms may help reduce inflammation.

MEDICAL TREATMENT:

- Anti-inflammatory medications such as IBUPROFEN and NAPROXEN
- Wrist splints to keep the wrists in a neutral position
- Injection of anti-inflammatory medications to decrease swelling

Women who have symptoms associated with pregnancy may not need treatment, because the condition can resolve after delivery when fluid volume returns to normal; however, splints may relieve discomfort if needed.

SURGICAL TREATMENT:

CARPAL TUNNEL RELEASE may be appropriate for certain intractable cases.

PREVENTION

Carpal tunnel syndrome is considered a chronic overuse condition; interrupting continuous activities with a break or varying hand and wrist positions frequently during repetitive tasks may be helpful.

CATARACT

A cataract is an opacity, or clouding, of the crystalline lens of the eye that reduces visual function.

The lens of the eye, which helps to focus light onto the retina, is usually clear, but the clouding effect of a cataract scatters the incoming light, causing blurred vision.

CAUSES

Cataracts are usually associated with aging, but they can also occur in patients with certain diseases such as DIABETES. Drugs such as steroids and cortisone taken orally or topically can induce cataract. Cataracts can also occur after trauma to the eye or in association with a chronic inflammation.

SYMPTOMS

Cataract causes VISION DISTURBANCES including
- Altered color vision
- Diminished side vision or night vision
- Double vision in the affected eye

DIAGNOSIS

The diagnosis is made after a careful eye examination in which a microscope is used to examine the lens of the eye.

COMPLICATIONS

GLAUCOMA and inflammation can occur in rare cases.

TREATMENT

SELF TREATMENT:

None.

MEDICAL TREATMENT:

Pupil-dilating eye drops that allow the patient to see around the cloudy part of the lens.

SURGICAL TREATMENT:

CATARACT REMOVAL is indicated in some patients.

PREVENTION

Cataracts can be prevented in some cases by
- Promptly treating ocular inflammation
- Using eye protection in hazardous situations

CELLULITIS

The skin normally protects the body from invading bacteria, but small wounds and minor skin diseases can open the skin itself to infection and lead to more serious problems.

Cellulitis is a serious infection of the skin. However, the infection can spread through the lymph system to other parts of the body with potentially life-threatening consequences.

CAUSES

The cause of cellulitis is either streptococcal or staphylococcal bacteria. Cellulitis often occurs when the skin is not intact due to a wound or skin disease such as DERMATITIS.

SYMPTOMS

Cellulitis usually starts as broad sheets, or plaques, of red skin that are hot and tender. The skin symptoms may also be accompanied by general symptoms of infection such as FEVER, chills, HEADACHE, and malaise.

DIAGNOSIS

Cellulitis is usually diagnosed by the characteristic symptoms of red, hot, swollen, and painful skin in a site that has had or is prone to trauma. BLOOD COUNT may be helpful.

COMPLICATIONS

Without prompt treatment, the infection of the skin can spread to other areas of the body including internal organs.

TREATMENT

SELF TREATMENT:

Cool tap-water compresses may help decrease the pain.

MEDICAL TREATMENT:

Treatment consists of administration of antibiotics such as PENICILLIN and ERYTHROMYCIN.

SURGICAL TREATMENT:

None.

PREVENTION

- Moisturizing the skin to avoid drying and cracking
- For people with DIABETES, routinely inspecting the feet for injuries

CERVICAL CANCER

The cervix is that part of the uterus that protrudes into the vagina and dilates during labor. Cervical cancer can be formed from either the cells on the outside surface of the cervix (squamous cells) or the cells inside of the cervical canal (glandular or adenocarcinoma cells).

Cervical cancer is often presaged by a precancerous condition usually detectable only by Pap smear, highlighting the importance of this simple test.

CAUSES

Malignant cells in the cervix are thought to arise from a particular event or exposure. Risk factors associated with premalignant changes that can go on to form cancer include

- Early sexual intercourse
- Multiple sexual partners
- Infection with certain types of human papilloma virus (genital warts)
- Tobacco use

In addition, women who were exposed prenatally to a substance called diethylstilbestrol (DES)—a drug that until 1971 was given to some pregnant women to help prevent miscarriage—are at increased risk for a rare type of cervical cancer.

SYMPTOMS

Premalignant changes usually cause no symptoms. Once the cancer becomes invasive, however, patients may notice

- Unusual VAGINAL DISCHARGE, which may or may not be malodorous
- Bleeding or spotting after intercourse

Advanced cancer may be associated with

- Pain in the back or leg
- Blood in the urine
- Loss of urine through the vagina

DIAGNOSIS

Fortunately, there is a long premalignant phase for most cervical cancers. PAP SMEARS are screening tests for the presence of abnormal cells on the cervix. Once a PAP SMEAR is found to be abnormal, colposcopy is performed. This involves looking at the cervix with a special microscope and using special solutions such as acetic acid to highlight and visualize the areas of abnormality (see ENDOSCOPY).

Once these areas are seen, a BIOPSY may be performed to obtain a sample for pathologic analysis. Depending on the degree of abnormality, the area of abnormality (the lesion) may be destroyed, or another, larger BIOPSY may be performed so a pathologist can determine whether an actual invasive cancer exists.

COMPLICATIONS

Allowing the cancer to progress without therapy will likely result in life-threatening bleeding and blockage of the urine flow from the kidneys to the bladder with resultant KIDNEY FAILURE and death.

TREATMENT

SELF TREATMENT:

None.

MEDICAL TREATMENT:

Medical therapy for cervical cancer is reserved for patients with cancer that has spread. Chemotherapy is used but is not as effective as either surgery or radiation therapy.

SURGICAL TREATMENT:

A radical HYSTERECTOMY with removal of the lymph nodes from the pelvis is performed for patients with early cancer. Once the cancer has spread beyond the cervix to the tissue next to the uterus, radiation therapy is necessary.

PREVENTION

Cervical cancer has a long premalignant phase that can be treated with minimal surgical therapy and retention of reproductive function. However, in order for this to occur, the patient must have regular pelvic examinations and PAP SMEARS performed by a physician experienced in interpreting the results. The frequency of the examinations should be based on the individual woman's risk factors.

Lifestyle changes to help prevent the development of premalignant changes include

- Sexual abstinence unless in a mutually monogamous relationship
- Avoidance of smoking
- Use of barrier methods of contraception

CHOLECYSTITIS AND CHOLANGITIS

Cholecystitis and cholangitis are lumped together because the gallbladder and the bile ducts are connected and infection in one can spread to the other.

Cholecystitis is an inflammation in the gallbladder; the condition can be chronic or acute. Chronic cholecystitis is the inflammation that is found with symptomatic GALLSTONES. Acute cholecystitis is a complication of GALLSTONES that causes infection in the gallbladder wall and bile.

Cholangitis is an inflammation in the bile duct system. It is most often due to bacteria, but can be viral, parasitic, or chemical in nature.

CAUSES

The cause of chronic cholecystitis is not known, but it may be caused by mechanical irritation of the gallbladder or intermittent obstruction of the gallbladder by GALLSTONES.

Acute cholecystitis results when a GALLSTONE obstructs the duct emptying the gallbladder. Infection begins in the bile behind the stone and extends into the gallbladder wall.

Acute cholangitis occurs when bacteria are in bile and when the pressure increases in the bile duct system. The increase in pressure results from obstruction of the bile duct by a GALLSTONE, a bile duct narrowing, or a tumor of the bile duct, of the first part of the intestine (the duodenum), or of the pancreas (PANCREATIC CANCER), which the bile duct traverses to reach the intestine.

SYMPTOMS

Chronic cholecystitis causes

- Intermittent attacks of upper right ABDOMINAL PAIN
- Nausea and VOMITING
- Indigestion
- Increased flatulence

Acute cholecystitis causes

- Unremitting upper right ABDOMINAL PAIN
- FEVER
- Nausea and VOMITING

The symptoms of acute cholecystitis may be very similar to chronic cholecystitis, but the symptoms do not resolve spontaneously. They progress and worsen with time.

Acute cholangitis classically causes

- Jaundice
- Upper right ABDOMINAL PAIN
- FEVER

However, most patients have only one or two of the three symptoms.

Sometimes acute cholangitis can be very severe, in which case it is called *toxic cholangitis*. In this condition, the patient experiences CONFUSION and very low blood pressure. This is a life-threatening event and requires emergency treatment.

DIAGNOSIS

Chronic cholecystitis is diagnosed from the history of the symptoms and by documenting the presence of GALLSTONES with ULTRASOUND of the gallbladder. If ULTRASOUND is not helpful, X rays (RADIOGRAPHY) can be used.

Acute cholecystitis may be diagnosed by the symptoms, a PHYSICAL EXAMINATION, and by documenting the presence of GALLSTONES with ULTRASOUND of the gallbladder. NUCLEAR MEDICINE tests can be very useful in the diagnosis.

With both chronic and acute cholecystitis, blood levels of enzymes produced by the liver and bilirubin are measured (see BLOOD TESTS) to exclude liver disease and jaundice due to stones in the common bile duct.

Acute cholangitis is suspected from the symptoms and from elevated levels of liver enzymes and bilirubin (see BLOOD TESTS). Diagnostic tests are then directed toward defining the cause of the cholangitis. Endoscopic retrograde cholangiography is a test in which a flexible scope is passed from the mouth through the stomach and into the duodenum to find the opening of the common bile duct, (see ENDOSCOPY). A small tube is then placed into the opening and radiologic dye is injected while X rays (RADIOGRAPHY) are taken. COMPUTED TOMOGRAPHY of the abdomen is useful in some cases to exclude a tumor in the area of the bile duct, such as a PANCREATIC CANCER.

COMPLICATIONS

- Chronic cholecystitis can develop into acute cholecystitis.
- GALLSTONES can pass into the common bile duct causing jaundice (and possibly cholangitis) or PANCREATITIS.
- Acute cholecystitis can lead to perforation of the gallbladder with abscess formation or to generalized infection in the abdomen (peritonitis).

- Acute cholangitis can lead to systemic infection in the circulatory system (BLOOD POISONING). This is a life-threatening condition.
- Patients with bile duct obstruction and acute cholangitis become very dehydrated and experience circulation impairment leading to critically low blood pressure and possibly KIDNEY FAILURE.

TREATMENT

SELF TREATMENT:

Avoiding fatty meals may be helpful, but patients with symptomatic GALLSTONES should seek medical advice.

MEDICAL TREATMENT:

Asymptomatic GALLSTONES do not require treatment. The risk of observation is no higher than that of treatment.

Symptomatic GALLSTONES should be treated; the risk of complications increases significantly once symptoms are present. The orally administered bile salts, ursodeoxycholate or chenodeoxycholate, dissolve cholesterol GALLSTONES in selected patients. Dissolution requires 12 to 24 months, and stones recur in the majority of patients. Unfortunately, most patients have stones that are not amenable to this treatment.

SURGICAL TREATMENT:

For cholecystitis, GALLBLADDER REMOVAL can be performed. Antibiotics are usually administered in conjunction with the procedure.

For cholangitis, options include

- Endoscopic retrograde cholangiography (see above), papillotomy (increasing the size of the bile duct opening to allow the stone to pass), and removal of stones
- Direct operative bile duct drainage with or without removal of stone from the duct
- Stone removal using ULTRASONIC LITHOTRIPSY

PREVENTION

Early treatment of symptomatic GALLSTONES is the best preventive measure.

COLON POLYP

A polyp can develop in any area of the large bowel, although it most often affects the lower part of the large bowel or colon, an area easily accessible to physicians by simple instruments.

A colon polyp is a small outgrowth of tissue in the large bowel, or colon. It can resemble a pea or sometimes a small mushroom on a stalk. Polyps can be made up of various types of tissue, some of which carry no malignant potential and some that do. If the tissue of the polyp is an adenoma, it may represent an increased risk for COLORECTAL CANCER. Hyperplastic polyps do not carry risk for COLORECTAL CANCER.

CAUSES

The cause of colon polyps is unclear, although there may be genetic explanations for polyps in some patients, especially those with a family history of colon polyps or COLORECTAL CANCER. Polyps may occur frequently in the population, and perhaps it is only those people with a certain genetic profile or those who have large or multiple polyps that are at increased risk for the development of COLORECTAL CANCER.

SYMPTOMS

Polyps are usually too small to cause any symptoms; often they are only discovered during routine screenings by a physician. At times, especially if the polyp is larger, it can cause visible RECTAL BLEEDING or microscopic bleeding that can be detected only by an OCCULT BLOOD TESTING of stools.

DIAGNOSIS

Because there are often no readily apparent symptoms, the diagnosis of colon polyps can require several tests, including

- OCCULT BLOOD TESTING of stool samples for hidden blood
- Sigmoidoscopy or colonoscopy—forms of ENDOSCOPY in which a flexible lighted instrument can view the rectum or entire colon
- X-ray barium studies of the large bowel (also called lower gastrointestinal [GI] series or barium enema; see RADIOGRAPHY)

COMPLICATIONS

The most important complication of a polyp is the development of a COLORECTAL CANCER. If there is a strong family history of COLORECTAL CANCER or colon polyps, especially in parents or siblings, patients are advised to seek medical advice regarding screening for colon polyps. This is especially important if there is a history of COLORECTAL CANCER occurring at an age younger than 50 in close family members.

WARNING SIGNS:

- Visible RECTAL BLEEDING
- Change in the nature or frequency of bowel movements
- Development of iron-deficiency ANEMIA

TREATMENT

SELF TREATMENT:

None.

MEDICAL TREATMENT:

Some preliminary research suggests that ASPIRIN or aspirin-like substances may inhibit the growth of polyps, but this treatment option remains experimental.

SURGICAL TREATMENT:

RECTAL- OR COLON POLYP REMOVAL can usually be accomplished through a flexible instrument called a *sigmoidoscope* or *colonoscope* placed into the rectum and colon (see ENDOSCOPY). In the rare case when the polyp is very large, however, more traditional surgery may be needed to remove the polyp.

PREVENTION

- Avoidance of smoking may reduce the risk of abnormal growths in the colon.
- Diets high in soluble fiber and low in fat may carry some protection against the development of colon polyps.
- Once an adenoma type of polyp is discovered, periodic screening (every three to five years) with colonoscopy (ENDOSCOPY) may be needed. Because this type of polyp can recur and does carry some risk of developing into COLORECTAL CANCER, regular surveillance is important.

COLORECTAL CANCER

One in every 20 people living in the United States contracts cancer of the large intestine.

Most cancers of the colon originate in the left side of the colon. These cancers are usually discovered during routine screening sigmoidoscopy (a form of ENDOSCOPY) or after tests are performed to investigate changes in the pattern of the bowels (see RECTAL BLEEDING; OCCULT BLOOD TESTING).

CAUSES

The incidence of cancer of the colon is higher in families with hereditary polyp syndromes, in which family members have multiple polyps in the colon (COLON POLYP). The COLON POLYPS in this condition have a high chance of becoming malignant. Some of the syndromes can also be associated with the development of other forms of cancer.

Patients with ULCERATIVE COLITIS or CROHN DISEASE also have an increased risk of development of colorectal cancer.

A diet high in fat has also been identified as a risk factor in the development of colorectal cancer.

SYMPTOMS

Symptoms may include

- Change in the pattern of the bowels, such as in frequency, caliber, color, consistency, and smell (see STOOL, ABNORMAL APPEARANCE)
- Red streaks or dark jellylike stool related to bleeding (see RECTAL BLEEDING)
- Pain with bowel movements in rectal cancer
- Generalized ABDOMINAL PAIN or WEIGHT LOSS in advanced disease

DIAGNOSIS

Some of the symptoms noted above will prompt the performance of a sigmoidoscopy or a colonoscopy, a form of ENDOSCOPY in which a scope is introduced into the rectum and colon and any suspicious lesions can be tested by BIOPSY or excised.

Following a diagnosis of a malignancy, COMPUTED TOMOGRAPHY of the abdomen is performed to define the extent of disease and to check if the cancer has spread to other organs.

COMPLICATIONS

Potential complications of cancer of the colon or rectum include

- Bleeding resulting in ANEMIA or iron loss
- INTESTINAL OBSTRUCTION
- Bowel perforation
- ABDOMINAL PAIN, WEIGHT LOSS, and ABDOMINAL SWELLING in advanced disease

TREATMENT

SELF TREATMENT:

A well-balanced diet will assist in the maintenance of a stable weight during treatment for this malignancy.

MEDICAL TREATMENT:

Treatment with chemotherapy after surgery in some stages of colon cancer, and the combination of chemotherapy and radiation before surgery in rectal cancer have led to a higher rate of survival.

SURGICAL TREATMENT:

Early on, before cancer develops, RECTAL- OR COLON POLYP REMOVAL is a preventive surgery.

Resection of colon and rectal cancers offers the only chance for cure of this cancer (see SIGMOID COLON REMOVAL; COLOSTOMY). Removal of the tumor that has spread to the liver, when this is the only site of spread, may also result in the cure of this cancer.

PREVENTION

The maintenance of a low-fat diet and careful follow-up with routine screening sigmoidoscopies or colonoscopies for suspicious lesions lead to the prevention, early discovery, and potential cure of these cancers. This is especially important for patients at high risk of developing this cancer, such as patients with familial polyp syndromes (see COLON POLYP) or ULCERATIVE COLITIS.

COMMON COLD

The common cold is one of the most frequent reasons that people seek medical attention.

The average adult suffers three episodes of the common cold each year; children generally have five to seven. Despite the frequency of this infection and the costs to society from lost productivity, there is no specific therapy or preventative measures for the common cold.

CAUSES

More than 200 viruses are associated with the common cold. Two groups of viruses—the rhinoviruses and the enteroviruses—are the most frequent causes. Most infections are spread by direct contact with the respiratory secretions of infected persons. It is well documented that the virus is spread by direct contact within households. In addition, rhinoviruses are very hardy and remain infectious on environmental surfaces for many hours.

SYMPTOMS

The incubation period for most respiratory viruses is one to four days, meaning symptoms may not arise during this period even though the infection is already in place. Some patients develop a chill prior to the onset of symptoms. The most common initial complaints are usually

- Sore throat (THROAT, SORE)
- Runny nose and congestion (NOSE, STUFFY OR RUNNY)
- Sneezing

Other manifestations include

- FEVER
- FATIGUE
- HEADACHE
- Muscle aches

High FEVER rarely occurs with the common cold.

DIAGNOSIS

The diagnosis of the common cold is made based on the symptoms. The specific virus that is causing the infection is not important. If sore throat (THROAT, SORE) is present, a test for strep throat may be indicated (see CULTURE). During the winter or when INFLUENZA is present in the community, a rapid test for INFLUENZA can be performed but may not be necessary.

COMPLICATIONS

The most common complications of the common cold are sinusitis (inflammation of the sinuses) and otitis media (middle ear infection). These complications should be suspected if a person develops FEVER three to five days after the cold starts. In children, these are often bacterial infections, which, unlike the common cold, respond to antibiotics. Common colds can also precipitate ASTHMA in children or adults.

TREATMENT

SELF TREATMENT:

There is no specific treatment for the common cold. Symptomatic relief can be achieved with any of the various over-the-counter cold remedies. ASPIRIN should not be given to children because of the increased risk of Reye syndrome—a rare, but deadly condition associated with ASPIRIN use in children with viral infections. Oral decongestants such as phenylpropanolamine can be used to relieve nasal stuffiness. Nasal sprays should be avoided because symptoms may worsen when therapy is stopped. Antihistamines such as chlorpheniramine may help dry secretions.

MEDICAL TREATMENT:

If influenza is suspected, then AMANTADINE or rimantadine can be given.

SURGICAL TREATMENT:

None.

PREVENTION

There are no vaccines that can prevent the common cold. Because of the large number of viruses that can cause this condition, it is unlikely that a vaccine will be developed. However, there are preventive measures:

- Frequent hand washing may help limit the spread of the illness.
- Good general health habits and good nutrition may decrease susceptibility.
- Stress-reduction techniques may also help prevent the illness.

CONGESTIVE HEART FAILURE

Congestive heart failure is a condition in which, for various reasons, the heart cannot pump efficiently enough to keep up with the body's circulatory demand.

When the heart does not pump enough blood to meet the needs of the body, the kidneys begin to retain fluid. In an attempt to make the heart catch up with circulatory demands, the adrenal glands release hormones that cause the blood vessels to constrict and the heart to increase its rate of pumping. The constriction of blood vessels caused by the adrenal glands may contribute to the worsening of heart failure over time by increasing the workload on the heart because of the increased resistance.

In some cases, the heart contracts well but fails to fill well (called stiffness) in between heartbeats and leads to a backup of blood and congestion in the lungs, liver, and legs. The fluid retention causes congestion leading to many of the symptoms of heart failure.

CAUSES

Anything that damages the heart's ability to contract or fill well in between heartbeats can lead to congestive heart failure. Major causes include

- HEART ATTACK (myocardial infarction)
- HEART VALVE DISEASE
- HYPERTENSION
- CARDIOMYOPATHY
- Congenital heart disease
- Pericardial diseases

SYMPTOMS

FATIGUE and progressive shortness of breath (BREATHING DIFFICULTY) with exertion are early signs of congestive heart failure. The shortness of breath may be associated with a COUGH or with wheezing. Fluid accumulation may lead to visible swelling in the legs (edema; see ANKLE SWELLING) and a loss of appetite from congestion in the liver (see APPETITE, LOSS OF).

As the process progresses, the patient may wake up hours after falling asleep and have to sit up to breathe or even spend the night in a chair to breathe easier.

DIAGNOSIS

Diagnosis can involve many facets. An individual's MEDICAL HISTORY and description of certain symptoms, such as shortness of breath, provide many important clues. A PHYSICAL EXAMINATION may reveal signs of congestion, including distended neck veins and fluid in the lungs, liver, and legs. A heart examination also may detect valve problems and signs of stiffness or weakness.

The chest X ray (RADIOGRAPHY) may confirm a diagnosis of congestive heart failure. An ELECTROCARDIOGRAPHY and echocardiography (ULTRASOUND) may help determine the cause. Ultimately, a CARDIAC CATHETERIZATION may be part of the diagnostic process.

COMPLICATIONS

The weakened heart is prone to ARRHYTHMIAS that could lead to FAINTING OR FAINTNESS or even sudden cardiac death. Because blood is allowed to pool, clots are more likely to form both in the heart and in the veins in the legs. These clots can travel to the brain causing a STROKE or to the lungs causing a PULMONARY EMBOLISM.

TREATMENT

SELF TREATMENT:

Physical activity may initially have to be limited, but in many cases, cautious mild exercise can be resumed when recommended and supervised by a physician. Salt intake should be restricted, and alcohol should be avoided.

MEDICAL TREATMENT:

Treatment varies depending the underlying circulatory or cardiac problem and the immediate cause that brought on the current episode of congestive failure (for example, medication or diet problems).

Drugs that are commonly used include

- Diuretics (such as FUROSEMIDE) to reduce fluid accumulation
- Digitalis (DIGOXIN) to strengthen the heartbeat and improve heart rhythm
- ACE inhibitors (such as CAPTOPRIL or ENALAPRIL) or alternatives to ACE inhibitors (such as HYDRALAZINE or NITROGLYCERIN) to open constricted blood vessels

Other medications may be used to treat or prevent complications, including

- Anticoagulants, such as WARFARIN
- Antiarrhythmics, such as PROCAINAMIDE and amiodarone

Drugs may also be needed to treat the underlying causes of heart failure such as HYPERTENSION and HYPERLIPIDEMIA.

SURGICAL TREATMENT:

- Open heart surgery can repair or replace a faulty valve (HEART VALVE REPLACEMENT) or bypass blocked vessels (CORONARY ARTERY BYPASS GRAFT SURGERY).
- Balloon catheter procedures (ANGIOPLASTY) may be used to open arteries or valves.
- Heart transplantation may be the best alternative for some advanced cases.

PREVENTION

- Avoidance of smoking (see ATHEROSCLEROSIS and HEART ATTACK)
- Avoidance of excessive alcohol intake (see CARDIOMYOPATHY)
- Appropriate treatment of strep throat infections to prevent heart valve and muscle damage from rheumatic heart disease
- With the advice and help of a physician, control of the problems that can otherwise progress to congestive heart failure (for example HYPERTENSION, HYPERLIPIDEMIA, and ATHEROSCLEROSIS)
- A diet low in salt, fat, and cholesterol

CONSTIPATION

Constipation is not really a disease, but it can be a symptom of many diseases. Overall, it is a very common condition, affecting all age groups and both sexes.

Constipation has different meanings for different people. The term can mean that stools are too small, too hard, too difficult to pass, or too infrequent. Patients may also experience a sense of straining and incomplete evacuation. The old adage that a daily bowel movement is the norm is not true, and patterns of bowel movements can be quite variable. It is completely normal for some people to have a bowel movement only every five to seven days.

CAUSES

The cause of constipation is frequently related to temporary changes in lifestyle or habits. Travel, changes in diet, and reduction of normal activity level can all bring on a case of constipation. The use of some medications can cause constipation as a side effect. On the more serious side, underlying metabolic and endocrine diseases, such as DIABETES or HYPOTHYROIDISM, can result in constipation. Neurologic problems in which there is nerve damage in the muscle groups related to the bowel may also result in constipation. Rarely, constipation can be caused by narrowing of the intestines or by an INTESTINAL OBSTRUCTION.

SYMPTOMS

- Hard, rounded, pebblelike bowel movements
- Incomplete, difficult, or painful evacuation
- Sense of rectal fullness with inability to pass stool

DIAGNOSIS

If constipation is limited and occasional and there are no other symptoms, no testing may be necessary. However, if the problem is persistent or severe, the following diagnostic tests may be in order

- BLOOD TESTS to check thyroid function and calcium or magnesium levels
- Sigmoidoscopy (a form of ENDOSCOPY of the rectum)
- X-ray barium studies of the large bowel (also called a lower gastrointestinal [GI] series or barium enema; see RADIOGRAPHY)
- Tests of motor function (anorectal motility)
- Tests of colonic transit using radio-opaque markers that the patient swallows

COMPLICATIONS

Complications are rarely seen with simple constipation. In the elderly or bedridden, however, an impaction may develop where the stool becomes so hard that it physically obstructs the large bowel (INTESTINAL OBSTRUCTION) and can lead to lower ABDOMINAL PAIN, ABDOMINAL SWELLING, and occasionally VOMITING.

TREATMENT

SELF TREATMENT:

- Regular daily exercise
- A diet that is high in fiber (breads, cereals, and fresh fruits and vegetables)
- Adequate fluid intake (at least eight eight-ounce glasses of fluid per day)

MEDICAL TREATMENT:

If dietary and lifestyle measures do not help, laxatives or small-volume rectal enemas can be used. Patients should use stimulant laxatives or enemas only very rarely because over time these medications can paradoxically cause the large bowel to become even more sluggish and less responsive. Bulking agents (for example, psyllium, methyl cellulose, calcium polycarbophil) that increase the volume and soften the consistency of stools are safe for long-term use and are the recommended agents to treat constipation.

SURGICAL TREATMENT:

Surgical treatment of constipation is very rare and used only for specific problems of constipation, such as INTESTINAL OBSTRUCTION or narrowing or Hirschsprung disease (congenital absence of nerve fibers in the rectum).

PREVENTION

The best preventive measure is to ensure adequate bulk and fiber in the diet. Although the dosage requirements are not well studied, increasing soluble fiber to approximately 20 grams daily either in the diet or by supplementing with bulking agents such as psyllium, methyl cellulose, and calcium polycarbophil is a good strategy.

CROHN DISEASE

Crohn disease, sometimes called granulomatous colitis, can afflict people of all ages, but tends to be a disease of the young.

Crohn disease is an inflammatory disease of the intestine that can involve the lower part of the small intestine, the large intestine, and other parts of the digestive tract. Crohn disease tends to be patchy in its distribution and may skip large areas of the intestine. Inflammation, however, does involve all layers of the intestinal wall—from the inner lining to the outside wall. When Crohn disease involves the lower part of the small intestine, it is called *ileitis*, or *regional enteritis*.

CAUSES

Crohn disease is a chronic illness and its cause remains unknown. It is *not* caused by emotional stress, food, or by anything transmitted from person to person. Research suggests that Crohn disease may result from an immunologic imbalance; the interaction of an infectious agent with the body's immune system might trigger the immune system, and the stimulated immune system causes constant or intermittent intestinal inflammation.

SYMPTOMS

There are many varied symptoms associated with Crohn disease, including

- ABDOMINAL PAIN, frequently in the right lower abdomen, especially after meals
- DIARRHEA
- Sores or recurrent BOILS in the anus
- Fissures or drainage in the anus
- Joint pain
- Loss of appetite (APPETITE, LOSS OF)
- WEIGHT LOSS
- Skin fistulae (abnormal openings from the intestine to the skin)
- Frequent canker sores of the mouth

DIAGNOSIS

There is no single test that provides a clear diagnosis of Crohn disease, but screening BLOOD TESTS can provide clues. In addition to a thorough PHYSICAL EXAMINATION, barium X rays of the lower bowel and barium X rays of the stomach and small intestine are generally performed (see RADIOGRAPHY). Sigmoidoscopy or colonoscopy—forms of ENDOSCOPY that permit direct examination and BIOPSY of the large bowel through a lighted flexible tube or video camera—are very frequently used in the diagnosis of Crohn disease and similar disorders.

COMPLICATIONS

On rare occasion, the inflammation in Crohn disease can be severe enough to cause an abscess outside the bowel wall in the abdomen. This complication results in high FEVER and persistent ABDOMINAL PAIN. The inflammation may also burrow through the intestine and cause abnormal connections (fistulae) with other organs such as

- Other parts of the intestinal system
- The skin
- The vagina
- The urinary bladder

If the inflammation does not respond to treatment, there may be enough intestinal scarring in some patients to cause a stricture or narrowing of the intestine. This condition can lead to INTESTINAL OBSTRUCTION with persistent ABDOMINAL PAIN and intractable VOMITING.

Occasionally, the liver and bile ducts are affected by an inflammatory condition called *sclerosing cholangitis*. This process is primarily detected by abnormal liver enzymes noted on BLOOD TESTS.

TREATMENT

SELF TREATMENT:

Good nutrition is essential. While specific foods play no role in causing Crohn disease, soft, bland foods may be better tolerated and cause less discomfort when the disease is active. If patients have substantial narrowing of the intestine, such poorly digestible foods such as nuts, raw fruits, and raw vegetables should be limited.

Emotional stress can influence the course of Crohn disease, and the family and medical professionals involved with these patients should be ready to provide understanding and support.

MEDICAL TREATMENT:

Several pharmaceutical options are available to lessen symptoms including

- SULFASALAZINE
- Corticosteroids such as PREDNISONE and METHYLPREDNISOLONE (pill and enema formulations)
- AZATHIOPRINE
- METRONIDAZOLE
- Mesalamine (pill and enema formulations)
- Olsalazine
- 6-mercaptopurine

SURGICAL TREATMENT:

Surgery for Crohn disease is reserved only for complications that do not respond to conservative treatment. Surgery is never curative, but it may allow for prolonged symptom-free periods. Usually, surgery involves removing a diseased segment of the bowel and two healthy ends of bowel are reattached (anastomosis).

At times, an abscess within the rectum, skin, or abdomen needs to be drained. If the abscess is in a "favorable" location, it sometimes can be drained by a radiologist using imaging such as ULTRASOUND or COMPUTED TOMOGRAPHY to guide a needle or catheter to the abscess, thus avoiding open surgery.

PREVENTION

Medical therapy has not been proved unequivocally to be of benefit in preventing flare-ups of Crohn disease, but some physicians feel that there is a benefit to long-term treatment with such agents as

- SULFASALAZINE
- AZATHIOPRINE
- Mesalamine
- 6-mercaptopurine
- Corticosteroids (in small doses)

CUSHING SYNDROME

Cushing syndrome is an endocrine disorder caused by excess adrenal hormones.

Cushing syndrome is a collection of problems associated with elevated levels of cortisol, a hormone produced by the adrenal gland. The problem can be in the adrenal glands themselves or in another area, such as the pituitary gland in the brain, that regulates or influences the adrenal glands.

CAUSES

High levels of cortisol in the body can have a number of causes, including

- A tumor or overgrowth of the adrenal glands, causing them to produce excess cortisol
- The pituitary gland's overstimulation of the adrenal glands (called Cushing *disease*)
- A pituitary tumor that overstimulates the adrenal glands
- Rarely, tumors in other parts of the body, particularly the lungs (LUNG CANCER), that can overstimulate the adrenal gland
- PREDNISONE and other medications used to treat inflammatory diseases and ASTHMA, because the levels used for medical purposes are usually high enough to eventually bring on problems

SYMPTOMS

Common symptoms of Cushing syndrome include

- Generalized fluid accumulation (see ANKLE SWELLING)
- Increased fat deposits between the shoulder blades near the base of the neck and in the face
- High blood pressure (HYPERTENSION)
- Muscle wasting, particularly in the shoulders and thighs, that can lead to FATIGUE and weakness
- Sudden changes in mood, such as DEPRESSION or euphoria
- Softening of the bones (OSTEOPOROSIS) that can lead to BONE FRACTURES, particularly in the vertebrae of the back or the small bones of the hand
- Skin changes such as easy bruising (see BRUISING, UNEXPLAINED), acne, and stretch marks, particularly on the abdomen and breasts and around the eyes.

DIAGNOSIS

The diagnosis is usually suspected clinically from the symptoms and the findings of a PHYSICAL EXAMINATION. It is confirmed with BLOOD TESTS and URINALYSIS to measure elevated levels of adrenal hormones or to look for excess stimulation by the pituitary gland. COMPUTED TOMOGRAPHY or MAGNETIC RESONANCE IMAGING may be used to identify tumors in the adrenal or pituitary glands.

COMPLICATIONS

The excess levels of cortisol can lead to

- BONE FRACTURES
- High blood pressure (HYPERTENSION)
- DIABETES

TREATMENT

SELF TREATMENT:

Following a strict diet that is low in salt and total calories can be helpful.

MEDICAL TREATMENT:

Medications that inhibit the secretion of the cortisol hormone such as aminoglutethimide and ketoconazole may be prescribed.

SURGICAL TREATMENT:

Surgery is generally the best treatment when the cause of the syndrome is either a pituitary or adrenal tumor; in these cases, the tumor is simply removed. Radiation therapy may also be used to treat these tumors.

PREVENTION

Patients taking PREDNISONE or related medications should work with their doctor to be on the lowest possible dose. Minimizing the amount of this kind of medication is the best way to prevent or minimize the risk of Cushing syndrome.

DEHYDRATION

Severe dehydration is a life-threatening condition. Mild, temporary dehydration is relatively common and not dangerous in the short term, but chronic dehydration could be detrimental in the long term.

Dehydration is a lack of water and salt in the tissues and bloodstream that can affect the entire body. The kidneys are particularly vulnerable to damage when there is not enough water to use in the elimination of wastes.

CAUSES

The causes include any excessive fluid loss or decreased fluid intake. Excessive losses can result from

- VOMITING
- DIARRHEA
- High FEVER causing excessive sweating (SWEATING, EXCESSIVE)
- Excessive loss of fluid through the kidneys because of diuretic medication or, occasionally, certain types of kidney disease or DIABETES

SYMPTOMS

Some of the earliest signs are increased thirst and dry mouth. As dehydration progresses, the skin may become wrinkled. Blood pressure may decrease and CONFUSION and coma can develop.

Except when the kidneys are to blame for the dehydration, the kidneys usually attempt to save fluid, leading to a marked decrease or absence of urination.

DIAGNOSIS

The patient's MEDICAL HISTORY and a PHYSICAL EXAMINATION, including BLOOD PRESSURE TESTING while laying and standing, can make the diagnosis of dehydration. BLOOD TESTS including kidney function and mineral balance tests can confirm the diagnosis and help estimate its severity.

COMPLICATIONS

With moderate dehydration kidney function may be impaired. With more extreme dehydration, drops in blood pressure can cause shock, loss of consciousness, and even death.

TREATMENT

SELF TREATMENT:

An appropriate amount of liquids, particularly electrolyte solutions, can treat mild dehydration. (See Prevention below.)

MEDICAL TREATMENT:

More severe dehydration may need to be treated with intravenous fluids. If an underlying condition such as DIABETES, a kidney disorder, or a gastrointestinal disorder has led to the dehydration, then a specific treatment for that problem will also help.

SURGICAL TREATMENT:

None.

PREVENTION

In general, one should drink at least eight eight-ounce glasses of fluid per day to stay well hydrated.

In some cases of excessive loss from heavy sweating (SWEATING, EXCESSIVE) or DIARRHEA, increasing fluid intake can prevent severe dehydration. A number of electrolyte solutions are available commercially or can be made up for adults by adding one teaspoon of sugar and one-half teaspoon of salt to one pint of water.

DEPRESSION

Depression is the most common psychiatric disorder. It affects 10 to 25 percent of women and 5 to 12 percent of men at some point in their lives.

People of all ages can suffer from depression, but the highest rates occur in people 25 to 45 years old. The rate of depression is not affected by ethnic group, education, income, or marital status.

CAUSES

The main cause of depression is not known. There is a genetic association, and relatives of people who have had depression, manic-depression, or ALCOHOLISM are at higher risk.

Alcohol or drug abuse can cause symptoms of depression, as can certain prescription medications such as PREDNISONE and some blood pressure medications.

Various medical conditions, such as HYPOTHYROIDISM, systemic infections, CONGESTIVE HEART FAILURE, autoimmune diseases, cancers, and neurologic disorders, can also cause symptoms of depression.

A difficult or tragic life circumstance may bring on depression, but often there is no triggering life event.

SYMPTOMS

The main symptoms of depression are either a depressed, saddened mood or the inability to enjoy things normally enjoyed. Other common symptoms include

- SLEEP PROBLEMS or sleeping too much
- Eating too little or too much (see APPETITE, LOSS OF)
- Difficulty concentrating or making decisions
- FATIGUE
- Feelings of guilt or worthlessness
- Feeling physically either slowed down or sped up
- Recurrent thoughts of death or wanting to be dead

DIAGNOSIS

Diagnosis is based on the presence of a combination of the common symptoms in the absence of a medical disorder, a medication side effect, or substance abuse that can adequately explain the symptoms. There is no specific test that can be used to detect depression.

COMPLICATIONS

The most severe complication of depression is suicide, the possibility of which makes depression a potentially fatal illness. Less severe but more common are impairments of one's ability to work and interact socially. Missed days of work, inefficiency at work, lost jobs, arguments with family and friends, divorce, and social isolation are all potential complications of depression.

TREATMENT

SELF TREATMENT:

- Reducing or eliminating use of alcohol, prescription sedatives, or recreational drugs
- Eating properly
- Getting regular exercise
- Using the appropriate therapies for any medical conditions

MEDICAL TREATMENT:

Psychotherapy and antidepressant medication can be used individually or together. Both have proved effective in the treatment of depression. The medicines most commonly used for depression are the selective serotonin-reuptake inhibitors (SSRIs), such as FLUOXETINE, and the tricyclic antidepressants, such as AMITRIPTYLINE.

Severe depression that is not manageable with medication is occasionally treated with electroconvulsive therapy.

SURGICAL TREATMENT:

None.

PREVENTION

Depression is difficult to anticipate, but those who have a family history should be acquainted with the symptoms. Suicide is preventable by seeking professional help promptly at the first hint of suicidal thoughts. Strong suicidal impulses warrant an immediate visit to an emergency department.

DERMATITIS

Dermatitis includes erythema (redness), pin-point vesicles (little tiny water blisters under the skin), scale, and severe itching. Poison ivy is a classic example of acute contact dermatitis.

Dermatitis is not a single disease. It is a pattern of skin inflammation that can be due to a number of causes. Another word for dermatitis is *eczema*. When eczema is chronic and long-standing, skin may have other changes and the pin-point vesicles may be much less obvious or even absent. Other changes include increased or accentuated skin lines (due to scratching), darkening of the skin, and sometimes a thickening or heaping up of the skin in the area.

CAUSES

Eczema can be caused by an external source or an internal source. External sources are those substances, such as poison ivy, that get on the patient's skin and either directly irritate it or cause an allergic reaction.

Internal reasons for eczema are probably genetic in nature. One kind of common eczema is seen in some families and is associated with ASTHMA and hay fever; it is called *atopic eczema*.

Many people have hand eczema that has no discernible cause. Some of these people may have poor hand-care habits, which lead to irritation of the hands or exacerbate the intrinsic problem. Some of these people have atopic eczema that is limited to the hands.

There are, however, some patients who have an allergy to something that gets on their hands and have true allergic eczema. These people may need ALLERGY TESTING to know what chemicals cause an allergic reaction, so that they may avoid these substances.

SYMPTOMS

- Hands that are easily irritated by a number of external agents such as soaps, detergents, fruit juices, vegetables, and oils
- ITCHING
- Red, scaly skin
- Pin-point tiny water blisters (see RASH) in groups just under the skin of the most severely involved areas

DIAGNOSIS

It is important to rule out or isolate an external cause with a careful MEDICAL HISTORY, usually via directed questions from a physician who is aware of the common culprits such as nickel, ethylenediamine, paraphenylenediamine, dichromates, parabens, vulcanizing ingredients, rubber products, formaldehyde, fabric softeners, and fragrances. Selected patch testing (ALLERGY TESTING) should be performed to confirm the suspected allergy. Sometimes a product use test is in order.

Fungal infections need to be ruled out by examining the scale with a microscope. Sometimes a CULTURE must be performed to make the determination.

Sometimes an already existing eczema may be infected by bacteria—a so-called *infectious eczematoid*—usually the bacteria *Staphylococcus aureus* or, less commonly, *Streptococcus* organisms. This infection can be confirmed by CULTURE.

New onset eczema in a middle-aged to elderly person with no obvious explanation may indicate cutaneous T-cell lymphoma and Sezary syndrome. In this situation, the patient must undergo BIOPSY at multiple sites of the eczema and the specimens are sent to a dermatopathologist to rule out lymphoma (see LYMPHOMA, NON-HODGKIN).

Sometimes chronic eczema can change so much in appearance from the patient's scratching, manipulations of the skin, and trials of topical agents that the eczema may have the features of a whole other group of skin diseases such as PSORIASIS. In these cases, a BIOPSY to rule out these other diseases may be needed.

COMPLICATIONS

Secondary infection is common, possibly causing an acceleration of the eczema, ITCHING (painful at times), pus pockets under the scale, glazing of blood and pus over the scale, red skin, and even oozing.

TREATMENT

SELF TREATMENT:

Cool wet compresses applied for one or two hours, three to five times a day can be helpful in alleviating the itching and redness. The application of HYDROCORTISONE cream to the areas and then wet compresses over the cream is often very effective, too.

Over-the-counter antihistamines, such as DIPHENHYDRAMINE or chlorpheniramine taken approximately every six hours can help to take the edge off of the ITCHING.

Topical preparations related to lanacaine or antihistamines can be helpful, but there is a relatively high incidence of contact allergy associated with these agents. Therefore, it is recommended that these agents be avoided if possible.

MEDICAL TREATMENT:

Low-, medium-, and high-potency topical steroids such as TRIAMCINOLONE are the cornerstone of the treatment of skin eczemas. In general, cool wet compresses applied over the topical steroids are a highly effective adjunct.

If an acute eczema is very weepy or infected, aluminum acetate solution soaks are very effective. For acute eczemas, topical steroid creams are advisable over ointments because the latter may occlude the weeping lesion and trap the inflammatory material being extruded.

Sometimes, a very brief course of oral corticosteroids is in order in addition to intensive topical care.

SURGICAL TREATMENT:

None.

PREVENTION

Avoiding substances that induce repeated irritation, redness, or ITCHING of the skin is the best preventive strategy for contact dermatitis. Good hygiene habits and prompt attention to skin problems can decrease the risk of complications.

DIABETES

Insulin, a hormone produced by the pancreas gland, helps blood sugar (the body's fuel) enter the cells and provide energy. In diabetes, the blood sugar, or glucose, cannot get into the cells properly. There are probably a number of mechanisms of diabetes, but two general types are recognized: type I diabetes (called insulin-dependent diabetes or juvenile diabetes) and type II diabetes (called non–insulin-dependent diabetes or adult-onset diabetes).

In insulin-dependent diabetes, the pancreas does not produce enough insulin. Because the blood sugar cannot get into the cells without the insulin, sugar levels rise in the bloodstream. In adult-onset (non–insulin-dependent) diabetes, the pancreas gland generally produces a reasonable amount of insulin, but the insulin is poorly timed and the body's cells seem to be resistant to insulin's effects. This also leads to elevated blood sugar levels.

Diabetes is a relatively common problem that leads to excessively high levels of blood sugar.

CAUSES

Insulin-dependent diabetes is probably related to the immune system attacking the pancreas gland, making it unable to produce as much insulin. Other diseases such as PANCREATITIS can also attack the pancreas gland. Of course, surgical removal of the pancreas, which is required for conditions such as PANCREATIC CANCER, will lead to a lack of insulin production.

Genetic causes are fairly important in non–insulin-dependent diabetes. OBESITY and receiving high levels of CORTISONE or drugs like PREDNISONE can also increase the risk.

SYMPTOMS

The most common symptoms related to high blood sugar levels are frequent urination (URINATION, FREQUENT) and excessive thirst. The appetite may be increased but despite this, WEIGHT LOSS will still occur when diabetes is out of control. High sugar levels also cause VISION DISTURBANCES. When blood sugar levels are extremely high, patients may experience

- Nausea and VOMITING
- CONFUSION
- Weakness
- Coma in severely neglected cases

Complications of diabetes can also cause symptoms.

DIAGNOSIS

An elevated blood sugar level is the most common way of diagnosing diabetes in a patient with a MEDICAL HISTORY and PHYSICAL EXAMINATION consistent with the disease. BLOOD TESTS that look for prolonged elevations of blood sugar can also be done and further support the diagnosis in cases where the blood sugar results are unclear. In men, URINALYSIS can also detect inappropriate amounts of glucose in the urine characteristic of diabetes.

COMPLICATIONS

Diabetes affects many parts of the body. After years of high blood sugar levels, almost all parts of the body can be damaged. The main parts of the body that are affected are

- The eyes
- The kidneys
- The nervous system

Eye problems include excessive growth of small blood vessels in the retina (the back part of the eye) that can lead to VISION DISTURBANCES and blindness. People with diabetes are more likely to get GLAUCOMA, too.

Nervous system problems can take years to develop and usually cause

- NUMBNESS
- Sudden weakness
- Shooting pains, particularly in the legs

After years of diabetes, the kidneys begin to leak protein and can progressively fail (KIDNEY FAILURE), leading to the need for dialysis. These complications usually take 10 to 20 years to develop.

People with diabetes are also predisposed to

- ATHEROSCLEROSIS
- HEART ATTACK
- Claudication (a pain in the calf that appears when walking and that is relieved by rest)

TREATMENT

SELF TREATMENT:

Self-care is crucial in the treatment of diabetes. Careful control of diet is very important and can minimize or eliminate the need for medication.

For patients who are overweight, appropriate weight loss may lead to resolution of diabetes and eliminate or minimize the need for medications.

MEDICAL TREATMENT:

Regular INSULIN injections are generally required for insulin-dependent diabetes.

For non–insulin-dependent diabetes, medication may be necessary. Oral hypoglycemic drugs such as GLIPIZIDE, glyburide, CHLORPROPAMIDE, or metformin can be used alone or in combination with INSULIN.

For difficult cases, INSULIN may be injected with a pump placed under the skin that can allow for more frequent dosing and potentially tighter control. It is becoming more and more clear that tight control—that is, attempting to keep blood sugar levels as normal as possible—can significantly decrease the chance of complications.

SURGICAL TREATMENT:

None.

PREVENTION

Avoiding excess weight decreases the chance of adult-onset diabetes.

For people who already have diabetes, preventive measures can help avoid complications. Periodic eye exams can be helpful in detecting problems before they lead to more severe VISION DISTURBANCES. Because of the NUMBNESS in the legs and the possibility of circulation problems in the legs, people with diabetes can be prone to injuries and infection that progress without their knowledge initially. A daily foot self-exam can be helpful in catching skin breakdown early and avoiding severe infections and GANGRENE.

DISLOCATION

A dislocation is an orthopedic emergency, and immediate evaluation and treatment will limit permanent damage to the joint and soft tissue.

A dislocation of a joint occurs when the normal alignment of the joint is disrupted traumatically, and the two joint surfaces become disconnected. This happens most frequently in the shoulders, elbows, wrists, fingers, and ankles. The hip and knee are less often affected because of the high energies required to dislocate these joints.

CAUSES

Almost all dislocations occur because of trauma. Occasionally, joints become loose because they have experienced multiple dislocations in the past, and it may take only minor pressure or stress to dislocate them again; this type of re-injury is most frequently seen in the shoulder or elbow.

RHEUMATOID ARTHRITIS and congenital conditions can also predispose some people to dislocations.

SYMPTOMS

The most common symptoms are severe pain and the inability to move the joint in the normal range of motion. Joints in the dislocated position may stretch the surrounding nerves and blood vessels and cause NUMBNESS, tingling, weakness, or pain farther down the affected arm or leg.

DIAGNOSIS

The diagnosis of a joint dislocation is made from the history of trauma and the loss of range of motion. In joints that do not have very much soft tissue covering, the malalignment can sometimes be seen and felt.

The definitive diagnosis is made by X ray (RADIOGRAPHY), which may also show if there are any associated BONE FRACTURES, as well.

COMPLICATIONS

In the dislocated position, soft tissues, nerves, and blood vessels are stretched and may cause injury to surrounding tissues or even tissues farther down the leg or arm.

Treatment

SELF TREATMENT:

Early recognition of the dislocation and seeking professional help immediately is the extent of self treatment for this injury.

MEDICAL TREATMENT:

Reduction—putting the joint back into its normal position—is the only real treatment for dislocation. The sooner this is done, the better, but only a trained professional should attempt it because improper reduction can cause further damage.

After the joint is returned to the proper position, it is then immobilized for a period of healing. The immobilization may be followed by rehabilitation therapy to improve muscle strength and blood flow.

The only medication given for dislocation would be pain medication such as ACETAMINOPHEN AND CODEINE COMBINATION if needed.

SURGICAL TREATMENT:

Open surgical reduction may be needed for difficult dislocations.

For cases of repeated dislocation in the same joint, a surgical procedure to tighten the ligaments may help prevent future dislocations.

Prevention

Dislocations usually occur accidentally in falls, motor vehicle crashes, and sports injuries and are, therefore, difficult to prevent. However, using appropriate safety gear when playing sports and wearing safety belts in cars may help prevent some dislocation injuries.

DIVERTICULAR DISEASE

Diverticula can be found in the majority of patients over the age of 55 and often cause no symptoms, but they can cause complications.

Diverticula are small marble-sized outpockets in the wall of the large bowel. When uncomplicated and asymptomatic, their presence is described as *diverticulosis*. When complicated by infection or inflammation, patients develop symptoms, and the condition is called *diverticulitis*. By far, the most common site within the large bowel for diverticula is the left or sigmoid colon.

CAUSES

Diverticula form in clefts of muscle where nourishing blood vessels penetrate the wall of the large bowel. With advancing age, the elasticity of the colon wall decreases, rendering the tissue less flexible and reducing its tensile strength. As pressure builds within the large bowel from muscle contraction, the weakest point of the large bowel muscle wall (the cleft with the blood vessel) balloons outward forming the diverticulum.

Diverticular disease is an illness of the developed world and its refined carbohydrate diet. It is virtually unknown in developing countries where insoluble cereal fiber is the primary dietary constituent. This suggests that increased stool weight, increased stool consistency, and faster transit (reducing intestinal wall tension) protect against the development of diverticular disease.

SYMPTOMS

Uncomplicated diverticulosis usually causes no symptoms, but at times, the patient may experience some mild cramping or bloating in the left lower part of the abdomen (see ABDOMINAL PAIN; ABDOMINAL SWELLING).

When stool or indigestible material gets caught in the diverticulum, inflammation and infection may develop. This condition can cause

- Severe ABDOMINAL PAIN, usually in the left lower abdomen
- Acute CONSTIPATION
- More rarely, DIARRHEA
- FEVER and chills, if the inflammation is severe enough

DIAGNOSIS

Diverticular disease is usually diagnosed with barium X rays of the large bowel (RADIOGRAPHY) or with sigmoidoscopy or colonoscopy (forms of ENDOSCOPY). If a patient experiences severe ABDOMINAL PAIN or FEVER it may be best, in certain circircumstances, to delay diagnostic studies until the inflammation settles down.

Diverticulosis develops in many people, and the mere presence of these pockets on a diagnostic study such as an X ray does not indicate a significant problem. The findings are always be interpreted with the patient's symptoms in mind.

COMPLICATIONS

If the inflammation within a diverticulum is severe enough, it may result in perforation of the colon, the formation of an abscess within the wall of the large bowel, or even an abscess in the abdomen itself.

Since the diverticula tend to form where blood vessels penetrate the wall of the large bowel, these blood vessels at times may rupture, causing serious RECTAL BLEEDING. (The bleeding tends to be painless because there is little inflammation involved with this complication.)

Fortunately, inflammation of the diverticulum usually results in THROMBOSIS of these blood vessels, reducing the risk of bleeding.

TREATMENT

SELF TREATMENT:

When symptoms are intermittent and chronic, prevention is in order (see Prevention below).

When the symptoms are acute and painful, especially if there is FEVER, avoiding solid food and restricting the diet to clear liquids may make the episode less uncomfortable by easing the stress placed on the digestive tract.

MEDICAL TREATMENT:

Medications that can be useful in the treatment of diverticular disease include

- Antispasmodic or anticholinergic drugs, such as DICYCLOMINE or hyoscyamine
- Stool softeners and bulking agents such as psyllium, docusate, methylcellulose
- For bacterial infection, antibiotics such as AMOXICILLIN, clavulanic acid, CLINDAMYCIN, TRIMETHOPRIM, METRONIDAZOLE, and sulfonamide antibiotics

SURGICAL TREATMENT:

In severe cases of diverticulitis, removal of the affected part of the large bowel may be needed. If surgery is done in an emergency, patients may require a temporary COLOSTOMY with reconnection of the bowel at a future date.

PREVENTION

The best preventive measure is insuring adequate fiber in the diet. Although the dosage requirements are not well studied, the propensity for diverticular disease may be reduced by increasing soluble fiber intake to approximately 20 to 30 grams daily either with high-fiber foods such as

- Fresh fruits and vegetables
- Bran cereals
- Unprocessed bran
- Whole-grain products

or with fiber supplements such as

- Psyllium
- Methylcellulose
- Calcium polycarbophil

Avoiding nuts, popcorn, and foods with small seeds and pits may help. Although it has not been clearly proved, these foodstuffs may get caught in the diverticula and lead to inflammatory problems.

EMPHYSEMA

In more than 80 percent of the cases, emphysema is directly attributable to cigarette smoking.

Emphysema is a condition of the lung characterized by permanent enlargement of the air sacs (called *alveoli*). The alveoli are located at the ends of the bronchial tubes and are bunched in groups like a bunch of grapes.

In healthy people, oxygen crosses the thin elastic walls of the alveoli into the bloodstream, and carbon dioxide from the blood enters the air sac to be exhaled. In emphysema, the walls of the alveoli are damaged or dissolved, creating a larger air sac—essentially a hole. This damage and the tendency of smaller bronchial tubes to collapse more easily interfere with the exhalation of air, trapping air in the enlarged air sacs. The next breath is taken on top of this trapped air, resulting in overinflation of the lung.

CAUSES

Cigarette smoking is *the* major cause of emphysema. The risk of developing emphysema is directly related to the amount and duration of smoking. Most patients have smoked at least an average of one pack of cigarettes per day for 30 years before developing symptoms in their 50s or 60s.

In rare cases, emphysema can occur in young adults who have an inherited deficiency of a protein called *alpha$_1$-antitrypsin* that protects healthy lung tissue.

Rare environmental exposures, such as inhaled cadmium, may also result in emphysema.

ASTHMA does not cause emphysema.

SYMPTOMS

Emphysema results in gradual development of BREATHING DIFFICULTY. With mild to moderate disease, BREATHING DIFFICULTY occurs only during significant exertion, but as the disease progresses, BREATHING DIFFICULTY occurs with less and less exertion. Finally, the symptom occurs when the patient is at rest. Often in the initial stages, the symptom is masked by the patient's more and more sedentary lifestyle.

COUGH, excess mucus production, and wheezing are features of chronic bronchitis (BRONCHITIS, CHRONIC) or respiratory tract infection, both of which may coexist with emphysema.

DIAGNOSIS

Emphysema is suspected in patients with a significant history of cigarette smoking who develop BREATHING DIFFICULTY in their 50s or 60s. PHYSICAL EXAMINATION usually reveals an enlarged chest (barrel-shaped) due to lung overinflation and possibly the overdevelopment of the muscles of the neck and chest trying to compensate for BREATHING DIFFICULTY. Breath sounds may be found to be diminished, and there is a delay in the exhalation of air.

Other tests that may be used to confirm the diagnosis include

- Chest X ray (RADIOGRAPHY)
- COMPUTED TOMOGRAPHY of the chest
- PULMONARY FUNCTION TESTING

COMPLICATIONS

The increasingly sedentary lifestyle adopted by many emphysema patients can result in general deconditioning, leading to even more BREATHING DIFFICULTY. WEIGHT GAIN may result from the lifestyle changes, especially if patients are receiving corticosteroid treatment; however, emphysema can also cause WEIGHT LOSS perhaps because of the increased labor of breathing.

Many patients experience psychological complications such as DEPRESSION from the isolation of a sedentary lifestyle and episodes of panic during periods of breathlessness, which can be alarming.

The disease has secondary effects on the heart. It becomes increasingly difficult for the right ventricle to pump blood through the diseased lungs, resulting in right heart failure in severe cases (see CONGESTIVE HEART FAILURE).

Occasionally, the air sacs may rupture, allowing air to escape into the chest cavity—a condition called *pneumothorax*. This condition can cause the lung to collapse because air can enter the chest cavity but it can't get back out, leading to serious BREATHING DIFFICULTY and requiring emergency treatment.

Routine respiratory tract infections can produce serious problems for people with emphysema. PNEUMONIA is life-threatening for emphysema patients.

TREATMENT

SELF TREATMENT:

Self treatment consists of

- Quitting smoking
- Embarking on a sensible exercise program
- Ensuring proper nutrition to maintain ideal body weight
- Washing hands frequently to decrease the risk of infection

MEDICAL TREATMENT:

Drug therapy may involve

- Oxygen for patients whose blood oxygen level is not adequate
- Inhaled bronchodilators such as ALBUTEROL and ipratropium bromide and oral bronchodilators such as THEOPHYLLINE to improve airflow
- Corticosteroids (PREDNISONE) to reduce swelling and inflammation in the bronchial tubes
- Antibiotics to address infections promptly
- Mucolytic agents such as guaifenesin to loosen mucus

INFLUENZA vaccine given in the fall can protect against the usual outbreak of INFLUENZA seen in the winter months. Pneumococcal vaccine offers protection against one of the most common causes of PNEUMONIA.

SURGICAL TREATMENT:

In select patients, a surgical procedure known as *volume-reduction surgery* may be beneficial (see LUNG RESECTION).

PREVENTION

Avoidance of smoking and exposure to smoke and pollutants is the most important preventive step.

ENDOMETRIOSIS

Because endometriosis is stimulated by estrogen, symptoms of endometriosis are unlikely before puberty, during pregnancy, or after menopause.

Endometriosis is the condition in which tissue from the inner lining of the uterus (the endometrium) becomes implanted outside the uterus. The areas most commonly affected include the ovaries, the ligaments supporting the uterus, and the space behind the uterus called the *posterior cul-de-sac*. Occasionally the bowel and the bladder can also be involved.

CAUSES

The specific cause of endometriosis is unclear, but theories include

- Endometrial tissue flows out through the fallopian tubes at the time of menstruation and becomes implanted outside the uterus.
- Embryonic cells that are present from birth are transformed into endometrial implants through hormone stimulation.
- Poor immune response allows the misplaced cells to grow outside the uterus.

Most investigators believe that the cause of endometriosis is a combination of all three.

Risk factors of endometriosis include

- Family history of the disease
- Short cycles and heavy flow (see MENSTRUAL IRREGULARITIES)
- Nulliparity (having never given birth to a live infant)

SYMPTOMS

Although many women with endometriosis are symptom free, for those who have symptoms the most common are

- Painful periods, especially if pain begins after years of pain-free menstruation
- Painful intercourse, especially in instances of deep penetration
- Lower back pain (BACKACHE)
- Infertility, with no other obvious cause

DIAGNOSIS

Diagnosis is based on

- Clinical history—MEDICAL HISTORY and reported symptoms
- Findings on PHYSICAL EXAMINATION
- Findings at the time of surgery (Surgery—either open surgery or surgery using ENDOSCOPY—is the only definitive means of diagnosis of endometriosis.)

COMPLICATIONS

Complications include

- Acute and/or chronic ABDOMINAL PAIN
- Infertility

TREATMENT

SELF TREATMENT:

Over-the-counter pain relievers such as acetaminophen and IBUPROFEN can be used for milder symptoms.

MEDICAL TREATMENT:

Nonsteroidal anti-inflammatory drugs (NAPROXEN, IBUPROFEN) are often used for relief of symptoms. Danazol, progestin, and leuprolide may help to shrink the tissue.

SURGICAL TREATMENT:

Surgical removal (using either ENDOSCOPY or open technique) of the tissue may be necessary for severe symptoms that do not otherwise respond to medical treatment. Removal may help improve fertility.

PREVENTION

No preventive strategies exist, but routine pelvic examinations done at the time of PAP SMEARS may detect endometriosis early, which can be helpful in family planning.

FIBROCYSTIC BREAST DISEASE

The nodules associated with fibrocystic breast disease are problematic because they make breast examination difficult and because they can mimic the findings of breast cancer. They do not, however, increase a woman's risk of breast cancer.

Fibrocystic breast disease refers to a group of entities which cause breast pain, breast masses, and breast cysts in women. Although the symptoms can be quite variable, most women with fibrocystic changes of the breast have some degree of pain related to their menstrual cycles. They also develop areas of nodularity and firmness in their breast, which are difficult to distinguish from breast tumors.

Some women develop large palpable fluid-filled cysts that can resolve spontaneously. When they do not, aspiration of the fluid with a fine needle can distinguish a breast cyst from a solid mass suspicious for BREAST CANCER.

CAUSES

The cause of fibrocystic changes of the breast are not known, but it appears to run in families, and there is probably a hereditary predisposition to the condition.

Dietary factors including high-fat and high-sodium diets have been implicated.

SYMPTOMS

Patients note pain in their breasts, often related to their menstrual cycle. Episodes of pain are most often intermittent, waxing and waning, and although troublesome, do not interfere with daily activities. However, many women become quite concerned because they believe that the pain is a symptom of a more serious problem, especially BREAST CANCER. (This fear is unfounded, as BREAST CANCER is manifest by a *painless* mass.) A minority of women have constant, severe pain that does impact greatly on their life.

Patients may also notice change in the consistency and nodularity of part or all of their breast tissue. Discrete masses are also common.

DIAGNOSIS

The diagnosis of fibrocystic breast disease is a clinical one based on the patient's symptoms and PHYSICAL EXAMINATION.

Mammography (a form of RADIOGRAPHY) is useful in excluding BREAST CANCER, but fibrocystic changes in the breast can make mammographic interpretation more difficult.

Aspiration of a suspicious mass with a fine needle to see if it contains fluid or to obtain aspirate for CYTOLOGY can be quite helpful. A fluid-filled cyst that disappears when aspirated requires no further evaluation.

If a mammogram and aspiration are not able to establish that a lump is due to fibrocystic changes, the lump should undergo surgical BIOPSY. The pathologist can then distinguish the finding of cancer from those of fibrocystic changes.

COMPLICATIONS

None.

TREATMENT

SELF TREATMENT:

Patients should perform regular breast self-examinations. Significant changes or the development of a discrete breast lump should be evaluated by a physician.

Women with pain may find relief by

- Finding reassurance from her doctor that she does not have a serious problem
- Wearing supportive, but not tight, clothing
- Taking ASPIRIN and IBUPROFEN for severe pain
- Taking vitamin E (400 to 800 IU per day)

About half of the women affected obtain relief if they avoid caffeine and too much sodium, but it takes several months before relief is noted.

MEDICAL TREATMENT:

Danazol has been used to treat pain associated with fibrocystic disease. It is rarely used today, because it causes side effects such as development of male characteristics (hair pattern, voice change, and MENSTRUAL IRREGULARITIES).

SURGICAL TREATMENT:

Surgical therapy is usually limited to BIOPSY of suspicious lesions.

PREVENTION

There is no known way to prevent the condition, but symptoms can sometimes be avoided or lessened (see Self treatment above).

FIBROID TUMORS

Fibroids are common benign tumors. One third to one half of all women have them at some point in their lives.

Fibroid tumors, also known as leiomyoma or myoma, are small benign growths in the uterus. The growths look like white marbles growing in the uterus; they are only rarely found in other parts of the body.

CAUSES

Fibroids are overgrowths of smooth muscle cells. While no specific cause is known, they are thought to grow in response to certain hormones. For many years, estrogen, the major female hormone, was believed to be the culprit. More recently, though, studies have shown progesterone to be the stimulating hormone.

SYMPTOMS

A large percentage of women with fibroids have no symptoms. However, depending on their size and location, fibroids can cause symptoms, including

- ABDOMINAL SWELLING and a heavy feeling when fibroids are large (Some women complain that their clothes no longer fit at the waistline.)
- CONSTIPATION when the fibroids press on the intestines
- Frequent urination (URINATION, FREQUENT) when the fibroids press on the bladder
- MENSTRUAL IRREGULARITIES such as bleeding between periods
- ABDOMINAL PAIN, MENSTRUAL IRREGULARITIES (heavy bleeding), and pain during sexual intercourse

It is very rare for fibroids to be a cause of infertility. During pregnancy they may cause uterine contractions, but generally do not cause premature labor.

DIAGNOSIS

The diagnosis of uterine fibroids is usually made during a pelvic examination by a primary care physician or a gynecologist and may be confirmed by ULTRASOUND. Fibroids may also be discovered during abdominal surgery, such as cesarean section or appendectomy, or during hysteroscopy (a form of ENDOSCOPY) performed to assess abnormal VAGINAL BLEEDING.

COMPLICATIONS

The complications of fibroids relate to the symptoms they cause. Large fibroids may compress other intra-abdominal organs such as the ureter, which carries urine from kidney to bladder.

Fibroids may also prevent the detection of other medical problems. For example, a uterus enlarged by fibroids hides growths on the ovaries (such as OVARIAN CANCER) or confuses a physician's attempts to discover the cause of intestinal complaints of CONSTIPATION or increased gas. ANEMIA can result from fibroids that cause excessive blood loss.

TREATMENT

SELF TREATMENT:

None.

MEDICAL TREATMENT:

Some medications can alleviate symptoms for a short amount of time, but they do not cure fibroids. Nonsteroidal anti-inflammatory drugs such as IBUPROFEN can help with pain and bleeding. Leuprolide given in monthly injections for three to six months may decrease fibroid size and symptoms. However, these effects reverse when the medicine is stopped; therefore it is only given preoperatively to facilitate surgery.

SURGICAL TREATMENT:

HYSTERECTOMY is the operation to remove the entire uterus, thus removing fibroids as well.

FIBROID TUMOR REMOVAL (called *myomectomy*) is a procedure to remove the fibroids from the uterus, which is then repaired and left in place. Myomectomy is generally performed in younger women who desire future fertility. It is not recommended for women who have completed childbearing as fibroids will grow back requiring surgery again in the future.

PREVENTION

There are no known methods to prevent the development of fibroid tumors.

GALLSTONES

Gallstones occur in as many as ten percent of the population, but most of the cases cause no symptoms.

Gallstones are concretions of cholesterol, bile pigments, and calcium salts that precipitate from bile in the gallbladder. Gallstones sometimes pass into the bile duct, which drains bile from the liver into the intestine. Less commonly, stones form in the bile duct instead of the gallbladder.

CAUSES

Gallstones are common in patients with no predisposing factors, but there are populations at higher risk, including

- Women, especially after multiple pregnancies
- Obese patients (see OBESITY)
- Native Americans

Dietary factors clearly influence gallstone formation and the high-fat, high-cholesterol diet consumed in Western society is associated with a high incidence of gallstones.

SYMPTOMS

Gallstones usually cause no symptoms. However, the characteristic symptoms, referred to as *biliary colic,* include

- Indigestion
- Flatulence
- Mild to severe intermittent attacks of upper right ABDOMINAL PAIN
- Nausea and VOMITING

Biliary colic may also be associated with pain in the right shoulder. Pain from gallstones is sometimes felt in the middle of the abdomen or chest. Gallstones can also mimic symptoms of ULCER disease or a HEART ATTACK.

DIAGNOSIS

Symptomatic gallstones can usually be suspected from the patient's description of the symptoms. Gallstones are most often documented by ULTRASOUND of the gallbladder. If ULTRASOUND is not helpful, an X-ray test (RADIOGRAPHY) in which the patient is given an iodinated agent that collects in the normal gallbladder may be performed. Other radiographic tests are required in selected patients to eliminate peptic ULCER disease.

Blood levels of enzymes produced by the liver and bilirubin are measured to exclude jaundice due to stones in the common bile duct and liver disease (see BLOOD TESTS).

COMPLICATIONS

- Acute cholecystitis (see CHOLECYSTITIS AND CHOLANGITIS) results in unremitting ABDOMINAL PAIN similar to biliary colic and FEVER.
- Obstructive jaundice can be caused by gallstones in the common bile duct. Infection is then a possibility (see CHOLECYSTITIS AND CHOLANGITIS).
- Common bile duct stones may also cause PANCREATITIS. Gallstone PANCREATITIS ranges from a very mild, self-limiting problem to a life-threatening disease.

TREATMENT

SELF TREATMENT:

Although gallstone formation and growth are related to dietary factors, the exact dietary causes of gallstones have not been defined, and recommendations are not yet available.

MEDICAL TREATMENT:

Asymptomatic gallstones require no treatment. The risk of observation is less than that of medical or surgical treatment. Symptomatic gallstones should be treated; the risk of complications increases significantly once symptoms begin.

The orally-administered bile salts, ursodeoxycholate or chenodeoxycholate, dissolve cholesterol gallstones in selected patients. Unfortunately, most patients have stones that are not amenable to this treatment, dissolution requires from 12 to 24 months, and stones recur in the majority of patients.

Gallstones have also been fragmented with sound waves (ULTRASONIC LITHOTRIPSY). Again, this has only been effective in a minority of patients, and recurrence rates are high.

SURGICAL TREATMENT:

GALLBLADDER REMOVAL.

PREVENTION

No reliable method of prevention is yet available.

GANGRENE

Gangrenous infection can be very dangerous, as it can spread quickly and have dire consequences.

Dead tissue resulting from a lack of blood flow is called *gangrene.* Gangrene can happen in many parts of the body but typically the toes, feet, legs, fingers, arms, and the bowels are the affected areas.

CAUSES

Many conditions and events can interrupt blood flow to an area long enough to lead to gangrene. Examples include

- Blood clots
- Infection of the area with the bacteria *Clostridium perfringens*
- Trauma from accidents
- Severe, advanced ATHEROSCLEROSIS, especially in smokers and people with DIABETES
- Prolonged frostbite

SYMPTOMS

The skin and tissue of the affected area may turn dark or even black. It may begin to smell or be painful and swollen, and small gas bubbles may even form under the skin. A FEVER may also be present.

If the bowel becomes gangrenous, it is heralded by rapidly progressive ABDOMINAL PAIN.

DIAGNOSIS

The diagnosis of gangrene can be apparent from the typical appearance. CULTURES may help target antibiotic treatment by identifying any infectious organisms. Angiograms (RADIOGRAPHY) may be done to evaluate the adequacy of the blood flow and arteries to the area and to plan possible corrective surgery.

COMPLICATIONS

- Loss of the body part
- Rapidly spreading infection, possibly leading to death

TREATMENT

SELF TREATMENT:

- Resting the area
- Avoiding smoking, because smoking further limits blood flow
- Keeping a sterile dressing on the area, and changing it often
- Increasing calorie and protein intake to help with repair and healing

MEDICAL TREATMENT:

- Antibiotics, such as CLINDAMYCIN, PENICILLIN, and gentamicin, are used to treat infection.
- Anticoagulants such as HEPARIN may help if blood clots are contributing to the problem.
- A hyperbaric (high-pressure) chamber with high concentrations of oxygen may help certain types of gangrene that are caused by the *Clostridium perfringens* bacteria.

SURGICAL TREATMENT:

- Vascular surgery to improve the blood flow to the area may help minimize the area of gangrene and ultimate tissue loss.
- AMPUTATION is necessary if infection threatens other areas.

PREVENTION

Tetanus vaccine may help prevent Clostridial gangrene.

In patients with DIABETES and ATHEROSCLEROSIS of the limbs, extra care should be taken to avoid injury from nail clipping, ill-fitting shoes, and other trauma. Careful inspection to catch problems early, especially on the toes and feet, can lead to early treatment to halt the progression to gangrene.

Prevention of ATHEROSCLEROSIS can help to prevent the development of gangrene caused by vascular disease.

GASTROENTERITIS

Gastroenteritis is an inclusive term for many types of intestinal infections. It is a very common illness, affecting all age groups, but especially young people.

Gastroenteritis is any acute inflammation of the lining of the stomach and small intestines. Although it can cause many difficult symptoms, it is usually not serious.

CAUSES

Viruses, such as rotavirus and Norwalk virus, are the most common causes of gastroenteritis, but bacteria can also be the agent. Some bacteria, such as *Shigella, Campylobacter, Yersinia,* and *Aeromonas* species, can directly invade the intestine causing ulceration, DIARRHEA, and VOMITING. Other bacteria, such as *Salmonella* species, *Vibrio cholerae* (the cause of cholera), and toxigenic *Escherichia coli*, or *E. coli* (the cause of traveler's diarrhea), cause disease by stimulating the intestine to secrete excessive amounts of fluid. Still other bacteria, such as *Staphylococcus*, are lumped into the category of food poisoning and produce a toxin that induces a short-lived illness.

SYMPTOMS

- Nausea and VOMITING
- DIARRHEA
- FEVER
- ABDOMINAL PAIN or cramps
- HEADACHE
- Muscle aches

DIAGNOSIS

Most episodes of gastroenteritis are self-limited and not dangerous and do not need laboratory investigation. The symptoms are quite typical and strongly suggest the diagnosis. However, if the illness is severe or prolonged, stools may be examined for the presence of infection. CULTURE of the stool can be used to identify the responsible organism if bacteria are involved.

COMPLICATIONS

Gastroenteritis tends to run its course in three to five days and complications are rare. DEHYDRATION from the VOMITING and DIARRHEA may be a problem in the aged or very young.

On very rare occasion in bacterial gastroenteritis, bacteria can invade the bloodstream and cause a severe systemic infection (see BLOOD POISONING).

TREATMENT

SELF TREATMENT:

Drinking plenty of clear liquids ensures proper hydration. Liquids should contain some sodium; soft drinks, juices, or bouillon are good choices. Beverages with caffeine or alcohol should be avoided. Avoiding solid food will prevent stimulation of the intestine and lessen the symptoms of VOMITING and DIARRHEA.

Over-the-counter medications, such as bismuth subsalicylate, pectin, phosphorated carbohydrate solution, and attapulgite, can be somewhat helpful.

MEDICAL TREATMENT:

Prescription agents include

- Antinausea medication (PROCHLORPERAZINE, promethazine, TRIMETHOBENZAMIDE, METOCLOPRAMIDE, or thiethylperazine)
- Antidiarrheal medication (diphenoxylate and atropine combination or LOPERAMIDE)
- Antispasmodic, or anticholinergic medication (DICYCLOMINE)
- Antibiotics (TRIMETHOPRIM, AMPICILLIN, or CIPROFLOXACIN)

SURGICAL TREATMENT:

None.

PREVENTION

The unique instance of traveler's diarrhea associated with travel to underdeveloped countries can sometimes be prevented by the use of antibiotics or bismuth subsalicylate during the visit to an area at high risk. The benefits of this approach should be discussed with medical professionals before travel.

GINGIVITIS

Gingivitis is preventable and completely reversible once the cause of the inflammation is eliminated, but it can lead to irreversible damage if not attended to.

Gingivitis is inflammation of the gum tissue, or gingiva, that surrounds the teeth. If left unchecked, gingivitis can mature into the more destructive form of gum disease, PERIODONTITIS, in which actual bone loss around the teeth occurs.

CAUSES

Gingivitis is caused by a number of factors, including

- Plaque (collections of bacteria)
- Tartar
- Systemic disease such as DIABETES
- Hormonal changes
- Certain medicines such as oral contraceptives
- Dry mouth

Stress and smoking have also been shown to contribute to this disease process. In the majority of cases, however, the primary cause of gingivitis is accumulation and retention of plaque around the necks of the teeth.

SYMPTOMS

Bleeding is the cardinal sign of gingivitis. This bleeding is easily seen after flossing; blood in the rinse water or on the toothbrush after use can reveal the condition. Direct examination of the gingiva itself can lead to discovery of blood around the crevice of the gum. Bad breath (BREATH, BAD SMELLING) or a bad taste in the mouth can also be a warning that gingivitis is present.

DIAGNOSIS

Clinical evaluation of the mouth is the chief means of confirming whether a patient has gingivitis. The clinician evaluates the tissue, looking for signs of swelling, puffiness, redness, and a smooth shiny surface—all characteristics of gingivitis. The insertion of a probe in the gum cuff around the tooth with bleeding in the crevice upon removal is also another clinical sign of gingivitis.

COMPLICATIONS

The single most significant adverse outcome of gingivitis is it can progress into PERIODONTITIS. This subsequent disease process causes loss of bone and deepening of the gingival pockets around the teeth. Moreover, this secondary disease is not reversible like gingivitis. When the early warning signs of gingivitis are noted, an appointment with a dentist for a thorough cleaning is the best remedy.

TREATMENT

SELF TREATMENT:

The best treatment for gingivitis is prevention. If the tooth surface is clean and clear of plaque, the gum tissue will remain healthy. The tooth surface will remain clean if brushed after every meal and if the teeth are flossed daily. In conjunction with oral home care, a cleaning by a dental professional every six months will help ensure that all areas of the teeth remain tartar free. If gingivitis is present, a visit for a professional cleaning will clear up the inflammation.

MEDICAL TREATMENT:

Some people accumulate more plaque than others do in spite of their efforts at good oral hygiene. Various mouthwashes (most notably, Listerine) are effective in reducing the amount of plaque-causing bacteria. A prescription drug, chlorhexidine, inhibits the ability of bacteria to bind to the tooth. Chlorhexidine is also a mouth rinse, but its use must be monitored because, like most medications, it may produce side effects.

SURGICAL TREATMENT:

Generally, a professional cleaning is enough to eliminate the gingival inflammation and allow for the return of the gum to its normal contour and shape. When, however, the source of the gingivitis is exacerbated by systemic disease, hormonal changes, or adverse medication effects, removal of the tissue (PERIODONTAL SURGERY) is occasionally indicated.

PREVENTION

As in most aspects of good oral health, the most important, cost-effective, and time-saving way to avoid gingivitis is with daily flossing, brushing after eating, and dental visits every six months.

GLAUCOMA

Glaucoma is the number one cause of blindness in the United States, but it is treatable if discovered early.

Glaucoma is an eye condition that results from an elevated fluid pressure in the eye. The optic nerve, which carries the visual information from the eye to the brain, is prone to permanent damage when the eye pressure is elevated. The amount of damage is related to

- The degree of pressure elevation
- The length of time the pressure has been elevated
- The underlying health of the nerve

CAUSES

The front of the eye is filled with a clear fluid called aqueous. Normal eye pressure is maintained because of a balance between aqueous produced in the eye and aqueous leaving the eye through its outflow mechanism. Glaucoma is usually caused by a defect or obstruction in this fluid outflow mechanism. Because fluid continues to be produced, but is unable to exit the eye, the eye pressure goes up.

Risk factors for the development of glaucoma include a family history of the condition, glaucoma in the other eye, and nearsightedness.

DIABETES, HYPERTENSION, and other diseases that affect circulation of blood to the optic nerve, such as ATHEROSCLEROSIS make it more susceptible to pressure damage.

Ocular injuries and chronic inflammation of the eye can damage the fluid outflow mechanism, resulting in elevated pressure. Farsightedness, an abnormally small eye, progressive CATARACT, or other abnormalities can block the fluid outflow apparatus. Finally, advancing age is associated with an elevation in the pressure within the eye.

SYMPTOMS

In the majority of cases glaucoma causes painless loss of side vision. The patient is often unaware of this irreversible loss in vision until it is so severe that it encroaches on the line of sight.

In the relatively rare cases of sudden elevations in eye pressure, a patient may notice

- Aching EYE PAIN
- Blurred vision (see VISION DISTURBANCES) with haloes around street lights
- Redness of the eye

DIAGNOSIS

The ophthalmologist makes the diagnosis of glaucoma by detecting an elevated intraocular pressure in the presence of glaucomatous optic nerve damage and loss of side vision on visual field testing.

COMPLICATIONS

The risk of undetected glaucoma is progressive loss of side vision. Ultimately, total blindness can result. In the majority of cases, there are no warning signs such as pain, redness, or blurred vision. For this reason, it is recommended that patients over 40 have their eye pressure measured at least every two years. When risk factors for glaucoma are present, closer monitoring is warranted.

TREATMENT

SELF TREATMENT:

Except for seeking professional evaluation as soon as possible, there is no self treatment for glaucoma.

MEDICAL TREATMENT:

Medical treatment consists of eyedrops and/or pills. The drops are used to improve the outflow or decrease the production of aqueous fluid. Some drops have both capabilities. The pills act to reduce production of the fluid. The ophthalmologist and patient together determine the right combination of medications such as acetazolamide and pilocarpine to control the eye pressure.

SURGICAL TREATMENT:

- A laser can be used to improve the outflow function or to improve the circulation of aqueous fluid within the eye.
- Glaucoma filter surgery creates a new outflow capability by bypassing the natural path.

PREVENTION

In most cases there is no way to prevent glaucoma. The key is early detection with regular ophthalmologic examination.

HEART ATTACK

Heart disease kills more than 500,000 people in the United States every year. Most of these deaths are attributable to heart attacks. Many people who have a heart attack never make it to the hospital, but of those who do, generally 90 to 95 percent are able to return home.

A heart attack (called a *myocardial infarction*) occurs when the heart muscle is damaged. Usually this damage is a result of a lack of blood flow to the affected area. Without the blood supply, the muscle does not get the oxygen it needs and part of it dies.

CAUSES

The main cause of the lack of blood flow to an area of the heart muscle is coronary artery disease (ATHEROSCLEROSIS). Rarely, a spasm of the coronary artery—the blood vessels feeding the heart muscle—can cause a lack of blood flow temporarily, long enough to cause a clot to form and block the flow entirely. Spasm has been seen under conditions of severe emotional stress and drug abuse (including cocaine use and cigarette smoking).

The general risk factors for ATHEROSCLEROSIS, and hence heart attack, include

- Smoking
- High blood pressure (HYPERTENSION)
- DIABETES
- Increased blood cholesterol levels (HYPERLIPIDEMIA)
- Family history of heart disease

Men are more prone to heart disease than women, but after menopause, women begin to have the same rate as men.

SYMPTOMS

Approximately one third of heart attacks cause no symptoms at all and may be detected incidentally by ELECTROCARDIOGRAPHY done for some other purpose. Symptoms generally include CHEST PAIN, which can be a pressure or heaviness or a squeezing type of pain in the center of the chest, but the pain can also be located as high as the jaw or as low as the upper abdomen. It can be in the right or left arm. ANGINA is a similar feeling and usually precedes a heart attack by weeks or years. The pain of a heart attack, however, generally lasts significantly longer, ranging from approximately 20 minutes to a few hours. Associated symptoms include

- Nausea
- BREATHING DIFFICULTY
- Profuse sweating

In the elderly, the symptoms can be more vague and can include sudden weakness and FAINTING OR FAINTNESS.

DIAGNOSIS

BLOOD TESTS are often used to detect signs of heart muscle damage by measuring the levels of certain enzymes in the blood. ELECTROCARDIOGRAPHY almost always reveals something abnormal. Echocardiography (ULTRASOUND) can reveal an area of the heart muscle that is not functioning normally because of a heart attack. Certain NUCLEAR MEDICINE studies can also show damage to the heart muscle. Ultimately, a CARDIAC CATHETERIZATION may be performed to locate the blocked artery and document the heart muscle damage.

COMPLICATIONS

A heart attack is very serious in itself, but it can also precipitate further life-threatening problems including

- CONGESTIVE HEART FAILURE
- Mitral regurgitation (a form of HEART VALVE DISEASE)
- Sudden cardiac death

TREATMENT

SELF TREATMENT:

The safest thing to do when one suspects that he or she is having a heart attack is to call 911 or other emergency services in their area. There is no way to self-treat a heart attack.

After a heart attack, a survivor may be involved in rehabilitation which can assist him or her in getting back to work and in reducing the risk of future heart attacks. The American Heart Association can also link people to support groups if necessary.

MEDICAL TREATMENT:

Many different drugs are used in the early hours and days of a heart attack. The most dramatic include the thrombolytic drugs—streptokinase and tissue plasminogen activator (TPA)—which help dissolve the blood clots that usually interfere with the blood flow to the heart muscle and cause the heart attack. For these drugs to be most effective, they need to be given within four to six hours of the onset of symptoms. This highlights the need for prompt medical attention if a heart attack is suspected.

Drugs comonly prescribed for heart attack include

- NITROGLYCERIN
- Beta-blockers such as ATENOLOL and METOPROLOL
- MORPHINE
- HEPARIN
- ASPIRIN

Because ARRHYTHMIAS may develop during a heart attack, certain medications such as lidocaine may be necessary. Defibrillation by medical personnel, in which an electrical charge is used to restore a steady rhythm to the heart muscle, may be necessary to treat sudden cardiac death.

SURGICAL TREATMENT:

Surgery is rarely needed in the early phase of a heart attack; however, emergency CORONARY ARTERY BYPASS GRAFT SURGERY may be needed to improve the blood flow to the heart and to treat some of the complications of a heart attack.

Emergency percutaneous transluminal coronary ANGIOPLASTY may also be used in the early hours of a heart attack. PACEMAKER INSERTION is occasionally needed to treat the complications of a heart attack.

In select patients under rare circumstances when a very large amount of heart muscle has been damaged, cardiac transplantation may be the best option.

PREVENTION

Avoidance of smoking is the single most powerful preventive measure. Also important is

- Control of high blood pressure (HYPERTENSION)
- Control of blood cholesterol levels with a low-fat, low-cholesterol diet and possibly drug therapy
- Regular aerobic exercise

ASPIRIN therapy for patients at significant risk for coronary artery disease and hormone replacement therapy for some postmenopausal women can also be useful in preventing heart attacks.

HEART VALVE DISEASE

Heart valves are, in a sense, one-way doors between the different chambers and exits. These valves can become damaged during the development of the fetus (in which case it is called *congenital* heart valve disease) or, more commonly, in childhood or adult life (called *acquired* heart valve disease). The disease can result in two types of problems: 1) if a valve becomes narrowed by scarring or a buildup of calcium deposits, it can partially block the flow of blood to the body and is said to be *stenotic;* or 2) if a valve becomes weak and leaky, it can allow blood to flow backward and is said to be *insufficient* or *regurgitant.*

There are four valves in the heart: the aortic, the mitral, the pulmonic, and the tricuspid. These valves ensure that blood flows through the heart in the proper direction.

CAUSES

Congenital heart valve disease is a result of either genetic abnormality or some problem during the pregnancy. Acquired valve disease can result from many factors including infections (such as rheumatic heart disease or endocarditis) and degenerative causes. HYPERTENSION, coronary artery disease (ATHEROSCLEROSIS), and other conditions such as CARDIOMYOPATHY that weaken the heart muscle can also cause a valve to malfunction.

SYMPTOMS

- Progressive BREATHING DIFFICULTY, fluid retention (ANKLE SWELLING), FATIGUE, and FAINTING OR FAINTNESS (symptoms similar to CONGESTIVE HEART FAILURE)
- Persistent unexplained FEVERS (possibly caused by heart valve infection—endocarditis)
- Heart rhythm abnormalities or palpitations (ARRHYTHMIA)

DIAGNOSIS

A physician can detect most cases by careful PHYSICAL EXAMINATION of the heartbeat and pulse, especially by listening with a stethoscope. A certain ULTRASOUND technique called *Doppler echocardiography* can identify and assess the severity of valve disease. CARDIAC CATHETERIZATION and angiocardiography may ultimately be needed to confirm the diagnosis of valve disease.

COMPLICATIONS

Blood clots can form near the malfunctioning valve and then travel in the bloodstream to other parts of the body potentially causing STROKE or, rarely, PULMONARY EMBOLISM.

Damaged valves can become infected (endocarditis) when bacteria are present in the bloodstream—an occurrence sometimes associated with recent dental work.

Valve malfunction can lead to CONGESTIVE HEART FAILURE.

TREATMENT

SELF TREATMENT:

Severe disorders may require restrictions on activity. Checking with a physician before any surgical procedure, including dental work, is important because of the risk of valve infection; prophylactic antibiotics may reduce this risk.

MEDICAL TREATMENT:

A physician may prescribe

- Antibiotics such as PENICILLIN to treat infected valves
- Anticoagulant drugs such as ASPIRIN and WARFARIN to remove risk of clot formation
- Drugs that remove the workload of the heart and resistance to forward flow of blood (NIFEDIPINE, ACE inhibitors such as ENALAPRIL and CAPTOPRIL)
- Drugs to treat congestive heart failure (DIGOXIN, diuretics such as HYDROCHLOROTHIAZIDE and FUROSEMIDE)

SURGICAL TREATMENT:

- HEART VALVE REPLACEMENT or heart valve repair
- Balloon expansion of a narrowed valve (a form of ANGIOPLASTY)

PREVENTION

- Appropriate treatment of strep throat infections significantly decreases the risk of rheumatic heart disease and, therefore, heart valve damage.
- Control of HYPERTENSION and avoidance of excessive alcohol consumption can help prevent damage to the heart muscle and subsequent valve malfunction.

HEMORRHOIDS

Hemorrhoids, often called *piles*, are a common affliction of the anal canal that can cause severe inflammation and discomfort.

Hemorrhoids are varicose veins in the lower rectum or anal canal. They are classified into internal hemorrhoids, which arise in the lower rectum, and external hemorrhoids, which arise at the end of the anal canal.

CAUSES

Hemorrhoids are frequently associated with CONSTIPATION. The straining during bowel movements puts pressure on the blood vessels of the area, thus slowing blood flow and causing the veins to swell. In developed countries, where a low-fiber diet is common, the population is more susceptible to hemorrhoids because adequate fiber can speed elimination and prevent CONSTIPATION and straining.

There may be a hereditary predisposition to hemorrhoids, but shared dietary habits could account for some of the apparent familial connections.

In women, hemorrhoids often develop or worsen during pregnancy. This occurs because the growing fetus presses on the pelvic veins.

SYMPTOMS

Hemorrhoids may cause

- ITCHING and mild perianal discomfort (Severe anal pain indicates another problem or complications of hemorrhoids.)
- Most commonly, painless, bright red RECTAL BLEEDING with bowel movements (Blood may be noted in the toilet water and coating the stool; it never mixes with the stool, however.)
- A soft mass that protrudes from the anus, a so-called *prolapsed* hemorrhoid

DIAGNOSIS

The diagnosis is made on the basis of the symptoms and a PHYSICAL EXAMINATION. A rectal examination should be performed and followed by examination of the anal canal and lower rectum with an anoscope (a form of ENDOSCOPY) to visualize the hemorrhoids. Examination of the entire rectum and lower colon with flexible sigmoidoscopy (another form of ENDOSCOPY) is also required in many circumstances to exclude other causes of bleeding. A complete BLOOD COUNT is usually performed to evaluate the patient for ANEMIA.

COMPLICATIONS

THROMBOSIS of an external hemorrhoid is the development of a blood clot in the hemorrhoid. It is very painful and causes a firm mass and swelling in the perianal area.

Prolapsed hemorrhoids are internal hemorrhoids that protrude from the anus. They can easily become irritated and cause soiling of anal secretions which, in turn, cause discomfort and perianal ITCHING.

TREATMENT

SELF TREATMENT:

Patients may obtain relief with warm baths (sitz baths), which soothe and cleanse the perianal area. (See also Prevention below.)

MEDICAL TREATMENT:

Dietary changes and fiber supplements are instituted to control bowel habits. Anal suppositories with or without cortisone may ameliorate symptoms.

SURGICAL TREATMENT:

- HEMORRHOID BANDING
- HEMORRHOID REMOVAL
- Infrared or electrocoagulation of hemorrhoids

PREVENTION

The development and progression of hemorrhoids can be avoided or impeded by avoiding CONSTIPATION and straining with bowel movements. A high-fiber diet is best for long-term control of bowel habits, but many patients require fiber supplements to control the consistency of bowel movements.

HEPATITIS

Hepatitis is an infectious or inflammatory condition of the liver caused by a variety of conditions. It most often is an acute self-limited event, although patients may be ill for weeks. Some forms of hepatitis may linger chronically and occasionally progress to substantial scarring or cirrhosis of the liver.

Most of the forms of hepatitis are self-limited and the patient recovers without difficulty, but some can result in a more chronic condition and complications.

CAUSES

Hepatitis may be caused by a variety of viruses including, hepatitis A, hepatitis B, hepatitis C, hepatitis delta, cytomegalovirus, and Epstein-Barr. A parasite, *Toxoplasma*, can also cause infectious hepatitis. Not all viral hepatitis has a demonstrable virus and unknown viruses responsible for hepatitis remain to be discovered.

Most viral hepatitis is transmitted silently from person to person. Hepatitis C, B, and delta may be transmitted by blood products or the sharing of needles in illicit use of injectable drugs. Hepatitis B can be transmitted sexually.

A wide variety of prescription and over-the-counter medications can also cause hepatitis. This form is self-limited when discovered early and does not usually progress to a chronic state.

Alcohol, when used excessively and chronically, can cause hepatitis. Toxins such as carbon tetrachloride and food poisoning from certain rare mushrooms may also result in acute hepatitis.

SYMPTOMS

- Malaise
- Loss of appetite (see APPETITE, LOSS OF)
- FEVER
- Nausea and occasionally VOMITING
- Upper right ABDOMINAL PAIN or ache
- Yellowing of the eyes and skin (jaundice)
- Dark urine (see URINE, ABNORMAL APPEARANCE)
- Diffused ITCHING

DIAGNOSIS

A diagnosis of hepatitis may be suspected in a patient with jaundice (yellowing of the skin and eyes) when other appropriate symptoms are present. The diagnosis is corroborated with blood tests that measure the activity of liver enzymes and bilirubin. BLOOD TESTS to measure exposure to hepatitis A, B, C, and delta, cytomegalovirus, Epstein-Barr virus, and *Toxoplasma* are available and will confirm the cause of infectious hepatitis in most instances.

If the diagnosis is unclear, ULTRASOUND or COMPUTED TOMOGRAPHY of the liver may be performed. On rare occasion, in cases without clear cause, a liver BIOPSY may be needed.

COMPLICATIONS

Most hepatitis is a self-limited condition, and after a period of several weeks, the patient fully recovers. On very rare occasion, viral hepatitis can be quite severe, even resulting in liver failure with coma.

Some forms of hepatitis (hepatitis B, C, and delta) can progress to a chronic condition that causes continued inflammation of the liver for months or years and may eventually even result in cirrhosis of the liver or LIVER CANCER. Follow-up with a physician and periodic evaluation of liver enzyme BLOOD TESTS will help in recognition and treatment of these complications.

TREATMENT

SELF TREATMENT:

- The need for prolonged bed rest in hepatitis is no longer considered essential; the patient should undertake only that activity that does not cause undue fatigue.
- Nutrition is important and the diet should be liberal; patients frequently will have a poor appetite and may find sweets and carbohydrates more palatable.
- Alcohol should be strictly avoided.
- The use of over-the-counter or prescription medication should be discussed with a physician.

MEDICAL TREATMENT:

- There is no nonexperimental treatment for acute viral hepatitis. Like other viral diseases, it is usually a self-limited illness that the patient's own immune system overcomes.
- Treatment with injectable interferon-alpha may be used in chronic hepatitis (more than six months of illness) caused by hepatitis B or C.
- Withdrawal of offending drugs, toxins, or alcohol is usually all that is required when these agents are the cause of hepatitis.

SURGICAL TREATMENT:

Liver transplantation has been used in cases of unremitting liver failure in patients who become desperately ill.

PREVENTION

Public health measures and modern sanitation have severely curtailed outbreaks of hepatitis in the United States and the industrialized world. Routine screening for hepatitis B and C in donated blood has virtually eliminated the risk of transfusion-related hepatitis. Hepatitis can still be spread within groups of illicit drug users who share needles, however. Hepatitis B can be spread sexually, and partners of patients should take precautions with protected sex.

Vaccines against hepatitis B are available and recommended for most children and groups of adults at higher risk for acquiring hepatitis B, including

- Medical professionals
- Patients on hemodialysis
- Patients with hemophilia or thalassemia requiring transfusion
- Morticians
- Homosexually active men
- Intimate contacts of persons with active hepatitis B

In the rare event that a patient is exposed to blood from a patient with active hepatitis B, injectable hepatitis B immune globulin may reduce the risk of acquiring hepatitis B. Immune gamma globulin is recommended for close household contacts of persons with hepatitis A.

HERNIA

Hernias can theoretically occur almost anywhere in the body, but the abdominal wall is the most common site.

A hernia is a defect in the abdominal wall that allows internal structures to protrude through the wall. The most common type of hernia, inguinal hernia, occurs in the groin, but a hernia can occur anywhere in the abdominal wall. A hernia in the naval (umbilical) or above it (epigastric) is also very common. A hernia can also occur at the site of a previous surgical incision.

CAUSES

Inguinal, umbilical, and epigastric hernias occur at a weak site in the abdominal wall that formed as the abdomen developed. Children who develop a hernia early in life are probably born with the defect. Adults who develop a hernia later in life are most likely born with a minimal defect that enlarges as tissues age and weaken. Increased pressure in the abdomen from lifting and straining may contribute to the development and enlargement of a hernia.

Healed abdominal incisions are never as strong as the normal abdomen tissues, and a hernia may develop in the wound. An incisional hernia is more likely to occur in patients with

- ABDOMINAL SWELLING
- Wound infection
- OBESITY
- Critical illness
- Malnourishment

All of these factors are thought to interfere with normal wound healing.

SYMPTOMS

A hernia most often appears as a mass that causes only mild discomfort. If the hernia becomes trapped, or incarcerated, in the defect, it may cause significant, unremitting pain, especially if the blood supply to the contents of the hernia has been cut off—a so-called *strangulated* hernia. These complications require prompt medical attention.

DIAGNOSIS

The PHYSICAL EXAMINATION alone is used to diagnose a hernia in almost all cases. In rare cases, COMPUTED TOMOGRAPHY or ULTRASOUND may be used.

COMPLICATIONS

- An incarcerated hernia is one in which the mass cannot be pushed back into the abdomen.
- A strangulated hernia occurs when the blood supply to the contents of the hernia is compromised. If the blood supply is cut off for too long, GANGRENE can result.

TREATMENT

SELF TREATMENT:

None. Some patients use trusses to hold their hernia in place and claim that they improve comfort, but there is no evidence that a truss is beneficial.

MEDICAL TREATMENT:

None.

SURGICAL TREATMENT:

HERNIA REPAIR, either open or laparascopic, is the only treatment. Small hernias that are not progressing and are not causing serious symptoms may be observed without treatment, holding surgery in reserve for any problems that might develop.

PREVENTION

None.

HERNIATED DISK

A herniated disk, sometimes known as a slipped disk, is usually the result of an injury and can cause debilitating pain.

A herniated disk is a rupture or bulging of the intervertebral disks (soft tissue spacers) located between the bones of the spine. When the bulging causes pressure or irritation of the nerve roots that provide the sensation and motor power of the legs, there may be NUMBNESS, TINGLING, weakness, and radiating pain in the affected leg or arm.

CAUSES

A herniated disk is most often caused by a combination of wear and tear changes in the disk that allow a portion of the disk to press on the nerve roots that run out of the spine. When this process is present, an inciting event—a fall, a heavy lifting episode, or a twisting injury—may be a contributing factor.

Repetitive spinal injuries, exposure to vibration in the workplace, OBESITY, and smoking have been demonstrated to increase the risk of a disk herniation.

SYMPTOMS

Patients with a disk herniation frequently notice

- A radiating pain from the buttock and thigh area into the calf or foot
- NUMBNESS or tingling in the same area
- Muscle weakness or fatigue in the affected limb

Much less frequently, a herniated disk in the neck can cause these symptoms in an arm.

DIAGNOSIS

The diagnosis of a herniated disk is made by a combination of specific symptoms and objective evidence of motor weakness, reflex loss, and decreased sensation noted during the PHYSICAL EXAMINATION. Plain X rays (RADIOGRAPHY) are not usually helpful; special radiologic studies such as MAGNETIC RESONANCE IMAGING, COMPUTED TOMOGRAPHY, and myelography (a form of RADIOGRAPHY) may be needed to confirm the diagnosis in patients whose symptoms are worsening. Electrical testing is occasionally useful in identifying the specific nerve root that is irritated.

COMPLICATIONS

While the vast majority of patients with disk herniation recover with patience and nonsurgical treatment, changes in bowel or bladder function or progressive extremity weakness should be evaluated as soon as possible, as these may lead to permanent nerve deficits.

TREATMENT

SELF TREATMENT:

- Depending on severity of symptoms, a decrease in activity is usually in order.
- Minor pain can be treated with over-the-counter analgesics and anti-inflammatories such as ASPIRIN, acetaminophen, or IBUPROFEN.

MEDICAL TREATMENT:

More severe pain can be managed by prescription oral analgesics and anti-inflammatories, such as an ACETAMINOPHEN AND CODEINE COMBINATION, or by epidural anti-inflammatory injections.

SURGICAL TREATMENT:

Diskectomy (see LUMBAR DISK REMOVAL).

PREVENTION

The chance of a disk herniation can be reduced by avoiding the risk factors such as

- Vibrations in the workplace
- OBESITY
- Smoking
- Improper lifting techniques

However, as degenerative changes of the disk occur in everyone with time, there is no preventative tactic that can completely eliminate the risk.

HODGKIN DISEASE

Although the disease sounds ominous and treatment can be difficult, 80 percent of patients with Hodgkin disease can be cured.

Hodgkin disease is a type of lymphoma. Lymphomas are cancers that arise from the lymph system, a network of small nodes and vessels that help to fight infections by filtering lymph fluid. Small lymph nodes may sometimes normally be felt in the neck or groin. In Hodgkin disease, lymph nodes become enlarged due to the presence of a tumor. Lymph nodes in the neck region are often involved.

CAUSES

The cause of Hodgkin disease is unknown. Some researchers believe that Epstein-Barr virus, the virus that causes mononucleosis, may be involved in the development of Hodgkin disease.

Immunosuppressant drugs used after transplantation surgery (see KIDNEY TRANSPLANT) may also be a factor in rare cases.

SYMPTOMS

Symptoms include

- Persistent swelling of a lymph node or nodes
- FEVER
- Night sweats (see SWEATING, EXCESSIVE)
- Unintended WEIGHT LOSS
- Generalized body ITCHING

DIAGNOSIS

Diagnosis is made by surgically removing an involved lymph node and examining it under the microscope. Once the diagnosis is made, other tests, such as bone marrow BIOPSY and COMPUTED TOMOGRAPHY of the chest and abdomen, are used to evaluate the extent of the disease and plan treatment strategies.

COMPLICATIONS

Without treatment, the immune system becomes progressively impaired, resulting in serious infections that can become life threatening.

TREATMENT

SELF TREATMENT:

None.

MEDICAL TREATMENT:

The use of chemotherapy and radiation therapy is determined by the stage of disease. One or the other or a combination of the two are options. With modern therapy, about 80 percent of patients with Hodgkin disease can be cured of their malignancy.

SURGICAL TREATMENT:

SPLEEN REMOVAL, also called splenectomy, is sometimes performed if the spleen—part of the lymphatic system—becomes dangerously enlarged, unresponsive to other therapies and a potential source of complications.

PREVENTION

Any persistently swollen lymph node greater than one centimeter in diameter (the size of a marble) should be evaluated by a physician. Early detection is the key to successful treatment.

HYPERLIPIDEMIA

The elevated level of lipids in the blood is a major risk factor for cardiovascular disease and one of the precursors to potentially life-threatening atherosclerosis.

Hyperlipidemia involves elevated blood levels of fats such as cholesterol and triglycerides. These high levels are associated with the formation of fat deposits on the inner surface of blood vessels (see ATHEROSCLEROSIS).

A related problem is abnormally low high-density lipoprotein (HDL) cholesterol—the so-called "good" part of total cholesterol—which is believed to help remove fat deposits from the lining of the blood vessel walls.

CAUSES

Risk factors for hyperlipidemia include

- OBESITY
- High-fat diet
- Lack of exercise
- Family history of the condition

Other conditions that can contribute to the problem include

- Thyroid disorders (HYPOTHYROIDISM)
- DIABETES
- Certain kidney and liver disorders

SYMPTOMS

The disease is relatively silent as far as what the patient can notice on his or her own. Only rarely do fatty skin deposits appear around the eyes or the ankle tendon above the heel. Other symptoms are related to the complications of ATHEROSCLEROSIS.

DIAGNOSIS

The characteristic fatty skin deposits may be detected by PHYSICAL EXAMINATION, but a BLOOD TEST of fasting lipid levels, including total cholesterol, triglycerides, and HDL cholesterol are necessary to make the diagnosis. Since random variation is significant, most physicians require two or three measurements over time to label a patient as having a problem.

COMPLICATIONS

The main danger of hyperlipidemia is its association with the formation of fatty deposits on the walls of blood vessels (ATHEROSCLEROSIS), which can lead to HEART ATTACK or STROKE.

Extremely high levels of triglycerides in the blood can cause PANCREATITIS.

TREATMENT

SELF TREATMENT:

- A diet low in cholesterol and fat (especially saturated fat)
- Regular exercise
- Maintenance of a healthy weight

MEDICAL TREATMENT:

CHOLESTYRAMINE, LOVASTATIN, GEMFIBROZIL, and niacin are examples of drugs commonly used to lower blood lipid levels. These have the most impact on patients with existing ATHEROSCLEROSIS.

Patients with multiple risk factors for ATHEROSCLEROSIS may also receive significant benefits from these drugs depending on their lipid levels after all dietary efforts have been pursued. Drug therapy for others is generally reserved only in rare instances.

SURGICAL TREATMENT:

A procedure to divert fats from the body into the bowel (called an *ileal bypass*) can be quite effective in severe cases.

PREVENTION

The same measures listed under Self treatment above may help avert hyperlipidemia.

HYPERTENSION

Hypertension is sometimes known as the silent killer because it causes no noticeable symptoms but it can be deadly.

Hypertension is abnormally high blood pressure. It is, unfortunately, very common in the United States, but because it usually causes no noticeable symptoms, the condition is only diagnosed by regular BLOOD PRESSURE TESTING.

CAUSES

In most cases, the cause of the high blood pressure is not clear. Multiple factors probably play a role, including family history and salt intake. Blacks and men are more commonly affected. Other factors include

- Emotional stress
- OBESITY
- Excessive alcohol intake
- Smoking
- A sedentary lifestyle

In rare cases, hypertension results from specific diseases; adrenal gland tumors, kidney diseases, and congenital abnormalities of the aorta, (the largest vessel coming out of the heart) can be the cause.

SYMPTOMS

Most patients with hypertension are without any symptoms. Some may experience HEADACHES, DIZZINESS, or nosebleeds, but these symptoms usually have other causes.

Unfortunately the first symptoms of hypertension are usually from a complication. That's why periodic BLOOD PRESSURE TESTING is valuable.

DIAGNOSIS

Healthy people may have temporarily elevated blood pressure (for example, when they are under stress). Hypertension is diagnosed, though, when an individual has persistently elevated blood pressure—measured on two or three occasions.

Although the cutoff is somewhat arbitrary, the usual definition of "abnormally high" is blood pressure greater than 140/90 mm Hg. Some patients' blood pressure is so variable that a 24-hour ambulatory blood pressure monitor or frequent home BLOOD PRESSURE TESTING may be needed.

COMPLICATIONS

Hypertension promotes ATHEROSCLEROSIS, KIDNEY FAILURE, CONGESTIVE HEART FAILURE, and STROKE. Any symptoms related to these complications can be a clue to hypertension too, including

- BREATHING DIFFICULTY
- ANGINA
- Claudication (pain during activity, relieved by rest)
- Swelling (see ANKLE SWELLING)
- NUMBNESS or weakness on one side of the body

TREATMENT

SELF TREATMENT:

Measures that may aid in lowering blood pressure include

- Limiting sodium intake
- Avoiding excessive alcohol
- Weight loss (if appropriate)
- Exercise (if hypertension is reasonably controlled)
- Relaxation techniques for stress reduction

MEDICAL TREATMENT:

If lifestyle changes don't improve hypertension enough or if the blood pressure is seriously elevated at the time of diagnosis, many types of medication can be used, including

- Diuretics such as HYDROCHLOROTHIAZIDE
- Beta-blockers such as ATENOLOL, METOPROLOL, and PROPRANOLOL
- Calcium channel blockers such as NIFEDIPINE, DILTIAZEM, VERAPAMIL, and AMLODIPINE
- ACE inhibitors such as CAPTOPRIL and ENALAPRIL
- Alpha-blockers such as PRAZOSIN and TERAZOSIN

SURGICAL TREATMENT:

For the rare cases where kidney or adrenal gland disorders are the cause, surgery may be necessary on those organs.

PREVENTION

Regular exercise, avoiding excess weight, moderation of salt intake, and limiting alcohol to no more than two drinks a day may help prevent hypertension.

HYPERTHYROIDISM

Thyroid hormone affects the entire body, and a wide variety of problems can be related to the excess amount of hormone produced in this disorder.

Hyperthyroidism is a disorder caused by excessive levels of thyroid hormone. Generally, excessive levels are caused by an overactive thyroid gland either acting on its own or being overstimulated by the pituitary gland.

CAUSES

- In some cases, excess thyroid hormone can be caused by an autoimmune disease in which antibodies attack thyroid tissue and lead to an overproduction of the hormone.
- Infections may occasionally cause an overstimulation of the thyroid gland, leading to excessive amounts of thyroid hormone in the bloodstream temporarily.
- Genetics seem to play a factor, because thyroid diseases tend to run in families and are more common in women.

SYMPTOMS

Excess thyroid levels can develop quite slowly or very quickly; the symptoms, therefore, may develop insidiously or rapidly. Symptoms include

- ANXIETY and restlessness
- Rapid heart beat (see ARRHYTHMIA)
- TREMBLING of the fingers
- Intolerance to the heat
- WEIGHT LOSS despite an increased appetite
- FATIGUE
- Weakness of the muscles, particularly the shoulders and thighs
- MENSTRUAL IRREGULARITIES

The thyroid gland may be noticeably swollen (a condition known as *goiter*), and when the autoimmune disease, called *Grave disease*, is the cause of excess thyroid stimulation, deposits behind the eyes may also develop, causing a bulging of the eyeballs.

DIAGNOSIS

The PHYSICAL EXAMINATION may lead to the initial suspicion of hyperthyroidism and BLOOD TESTS confirming high levels of hormone or suppressed levels of the pituitary hormone will confirm the diagnosis. A thyroid scan (a form of NUCLEAR MEDICINE) or ULTRASOUND may also be used to examine the thyroid gland.

COMPLICATIONS

- Excess thyroid hormone can lead to overstimulation of the heart muscle and may, rarely, cause a HEART ATTACK.
- Long-term hyperthyroidism may also lead to softening of the bones (OSTEOPOROSIS).
- The deposits behind the eyes, if allowed to progress, can lead to VISION DISTURBANCES.

TREATMENT

SELF TREATMENT:

None.

MEDICAL TREATMENT:

Radioactive iodine, which collects in the thyroid gland can be used to destroy enough of the thyroid gland so that it produces less thyroid hormone.

Other medications that may interfere with the production of thyroid hormone and can be used treatment include propylthiouracil and methimazole.

SURGICAL TREATMENT:

In some occasions, very large thyroid glands or portions of the thyroid gland may be removed to control thyroid hormone production with both surgery (THYROIDECTOMY) and radioactive iodine.

Removing too much is not uncommon, causing the gland to produce too little thyroid hormone (HYPOTHYROIDISM), but this condition is relatively easily treated with the appropriate amount of thyroid hormone medication.

PREVENTION

None.

HYPOTHYROIDISM

Thyroid hormone affects the entire body and a wide variety of problems can be related to the reduced amount of hormone produced in this disorder.

Hypothyroidism is when the thyroid gland fails to make an adequate amount of thyroid hormone. Because the hormone is integral in the regulation of metabolism, this disorder has widespread effects on the body's function.

CAUSES

- The cause of hypothyroidism is frequently the end stage of an autoimmune disorder in which the body's immune system has attacked the thyroid gland tissue over a period of years.
- Also common is the understimulation of the thyroid gland by hormones from the pituitary gland, which helps regulate thyroid hormone production.
- Rarely, some viral infections may cause a temporary excess and then a temporary inadequacy of thyroid hormone.
- Genetics seem to play a role; hypothyroidism can run in families.
- Lack of dietary iodine can cause a decrease in thyroid function, but such a deficiency is very uncommon today.

SYMPTOMS

Symptoms of hypothyroidism include

- FATIGUE
- Intolerance to cold
- Unexplained WEIGHT GAIN
- A hoarse voice
- Puffiness around the eyes
- Dry skin
- Hair loss
- Slowing of mental function (see CONFUSION; MEMORY PROBLEMS)
- CONSTIPATION
- MENSTRUAL IRREGULARITIES, particularly abnormally heavy, prolonged periods

DIAGNOSIS

The diagnosis is usually suspected from the symptoms and a PHYSICAL EXAMINATION, and it is confirmed by a BLOOD TEST of blood level of thyroid hormone.

COMPLICATIONS

If hypothyroidism is left untreated it can progress to coma and even death. If left untreated during infancy, it can result in permanent mental retardation and cretinism.

TREATMENT

SELF TREATMENT:

None.

MEDICAL TREATMENT:

Hypothyroidism is usually treated with thyroid hormone (thyroxine).

SURGICAL TREATMENT:

Without adequate iodine, the thyroid gland enlarges. If the thyroid gland is large enough to interfere with breathing or swallowing, THYROIDECTOMY may be required.

PREVENTION

Most parts of the United States now have an adequate amount of iodine in the diet—most of it from iodized salt. Before this became a widespread practice, insufficient dietary intake of iodine was a cause of hypothyroidism.

IMPOTENCE

Impotence is a very common condition. Almost all men experience it at some point in their lives, albeit usually a temporary case.

Impotence is the inability to achieve or maintain an erection satisfactory for intercourse. Erection depends on many factors including the proper functioning of the

- Circulatory system
- Endocrine system
- Nervous system

The penis is mostly made up of spongy erectile tissue that fills with blood to become erect. This event requires each of these systems to work together in ways that are still not fully understood.

CAUSES

The causes of impotence are as varied as the systems involved in proper erectile functioning. The most common causes are psychological. Performance anxiety is a common cause even in stable, loving relationships. Other common psychological factors that can lead to impotance include

- General ANXIETY
- Stress
- DEPRESSION

Loss of function can be caused by disorders involving the actual erectile mechanisms. Risk factors for this type of impotence include

- DIABETES
- Vascular disease (ATHEROSCLEROSIS)
- Smoking
- High blood cholesterol levels (HYPERLIPIDEMIA)

Hormonal imbalances and the side effects of certain medications such as beta-blockers (PROPRANOLOL) and antihistamines can also cause impotence. Rarely, nerve damage from surgery in the area, STROKE, or MULTIPLE SCLEROSIS can be the cause.

DIAGNOSIS

Diagnosis of impotence includes determining the cause. An individual's MEDICAL HISTORY is a vital clue. A BLOOD TEST to determine circulating hormone levels and a general PHYSICAL EXAMINATION can also be useful.

TREATMENT

SELF TREATMENT:

See Prevention below.

MEDICAL TREATMENT:

- Medication that is suspected of causing the problem can be withdrawn.
- Hormone medication such as BROMOCRIPTINE and testoreroneis is used as treatment for men with hormone imbalances.
- In men for whom the difficulty cannot be resolved, self-injection of vasoactive agents into the penis can provide temporary erection.
- A special vacuum device placed over the penis can also help engorge the penis to allow a temporary erection.

SURGICAL TREATMENT:

For permanent cases of impotence, PENILE IMPLANTATION is an option.

PREVENTION

- Avoidance of smoking
- Control of blood cholesterol levels through diet and exercise
- Avoidance of alcohol and depressant drugs which can interfere with proper functioning

INCONTINENCE

Incontinence is a condition that becomes more common with age. For various anatomic reasons, it is more often seen in women than it is in men.

Incontinence is the involuntary loss of urine from the bladder. The severity can range from minor leakage to near complete loss of all bladder control. The most common forms are either *urgency incontinence,* in which urine is lost because of a sudden urge to urinate, and *stress incontinence,* in which any sudden strain such as a cough or sneeze causes a loss of some urine.

CAUSES

Stress incontinence can be caused by the weakening of the muscles of the pelvic floor. These muscles, which are responsible for closing off the opening to the bladder and holding the urine in, can become weaker and looser with age, especially in women after childbirth; menopause also contributes because of the effects of decreased hormonal levels on the mucous membranes lining the urethra.

Sometimes another disorder is the cause of stress incontinence; cystocele and urethrocele are common culprits.

Urge incontinence can be caused by intrinsic bladder problems such as BLADDER INFECTION.

Damage to the nervous system, such as that caused by STROKE, can also lead to incontinence.

DIAGNOSIS

To determine the type and cause of incontinence, a PHYSICAL EXAMINATION and a complete MEDICAL HISTORY are useful. A catheter is sometimes used to determine the adequacy of bladder emptying. A CULTURE to detect the presence of any infection may also be performed.

COMPLICATIONS

Leaked urine can cause skin irritation, but this is not a very serious problem. The biggest problem caused by incontinence is the social stigma that accompanies it. Incontinence or fear of it can lead to a gradual withdrawal from social situations and activities.

TREATMENT

SELF TREATMENT:

- Moderation of excessive fluid intake can decrease episodes.
- Completely emptying the bladder as much as possible with each urination can help.
- Kegel exercises (repeated contraction of the muscles of the pelvic floor) can strengthen the muscles and lead to better bladder control.

MEDICAL TREATMENT:

- Anticholinergic drugs such as oxybutynin and hyoscyamine can help with incontinence by acting on certain nerve pathways and decreasing the frequency of urination.
- Biofeedback, using electrical equipment, can help increase awareness and control of muscles involved in control of the bladder.

SURGICAL TREATMENT:

Bladder suspension is a surgical technique that can repair the muscles of the pelvic floor and prevent leakage from stress incontinence.

PREVENTION

Hormone replacement therapy may prevent incontinence in some postmenopausal women whose incontinence relates to changes in the urethra's lining.

INFLUENZA

Influenza is a seasonal illness and occurs during the winter months. It is uncommon before November 15th or after March 15th.

Influenza (commonly known as the flu) viruses have been an important cause of respiratory tract infections for centuries. The virus can cause worldwide outbreaks (pandemics), local outbreaks (epidemics), or sporadic cases (endemic). The different strains of the virus have the unique ability to change their outer coat, resulting in more severe infections in individuals not previously exposed. Global pandemics generally occur every 20 to 30 years.

CAUSES

The cause of influenza is a virus that frequently changes its genetic material. Although there are three viruses—A, B, and C—types A and B account for the vast majority of all.

SYMPTOMS

Influenza is characterized by

- FEVER (often very high)
- COUGH
- HEADACHE
- Muscle aches
- Weakness and FATIGUE

A characteristic finding that helps distinguish influenza from the COMMON COLD is that patients with influenza often have severe FATIGUE requiring bed rest. The FEVER and FATIGUE usually last three to four days, but the COUGH, weakness, and muscle aches may persist for weeks. Influenza may be indistinguishable from other viral infections in young children.

DIAGNOSIS

The diagnosis of influenza is generally made on the basis of the clinical symptoms. However, there are tests that can confirm the diagnosis.

- A CULTURE of oral secretions can identify the virus, but this takes several days.
- Recently, a rapid diagnostic test was developed that can give doctors the diagnosis in 24 hours.
- There are also BLOOD TESTS available, but they require confirmation two to four weeks later and are rarely helpful clinically.

COMPLICATIONS

Influenza is usually a self-limited disease, but complications can occur. Although influenza rarely causes PNEUMONIA, when it does, the mortality is high. The virus can also damage the heart muscle (MYOCARDITIS) and cause disease in the nervous system. Influenza B is an important cause of Reye syndrome, which can be fatal in children.

TREATMENT

SELF TREATMENT:

Individuals with influenza infection should adhere to the instructions of Mom, including

- Drinking plenty of fluids
- Getting plenty of rest
- Taking acetaminophen to reduce FEVER and aches

Fluid intake is especially important to prevent DEHYDRATION. ASPIRIN should be avoided, particularly in children; ASPIRIN use during viral infection is associated with the often fatal condition, Reye syndrome.

MEDICAL TREATMENT:

There are two antiviral medications that are effective against influenza. AMANTADINE is effective for both the treatment and prevention of influenza, but is associated with nervous system side effects, especially in the elderly. Rimantadine, a recently approved medication, is less toxic but more costly. Both of these medications must be administered within 48 hours of symptoms for maximum efficacy.

SURGICAL TREATMENT:

None.

PREVENTION

The most effective method of preventing influenza is vaccination. A new influenza vaccine is developed every fall to immunize people against the most commonly encountered strains in the community. Patients who are allergic to eggs should not receive the vaccine. For patients who do not get vaccinated, AMANTADINE and rimantadine can be given to prevent infection. Treatment with either medicine is about 70 percent effective in preventing the illness.

INTESTINAL OBSTRUCTION

Intestinal obstruction may occur anywhere in the gastrointestinal tract from the esophagus to the anus.

Intestinal obstruction occurs when the normal movement of intestinal contents through the digestive tract is interrupted. Intestinal obstruction usually refers to a lesion that mechanically blocks the intestine, but movement of intestinal contents can also be impeded when the normal contractions (motility) of the bowel are impaired.

CAUSES

Intestinal obstruction can be caused by

- Scars from previous operations (most commonly)
- Tumor (see COLORECTAL CANCER)
- Incarcerated HERNIA
- Twisting of the bowel (called *volvulus*)
- Telescoping of the bowel into itself
- Intra-abdominal abscesses pressing on the bowel
- Inflammatory diseases of the intestines

Bowel obstruction can sometimes result from impacted fecal material, parasites, and foods that cannot be completely digested, and occasionally by large GALLSTONES.

SYMPTOMS

The symptoms of intestinal obstruction depend on the level of the obstruction. Obstruction high in the gastrointestinal tract causes nausea and VOMITING early. The food is undigested or only partially digested. Lower obstruction is manifest by crampy ABDOMINAL PAIN and ABDOMINAL SWELLING. Nausea and VOMITING are later symptoms.

Although patients with complete intestinal obstruction may have bowel movements early as the contents of the bowel farther on than the obstruction are eliminated, they are usually unable to pass stool and flatus. Patients with partially obstructed intestines will continue to pass small amounts.

DIAGNOSIS

The diagnosis of obstruction is based largely on the history of the illness and the PHYSICAL EXAMINATION. It is confirmed by abdominal X rays (RADIOGRAPHY), which show distended intestinal loops filled with fluid and gas.

Laboratory tests including complete BLOOD COUNT, and other BLOOD TESTS are performed to assess kidney function and the amount of fluid lost into the obstructed bowel.

COMPLICATIONS

The most serious complication from a bowel obstruction occurs when obstruction compromises blood supply to the involved intestine resulting in bowel death (GANGRENE) and perforation. The patient can develop infection of the abdominal cavity (peritonitis). This is a potentially life-threatening complication.

They can also suffer from severe DEHYDRATION and may develop KIDNEY FAILURE.

TREATMENT

SELF TREATMENT:

None.

MEDICAL TREATMENT:

Fluid and electrolyte imbalances must be corrected with intravenous fluids before the obstruction can be addressed.

The obstruction may resolve spontaneously if it

- Occurs shortly after another operation
- Is the result of an inflammatory disease of the bowel such as CROHN DISEASE or DIVERTICULAR DISEASE
- Is a partial, rather than a complete, obstruction

In other cases, the patient may be treated initially with a nasogastric tube placed on suction.

SURGICAL TREATMENT:

If the cause of obstruction is an incarcerated HERNIA, prompt HERNIA REPAIR may be required. If the bowel is found to have a compromised blood supply during HERNIA REPAIR, the bowel must be removed.

Patients with other causes of intestinal obstruction may require exploratory surgery to find the problem. The obstruction may be relieved by cutting or destroying adhesions or by removing or by-passing a severely scarred portion of intestine or intestine involved with tumor. Bowel with compromised blood supply also must be removed.

PREVENTION

None.

IRRITABLE BOWEL SYNDROME

Irritable bowel syndrome is a very common affliction. It is often a frequently recurring condition. For reasons that are not clear, it affects women much more often than men.

In general, irritable bowel syndrome (IBS) is an increased sensitivity of the large intestine—and possibly the small intestine as well—to certain stimuli such as food, stress, and hormones. In IBS, nerve impulses to the intestine generate higher and more prolonged pressure within the bowel wall, resulting in changes of bowel habits, ABDOMINAL PAIN, and bloating.

IBS has many synonyms, including *spastic colon* and *mucous colitis*. *Colitis* is not a good term, though, because it is actually a different condition, one that involves inflammation. There is no visible or microscopic inflammation or damage associated with IBS.

CAUSES

The cause of IBS is unclear. Some studies indicate that the pressure generated within the colon in patients with IBS is higher than in other healthy individuals. The colon relaxes more slowly in IBS, as well. Patients also seem to have a lower pain threshold within the intestine—even small increases in the amount of gas or stool can cause substantial discomfort.

SYMPTOMS

- Sense of incomplete evacuation of bowel movements
- ABDOMINAL SWELLING and gas
- ABDOMINAL PAIN
- Sense of CONSTIPATION, at times even alternating with DIARRHEA
- Rectal discharge of mucus

These symptoms are frequently improved, at least temporarily, after a bowel movement.

DIAGNOSIS

There is no specific test that will diagnose this condition; it remains largely a diagnosis of exclusion. It can be diagnosed if the typical symptoms are present and the results of a PHYSICAL EXAMINATION are normal. Other tests, if done, are usually used to exclude other conditions.

COMPLICATIONS

Although the symptoms can be quite distressing to the patient, this condition does not progress into a situation where significant complications develop. RECTAL BLEEDING, WEIGHT LOSS, persistent DIARRHEA, or other unremitting symptoms, however, should guide the patient to seek medical advice.

TREATMENT

SELF TREATMENT:

- Partaking in regular exercise
- Eating a diet rich in fiber (whole-grain breads, bran, vegetables)
- Avoiding fats and fried food
- Avoiding laxatives
- Limiting dairy products (IBS is often associated with lactose intolerance)

MEDICAL TREATMENT:

- Fiber supplements, such as methylcellulose or psyllium
- Antispasmodic or antimotility agents such as DICYCLOMINE or hyoscyamine.
- Rarely, antidepressants such as AMITRYPTILINE

SURGICAL TREATMENT:

None.

PREVENTION

There is no specific prevention strategy although a high-fiber, low-fat diet may reduce the severity of symptoms. For those with lactose intolerance, avoidance of dairy products is also helpful.

KIDNEY FAILURE

The kidneys are the body's waste-treatment facility, filtering the excess water and metabolic wastes from the blood to make urine. Their failure can have devastating effects.

Kidney failure describes the loss of the kidney's ability to eliminate the excess water and bodily wastes from the blood stream. This can happen over a period of hours (as in BLOOD POISONING or the very low blood pressure of shock), over a period of days (as in the toxic effects of medication such as gentamicin, anticancer drugs, and amphotericin B), or over a period of years (as in DIABETES, uncontrolled HYPERTENSION, excessive use of pain killers, or ATHEROSCLEROSIS).

CAUSES

High blood pressure (HYPERTENSION) and DIABETES are the most common causes of kidney failure. Other less common factors that can damage the kidneys and lead to failure include

- Prolonged low blood pressure (shock)
- Persistent urinary obstruction from KIDNEY STONES, BLADDER STONES, or enlarged prostate (PROSTATE, ENLARGED)
- Infection
- Hereditary diseases
- Massive muscle damage or certain forms of LEUKEMIA, which can release protein in the blood that "plugs up" the kidneys
- CONGESTIVE HEART FAILURE, in which the heart cannot pump enough blood through the kidneys to make them effective
- Autoimmune diseases, such as systemic LUPUS ERYTHEMATOSUS

Some commonly used drugs can precipitate kidney failure, especially in the elderly. Nonsteroidal anti-inflammatory drugs such as IBUPROFEN and INDOMETHACIN are the main culprits, but they rarely lead to to severe kidney failure.

SYMPTOMS

Early in kidney failure there are usually no symptoms at all. In advanced cases, though, the usual symptoms include

- Weakness
- Lethargy and FATIGUE
- Swollen or puffy extremities (ANKLE SWELLING)
- Nausea

In some cases, decreased urinary output and blood in the urine may be noted.

DIAGNOSIS

A PHYSICAL EXAMINATION may show edema (swelling) and enlarged kidneys in some cases, but the majority of a diagnosis of kidney failure depends on

- BLOOD TESTS for creatinine and blood urea nitrogen
- URINALYSIS to detect inflammation of the kidneys or any metabolic abnormalities
- ULTRASOUND of the kidneys to reveal their size and the presence of any obstruction

COMPLICATIONS

- HYPERTENSION can result from kidney failure.
- CONGESTIVE HEART FAILURE can be precipitated by the kidney's inability to eliminate excess fluid and salt.
- Potassium buildup, acid buildup, and pericarditis are potentially life-threatening complications.
- Calcium imbalances can lead to OSTEOPOROSIS.

TREATMENT

SELF TREATMENT:

A carefully selected and prescribed diet can be helpful in slowing the progression of kidney failure. Usually, the diet is a low-sodium, low-potassium, low-protein diet.

MEDICAL TREATMENT:

Treatment is aimed at the underlying condition, such as HYPERTENSION. Tight control of DIABETES is also important. Early in kidney failure, ACE inhibitors such as CAPTOPRIL and ENALAPRIL may slow the progression of failure in some cases.

SURGICAL TREATMENT:

- Dialysis
- KIDNEY TRANSPLANT

PREVENTION

- Control of HYPERTENSION
- Tight control of DIABETES
- Early relief of urinary obstructions such as BLADDER STONES and KIDNEY STONES

KIDNEY STONES

For reasons that are not entirely understood, middle-aged men and people with recurrent urinary tract infections are more susceptible to the development of kidney stones.

Kidney stones are deposits of mineral or organic substances from urine that form in the kidneys. The stones can be very tiny or as large as a walnut.

CAUSES

Stones can form because of metabolic abnormalities that change the chemistry of the urine. This abnormality can be no more than a constant predisposition or it can be a definitive metabolism problem. Examples of predisposing problems include CROHN DISEASE and an overactive parathyroid gland.

Bacterial infections of the urine can also contribute to stone formation.

SYMPTOMS

The symptoms of kidney stones are usually unmistakable. The stones cause severe, colicky flank pain. Occasionally, they can also cause blood in the urine, which can turn urine bright red or the color of tea, depending on the amount of blood (see URINE, ABNORMAL APPEARANCE).

DIAGNOSIS

Apart from consideration of the typical symptoms, diagnosis can involve

- BLOOD TESTS to check kidney function
- URINALYSIS
- CULTURE
- Intravenous pyelogram (RADIOGRAPHY)
- ULTRASOUND

COMPLICATIONS

Without proper treatment or with delayed treatment, a stone can cause an obstruction in the kidney or the urinary tract; an obstruction can lead to loss of kidney function (KIDNEY FAILURE). Another danger is a complicating infection, heralded by worsening pain and a FEVER.

TREATMENT

SELF TREATMENT:

See Prevention below.

MEDICAL TREATMENT:

- Some kidney stones will dissolve with medication, but most will not.
- Sometimes antispasmodic medications can encourage passage of the stone.

SURGICAL TREATMENT:

Extracorporeal shock-wave lithotripsy (ULTRASONIC LITHOTRIPSY) is a technique in which the patient is placed in a bath and tiny shock waves are pulsed through the water and the body to break up the stones. Once the stones are pulverized, they can pass through the urinary tract.

Another surgical option is kidney stone removal, which can be performed open (traditional surgery) or with a special flexible scope threaded up the ureter or inserted directly in from the side (see ENDOSCOPY).

PREVENTION

- Adequate fluid intake (at least eight eight-ounce glasses of fluid per day) may help discourage stone formation.
- Dietary changes to decrease intake of calcium, uric acid, and oxalates (depending on the type of stone) may help prevent recurrences.
- Diuretic medication (such as HYDROCHLOROTHIAZIDE), medication to lower uric acid levels (such as ALLOPURINOL), or other drugs that affect salts and change the acid balance of the urine may help prevent recurrence in some patients.

LARYNGEAL CANCER

Although the disease is certainly not limited to this group, the peak incidence of this disease occurs in men in their 60s.

Laryngeal cancer is a tumor of the larynx, or voice box. The disease most commonly affects middle-aged or older men who have a history of smoking and excessive alcohol consumption.

CAUSES

Laryngeal cancer is most consistently associated with smoking and heavy alcohol intake. Other possible factors include

- Chronic laryngitis
- Chronic gastric reflux (heartburn)
- Exposure to nitrogen mustard, asbestos, and ionizing radiation

SYMPTOMS

Hoarseness of the voice is the most common symptom. Heavy smokers are often hoarse, anyway, which can lead to a masking of the telltale initial symptom and delay diagnosis and treatment. Any change in voice that does not resolve in a few weeks warrants a laryngeal examination.

WEIGHT LOSS without reduced caloric intake may also be one of the initial symptoms.

Cancers of the supraglottic larynx (the area above the vocal cords) do not produce early symptoms and signs, and it is not uncommon to see enlargement of the lymph nodes—a sign that the cancer may have spread to the lymph system—as the first sign. Early subtle symptoms include alteration of one's tolerance for hot and cold foods and scratchy sensations when swallowing.

DIAGNOSIS

The typical symptoms (hoarseness or change in voice associated with WEIGHT LOSS) in a person with a significant history of alcohol intake and smoking raises the index of suspicion for laryngeal cancer. Flexible laryngeal ENDOSCOPY can be done to inspect the area, while direct laryngoscopy (another form of ENDOSCOPY) is reserved for BIOPSY. COMPUTED TOMOGRAPHY is performed to evaluate the extent and stage of the disease.

COMPLICATIONS

Upper airway obstruction can develop due to soft-tissue swelling around the tumor. Patients can develop shortness of breath and the sensation of inability to breathe (BREATHING DIFFICULTY). Speech and SWALLOWING DIFFICULTIES are often related to the cancer, but sometimes to the treatment side effects as well.

TREATMENT

SELF TREATMENT:

Tobacco smoking and alcohol use should be discontinued immediately.

MEDICAL TREATMENT:

Early stage disease is highly curable by radiation therapy or surgery. Advanced stage disease is usually treated with combined chemotherapy, radiation, and surgery.

SURGICAL TREATMENT:

Supraglottic laryngectomy, hemilaryngectomy, and total laryngectomy are considered—surgeries to remove various parts of the larynx—based on the stage of cancer. The ability to speak can sometimes be preserved in early cases.

PREVENTION

Abstinence from alcohol and smoking is important. Ongoing clinical trials will determine if retinoic acid (a vitamin A–like compound) has a role in the prevention of second primary cancers.

LEUKEMIA

High-dose chemotherapy with bone marrow transplantation can cure some types of leukemia, but the acute forms of leukemia are difficult to treat and are often fatal.

Leukemia is a cancer of the bone marrow causing an abnormal proliferation of white blood cells. Leukemia can be divided into acute and chronic forms. In acute leukemia, immature white blood cells proliferate. In chronic leukemia, mature white blood cells proliferate.

CAUSES

The cause of leukemia is unknown. Risk factors for developing leukemia include

- Radiation exposure
- Chemotherapy, especially for HODGKIN DISEASE, lymphoma (LYMPHOMA, NON-HODGKIN), multiple myeloma, or OVARIAN CANCER
- Chemical exposure such as exposure to the solvent benzene

SYMPTOMS

The symptoms of leukemia are very diverse. They can include

- FATIGUE
- Pallor (see ANEMIA)
- Easy bruising (BRUISING, UNEXPLAINED) or easy bleeding
- Shortness of breath (BREATHING DIFFICULTY)
- FEVERS
- Recurrent infections
- WEIGHT LOSS
- Loss of appetite (APPETITE, LOSS OF) or feeling full soon after eating

DIAGNOSIS

Diagnosis of leukemia is suspected by an abnormal complete BLOOD COUNT. To confirm the diagnosis, a bone marrow BIOPSY must be performed. Chromosomes are also analyzed at that time.

PHYSICAL EXAMINATION may show fast heart rate, pallor, bruises (BRUISING, UNEXPLAINED), RASH, and enlarged spleen, liver, or lymph nodes. There may also be evidence of infection.

COMPLICATIONS

Complications include

- Bleeding—most patients diagnosed with leukemia are at risk of bleeding or bruising (BRUISING, UNEXPLAINED) due to low platelet counts.
- Infection—although there are numerous white blood cells available, they do not function normally. Patients are susceptible to bacterial, viral, and fungal infections.
- The transformation of chronic forms of leukemia into acute forms of leukemia or lymphoma (LYMPHOMA, NON-HODGKIN)—these are difficult to treat and are usually fatal.

TREATMENT

SELF TREATMENT:

None.

MEDICAL TREATMENT:

- Chemotherapy is given to treat leukemia. (The type of medication and duration of treatment depends on the form of leukemia.)
- Transfusions of platelets and red blood cells are given as needed.
- Prevention of infection with vaccines and antibiotics is crucial.
- High-dose chemotherapy with bone marrow transplantation is done for many types of leukemia with a goal of curing the disease.

SURGICAL TREATMENT:

With some types of leukemia, splenectomy (SPLEEN REMOVAL) may be helpful, but in general, there is no surgical intervention available for leukemia.

PREVENTION

Avoidance of unnecessary exposure to radiation and chemicals that can cause the disease is the only preventive strategy.

LIVER CANCER

Although relatively rare in the United States, liver cancer is one of the most common fatal malignancies in the world, causing more than one million deaths a year. It is most common in Africa and Asia.

The prognosis for this cancer is usually quite poor with progression to death usually in 6 to 12 months.

CAUSES

Risk factors for the disease include long-standing HEPATITIS B infection, cirrohosis of the liver, and ALCOHOLISM.

SYMPTOMS

Liver cancer can cause ABDOMINAL PAIN, ABDOMINAL SWELLING, jaundice, FATIGUE, internal bleeding (possibly RECTAL BLEEDING), and generalized ITCHING.

DIAGNOSIS

COMPUTED TOMOGRAPHY and ULTRASOUND of the abdomen can detect even small liver cancers. A BLOOD TEST for a substance called *alpha-fetoprotein* may be helpful. Ultimately the diagnosis is made by BIOPSY of the liver.

COMPLICATIONS

Complications are most commonly seen in relation to chronic liver disease or cirrhosis of the liver.

TREATMENT

SELF TREATMENT:

A well-balanced diet should be maintained.

MEDICAL TREATMENT:

Chemotherapy does not appear to offer any advantage in the treatment of this cancer.

SURGICAL TREATMENT:

Resection of this tumor offers the only reliable cure for this cancer. Liver transplantation is curative in few patients.

PREVENTION

Abstinence from alcohol consumption and the screening and prevention of chronic HEPATITIS B infections can go a long way in the prevention of this cancer.

LUNG CANCER

Lung cancer is an overgrowth of cells originating in the lung. This cell growth proceeds outside of the body's normal control mechanisms. It commonly spreads to the lymph nodes, bone, liver, brain, and adrenal glands.

Lung cancer is the most common form of cancer, and 80 to 90 percent of newly diagnosed cases are caused by tobacco smoking.

CAUSES

Tobacco smoking is the most common cause of lung cancer, but it is not the only cause. An increased risk of lung cancer is also seen after occupational exposure to

- Asbestos
- Chromium
- Nickel
- Radon
- Hydrocarbons
- Arsenic
- Ether

There may also be a genetic predisposition to developing lung cancer, but this has not been shown definitively.

SYMPTOMS

Symptoms of lung cancer include

- BREATHING DIFFICULTY
- CHEST PAIN or pressure
- FATIGUE
- WEIGHT LOSS
- Loss of appetite (APPETITE, LOSS OF)
- Bloody sputum

DIAGNOSIS

Diagnostic tests include

- Chest X ray (RADIOGRAPHY)
- COMPUTED TOMOGRAPHY of the chest to locate the tumor precisely and to check for the spread of the disease to the lymph nodes, liver, and adrenal glands
- BIOPSY of the tumor, to determine the exact type of cancer, which is done with either bronchoscopy (a form of ENDOSCOPY) or COMPUTED TOMOGRAPHY–guided fine needle aspiration (Rarely is a surgical procedure needed for BIOPSY.)
- Sputum testing, for evidence of cancer (CYTOLOGY)

- BLOOD TESTS to evaluate liver function, calcium level, and electrolytes
- Bone scan (NUCLEAR MEDICINE) and COMPUTED TOMOGRAPHY of the head and neck to determine the extent of the disease

COMPLICATIONS

Possible complications of lung cancer include
- PNEUMONIA
- High blood calcium levels
- Hoarseness
- SWALLOWING DIFFICULTIES
- Arm pain
- Facial swelling
- Fluid collection around the lung

Other complications related to tumor spread to other organs can occur.

TREATMENT

SELF TREATMENT:

Many people feel an improvement in their BREATHING DIFFICULTY and COUGH after they stop smoking, although it may have no effect on the tumor itself.

MEDICAL TREATMENT:

Some types of lung cancer are responsive to chemotherapy given in either oral or intravenous form. Most types of lung cancer, though, have either minimal or no response to chemotherapy. These tumors often benefit from radiation therapy.

SURGICAL TREATMENT:

Small tumors that have not spread are best treated by surgical removal (LUNG RESECTION). The size and location of the tumor determine the surgical procedure and amount of lung tissue removed.

PREVENTION

Tobacco smoking and occupational exposures should be avoided.

LUPUS ERYTHEMATOSUS

Lupus erythematosus is an inflammatory disease of the small blood vessels in various organs of the body, especially the joints, the kidneys, the lungs, the brain, and the skin.

Depending upon the site of the inflammation, the process can be damaging or of only temporary concern. The joint disease in lupus, for instance, is usually nondestructive; whereas the kidney disease, brain disease, and lung disease in lupus can cause life-threatening organ destruction.

Lupus erythematosus affects women ten times more often than it affects men, and it can afflict people of any age.

CAUSES

No cause is known. As in RHEUMATOID ARTHRITIS, there may be extrinsic, or environmental, factors, but none has been recognized. Some forms of lupus occur in response to medication; drugs such as PROCAINAMIDE (used for cardiac ARRHYTHMIAS), or phenytoin (used in the treatment of epilepsy) can precipitate lupus. Once these drugs are discontinued, however, the lupus process tends to correct itself.

Intrinsic factors involved in lupus are less well defined than they are in RHEUMATOID ARTHRITIS, but genetic features may be important. No specific genetic abnormality has thus far been determined, though.

SYMPTOMS

Symptoms depend upon the organs that are involved. In the skin, the usual symptoms include a RASH that causes a reddened, slightly thickened skin. The reaction is usually nondestructive and involves the areas on the nose and the cheekbones. Some patients experience a destructive skin RASH, which is called *discoid lupus*. This RASH occurs on the face and sun-exposed areas of the body, the scalp (where hair loss can take place), and in the ear canals.

Joint inflammations resemble the symptoms of RHEUMATOID ARTHRITIS. Multiple joints can be inflamed, but unlike RHEUMATOID ARTHRITIS, long-term damage is not likely.

Brain involvement is revealed by seizures, mental CONFUSION, MEMORY PROBLEMS, and in rare cases, coma. Restriction of lung expansion leads to BREATHING DIFFICULTY.

DIAGNOSIS

The diagnosis of lupus can be difficult at times because the disease takes many different forms; its manifestations vary widely. However, a diagnosis of lupus is usually made when all three of the following conditions are true:

- Inflammation of several of the signature organs (mentioned above)
- Positive results on certain laboratory tests (mentioned below)
- Absence of other causes of the inflammation

The laboratory tests that are involved are BLOOD TESTS for the antinuclear antibody (ANA) and its subsets. The presence of ANA is very characteristic of this disease, but it can also appear in several other conditions but with a weaker reaction.

COMPLICATIONS

The list of complications is extraordinarily large in lupus because so many organ systems can be involved. (See Symptoms above.)

TREATMENT

SELF TREATMENT:

The patient's help in managing the disease is critical. Drug compliance is particularly important. The patient needs to take medications, even at times when it seems as though they have little effect.

The patient must be alert to the disease's progression in critical areas of the body. Regular visits for examination and tests are required to monitor the inflammatory process.

Many patients with lupus have an undue sensitivity to the sun. Direct exposure to certain ultraviolet rays can not only cause a sunburn, but can increase and accelerate the symptoms of the lupus process itself. Thus, all patients with lupus should avoid direct exposure to the sun, wear long sleeves and a hat when going out in the daytime, and apply sunscreen with a sun protection factor (SPF) of 15 or higher on sun-exposed areas of the body.

MEDICAL TREATMENT:

Routine tests to monitor the disease include

- BLOOD COUNTS (in part to check for ANEMIA)
- URINALYSIS is done to detect protein in the urine or red cells (a sign of kidney involvement)
- BLOOD TESTS to monitor whether liver or kidney damage is occurring either as a result of the disease or sometimes as a consequence of the treatment and to determine the activity level of the disease process

The need for medications to control inflammation are governed by two considerations. The first consideration is the activity of the disease. More activity requires larger doses and more potent drugs. The second consideration is knowledge of the particular organs that are under attack. If joints are involved with lupus, mild treatment only may be required, since damage is not likely to occur even on a long-term basis. On the other hand, if the kidneys are involved, more aggressive therapy must be applied early.

Unfortunately, aggressive therapy can have significant side effects. For example, corticosteroid drugs, such as PREDNISONE, in high doses can cause

- WEIGHT GAIN, especially around the face and trunk
- Thinning of the bones (OSTEOPOROSIS)
- DIABETES
- CATARACTS

Other drugs include hydroxychloroquine, which has a good safety record but requires eye checks one or more times a year, and CYCLOPHOSPHAMIDE, which is given intravenously each month in cases of severe kidney, brain, or lung disease.

SURGICAL TREATMENT:

Surgical treatment is not ordinarily considered in the treatment of lupus; however, a KIDNEY TRANSPLANT may be performed if kidney function has become obliterated by lupus, particularly if dialysis treatment is not well tolerated.

PREVENTION

None.

LYMPHOMA, NON-HODGKIN

In the past, these forms of lymphoma were often caught too late for treatment, but newer methods have made long periods of remission possible.

Lymphomas are cancers that arise from the lymph system, a network of small nodes (especially in the neck, groin, and armpits) and vessels that help to fight infections. Lymphoma is divided into two major categories: HODGKIN DISEASE and non-Hodgkin lymphoma.

In lymphoma, lymph nodes become enlarged due to the presence of a tumor. Any area where there is lymphoid tissue, including the chest and abdomen, may be involved.

CAUSES

The cause of lymphomas is unknown, but some viral infections may be a contributing factor. Immunosuppressant drugs used after transplant surgery (see KIDNEY TRANSPLANT) to prevent organ rejection may also increase the risk of lymphoma.

SYMPTOMS

Symptoms of lymphoma include

- Persistent swelling of a lymph node or nodes
- FEVER
- Night sweats (SWEATING, EXCESSIVE)
- Unintended WEIGHT LOSS

DIAGNOSIS

The diagnosis can be suspected from the symptoms, but is made definitively only by surgical BIOPSY of an involved lymph node. The examination of the sample of lymphatic tissue permits a determination of the type and stage of lymphoma present (non-Hodgkin lymphomas are categorized as low grade, intermediate grade, or high grade).

Once the diagnosis is made, other tests such as COMPUTED TOMOGRAPHY of various areas are used to evaluate the extent of the disease.

BLOOD COUNT and chest X rays (RADIOGRAPHY) may also be useful.

COMPLICATIONS

Without treatment the immune system becomes progressively more and more impaired, resulting in serious infections that can be life threatening.

TREATMENT

SELF TREATMENT:

None.

MEDICAL TREATMENT:

Treatment depends on both the grade (low grade versus intermediate or high grade) and the degree to which the tumor has spread and involved other areas and other organs. Treatments presently used for the management of non-Hodgkin lymphomas are

- Chemotherapy
- Radiation therapy
- Bone marrow transplantation

SURGICAL TREATMENT:

None.

PREVENTION

Any lymph node greater than one centimeter in diameter (the size of a small marble) should be evaluated by a physician.

MIGRAINE HEADACHE

Migraines are more common in women, although there is a counterpart in men: the cluster headache.

Migraine headaches are an extremely frequent benign headache syndrome; they are sometimes called *vascular headaches*. Migraines can cause intense pain and other symptoms. They are often presaged by a phenomenon known as an *aura*.

CAUSES

The cause of migraines is unknown; however, there seems to be some hereditary connection, as a family history of the condition is not uncommon.

There do appear to be triggers for certain individuals. Some patients develop a headache related to physical exertion—for example while lifting weights or during sexual climax. Certain drugs and substances in food and drink may also play a role for some individuals.

SYMPTOMS

Not all migraines are preceded by preliminary symptoms, or auras, but if they are, the symptoms associated with an impending migraine usually involve some kind of VISION DISTURBANCE such as

- Bright or dark spots (sometimes resembling champagne bubbles)
- Tunnel vision
- Zigzag lines (called *fortification spectra*)

The aura is followed by an intense crescendo of a HEADACHE, frequently behind one eye or on one side of the head. The pain may be pounding, throbbing, viselike, or stabbing; frequently it feels like the head is going to explode from pressure. Other symptoms that can accompany the headache of a migraine, include

- Sensitivity to light
- Nausea
- VOMITING

DIAGNOSIS

The diagnosis of migraine can usually be made from the symptoms and a PHYSICAL EXAMINATION that reveals no neurologic problems.

Although many individuals experience the head pain predominantly on one side, if they have not had at least one instance involving the opposite side, there may be cause for concern. In cases of unilateral headache or those related to exertion, MAGNETIC RESONANCE IMAGING and ELECTROENCEPHALOGRAPHY may be indicated to rule out other possibilities.

COMPLICATIONS

There should be no lasting complications from a migraine, although some research indicates that patients who are prone to experience migraines may have an increased risk of STROKE.

TREATMENT

SELF TREATMENT:

Rest in a quiet, darkened room and an adequate fluid intake can help one weather a migraine. (See also Prevention below.)

MEDICAL TREATMENT:

Medications used to treat various aspects of episodes of migraine include

- ERGOTAMINE
- Isometheptene
- Butalbital
- ACETAMINOPHEN AND CODEINE COMBINATION
- Butorphanol nasal spray
- Antinauseants such as PROCHLORPERAZINE, CHLORPROMAZINE, or METOCLOPRAMIDE
- Certain nonsteroidal anti-inflammatory drugs such IBUPROFEN
- Corticosteroids such as PREDNISONE (limited use under strict supervision)
- Sumatriptan

(See also Prevention below.)

SURGICAL TREATMENT:

None.

PREVENTION

Prevention of migraines involves two approaches. The first is avoidance of potential triggers. Strategies include

- Regularizing intake of caffeine so as not to induce symptoms from caffeine withdrawal
- Avoiding food containing tyramine such as chocolate, ripe cheese, yogurt, nuts, sour cream, and onions
- Avoiding foods high in nitrates such as processed meats
- Avoiding certain food additives such as monosodium glutamate and aspartame
- Limiting or eliminating alcoholic beverages, especially red wine, champagne, and beer
- Avoiding overuse of pain-killing medication

The second preventive approach involves the use of medication to head off migraines. Medications used for prevention include

- PROPRANOLOL
- Antidepressant drugs such as AMITRIPTYLINE or IMIPRAMINE
- VERAPAMIL
- Anticonvulsants such as CARBAMAZEPINE, phenytoin, and divalproex
- Methysergide
- Cyproheptadine
- LITHIUM

MULTIPLE SCLEROSIS

Multiple sclerosis is an inflammatory disease of the central nervous system. It usually starts in young adulthood and its course is chronic but highly variable. It attacks different portions of the nervous system to a varying and unpredictable extent in episodes that remit and recur over many years.

Multiple sclerosis is most prevalent in temperate climates. It is almost twice as frequent in women as it is in men, and twice as frequent in whites as blacks.

CAUSES

The cause of multiple sclerosis is not known, but viruses have been implicated.

SYMPTOMS

The initial manifestations of the disease may be very minor and not enough to be brought to medical attention. Symptoms include

- Weakness
- VISION DISTURBANCES such as decreased or double vision
- Incoordination
- Tingling
- NUMBNESS

The symptoms may spontaneously subside, but after a variable interval (up to ten years), there may be a recurrence of the same or new symptoms. As the disease progresses, the deficits become more significant and irreversible. Some more severe symptoms include

- FATIGUE, especially in the summer months
- INCONTINENCE
- Spasticity, especially of the legs
- Trigeminal neuralgia—bouts of facial pain

DIAGNOSIS

Diagnosis of the disease is generally suspected from the characteristic course and symptoms, the patient's MEDICAL HISTORY, and a PHYSICAL EXAMINATION that focuses on neurologic function.

The most important test used for diagnosis today is MAGNETIC RESONANCE IMAGING of the brain and brain stem, which can reveal the characteristic inflammatory lesions.

Cerebrospinal fluid obtained by a LUMBAR PUNCTURE can be examined for proteins and immunoglobulin G, which is characteristic of multiple sclerosis.

Electrophysiologic tests of the central nervous system similar to ELECTROENCEPHALOGRAPHY may also be useful.

COMPLICATIONS

As symptoms continue to cause irreversible damage, many complications can arise in a wide variety of body systems. Infections of any sort can cause exacerbations of the disease; they must be detected and treated promptly. The most frequent infections are kidney infection, BLADDER INFECTION, and PNEUMONIA.

TREATMENT

SELF TREATMENT:

Patients find it helpful to minimize their exposure to hot environments.

MEDICAL TREATMENT:

- Steroids such as PREDNISONE and METHYLPREDNISOLONE are the mainstays of treatment. They function as anti-inflammatory agents and also suppress the immune system.
- Interferon-beta, a substance with antiviral properties that is produced by the body, is sometimes administered to decrease the frequency of relapses.
- Experimental treatments with plasmapheresis, immunomodulators, cytotoxics, copolymer-1, and other drugs are being studied, but none has proved to be beneficial.

SURGICAL TREATMENT:

None.

PREVENTION

None.

MYOCARDITIS

Myocarditis is the inflammation of the muscular walls of the heart (the thick middle layer of the heart wall is called the *myocardium*). Although the condition may subside when the underlying cause is treated, myocarditis—as with all conditions that affect the heart—can be dangerous, leading to CONGESTIVE HEART FAILURE.

Myocarditis is often associated with some underlying disease such as an infection. The degree of inflammation varies greatly and may cause little or no symptoms or progress to significant disability.

CAUSES

Many times the cause of a specific case is uncertain, but the most commonly identified causes include

- Viral infection
- Lyme disease
- Rheumatic fever
- Parasitic infections
- Excessive alcohol intake (ALCOHOLISM)
- Ingestion of a toxic substance such as cobalt

SYMPTOMS

Often the condition will produce no symptoms, but the inflammation can impair the heart muscle enough to cause FATIGUE, BREATHING DIFFICULTY, and swelling of the extremities (see ANKLE SWELLING). Heart rhythm abnormalities (ARRHYTHMIAS) caused by myocarditis can also lead to palpitations, FAINTING OR FAINTNESS, or even cardiac arrest.

DIAGNOSIS

Careful PHYSICAL EXAMINATION of the heart, lungs, neck veins, and legs can help support a diagnosis of CONGESTIVE HEART FAILURE. ELECTROCARDIOGRAPHY may provide clues that suggest myocarditis. Special BLOOD TESTS looking for signs of viral infections may also be performed. An echocardiogram (ULTRASOUND) can document the degree of muscle impairment. Occasionally, a BIOPSY can be performed by a special catheter passed through the veins; the small amount of tissue obtained can document the inflammation and sometimes suggest the cause.

COMPLICATIONS

Myocarditis can lead to serious complications including

- CONGESTIVE HEART FAILURE leading to severe BREATHING DIFFICULTY
- ARRHYTHMIAS leading to FAINTING OR FAINTNESS
- Even sudden cardiac death

TREATMENT

SELF TREATMENT:

Decreased physical activity may be important particularly early in the course of myocarditis. A low-salt diet and avoidance of alcohol are also strongly recommended.

MEDICAL TREATMENT:

The general treatment of CONGESTIVE HEART FAILURE includes diuretics (such as FUROSEMIDE), DIGOXIN, and ACE inhibitors (ENALAPRIL and CAPTOPRIL).

Antibiotics for particular infections such as Lyme disease or parasitic infections may be used in some cases.

Drugs used to suppress the immune system such as PREDNISONE may be warranted in selected patients.

SURGICAL TREATMENT:

In very severe cases for appropriate patients, heart transplantation may be required.

PREVENTION

The risk of myocarditis can be reduced by

- Limiting alcohol consumption to moderate levels
- Seeking appropriate treatment for strep throat infections to avoid damage to the heart muscle
- Receiving a full series of childhood vaccinations

OBESITY

Obesity is generally defined as an excess amount of fat leading to a body weight that is more than 20 percent over what is accepted as ideal for that person's body type and height.

Obesity is associated with a large number of diseases; therefore, it is considered more of a risk factor than a disease itself.

CAUSES

If energy intake exceeds energy expenditure, then the body stores the energy as fat deposits and weight goes up. Usually, obesity develops from a habit of modestly excessive food intake combined with limited physical activity.

A person's metabolic rate—the rate at which the person burns energy for resting metabolic processes such as breathing and pumping blood—may also be a factor (see HYPOTHYROIDISM). In rare cases, CUSHING SYNDROME is the underlying cause.

Heredity and psychological factors seem to play a role in obesity. In recent years at least two types of genes that contribute to obesity symptoms have been isolated.

SYMPTOMS

Obesity is defined as body weight more than 20 percent greater than the recommended ideal body weight. This could be considered its defining symptom.

DIAGNOSIS

Excess fat can be measured with special calibers around the flank or under the upper arms. Generally, height and weight can be compared to standard tables to decide the percent of ideal body weight a person is at.

COMPLICATIONS

The main reasons to avoid obesity are the long-term complications. Obesity is associated with a higher risk of

- High blood pressure (HYPERTENSION)
- ATHEROSCLEROSIS
- HEART ATTACK
- CONGESTIVE HEART FAILURE
- DIABETES
- Certain types of cancer such as UTERINE CANCER

Obesity also places a greater stress on the bones and can

aggravate RHEUMATOID ARTHRITIS. In our society, obesity may also lead to a poor self image and can lead to a vicious cycle of less activity and further weight gain.

TREATMENT

SELF TREATMENT:

Reducing total caloric intake and increasing exercise are the mainstay of the treatment of obesity.

MEDICAL TREATMENT:

In rare cases, medications to suppress appetite such as FENFLURAMINE and FLUOXETINE may be used for short periods of time. These drugs and others are generally considered to have only short-term effectiveness.

A very-low-calorie diet (800 calories per day) can be attempted but only under close supervision to insure proper nutrition.

SURGICAL TREATMENT:

Stomach bypass procedures are probably the most common surgical treatment, although many variations have been developed. Surgery is somewhat controversial and generally limited to the most severe and resistant cases of obesity.

Liposuction may be used to remove excess fat, but this is generally done for cosmetic reasons.

PREVENTION

Except in the rare case of a strong hereditary predisposition to weight gain or a metabolic disorder, moderate caloric intake combined with moderate physical activity should be enough to prevent obesity.

ORAL CANCER

Oral cavity cancer includes cancer of the various anatomic structures of the mouth such as the

- Lip
- Tongue
- Floor of the mouth
- Palate

Cancers of the mouth most commonly affect men older than 45 who have some history of having either chewed or smoked tobacco.

At one time, cancer of the mouth was often a disfiguring, if not deadly, disease. Now, cosmetic surgery techniques have minimized this and made rehabilitation easier, but prevention or early detection are still the best measures.

CAUSES

Cigarette smoking is the major cause. A clear relationship has been identified between the extent of tobacco exposure and the risk of oral cancer.

Additional risk factors include

- Vitamin A deficiency
- Alcohol abuse (ALCOHOLISM)
- Chronic irritants, such as poor dental hygiene
- Syphilis

SYMPTOMS

Common symptoms are based on anatomic location of the tumor, including

- Lip—ulcerative lesion of the lower lip or NUMBNESS of the skin of the chin
- Tongue—difficulty in speech and swallowing (SWALLOWING DIFFICULTIES) and greater likelihood of spreading to the lymph nodes
- Insides of the cheeks (buccal mucosa)—pain, difficulty chewing, and bleeding
- Floor of the mouth—pain
- The bone beneath the teeth (alveolar ridge)—pain exacerbated by chewing, loose teeth, and bleeding

A sore anywhere in the mouth that does not heal in a few weeks should be evaluated by a physician or dentist.

DIAGNOSIS

PHYSICAL EXAMINATION of the oral cavity typically reveals the tumor, which is either ulcerative or exophytic (growing on the surface of the structure from which it originated). Cervical lymph nodes can usually be felt. COMPUTED TOMOGRAPHY of the area, including the base of the skull, is necessary for staging purposes. A BIOPSY is necessary to confirm the diagnosis.

COMPLICATIONS

Bleeding from the ulcer is a common complication. Difficulties in speech and SWALLOWING DIFFICULTIES are also common complications.

TREATMENT

SELF TREATMENT:

Discontinue smoking and alcohol intake.

MEDICAL TREATMENT:

For advanced disease, a combination of chemotherapy, radiation, and surgery is standard therapy and may offer a cure for early-stage tumors.

SURGICAL TREATMENT:

For early cancers, surgical resection is the treatment of choice. Reconstructive surgery is based on the extent of the primary tumor.

PREVENTION

Avoidance of smoking and alcohol abuse can significantly reduce risk. Ongoing clinical trials are evaluating retinoic acid (a vitamin A–like compound) as a preventive agent for second tumors.

OSTEOARTHRITIS

Osteoarthritis is a chronic arthritis involving damage to the cartilage cushion that caps the bones at a joint. Later, secondary changes occur in the adjacent bone itself. This process begins insidiously, usually in middle age, and increases in extent as the person gets older.

Although injury may cause the degenerative process of osteoarthritis at an early age, most cases do not develop until after the age of 55.

CAUSES

Cartilage breakdown can be the consequence of either decreased formation of cartilage or increased breakdown of cartilage, or both. Ultimately, the two bones in the joint rub directly against each other. Bone formation increases at points where the two bones of the joint meet, forming spurs.

There are two possible causes of osteoarthritis:

- Excess strain caused by repetitive trauma or a muscle imbalance around the joint.
- A (often genetic) defect in the way cartilage is formed allows for increased breakdown of cartilage or decreased formation of new cartilage.

SYMPTOMS

Major symptoms of osteoarthritis are

- Pain of the affected joint or joints, which is made worse by activity and improved by rest
- Inflammation (although this is less common in osteoarthritis than in RHEUMATOID ARTHRITIS)
- A bony enlargement, which appears as nodules at the last row of joints in the hand (Heberden nodes), at the middle row of joints of the fingers (Bouchard nodes), and at the joint at the base of the thumb
- Pain in the hip (often felt in the groin)
- Pain in the knee

Limitation of motion results when pain is severe.

DIAGNOSIS

No specific findings mark early osteoarthritis. When the disease is beginning, nondescript pain can appear. X rays (RADIOGRAPHY) at this point are normal. Occasionally, swelling in the hands begins before a Heberden node develops. Laboratory tests are not diagnostic of osteoarthritis either.

Later in the disease's progression, the loss of cartilage can be detected on X-ray films (RADIOGRAPHY).

COMPLICATIONS

Natural progression of the illness can limit the function of the involved joint.

TREATMENT

SELF TREATMENT:

Good body mechanics maintain normal bone and joint structure. Walking with a proper gait under good muscle control is beneficial. OBESITY has a role in causing abnormal posture in the patient, which in turn creates a greater strain on the joints. In this aspect, maintaining a healthy weight can be considered beneficial.

MEDICAL TREATMENT:

Pain relief is accomplished by medications including acetaminophen and various nonsteroidal anti-inflammatory drugs such as IBUPROFEN.

Supportive techniques are available for individual joints that are damaged by osteoarthritis, including splints, canes, and orthoses. Orthotics are particularly helpful in patients with foot osteoarthritis.

SURGICAL TREATMENT:

Although surgery has no place in the early phases of osteoarthritis, it is a dramatic and successful treatment for bone that is totally damaged and for which medical means are no longer effective. Joint replacement can be performed in which an artificial metal or plastic material replaces the damaged bone. KNEE ARTHROPLASTY and HIP ARTHROPLASTY can be very successful in this regard. Sometimes a joint or vertebrae can be fused. The amount of motion that is lost may be negligible and pain is eliminated.

PREVENTION

No successful prevention strategy is now available, although maintenance of good posture, good gait, and strong muscle development without OBESITY over the course of one's life ought to be helpful in retarding the progress of osteoarthritis.

OSTEOPOROSIS

Osteoporosis is a condition in which bone substance is lost from the bone found at the ends of long bones, the pelvis, and the ribs, or from the shaft of long bones in the arm or leg. Bone loss weakens the bone structure and makes it vulnerable to easy injury. BONE FRACTURE, even with little or no provocation, can result from a minor fall.

Osteoporosis is more common in women than men, and for reasons that are not entirely understood, white and Asian women are more likely to develop the disease than black women are.

CAUSES

Bone is a complex, dynamic tissue with an even balance between formation and removal. During periods of growth in childhood and in early adulthood, such remodeling is necessary to increase the size of the skeleton to reach its full maturity. After this time, density of the skeleton slowly decreases.

This thinning process continues over the course of a person's life span. In women, however, this thinning process is accelerated after menopause. If the skeleton is too small to begin with, bone has been lost at a faster rate than normal because of illness, drugs such as PREDNISONE and thyroid hormone, or alcohol use, bone damage can ensue.

SYMPTOMS

No symptoms are noted until the bone has become so weak that a BONE FRACTURE occurs even after a trivial insult. The vertebrae in the spine can be slowly compressed in height leading to rounding of the upper back.

DIAGNOSIS

The diagnosis is made accidentally in many cases when a routine X ray (RADIOGRAPHY) is taken for other purposes. Bone density measurements (BONE MINERAL DENSITY testing) can accomplish this objective, and by repeating them, the rate of bone loss over time can be determined.

COMPLICATIONS

Complications include BONE FRACTURES, especially hip fractures, and postural changes in the body, particularly rounding of the upper spine area.

TREATMENT

SELF TREATMENT:

(See Prevention below.)

MEDICAL TREATMENT:

For small-sized women who are postmenopausal and who have not had estrogen replacement therapy, constant intake of calcium over a lifetime is stressed. In addition, a source of vitamin D should be provided either in milk or in a daily multivitamin preparation that contains 100 percent of the adult requirement for vitamin D. Estrogen replacement therapy is recommended for postmenopausal women if there are no contraindications to its use.

If osteoporosis has been shown and particularly if BONE FRACTURES have occurred, medications are available that may retard further thinning of the bone and possibly increase the amount of bone in the skeleton. These medications include

- Calcitonin
- Etidronate
- Alendronate

SURGICAL TREATMENT:

No treatment is indicated except for treatment if a BONE FRACTURE should occur.

PREVENTION

Prevention of the complications of osteoporosis is possible. All individuals should maintain a lifestyle that encourages exercise and adequate intake of calcium and vitamin D. Estrogen replacement for select postmenopausal women completes the usual preventive measures.

Calcium intake should be approximately 1,500 mg daily. This amount of calcium is found in a quart of milk. If a person is not able to tolerate milk and cheese, cultured yogurt, calcium-fortified orange juice and vegetables such as spinach are also good sources that do not contain lactose. Calcium can be made up by any number of commercial supplements that are available over the counter.

Regular physical activity is a plus in maintaining a strong skeleton, particularly in the early years of life. Weight-bearing exercise such as walking or weight training are useful in maintaining a healthy skeleton.

OVARIAN CANCER

Cancer of the ovaries is the deadliest of the gynecologic cancers. It accounts for approximately 14,500 deaths per year compared with only around 5,000 each for UTERINE CANCER and CERVICAL CANCER.

Unfortunately, no appropriate screening method exists for ovarian cancer, so the disease is rarely caught in the early stages.

CAUSES

The exact cause of ovarian cancer cannot be pinpointed, but risk factors for the disease include

- Advancing age (The group at highest risk is between 75 and 79 years of age.)
- Nulliparity (having never given birth to a live infant)
- Personal history of endometrial cancer, COLORECTAL CANCER, or BREAST CANCER
- Family history of ovarian cancer

There appears to be no risk associated with the use of fertility drugs.

A very small number of women (less than 0.05 percent) are at significantly increased risk because of hereditary ovarian cancer syndromes.

SYMPTOMS

Symptoms are not noticeable in the early stages of the disease. The first symptoms usually appear after the cancer is advanced. They include

- Increasing abdominal girth
- Early satiety
- Changes in bowel or bladder habits
- Pelvic pressure
- VAGINAL BLEEDING

DIAGNOSIS

The diagnostic approach to ovarian cancer involves a complete PHYSICAL EXAMINATION including pelvic examination. If an enlarged ovary is suspected, ULTRASOUND can be used to determine the size of the tumor and the rate of bloodflow to the area.

A BLOOD TEST for CA-125 may be helpful in the diagnosis of the disease in some cases, especially in postmenopausal women.

COMPLICATIONS

Untreated ovarian cancer can lead to

- Internal bleeding
- Spread of the cancer to other parts of the body
- Continued WEIGHT LOSS

TREATMENT

SELF TREATMENT:

None.

MEDICAL TREATMENT:

After surgery, chemotherapy is required. The exact regimen depends on the type of tumor and the stage.

SURGICAL TREATMENT:

The first line of treatment for ovarian cancer is surgical removal. The extent of the operation depends on the stage and size of the tumor and on whether the woman would like to preserve her reproductive capabilities. In advanced cases, total hysterectomy with complete removal of the ovaries and fallopian tubes may be necessary, but some cases may only require removal of one ovary, leaving the rest of the reproductive system intact.

PREVENTION

Although there are no specific strategies to prevent ovarian cancer, there may be some protective factors, including

- Having more than one full-term pregnancy
- Using oral contraceptives for more than five years
- Breast-feeding

In women who have a hereditary ovarian cancer syndrome, the ovaries can be removed surgically to prevent the development of the disease. Prophylactic removal of the ovaries can be performed on women at risk who do not have the hereditary syndrome if they are undergoing abdominal surgery for another reason and do not desire children in the future. This preventive approach is not appropriate for women who do not have the hereditary syndrome and are not undergoing abdominal surgery for another reason.

OVARIAN CYSTS

An ovarian cyst is an abnormal growth consisting of various cell types within normal ovarian tissue.

Ovarian cysts are common, usually asymptomatic, and benign in the vast majority of cases.

CAUSES

Although some ovarian cysts may develop from gonadotropin stimulation or fertility medications, most cysts have no specific cause.

SYMPTOMS

Although many cysts of the ovary do not produce symptoms, some symptoms produced by ovarian cysts are

- Dull or pressure-like pain in the low abdominal or pelvic region (see ABDOMINAL PAIN), which may be chronic
- Abnormal uterine bleeding including spotting and MENSTRUAL IRREGULARITIES
- Acute severe low-abdominal or pelvic pain (see ABDOMINAL PAIN) if an ovarian cyst ruptures or torsion (twisting) occurs
- Dyspareunia (painful intercourse)
- Abdominal enlargement (ABDOMINAL SWELLING) with large ovarian cysts or ascites (fluid in the abdomen)
- Gastrointestinal symptoms
- Urinary tract obstruction (rarely)

DIAGNOSIS

Ovarian cysts may be detected during a pelvic exam either incidentally or when investigating suspicious symptoms that suggest the possibility of an ovarian cyst. However, to define the characteristics of an ovarian cyst more precisely, such as its size, location, and consistency, an ULTRASOUND may be required. This can be done either abdominally or vaginally.

In rare cases, COMPUTED TOMOGRAPHY or MAGNETIC RESONANCE IMAGING is useful for defining ovarian cysts. These two procedures may be useful in people suspected of having OVARIAN CANCER or those with ovarian cysts that cannot be seen adequately by ULTRASOUND, but at present, there is no reliable imaging technique to screen for OVARIAN CANCER.

COMPLICATIONS

Complications of ovarian cysts include

- Rupture or torsion (twisting) of the cyst, which may require immediate surgery
- Internal bleeding caused by cyst rupture
- Infection (rare)
- Malignant degeneration in which cancer develops in the cyst (very rare)

TREATMENT

SELF TREATMENT:

None.

MEDICAL TREATMENT:

- Nonsteroidal anti-inflammatory drugs such as IBUPROFEN may be used for mild to moderate pain.
- Narcotics may be required in cases of severe pain.
- Oral contraceptives may reduce development of new ovarian cysts in the future.

SURGICAL TREATMENT:

Indications for surgery include

- Persistent or enlarging ovarian cyst greater than six centimeters after four to six weeks of observation
- Cysts greater than eight to ten centimeters
- Postmenopausal cysts greater than five centimeters
- Cysts that occur before menstruation starts
- Complex characteristics on ULTRASOUND or pelvic examination
- Ascites (abdominal fluid collection)

The procedure of choice is an ovarian cystectomy or OVARIAN CYST REMOVAL. Oophorectomy (removal of the entire ovary) may be required in some cases.

PREVENTION

Ovarian cyst formation may be reduced with the use of oral contraceptives. In addition, oral contraceptives reduce the risk of epithelial OVARIAN CANCER.

PANCREATIC CANCER

Only 15 percent of pancreatic tumors can be fully removed, but cessation of cigarette smoking can greatly reduce the incidence of this fourth leading cause of cancer death.

The pancreas is an organ involved in endocrine functions, such as the secretion of insulin, and exocrine functions, such as the secretion of enzymes involved in digestion. It is located underneath the stomach and liver and adjacent to the duodenum (the first section of the small intestine).

CAUSES

The cause of this cancer remains unknown. The best established risk factor for the development of this cancer is cigarette smoking. Other less common risk factors are

- A high-fat diet
- DIABETES
- Chronic PANCREATITIS, generally related to high alcohol intake
- Workers in contact with organic chemicals

SYMPTOMS

When the cancer originates in the head of the pancreas, which is the closest area to the duodenum, patients suffer from jaundice and generalized ITCHING. If, on the other hand, the tumor originates in the area of the tail of the pancreas, which is furthest from the duodenum, the tumor can grow to larger sizes before causing symptoms. This condition can result in the obstruction of bile excretion leading to the development of

- Jaundice
- Pale-colored stools (see STOOL, ABNORMAL APPEARANCE)
- Generalized ITCHING
- ABDOMINAL PAIN
- WEIGHT LOSS
- A palpable mass

Many patients with pancreatic cancer also have symptoms of cancer that has spread to other organs.

DIAGNOSIS

Cancer of the pancreas can be easily seen with COMPUTED TOMOGRAPHY or ULTRASOUND of the abdomen. The diagnosis needs to be confirmed by obtaining a BIOPSY.

COMPLICATIONS

Complications arise from the spread (metastasis) of the cancer to other organs or from the physical size of the tumor causing obstruction of the bile duct or other internal structures.

TREATMENT

SELF TREATMENT:

An overall healthy lifestyle with a well-balanced diet is essential to maintain general health during the treatment for pancreatic cancer.

MEDICAL TREATMENT:

Although treatment with chemotherapy has not been very encouraging, promising new chemotherapy agents are always being investigated.

Combinations of treatment with chemotherapy and radiation therapy may help control symptoms in some cases of advanced cancer.

SURGICAL TREATMENT:

Removal of the tumor offers the only chance for cure of this type of cancer. Unfortunately, only about 15 percent of patients can have their tumors fully removed. The rest of the patients have cancers that have grown too extensive to remove completely.

PREVENTION

The only well-established risk for the development of pancreatic cancer is cigarette smoking. Smoking cessation should, therefore, result in a decreased chance of developing this type of cancer.

PANCREATITIS

Because excessive alcohol consumption is a major cause of this condition, many cases of pancreatitis are preventable.

The pancreas aids in the digestive process by secreting various enzymes that break down nutrients directly into the intestine. The pancreas also secretes insulin into the bloodstream. Pancreatitis occurs when the pancreas is inflamed and these potent digestive enzymes leak out of the gland and self-digest tissues close to the pancreas gland.

CAUSES

The most common causes of pancreatitis are GALLSTONES and excessive alcohol intake. Passage of small GALLSTONES from the gallbladder into the ductal system of the liver may lead to blockage of the pancreatic duct, resulting in pancreatitis.

Alcohol may directly damage the pancreas in some patients. Although this type of pancreatitis is somewhat unpredictable, it usually relates to excessive and prolonged alcohol abuse (see ALCOHOLISM).

Although rare, pancreatitis may also be caused by drugs such as AZATHIOPRINE and HYDROCHLOROTHIAZIDE, toxins (scorpion stings), blunt trauma to the abdomen, and metabolic conditions (severe HYPERLIPIDEMIA, elevated blood calcium).

SYMPTOMS

Pancreatitis may be acute, without prior symptoms, or chronic, if there are repeated episodes.

The symptoms of acute pancreatitis are sudden, severe mid-ABDOMINAL PAIN, made worse with food, frequently radiating directly into the patient's back. VOMITING and FEVER are not unusual.

Chronic pancreatitis causes symptoms similar to acute pancreatitis with repeated episodes of mid-ABDOMINAL PAIN. Also, DIARRHEA with foul, greasy stools and WEIGHT LOSS. The DIARRHEA is made worse with food, especially fats. At times, insulin release may be compromised and elevated blood sugar may cause the symptoms of DIABETES.

DIAGNOSIS

A diagnosis of pancreatitis may be suspected in any case of severe or recurrent mid-ABDOMINAL PAIN. It is corroborated by BLOOD TESTS that measure levels of pancreatic enzymes, amylase, and lipase. GALLSTONES as a cause of pancreatitis need to be ruled out with a gallbladder ULTRASOUND. In complicated or protracted cases, ULTRASOUNDS or COMPUTED TOMOGRAPHY of the pancreas may be performed.

COMPLICATIONS

Persistent pain beyond four or five days raises the possibility of inflammatory cysts within the pancreas. These cysts may become infected or bleed internally. If the pancreatitis is due to GALLSTONES or extensive, the main duct of the liver may become obstructed, resulting in jaundice. Rarely, and only with severe pancreatitis, the inflammatory substance released by the damaged pancreas may cause damage to the lungs, kidneys, and coagulation system. If the pancreatitis is chronic, some patients may develop chronic DIARRHEA, WEIGHT LOSS, and even DIABETES.

TREATMENT

SELF TREATMENT:

Patients with pancreatitis not due to GALLSTONES or a specific drug should avoid alcohol. Patients with chronic pancreatitis may benefit from less fat in the diet.

MEDICAL TREATMENT:

No direct medical therapy has been proved to be of obvious benefit. Patients with severe symptoms should be monitored in the hospital, and fasting or suctioning gastric secretions with a tube and introducing intravenous fluids and antibiotics may limit the course of pancreatitis.

SURGICAL TREATMENT:

If a GALLSTONE is blocking the common bile duct, removal of the stone may be attempted with ENDOSCOPY or surgery at an appropriate time (see GALLBLADDER REMOVAL). Open surgery is otherwise restricted to complications of pancreatitis.

PREVENTION

Limiting alcohol use eliminates this cause of pancreatitis. A low-fat diet to minimize HYPERLIPIDEMIA is also helpful.

PARKINSON DISEASE

About 20 percent of patients who seem to have Parkinson disease actually have something different. Some of these other conditions are amenable to treatment, but most are not.

Parkinson disease, named for the 19th century English physician James Parkinson, is a degenerative disease of the central nervous system. It is sometimes called *paralysis agitans*, especially when there is no readily apparent cause.

There are other syndromes and conditions that have similar features to those of Parkinson disease, but are not precisely the same. These conditions are often refered to as *Parkinsonism* or *Parkinsonism plus* if they share some of the same aspects but are not the strictly defined disease. (See Diagnosis below.)

The part of the brain that the disease mainly affects is a structure called the *substantia nigra*, which is located deep in the area of the brain called the *brain stem*. The disease slowly destroys the nerve cells in this area of the brain and can go unnoticed for a long time; it is believed that by the time the symptoms of the disease begin to be noticeable, about 75 to 80 percent of the nerve cells in the substantia nigra have already degenerated.

The degeneration of the cells in the substantia nigra causes changes in other parts of the brain, as well, because the substantia nigra is responsible for producing a substance called *dopamine*—a neurotransmitter that is needed for the proper communication between nerve cells. The other parts of the brain begin to suffer from the deficiency of dopamine caused by the damage in the brain stem.

CAUSES

In most cases, the cause is unknown. However, some cases can be caused by

- Hereditary factors
- Brain injury from infection or carbon monoxide poisoning
- Tumors

SYMPTOMS

The symptoms of Parkinsonism are generally related to the nervous system's inability to control movement normally. Voluntary muscle movement becomes affected. Specific, characteristic symptoms include

- Tremor of the muscles while they are at rest (TREMBLING)
- Slowness of movements
- Rigidity
- Shuffling gait
- A tendency to fall

DIAGNOSIS

The diagnosis of Parkinson disease is a clinical one, based on the MEDICAL HISTORY and a thorough neurologic examination. Nonetheless, in up to 20 percent of cases, the physician may later change the diagnosis from Parkinson disease to Parkinsonism or Parkinsonism plus, based on either

- Other symptoms that develop and that do not fit the profile for true Parkinson disease
- The fact that the condition does not seem to respond to specific treatments that would have an effect in Parkinson disease

Physicians may order COMPUTED TOMOGRAPHY or MAGNETIC RESONANCE IMAGING of the brain to look for changes in the brain's anatomy.

COMPLICATIONS

Progression in severe cases can lead to MEMORY LOSS and immobility. Even before severe progression, hazardous falls can lead to injury, and the condition can precipitate associated problems such as DEPRESSION.

TREATMENT

SELF TREATMENT:

Staying active with regular exercise can help optimize functioning.

MEDICAL TREATMENT:

The major treatment strategies for Parkinson disease are directed toward supplying or increasing the amount of dopamine or dopamine-like substances in the brain. Recent basic science discoveries have resulted in some newer approaches that may prove useful.

Drugs being used include

- Deprenyl, a drug that provides some symptomatic relief and is also thought to slow down the development of the disease (It is not entirely clear yet that the disease can be slowed.)
- Carbidopa-LEVODOPA, the mainstay of symptomatic treatment at all stages of the disease
- BROMOCRIPTINE and pergolide, which mimic the effect of dopamine in the brain (These can be used early or later in the disease, alone or as adjuncts to carbidopa-LEVODOPA.)
- Trihexyphenidyl and benztropine, anticholinergic drugs that work by a different mechanism "downstream" of where dopamine works in the brain
- AMANTADINE, better known as an antiviral agent

Physical and occupational therapy are beneficial.

Treatment of associated conditions (such as DEPRESSION) or supportive services for dementia or general disability should not be neglected.

SURGICAL TREATMENT:

Several surgical options are being studied. In very advanced cases, small destructive lesions in the brain are carried out with small needles rather than with major surgery. This is effective in treating disabling tremor. Implantation of fetal tissue appears to have some promise but is still highly experimental.

PREVENTION

None.

PELVIC INFLAMMATORY DISEASE

One million women per year are treated for pelvic inflammatory disease in the United States, with 150,000 undergoing surgical procedures for complications of the disease.

Pelvic inflammatory disease (PID) is a profound infection of the fallopian tubes, ovaries, and pelvis in women who have unchecked or untreated sexually transmitted diseases such as gonorrhea or chlamydia. Typically, the infection starts in the fallopian tubes, but it can sometimes involve the ovaries. Advanced infection can be diffusely disseminated throughout the pelvis.

CAUSES

Pelvic inflammatory disease is usually caused by sexually transmitted diseases such as gonorrhea and chlamydia, although sometimes the infection occurs spontaneously in women who are not sexually active. Infection in these women occurs from the normal organisms that live in the vagina.

Risk factors for PID include

- New or multiple sex partners
- Low socioeconomic status
- Being unmarried
- A history of sexually transmitted diseases
- The lack of barrier contraceptive use
- The use of an intrauterine device (IUD)

SYMPTOMS

Typical symptoms of acute PID include

- Acute lower ABDOMINAL PAIN
- Pain on pelvic examination
- VAGINAL DISCHARGE
- FEVER higher than 100°F
- MENSTRUAL IRREGULARITIES

However, some cases of PID can be asymptomatic, and usually laboratory tests can help make the diagnosis when the symptoms are not as pronounced.

DIAGNOSIS

The diagnosis of PID is based on a thorough MEDICAL HISTORY and PHYSICAL EXAMINATION. Patients undergo a careful pelvic examination, and CULTURES of the cervix are performed. BLOOD TESTS including a complete BLOOD COUNT are also necessary to make the diagnosis, and on occasion, an ULTRASOUND may be useful. In some cases, surgery may be required to confirm the diagnosis.

COMPLICATIONS

Acute complications include diffuse pelvic infection, which if unchecked can be life threatening. As with any serious infection, if this disease is not treated quickly and aggressively, diffuse sepsis (BLOOD POISONING) may ensue and death could result. Death from acute PID, however, is rarely seen in developed countries.

There are two major long-term complications of PID, both of which impact upon future reproduction. The first is tubal factor infertility and the second is an increased risk for ectopic pregnancy. Tubal factor infertility occurs in 20 to 60 percent of women who have PID. Ectopic pregnancy tends to increase by at least 15 percent for each time a woman has had an episode of PID. Other less common complications of PID include chronic pelvic pain, pain with intercourse, and pelvic adhesions.

TREATMENT

SELF TREATMENT:

(See Prevention below.)

MEDICAL TREATMENT:

There are a variety of antibiotic regimens available for treating PID. Depending on the severity of the disease, either outpatient therapies or inpatient therapies with intravenous antibiotics might be indicated. A decision to hospitalize depends on the severity of the infection.

SURGICAL TREATMENT:

Surgical treatments, including laparoscopy (a form of ENDOSCOPY) and laparotomy (open abdominal surgery), may be indicated in women with life-threatening infection; however, most of the time, the diagnosis can be made without surgery, and medical treatment can be instituted.

PREVENTION

The key to prevention of this disease is avoidance of sexual contact with infected partners. Abstinence or monogamous relationships are safer. For those women who are sexually active, use of the male or female condom may decrease the incidence of infection significantly.

PERIODONTITIS

Unlike gingivitis, which is often the precursor to this condition, periodontitis is not reversible.

Periodontitis is a chronic inflammation of the supporting structures of the teeth that leads to the formation of pockets in the gingiva—the gum tissue—and bone loss in tooth sockets. Loosening of the teeth is a late warning sign that advanced bone loss has already occurred.

CAUSES

The primary cause of periodontitis is poor oral hygiene. The accumulation of plaque (deposits of bacteria) and calculus (the hardened form of plaque) can lead to the development of GINGIVITIS and then proceed to periodontitis. Tobacco smoking has been shown to be a factor in the development of periodontitis since this habit increases irritation of the gingival tissues. It can be definitively shown that any habit that creates chronic gingival irritation, such as smoking does, makes a person more susceptible to periodontitis.

SYMPTOMS

Periodontitis is often asymptomatic in its early stages. The loosening of teeth is usually a sign of advanced, long-standing periodontal disease. In certain instances, an acute periodontal abscess may develop as a warning sign. A periodontal abscess is a localized painful swelling of the gingiva around the tooth. Occasionally, bad breath (BREATH, BAD SMELLING) can accompany periodontitis.

DIAGNOSIS

The diagnosis of periodontal disease is made by measuring the periodontal pocket depths over time. Pockets that have increased to deeper than three millimeters must be evaluated for periodontal breakdown. Bleeding on probing is also recorded to assess the amount of inflammation present. A measurement of the plaque index is often used to determine the effectiveness of the patient's home oral efforts.

Many practitioners advocate the use of a DNA analysis to identify the microorganisms in cases of periodontitis that do not respond to conventional periodontal therapy. This allows the dental professional to prescribe an antibiotic or combination of antibiotics that are highly active against the specific microorganism.

COMPLICATIONS

The primary complication of periodontitis is loss of teeth that occurs after loss of supporting bone. Many times the early symptom, loose teeth, is a sign that the disease is already advanced.

TREATMENT

SELF TREATMENT:

A patient with a diagnosis of periodontal disease must practice greatly improved oral hygiene consisting of brushing after every meal, daily flossing, and more frequent visits to the dentist office for a thorough professional dental cleaning.

MEDICAL TREATMENT:

Periodontal disease is first treated with a procedure called *scaling and root planing*—a nonsurgical deep cleaning of the roots of the teeth. If periodontal pocketing persists after scaling and root planing, treatment could consist of surgical intervention.

SURGICAL TREATMENT:

If the patient's periodontitis does not favorably respond to conventional nonsurgical techniques, PERIODONTAL SURGERY may be required. The primary purposes of periodontal surgery are to eliminate periodontal pockets and to allow a direct view of the tooth roots to ensure that all debris has been removed.

PREVENTION

Periodontal disease can be prevented by practicing good oral hygiene, which includes brushing after every meal and flossing once daily. In addition, visits to the dentist at least twice a year for professional cleaning aid in the early detection and management of any periodontal problems. Tobacco use should be stopped.

PNEUMONIA

Pneumonia can strike previously healthy individuals, but most often, patients have an identifiable risk factor such as alcoholism, diabetes, chronic heart or lung disease, neuromuscular weakness, or HIV infection.

Pneumonia is an infection of the lower respiratory tract, particularly of the air sacs, or alveoli, at the ends of the bronchial tubes. Infected alveoli fill with pus and fluid and interfere with the delivery of inhaled oxygen to the bloodstream.

CAUSES

Pneumonia can be caused by a variety of infectious agents. Most of the time, it is caused by a virus, bacterium, or some bacterium-like organism. The most commonly responsible organisms include

- *Streptococcus pneumoniae* (pneumococcal pneumonia)
- *Mycoplasma pneumoniae*
- Viruses such as INFLUENZA

Pneumonia caused by the bacteria *Pneumocystis carinii* is rare except in patients with AIDS.

SYMPTOMS

Bacterial pneumonia causes

- FEVER
- COUGH
- Excess mucus
- BREATHING DIFFICULTY
- CHEST PAIN

The symptoms get worse over the course of hours or days until they are severe enough for the patient to seek medical attention. Viral and mycoplasmal infections tend to cause less severe illness with more aches and pains.

DIAGNOSIS

Pneumonia is generally suspected after the MEDICAL HISTORY and the PHYSICAL EXAMINATION reveal FEVER and respiratory distress. The most useful diagnostic test is the X ray (RADIOGRAPHY), which can show the poorly aerated lung tissue and the area involved. Laboratory tests include

- Tests of blood oxygen level (see BLOOD TESTS)
- BLOOD COUNT
- Possibly CULTURE of blood or mucus

In particularly difficult cases, bronchoscopy (a form of ENDOSCOPY) may be needed to establish a definitive diagnosis.

COMPLICATIONS

Severe cases on pneumonia can lead to respiratory failure requiring mechanical ventilation. Lung tissue can be damaged, causing tissue death, internal bleeding, and possibly lung collapse. Infectious agents can spread to other specific organs, such as the brain, or throughout the bloodstream (see BLOOD POISONING).

TREATMENT

SELF TREATMENT:

General measures such as bed rest and adequate fluid intake are appropriate, but medical attention is necessary.

MEDICAL TREATMENT:

Bacterial pneumonia is primarily treated with antibiotics such as ERYTHROMYCIN, CLARITHROMYCIN, and AZITHROMYCIN. Frequently, more than one antibiotic is prescribed to cover all the likely organisms before the specific one is identified; often the organism is never identified, and the broad-spectrum antibiotics are used.

Viral infections are much less easily treated. General supportive therapy may be all that can be done, but some medications can be helpful against specific viruses. These include

- AMANTADINE
- Rimantadine
- Acyclovir
- Ganciclovir

SURGICAL TREATMENT:

None.

PREVENTION

Yearly INFLUENZA vaccination is the single most effective preventive strategy. Pneumococcal vaccine offers protection from pneumonia caused by *Streptococcus pneumoniae* (pneumococcal pneumonia). These vaccines are appropriate for people at high risk, including

- Those with chronic heart, lung, or kidney disease
- Those with DIABETES
- Those older than 65

PROSTATE CANCER

Prostate cancer is the second most common cancer in men, with over 85,000 new cases each year.

Prostate cancer is a growth of tumor cells within the prostate gland in men. This growth is stimulated by androgens (male sex hormones), especially testosterone.

CAUSES

The cause of prostate cancer is unknown. Several factors associated with an increased risk of prostate cancer include

- High-fat diet
- Cirrhosis of the liver
- Occupational exposure to rubber and cadmium
- Being married
- Certain demographics (high risk in Sweden and the United States; low risk in Asia), suggesting environmental factors
- A family history of the disease

SYMPTOMS

Often there are no symptoms at the time of diagnosis. Symptoms frequently indicate advanced disease and include

- Difficulty passing urine (URINATION, PAINFUL)
- Blood in the urine
- Frequent urination (URINATION, FREQUENT)
- Back pain (BACKACHE)
- Bone pain at any site

DIAGNOSIS

Routine blood work includes a complete BLOOD COUNT, kidney and liver function tests, and tests for calcium, phosphorous, and alkaline phosphatase levels (see BLOOD TESTS). A URINALYSIS and chest X ray (RADIOGRAPHY) are also performed. An acid phosphatase and prostate-specific antigen (PSA) are BLOOD TESTS that are relatively specific markers for prostate cancer. They are also used to follow the disease course. A needle BIOPSY of any nodules found during rectal examination is used to make the diagnosis and help determine the stage of the cancer. A bone scan (see NUCLEAR MEDICINE) and COMPUTED TOMOGRAPHY of the abdomen and pelvis are needed to determine the extent of the disease.

COMPLICATIONS

Complications of prostate cancer can include

- Spread (metastasis) of the cancer into bone, which can cause pain or BONE FRACTURES
- Spinal cord compression, which can result from metastasis of the cancer to the spine and may be accompanied by weakness, NUMBNESS, INCONTINENCE, and a loss of bowel control (BOWEL CONTROL, LOSS OF)
- IMPOTENCE as a result of therapy
- ANEMIA, in advanced disease, with associated symptoms of FATIGUE, BREATHING DIFFICULTY, and pallor
- KIDNEY FAILURE from obstruction of urine outflow by the prostate

TREATMENT

SELF TREATMENT:

None.

MEDICAL TREATMENT:

Very early stage disease may be treated by observation alone. Tumors confined to the prostate can be treated with radiation therapy. Hormone therapy can be useful. Chemotherapy is only used in patients with recurrent advanced disease.

SURGICAL TREATMENT:

The disease can be treated with PROSTATE GLAND REMOVAL surgery. Removal of the testicles can also cause prostate cancer to shrink.

PREVENTION

There is no established means to prevent prostate cancer. Regular rectal examinations can detect early stage disease and improve prognosis.

PROSTATE, ENLARGED

The benign growth and enlargement of the prostate gland occurs in the majority of men older than 40.

During puberty, the prostate gland goes through a growth spurt until it becomes the mature adult size and remains at this size through most of adulthood. Then, for reasons that are not entirely understood, around the age of 45 or 50, the prostate can go through another growth spurt causing the symptoms of enlarged prostate.

CAUSES

No specific cause or risk factors have been identified for the enlargement of the prostate in older men. Aging seems to be a contributing cause, and levels of male hormones are also a factor.

SYMPTOMS

When the gland enlarges, it can interfere with or obstruct the urinary tract, causing

- Diminished urinary stream pressure
- FREQUENT URINATION during the day and night
- Incomplete bladder emptying

DIAGNOSIS

An individual's MEDICAL HISTORY and a PHYSICAL EXAMINATION are usually sufficient to make a diagnosis. Additional tests may include cystoscopy (a form of ENDOSCOPY) and urodynamic testing of bladder function.

COMPLICATIONS

Urinary retention can lead to problems such as BLADDER INFECTION.

WARNING SIGNS:

- Infrequent urination
- Urination of small volumes
- Needing to strain to pass urine
- Urine leakage (INCONTINENCE)

TREATMENT

SELF TREATMENT:

None.

MEDICAL TREATMENT:

The drug finasteride can shrink the size of the prostate gland. The drugs TERAZOSIN and DOXAZOSIN can decrease the amount of urinary obstruction and relieve some of the annoying symptoms.

SURGICAL TREATMENT:

There are several surgical options for the treatment of an enlarged prostate. All involve removing part of the gland to reduce its size (see PROSTATE GLAND REMOVAL).

- Transurethral resection of the prostate involves using a cystoscope to pass an instrument up the urethra to the gland and then removing part of the gland.
- Transurethral incision of the prostate involves using a cystoscope to cut the gland in a key location to improve urine flow.
- Simple prostatectomy is a traditional open surgical technique to remove the gland.
- Laser ablation of the prostate involves destroying part of the gland with lasers.

PREVENTION

None.

PSORIASIS

Two to three percent of the population have psoriasis, a chronic skin condition.

Psoriasis is a chronic affliction of the skin featuring red plaques with thick scales. Characteristically, it involves the scalp, elbows, knees, and sacral area of the lower back.

CAUSES

The cause is unknown, although a genetic component is likely in some patients.

SYMPTOMS

Most of the time, psoriasis causes minimal ITCHING, except when it is in the scalp and skin folds. The patient will readily recognize red inflammatory plaques with thick scale on the scalp, elbows, knees, sacral area, and other sites.

Psoriasis can involve the entire skin surface in some severe cases and often involves fingernails and toenails, causing discoloration and pitting of the nails. Although it may involve the face in some cases, most of the time the face is spared.

Another kind of psoriasis occurs after an infected throat or upper respiratory tract infection. This condition occurs with the sudden onset of crops of salmon-pink or red half-inch-wide papules and small plaques with scale all over the body, especially the torso. This is called *guttate* (meaning teardrop–like) psoriasis.

DIAGNOSIS

The clinical presentation is usually highly suggestive to a trained professional and further testing may be unnecessary. Where confirmation is needed, a skin BIOPSY can be performed for a tissue diagnosis.

COMPLICATIONS

Normal-appearing skin in a patient with psoriasis is not really normal. If the skin is scraped or cut, psoriasis may form at the site of injury.

Persons with psoriasis may also have RHEUMATOID ARTHRITIS.

In some patients, psoriasis invokes a significant amount of emotional turmoil, dependency, anger, DEPRESSION, resentment, passive-aggressive behavior, and questions of self-esteem.

TREATMENT

SELF TREATMENT:

Trauma to the skin should be avoided. The skin should be kept well lubricated with topical emollients. Mild soaps should be used, and the patient should not overbathe.

MEDICAL TREATMENT:

Many medications can be used in the treatment of psoriasis, including

- Topical steroid creams and ointments
- Topical tar preparations
- Topical vitamin D
- Topical anthralin
- Short-wave ultraviolet light
- Long-wave ultraviolet light after the oral administration of 8-methoxypsoralen (a photosensitizer)
- Oral administration of vitamin A analogues
- Oral or intramuscular METHOTREXATE
- Oral CYCLOSPORINE A, a powerful immunosuppressive agent
- Oral administration of SULFASALAZINE, an agent used for inflammatory bowel disease
- Oral administration of hydroxyurea

SURGICAL TREATMENT:

None.

PREVENTION

None.

PULMONARY EMBOLISM

Over half a million people experience pulmonary embolism each year. Early appropriate treatment makes a major difference, because untreated, pulmonary embolism can have a mortality as high as 30 percent.

When a blood clot travels into the lung, it is called a pulmonary embolism. The clot may interfere with blood flow through a portion of the lung so that oxygen from the air spaces cannot be delivered to the blood by that portion of the lung. That area of the lung may even die (infarct). Pulmonary embolism is an extremely dangerous complication of other disorders of the circulatory system.

CAUSES

Clots can come from many portions of the body because all the blood from the legs, arms, and abdominal and pelvic organs drains into the right side of the heart and is pumped into the lungs.

The most common sites for clots to form are the deep veins of the legs (especially the thigh and groin region). Less often the clot may come from the veins draining the kidneys or the larger veins leading up to the right side of the heart.

Risk factors for these clots are varied, but they usually involve

- Prolonged immobility
- Damage to veins
- Drugs or cancers that increase the clotting of the blood in general

SYMPTOMS

The most common symptom is sudden shortness of breath (BREATHING DIFFICULTY). It may be associated with

- Sweating (SWEATING, EXCESSIVE)
- COUGH
- CHEST PAIN
- Coughing up blood
- FAINTING or FAINTNESS
- Signs of a clot in the leg (THROMBOSIS)
- Fast pulse
- FEVER

Almost always, the risk factors for THROMBOSIS will be apparent, including

- Immobility such as that after surgery or a STROKE
- Vein damage from hip, knee, or pelvic surgery or trauma

- An overactive coagulation system from smoking, estrogen therapy, a genetic predisposition, or cancer

DIAGNOSIS

The presence of risk factors and compatible symptoms raises the suspicion of pulmonary embolism.

ELECTROCARDIOGRAPHY or chest X ray (RADIOGRAPHY) may provide additional clues. Measurement of oxygen level in the blood (arterial blood gas) is usually done as a next step (see BLOOD TESTS).

Other new tests of coagulation may be helpful, but usually a NUCLEAR MEDICINE scan of the lungs is required to confirm the diagnosis. If this is not definitive, an angiogram (RADIOGRAPHY) may be necessary to see the clot, or serial blood flow studies, which involve ULTRASOUND to examine the dynamics of blood in vessels, of the leg may be done to assess risk of recurrent clot formation.

COMPLICATIONS

Cyanosis, a bluish coloring of the skin associated with dangerously low oxygen levels in the blood, may be seen in more severe pulmonary emboli. Even with treatment, pulmonary embolism can lead to

- Dangerously low blood pressure
- HEART ATTACK
- Death

TREATMENT

SELF TREATMENT:

(See Prevention below.)

MEDICAL TREATMENT:

- HEPARIN is the main initial treatment. (New forms of this drug may even be more effective and safer.)
- Clot-dissolving drugs like tissue plasminogen activator (TPA), streptokinase, and urokinase may be used for more life-threatening emboli.
- Oxygen is generally given to raise blood levels.

Longer-term prevention of recurrence is accomplished with WARFARIN or HEPARIN.

SURGICAL TREATMENT:

On rare occasion, for a life-threatening massive clot to the lungs, immediate surgical removal may be attempted.

For patients who cannot be on anticoagulants like HEPARIN or for whom the medication fails to work, the large vein in the abdomen that drains the blood from both legs and the pelvis (the vena cava) may be interrupted with a filter of some type. The filter can trap subsequent clots to help prevent a life-threatening recurrence. Nowadays these filters can be placed without major surgery by special catheters threaded through the veins with X ray (RADIOGRAPHY) guidance.

PREVENTION

Special compression stockings—some with inflatable compartments to keep blood from flowing too slowly and clotting—can be placed on the legs before and after high-risk times for clots to form, such as with hip or knee surgery, or during other times of immobility, such as after a STROKE. Low-dose anticoagulants are also given at these times to decrease the chance of THROMBOSIS.

Other strategies to help prevent clots or recurrences include

- Not smoking
- Maintaining an active lifestyle
- Maintaining a healthy weight
- Rapid rehabilitation after surgery
- Frequent leg movement on long trips by car, plane, or train

RHEUMATOID ARTHRITIS

Rheumatoid arthritis is an inflammation of the membrane lining the joint; this membrane is called the *synovium*. An inflammation called *synovitis* results in thickening of the membrane and the formation of extra fluid within the joint. As a consequence, the joints, tendons, or bursas—all of which have a synovial lining—become swollen and painful and experience a reduced range of motion.

Multiple joints are usually involved in a symmetrical fashion; that is, both wrists, both thumbs, both middle fingers, and so on.

Although often associated with aging, rheumatoid arthritis can affect people of any age. Climate conditions are not important. Women have a slightly greater frequency of the disease than men.

CAUSES

No cause has been recognized for this disease, but two factors are likely contributors: 1) extrinsic or environmental factors, and 2) intrinsic or genetic factors.

Although no specific extrinsic or environmental factors have yet been recognized, viruses or toxic factors in the environment could play a role in the development of the disease. Rheumatoid arthritis did not seem to exist before the industrial era several centuries ago, implying that toxic factors due to industry may be involved. At this point, however, these are only speculations.

More knowledge is available about intrinsic factors. These are some well-studied genetic abnormalities of the immune system involving a specific part of the human genetic code. Research in this area continues, but has not yet yielded any practical treatments.

SYMPTOMS

Rheumatoid arthritis usually involves morning stiffness lasting 15 minutes or more and an associated swelling of the joints. The patient begins to feel better late in the day, but then fatigue may set in.

Not only are the joints involved, but sometimes inflammation exists in other areas such as

- The whites of the eye
- The lungs—where increased fibrous scar tissue can form
- Near the elbows—where nodules can appear
- The blood vessels

DIAGNOSIS

The diagnosis of rheumatoid arthritis is usually made by observation of the symptoms: the persistent swelling of multiple joints that does not disappear in 6 to 12 weeks. If the symptoms do disappear in that time, other conditions that may mimic rheumatoid arthritis, including LUPUS ERYTHEMATOSUS or some viral disease, may be involved.

Laboratory tests are helpful in diagnosis. BLOOD TESTS are used to search for an elevation in the sedimentation rate which reflects the inflammatory process that underlies the disease, a slight ANEMIA, and rheumatoid factor. The rheumatoid factor test is positive in about 80 percent of the patients with rheumatoid arthritis.

COMPLICATIONS

In the joints, complications include damage by destruction of the cartilage and bone that underlies the cartilage. Natural cartilage and bone tissue are replaced by the inflamed synovium. Such joints become unstable and lack sufficient motion, interfering with function. Hand function or the ability to walk normally can be impaired. In some cases these complications can be life threatening. If bone erosion takes place high in the spine, the top joint in the neck becomes unstable and pressure can be exerted against the spinal cord with serious consequences such as paralysis.

In rare instances, rheumatoid arthritis can cause blood vessel inflammation that leads to damage in organs, peripheral nerves, or the skin—sometimes leading to GANGRENE in the tips of the fingers or in the intestines. Lung disease, seen in a small number of patients, is the result of an increase in fibrous tissue that impairs the lungs' ability to oxygenate the blood.

A few patients have a decreased white blood cell count and are vulnerable to infections. Lastly, some patients develop an inflammation of the glands that produce saliva and tears. When this happens, they experience dryness of the mouth and eyes. This complication is called *Sjögren syndrome*—a problem that can also exist independently of rheumatoid arthritis.

TREATMENT

SELF TREATMENT:

The patient's response to the illness is critical. Education about the disease helps the patient develop a realistic approach to his or her own particular case. Rest periods are beneficial. Exercise is encouraged, but should be moderated to suit the degree of illness. Compliance with medication intake is important.

MEDICAL TREATMENT:

Physical therapy is important. It can be accomplished through structured programs under the care of a physical therapist, or the educated patient can maintain such a program on his or her own.

Drug treatment is geared to the amount and type of drugs needed to control the inflammation. Almost all patients benefit from nonsteroidal anti-inflammatory drugs such as IBUPROFEN and NAPROXEN. Some joints can be treated by injection of corticosteroids such as TRIAMCINOLONE directly into the joint.

Long-term therapy with medications such as METHOTREXATE, SULFASALAZINE, AZATHIOPRINE, CYCLOPHOSPHAMIDE, hydroxychloroquine, and gold salts can prevent tissue damage from accelerating.

SURGICAL TREATMENT:

Surgical treatment is reserved for two circumstances:

- The removal of inflamed synovial tissue from joints or tendons to avoid damage to these structures
- Replacement of the total joint, particularly the knee (KNEE ARTHROPLASTY) and the hip (HIP ARTHROPLASTY)

In contrast to patients with OSTEOARTHRITIS, the bone structure of patients with rheumatoid arthritis is usually weaker. As a consequence, they may have less successful results. Even so, the results can be truly dramatic in selected patients.

PREVENTION

No known preventive techniques are available.

SCLERODERMA

Initially, scleroderma was thought to involve only the skin, but it is now known to affect many internal organs as well.

Scleroderma is a relatively rare disease in which the skin becomes thickened and fibrotic from deposits of fibrous connective tissue. Besides the skin, other internal organs such as the kidneys may also be involved. Although the disease is progressive and chronic, there are sometimes periods of remission in which the skin appears perfectly normal.

CAUSES

The causes of scleroderma are unknown. In healthy individuals, a connective tissue called *collagen* is produced rapidly when a wound must be healed, but as soon as it is closed, the collagen production ceases. In scleroderma, collagen production is out of control and does not let up. The disease seems to be in the family of autoimmune disorders.

One scleroderma-like disease called *eosinophilic myalgia syndrome,* which involves muscle pains and fibrotic, thickened skin, is due to a contaminant in the synthesis of tryptophan—an amino acid.

Other possible risk factors include exposure to silica dust and hydrocarbons.

SYMPTOMS

The most noticeable symptoms involve the progressive thickening of the skin, which becomes firm and sometimes feels bound down to deeper connective tissue. Some of the telltale symptoms include

- Fingers that are very sensitive to cold, which provokes changes in skin color (see SKIN CHANGES)
- Fingers that appear tapered
- Fingers that have taut overlying skin that feels bound to lower layers of tissue
- Areas of skin that are thickened in large plaque-like areas
- Difficulty opening the mouth
- SWALLOWING DIFFICULTIES
- ITCHING
- Symptoms of KIDNEY FAILURE

DIAGNOSIS

Besides the recognition of the characteristic symptoms, there are a number of BLOOD TESTS that support the diagnosis of scleroderma such as tests for antinuclear antibody, Scl 70, and anticentromere antibody. A BIOPSY of the skin is often very helpful for making the diagnosis, because under the microscope, one can see the increased fibrotic collagen in the skin impinging upon skin appendages such as sweat glands and oil glands.

COMPLICATIONS

Complications can affect almost every body system:

- Skin ulceration and subsequent infection can result as the blood supply to the outer layers of skin become strangulated by the thick collagen deposits.
- The lungs can become fibrotic, leading to progressive BREATHING DIFFICULTY and respiratory failure.
- The membrane around the heart may become replaced by fibrotic tissue, restricting its ability to pump and leading to CONGESTIVE HEART FAILURE.
- Deposits in the gastrointestinal tract can lead to malabsorption of nutrients and INTESTINAL OBSTRUCTION.
- The kidneys can become affected, leading to severe HYPERTENSION and possibly KIDNEY FAILURE.

TREATMENT

SELF TREATMENT:

None.

MEDICAL TREATMENT:

Many therapies are often tried to treat scleroderma, including immunosuppressive agents such as AZATHIOPRINE and penicillamine. So far, however, nothing has proved to be consistently very effective.

SURGICAL TREATMENT:

None.

PREVENTION

None.

SHINGLES

Shingles can be viewed as a recurrence of chicken pox virus in adults, usually the elderly, but it affects the skin in a different way from the chicken pox of childhood.

Shingles is a skin eruption that is usually localized within one or two areas of the skin. When a shingles eruption begins in adult life, it is thought that the dormant chicken pox virus becomes active again and escapes the person's immune system, which has kept the chicken pox virus dormant for many years. Common areas of involvement are linear segments of the trunk that follow the skin lines, along the arms or legs, over a linear area of the scalp, and around the eyes or nose.

CAUSES

Shingles is caused by the dormant chicken pox virus, varicella becoming activated and escaping the person's immune surveillance.

SYMPTOMS

Often before anything is seen on the skin, the patient will experience a localized area of skin that is painful, burning, or ITCHING. This is often in a linear distribution. Then, a day or two later, small clusters of small water blisters erupt on the skin, which is usually red and inflamed. These blisters pop and leave open sores (erosions) that eventually form thick, crusty scabs. The scabs may persist for 7 to 14 days before they fall off, leaving pink or white spots in a localized linear distribution.

There may be associated burning, ITCHING, and pain throughout the course of the active eruption. This pain may persist for a long time even after the skin lesions have completely healed.

DIAGNOSIS

The PHYSICAL EXAMINATION and the telltale symptoms usually provide enough clues to make the diagnosis of shingles. The physician can confirm this diagnosis in the office with a Tzanck Smear. In this test, the physician unroofs a blister or early crust, gently scrapes the blister roof and base, makes a thick smear on a slide, and examines it under the microscope. Alternatively, the physician can make a thick smear of blister and blister base fluids on a slide and send it for direct immunofluorescence at a laboratory, which can positively identify the chicken pox virus. Or, the physician can take the same fluid for viral CULTURE; the chicken pox virus, however, is notoriously difficult to CULTURE.

COMPLICATIONS

Secondary infection of the open erosions is common. Severe pain and continuous pain after the skin eruption has abated is another frequent complication.

When the eruption involves the eye, there may be injury and scarring of the eye as a severe complication.

In patients with weakened immune systems, shingles may become a widespread systemic infection rather than just a localized infection of the skin.

TREATMENT

SELF TREATMENT:

- Aluminum acetate solution on cool, wet compresses
- Antibacterial ointment on open erosions
- Chlorpheniramine or DIPHENHYDRAMINE antihistamines for ITCHING
- ASPIRIN for pain

MEDICAL TREATMENT:

If the patient is seen early, an antiviral drug such as acyclovir or valacyclovir can inhibit the virus and shorten the course of the eruption.

SURGICAL TREATMENT:

None.

PREVENTION

A new vaccine to prevent chicken pox entirely is being offered for children, but it is not helpful for adults who have already had chicken pox.

SKIN CANCER

Most skin cancers occur on the head, neck, and hands—the sun-exposed areas of the body.

The four essential types of skin cancer are

- Melanoma, a pigmented skin tumor that is quite serious and may be life-threatening
- Basal cell carcinoma, the most common skin tumor, which is locally invasive and destructive (it destroys tissue in the immediate area), but it usually does not spread or result in death
- Squamous cell carcinoma, which is three times more rare than a basal cell carcinoma but behaves in a similar manner
- Bowen disease, a cousin of the squamous cell carcinoma but more superficial, involving only the outermost layer of the skin

The typical basal cell carcinoma is an elevated round-oval, pearl-like bump with some red coloration due to fine red blood vessels going across or into it. Sometimes several small bumps form a circle. They bleed easily and sometimes ulcerate. The squamous cell carcinoma is less well-defined, has uneven, poorly visualized borders, and may be a scaly, crusted, red elevation with a rough surface. Bowen disease usually is a red or pink plaque-like elevation with very clear borders. Basal cell carcinoma and squamous cell carcinoma tend to occur on sun-exposed sites of the skin.

CAUSES

The cause of cancer is unknown. It is thought, however, that squamous cell carcinoma and basal cell carcinoma are related to an accumulation of sunlight over a lifetime. People with light complexions have these tumors more often than people with dark complexions.

Malignant melanoma is believed to be associated with numerous severe sunburns during childhood, adolescence, or young adulthood. It, too, occurs more commonly in lightly pigmented people, especially those with blue or green eyes, freckles, and almost white skin. A tendency to develop melanoma seems to run in families.

SYMPTOMS

- Skin lesions with persistent ulceration or bleeding
- Persistent skin lesion that changes size, shape, or color (SKIN CHANGES)

DIAGNOSIS

A BIOPSY should be done on any suspicious skin lesions. When evaluating pigmented skin lesions, the physician usually looks for good and bad signs. Bad signs include

- Uneven pigmentation or coloration of the lesion
- Irregular borders
- Asymmetry
- Marked elevation
- Large size (bigger than a pencil eraser)

TREATMENT

SELF TREATMENT:

None.

MEDICAL TREATMENT:

Skin cancer requires surgical treatment.

SURGICAL TREATMENT:

All of the skin cancers described above can be treated by means of excision and removal of the tumor. Surgical removal results in a better than 90 percent cure rate for nonpigmented tumors (basal cell carcinoma, squamous cell carcinoma, and Bowen disease). Alternative methods for destroying the cancer include using liquid-nitrogen freezing (cryosurgery) or scraping with a curette and burning the tissue with electric cautery (electrodesiccation and curettage).

The treatment of melanoma depends upon the thickness of the tumor and the depth of invasion when examined with the microscope. When the tumor is thin and superficial, excision may be all that is necessary. Deeper lesions may require an examination of the lymph nodes draining the skin area and chemotherapy (see MALIGNANT MELANOMA REMOVAL).

PREVENTION

Prolonged sun exposure increases the risk of skin cancer, so limiting exposure to the sun is the best prevention, particularly for those with fair complexions. Most skin cancers occur on the head, neck, and hands, so clothing (wide-brimmed hats, long sleeves) and use of sun block with a sun protection factor of 15 offers adequate protection.

STOMACH CANCER

Although stomach cancer was the leader among cancer deaths worldwide until 1988, its incidence has decreased dramatically in the last three decades, most likely due to changes in dietary habits.

Most stomach tumors occur in the lower third of the stomach, arising from cells in the lining of the stomach. A second tumor occurs in up to 20 percent of patients. The cancer is isolated to the stomach in only about 10 percent of cases. By the time it causes symptoms and is diagnosed, the cancer has usually spread to the adjacent tissues and lymph nodes.

CAUSES

Stomach cancer is associated with consumption of smoked or salty foods. There is an increased incidence of gastric cancer in

- Smokers
- Japanese and Chilean people (possibly related to dietary habits)
- Asbestos workers
- People with lower socioeconomic status
- Patients who have undergone stomach resection for the treatment of peptic ulcer disease (see PEPTIC ULCER SURGERY), as many as three decades after the operation
- People infected with *Helicobacter pylori*, a bacteria known to cause gastritis

SYMPTOMS

Most patients have symptoms similar to those of ULCER disease, such as

- Anorexia (APPETITE, LOSS OF)
- Stomach fullness
- Abdominal discomfort worsened by some foods and improved by antacids.

Patients may also experience painless gastrointestinal bleeding with black tarry stools. Less commonly, patients may experience symptoms related to the advanced nature of their tumor, such as early satiety and WEIGHT LOSS.

DIAGNOSIS

The diagnosis of stomach cancer is most commonly made by performing a stomach ENDOSCOPY with BIOPSY of a suspicious lesion. Barium-enhanced X rays (RADIOGRAPHY) of the upper gastrointestinal tract may also lead to the discovery of the disease. COMPUTED TOMOGRAPHY of the abdomen is later performed to determine the extent of the cancer at diagnosis.

COMPLICATIONS

Complications include

- Bleeding from the tumor, leading to ANEMIA
- Rupture of the tumor, resulting in ACUTE ABDOMINAL PAIN
- Other complications in advanced cancer

TREATMENT

SELF TREATMENT:

Abstinence from tobacco and alcohol and maintenance of a well-balanced diet will help during treatment of this disease.

MEDICAL TREATMENT:

Treatment with antacids and ulcer medications such as CIMETIDINE and RANITIDINE are most helpful in the control of pain.

At present there is no role for treatment with chemotherapy in early stomach cancer, but chemotherapy may be used to treat patients with advanced cancer. Its use may result in shrinkage of up to 50 percent of stomach cancer and may result in improved control of symptoms.

SURGICAL TREATMENT:

Total gastrectomy (removal of the entire stomach) offers the best chance of cure.

PREVENTION

Abstinence from tobacco and alcohol may help decrease the chance of stomach cancer.

Screening programs for gastric cancer have been instituted in Japan where this cancer is responsible for 40 percent of cancer deaths. Screening has resulted in improved survival.

STROKE

Stroke is the second most common cause of death in the United States, ranking behind only heart disease.

More than any other organ, the brain depends on an adequate supply of oxygen. If part of the brain is deprived of oxygen, it becomes damaged or dies—this is a stroke.

CAUSES

Some of the possible causes include

- HEART VALVE DISEASE, which can lead to the formation of blood clots that can break off and flow to the brain where they block smaller arteries
- ATHEROSCLEROSIS, which can cause build-up of plaque along the walls of the arteries, potentially blocking flow because of narrowing of the artery or plaque breaking off and causing blockages farther downstream
- ARRHYTHMIAS or ATRIAL FIBRILLATION
- Polycythemia
- Weak spots in the blood vessels of the brain that rupture (ANEURYSM)
- HYPERTENSION—the single most important cause

The major risk factors for stroke are

- Age older than 60 years
- Smoking
- High blood pressure (HYPERTENSION)
- DIABETES
- ATRIAL FIBRILLATION
- Previous stroke or transient ischemic attack

SYMPTOMS

The symptoms of stroke can be very diverse. They include

- Weakness in one part of the body
- Drooping of the face
- Difficulty walking
- VISION DISTURBANCES such as double vision.
- NUMBNESS of the face or an extremity

If any of these symptoms are temporary and resolve in a matter of minutes or hours, it is a transient ischemic attack, which can be a warning sign of an impending stroke. The fact that they resolve should *not* reassure the patient into delaying medical evaluation.

DIAGNOSIS

A MEDICAL HISTORY and PHYSICAL EXAMINATION are performed. Other tests include

- COMPUTED TOMOGRAPHY of the brain
- MAGNETIC RESONANCE IMAGING of the brain
- ULTRASOUND to evaluate the blood flow
- ELECTROCARDIOGRAPHY
- BLOOD COUNT

COMPLICATIONS

A stroke is as life-threatening as a HEART ATTACK and can cause permanent neurologic damage and death.

TREATMENT

SELF TREATMENT:

None.

MEDICAL TREATMENT:

The main course of treatment is the intravenous administration of powerful blood thinners such as HEPARIN. This treatment is appropriate in only certain types of strokes; it can be harmful in others.

SURGICAL TREATMENT:

(See Prevention below.)

PREVENTION

Reducing risk factors includes

- Avoiding smoking
- Eating a diet low in fat, cholesterol, and sodium
- Maintaining a healthy weight
- Avoiding excessive alcohol intake
- Taking steps to control HYPERTENSION

After a stroke or a transient ischemic attack has occurred, therapies can reduce the risk of another. Antiplatelet drugs, such as ASPIRIN or ticlopidine, and anticoagulants, such as HEPARIN and WARFARIN can reduce the risk of blood clot.

CAROTID ENDARTECTOMY, a procedure used to open carotid arteries that have become occluded, can be helpful in a select group of medically stable patients at high risk of stroke.

TEMPOROMANDIBULAR DISORDERS

The American Dental Association estimates that as many as ten million Americans suffer from some form of temporomandibular disorder.

The complex joints that connect the mandible to the skull are the temporomandibular joints. A temporomandibular disorder (TMD) is an abnormal, incomplete, or impaired function of the temporomandibular joint. The condition was once called *temporomandibular joint syndrome (TMJ).*

CAUSES

Historically, the development of pain in the temporomandibular joint and associated muscles of mastication (chewing) has been attributed to a variety of causes such as

- Loss of back teeth
- Malocclusion
- Stress
- Parafunctional habits, such as clenching or grinding of the teeth, which may happen unconsciously.
- Trauma to the head and neck area
- Anatomic internal problems

SYMPTOMS

- Pain on opening the jaw, with or without a "clicking" or "popping" sound
- A noticeable limitation in the range of opening because of muscular spasm and pain
- Occasionally, the locking of the jaw in an open or closed position because of a dislocation of the disk

The presence of joint noise on opening or closing does not indicate that a temporomandibular disorder has developed unless the other symptoms are also present.

DIAGNOSIS

The diagnosis of temporomandibular disorders is made primarily on a clinical evaluation by an experienced practitioner who evaluates the symptoms experienced by the patient together with clinical findings of

- Joint "clicking" or "popping"
- Shift of the mandible to one side on opening
- Painful opening or closing of the jaw
- Limitation of opening

RADIOGRAPHY is often performed to evaluate the joint for any bony anatomic abnormality. If a soft-tissue abnormality is suspected, MAGNETIC RESONANCE IMAGING may be useful.

COMPLICATIONS

Pain on movement of the lower jaw is the most common complication of TMD. The articular disk may become displaced, which leads to a limited opening or, in more severe cases, "locking" of the mandible where movement is not possible for a short period.

TREATMENT

SELF TREATMENT:

Patients who have parafunctional habits would benefit from identifying the habit and consciously trying to decrease its occurrence during the waking hours. The joint should be rested. Therefore, yawns should be stifled and wide openings to eat large bites of food should be avoided. Stress reduction techniques may also be appropriate.

MEDICAL TREATMENT:

The fabrication of a temporomandibular joint appliance by a dentist will act to reposition the mandible while sleeping, therefore taking pressure away from any sore areas within the joint. The appliance also acts to stretch the muscles, which may be spasming and painful. In addition, if the pain can be attributed to muscular discomfort, physical therapy may be of great benefit. Techniques that include deep massage, exercises, and heat application can be very beneficial for this discomfort. Biofeedback may also be helpful.

SURGICAL TREATMENT:

Surgical intervention to correct a temporomandibular disorder should only be considered if all conservative techniques have failed and the patient continues to have pain. In addition, the surgeon must have information that allows him to diagnose that there truly is something deranged in the joint that can be surgically corrected. Arthroscopy (a form of ENDOSCOPY) is a closed joint procedure that has been very beneficial diagnostically as well as therapeutically.

PREVENTION

Consciously trying to avoid grinding teeth or clenching the jaw in response to stress may help head off this disorder.

TENDINITIS

Although bothersome and potentially painful, tendinitis usually responds to early recognition, rest, and anti-inflammatory medication.

Tendinitis is an inflammatory condition involving a tendon, which is the specialized soft-tissue connection from the muscle to the bone. Inflammation of the tendon and its surrounding sheath (the tendon covering that helps with smooth gliding) causes pain when a patient moves the joint or stresses the tendon.

CAUSES

- Overuse of the joint or tendon in sports or occupational activities
- Minor trauma (occasionally)
- In children, mismatch growth of bone and soft tissues that causes the bones to grow too fast, stretching the tendons

SYMPTOMS

- Usually patients will notice pain when they perform certain activities that move joints.
- The tendon may be painful with direct pressure or when the muscle movement is resisted.
- In rare instances, there is some redness or swelling over the affected tendon.

DIAGNOSIS

The diagnosis of tendinitis is generally made by a MEDICAL HISTORY of overuse or minor trauma and PHYSICAL EXAMINATION findings consistent with the condition. Direct manipulation that causes pain with resisted motion of the specific tendon or tendon group provides the clinical diagnosis.

Laboratory tests are rarely necessary unless there is a concern that there may be an infection. X rays (RADIOGRAPHY) may be useful for assessing the joint, but will not show the tendinitis.

COMPLICATIONS

There are rarely complications to tendinitis other than the continued discomfort. If there is an associated cut or puncture wound, there is a risk of infection; these injuries should be assessed by a physician.

Long-standing tendinitis in some generalized inflammatory conditions may lead to rupture of the tendon and loss of the connection between the tendon and the muscle, but this is a very rare complication.

TREATMENT

SELF TREATMENT:

- Decreased activity and rest of the joint or tendon

MEDICAL TREATMENT:

- Anti-inflammatories and analgesics such as IBUPROFEN and acetaminophen
- Splinting to rest the joint or tendon
- Physical therapy

SURGICAL TREATMENT:

There is no special surgical procedure for tendinitis. In rare circumstances, surgery may be done for infection or tendon rupture.

PREVENTION

Tendinitis frequently occurs in conjunction with overuse or minor trauma injuries that happen with sports and occupational activities. Early recognition and treatment of the problem with rest and anti-inflammatory agents will usually resolve the condition.

TESTICULAR CANCER

Testicular cancer is the most common cancer in young men aged 15 to 35, affecting 2 out of 1,000 American men in that age group. Fortunately, through advances in treatment, 90 percent are cured.

Testicular cancer is a malignancy that arises in one of the testicles, the paired male reproductive organs that produce sperm and the hormone, testosterone.

CAUSES

The cause of testicular cancer is unknown. There is a higher risk of testicular cancer, though, in men with a history of undescended testes (cryptorchidism), but the reason for this conneciton is unknown.

SYMPTOMS

Testicular cancer usually occurs as a painless swelling or firm nodule in one testicle. This may be accompanied by a dull aching in the scrotum. In about 10 percent of patients, pain in the testicle is present (TESTICLES, PAINFUL OR SWOLLEN).

In occasional patients, symptoms may result from the metastatic spread of tumor to other locations, such as the lungs (LUNG CANCER).

DIAGNOSIS

ULTRASOUND examination of the testicle may assist the physician in determining whether a mass in the scrotum is within or outside of the testicle. In patients with a mass within the testicle, testicular cancer must be ruled out. Removal of the abnormal testicle (orchiectomy) through an incision in the groin is the only accepted method of diagnosing testicular cancer.

Once the diagnosis is made, other studies are used to determine whether the cancer has spread beyond the testicle include

- BLOOD TESTS
- X rays (RADIOGRAPHY)
- COMPUTED TOMOGRAPHY

COMPLICATIONS

Metastasis of the cancer to other areas in the body is a danger with all cancers.

TREATMENT

SELF TREATMENT:

None.

MEDICAL TREATMENT:

Chemotherapy and radiation therapy are most helpful. Because of advances in therapy, 90 percent of patients can be cured of their cancer.

SURGICAL TREATMENT:

Two surgical treatments are used: orchiectomy (removal of the testicle) and retroperitoneal lymph node dissection (removal of lymph nodes in the pelvic region where testicular cancer may spread).

PREVENTION

All men between the ages of 15 and 35 can perform monthly testicular self-exams. The normal coiled, slightly tender structure (the epididymis), found at one pole of each testicle, should not be a cause for concern. Any nodule or abnormal thickening of a testicle should be evaluated by a physician.

THROMBOSIS

There is a delicate balance in the blood between too much and too little clot formation. Too little can lead to bleeding problems; too much can lead to thrombosis.

Thrombosis, or blood clotting, is an essential protective mechanism of the body to help with daily trauma. However, clots can also be problematic. The most common problem is when they form in the deep veins of the legs (called *thrombophlebitis)* and travel downstream, potentially obstructing a blood vessel in the lungs (PULMONARY EMBOLISM). Other problems include clots that form on top of cholesterol plaques in arteries (ATHEROSCLEROSIS), which can lead to HEART ATTACKS, STROKES, or GANGRENE. Clots also form in the heart, in such circumstances as ATRIAL FIBRILLATION or HEART VALVE DISEASE, and can travel downstream to obstruct a blood vessel.

CAUSES

Inappropriate clots may form because of several major risk factors, including

- Vessel damage from ATHEROSCLEROSIS, hip or knee surgery, or trauma
- A slowing of blood flow from immobility on account of OBESITY, surgery, STROKE, or prolonged travel
- Overactivity of the clotting system because of familial disorders, smoking, cancer, or estrogen therapy

SYMPTOMS

Deep vein thrombosis only causes noticeable symptoms in about half of cases (swelling and leg pain). Once a clot breaks off and obstructs a downstream vessel, it usually causes symptoms (see STROKE; HEART ATTACK; PULMONARY EMBOLISM; and GANGRENE). Sometimes clots form in an area that is more apparent, such as in HEMORRHOIDS or in VARICOSE VEINS on the surface of the leg (superficial thrombophlebitis). These are not dangerous because of their location but are more often painful and recognized as a tender lump in a vein.

DIAGNOSIS

The diagnosis is based on clues from the MEDICAL HISTORY and PHYSICAL EXAMINATION. Usually, a blood flow study such as an ULTRASOUND is done to check the veins of the leg for signs of clotting. This can be definitive and therapy can be started. If it is inconclusive, then venography (RADIOGRAPHY) is performed, injecting contrast dye into the vein to help image the clot.

COMPLICATIONS

Deep-vein thrombosis of the leg can break off and travel to the lung, causing a PULMONARY EMBOLISM. Thrombosis in an artery can cause a STROKE, HEART ATTACK, or GANGRENE.

TREATMENT

SELF TREATMENT:

Warm compresses and leg elevation may help a superficial thrombophlebitis of the leg.

MEDICAL TREATMENT:

HEPARIN is the main initial treatment. Clot-dissolving drugs like tissue plasminogen activator (TPA), and streptokinase may be used for more life-threatening thrombosis. The risk of recurrence can be decreased with WARFARIN or HEPARIN.

ASPIRIN is used for patients at risk of thrombotic STROKE or HEART ATTACK to decrease the risk of thrombosis.

SURGICAL TREATMENT:

For patients who cannot be on anticoagulants like HEPARIN or for whom the medication fails to work, the large vein in the abdomen (the vena cava) may be interrupted with a filter of some type. The filter can trap subsequent clots to help prevent a life-threatening recurrence. Nowadays these filters can be placed without major surgery by special catheters via the veins with X ray (RADIOGRAPHY) guidance.

A clot in the artery of the leg can sometimes be "fished out" with special plastic tubes (catheters).

Painful clots in HEMORRHOIDS may be removed with a scalpel.

PREVENTION

- Minimizing risk factors of immobility with early mobilization after surgery
- Special elastic or compression stockings on the legs
- Low doses of anticoagulant drugs such as ASPIRIN, HEPARIN, or WARFARIN in patients at significant risk
- Frequent leg movements on long trips to help keep the blood circulating
- Avoiding smoking
- Avoiding OBESITY

ULCER

Although ulcers can be temporarily healed by reducing gastric acid, the permanent healing of ulcers requires eradication of the bacteria *Helicobacter pylori*.

An ulcer is a sore that develops in the lining of the stomach or duodenum and visually resembles an excavated crater. The more generic term *peptic ulcer* does not indicate the ulcer's location, whereas *gastric ulcer* and *duodenal ulcer* clearly describe anatomic location and are the preferred terms.

CAUSES

At least 90 to 95 percent of duodenal ulcers and 70 percent of gastric ulcers are associated with the bacteria called *Helicobacter pylori*. Other less frequent causes of ulcers are

- ASPIRIN or nonsteroidal anti-inflammatory drugs such as IBUPROFEN
- Excessive amounts of gastric acid secreted in response to hormonal stimulation by an intra-abdominal tumor (Zollinger-Ellison syndrome)

SYMPTOMS

Localized discomfort, typically a dull ache rather than a severe pain, just below the end of the breast bone, usually occuring one to two hours after meals. The discomfort may be temporarily alleviated with food or antacids. It may occur in the middle of the night, and it is typically intermittent, with days or weeks separating episodes of distress.

DIAGNOSIS

At times, the diagnosis may be made by the physician based on typical symptoms without need for diagnostic testing. However, further tests might include

- BLOOD TESTS to detect exposure to *Helicobacter pylori*
- Gastroscopy (a form of ENDOSCOPY), allowing the physician to biopsy tissue (BIOPSY), assessing for the presence of *Helicobacter pylori*
- Barium X rays (RADIOGRAPHY) of the stomach and duodenum
- Breath tests, where expired air from a patient is collected in a small bag after the patient consumes a pudding treated with minute amounts of radioactively labeled carbon, to diagnose *Helicobacter pylori* infection quickly (This test is under development and is not yet widely available.)

COMPLICATIONS

Complications are fairly rare. Ulcers may bleed internally, at times without prior symptoms. The bleeding may be noted as black, loose stool (STOOL, ABNORMAL APPEARANCE) or, more rarely, as VOMITING of dark, "coffee-ground" material or obvious blood.

If ulcers recur chronically, the outlet of the stomach and duodenum into the small intestine may become narrowed, causing obstruction. This results in the sensation of immediate fullness after meals, episodes of VOMITING or regurgitation, and at times VOMITING of undigested food, many hours after a meal.

Ulcers may also perforate into the abdominal cavity or adjacent organs, resulting in severe, intractable ABDOMINAL PAIN and FEVER, peritonitis and even BLOOD POISONING.

TREATMENT

SELF TREATMENT:

Dietary adjustments do not have a major impact on ulcer disease. The previously held belief that milk, cream, and bland foods are beneficial has not held up to medical scrutiny. Patients should avoid foods that upset their stomach and each individual may have different food sensitivities. A regular meal schedule (avoiding long periods of not eating) should be followed, simply because food within the stomach buffers stomach acid. Coffee and tea (both caffeinated and decaffeinated) and alcohol should be avoided. Tobacco should be totally avoided.

MEDICAL TREATMENT:

Oral antacids (many available over the counter) can help alleviate symptoms.

Antibiotics to eradicate *Helicobacter pylori* include

- METRONIDAZOLE
- AMOXICILLIN
- TETRACYCLINE
- AZITHROMYCIN
- Bismuth products (these are used in combination with antibiotics to eradicate *Helicobacter pylori;* use of bismuth alone is not effective)
- Pepto-Bismol

Histamine$_2$-receptor antagonists that suppress stomach acid production include

- CIMETIDINE
- RANITIDINE
- Famotidine
- Nizatidine

Proton pump inhibitors that suppress stomach acid production include

- OMEPRAZOLE
- Lansoprazole

Other effective agents include

- SUCRALFATE
- Misoprostol

SURGICAL TREATMENT:

Surgery (PEPTIC ULCER SURGERY) is primarily reserved for the complications of ulcer and is very rarely done today for symptoms not responding to medical treatment. Surgical procedures include

- Vagotomy and pyloroplasty
- Highly selective vagotomy
- Antrectomy with Billroth I or II anastomosis

PREVENTION

No good preventive measures are available. Since this is in large part a bacterial infection, improvement in general sanitation has decreased the incidence of ulcer in underdeveloped countries. Researchers are working on possible vaccines against *Helicobacter pylori,* which may be useful in areas of the nonindustrialized world where the infection seems to start at an early age.

ULCERATIVE COLITIS

Ulcerative colitis is an inflammatory condition that causes ulceration of the inner lining of the large intestine. When only the lower part of the large intestine is involved, it is called *ulcerative proctitis;* when the entire colon is involved, it is called *ulcerative colitis.* Unlike CROHN DISEASE, it does not involve the small intestine.

Although any age group can be affected by ulcerative colitis, it tends to begin between the ages of 15 and 40.

CAUSES

As in CROHN DISEASE, the specific cause of ulcerative colitis is not known. Most recent research suggests that the body's immune system is reacting against some substance in the digestive tract that induces the body's own defenses to produce an inflammatory response. It remains quite unclear as to what this foreign substance is, though.

SYMPTOMS

- Loose, frequently bloody stools (STOOL, ABNORMAL APPEARANCE)
- Urgency to have a bowel movement
- Sense of incomplete evacuation
- Crampy ABDOMINAL PAIN
- Skin RASH or painful lumps in the skin
- Pain in the lower back or joint pain

DIAGNOSIS

In addition to a thorough PHYSICAL EXAMINATION, barium X rays (RADIOGRAPHY) of the lower bowel or sigmoidoscopy or colonoscopy (forms of ENDOSCOPY) are needed to diagnose ulcerative colitis. A BLOOD TEST to detect antineutrophilic cytoplasmic antibody is being used by researchers in an attempt to learn more about various subtypes of ulcerative colitis.

COMPLICATIONS

On rare occasion, the ulcerative colitis may become severe and not respond to medical therapy, resulting in fulminant colitis. Patients with this condition are quite ill with

- FEVER
- Intractable DIARRHEA
- RECTAL BLEEDING
- ABDOMINAL SWELLING

A few patients may develop large nonhealing sores on the skin (pyoderma gangrenosum) or inflammation of the bile ducts of the liver (sclerosing cholangitis). (see CHOLECYSTITIS AND CHOLANGITIS).

Some people with chronic ulcerative colitis have an increased risk of developing COLORECTAL CANCER. This risk is primarily restricted to those patients with involvement of the entire colon who have had the disease for more than 10 years.

TREATMENT

SELF TREATMENT:

Good nutrition is essential. Although specific foods play no role in causing ulcerative colitis, soft, bland foods may be better tolerated and cause less discomfort when the disease is active. A unique association between discontinuing smoking and flare-ups of ulcerative colitis has been noted in several studies. The general health risks of smoking, however, greatly outweigh any potential benefit.

MEDICAL TREATMENT:

Medications that can be helpful in the condition include

- SULFASALAZINE
- Mesalamine (pill and enema formulations)
- Olsalazine
- Corticosteroids, such as PREDNISONE and METHYLPREDNISOLONE
- 6-mercaptopurine
- AZATHIOPRINE

SURGICAL TREATMENT:

Surgery is usually reserved for those patients with unremitting symptoms unresponsive to medical treatment or in instances of fulminant colitis. Unlike CROHN DISEASE, where surgery is not curative, removal of the entire colon will cure ulcerative colitis (see ILEOSTOMY).

PREVENTION

Very long-term use of such medications as SULFASALAZINE or mesalamine may keep the disease in remission, preventing relapses.

UTERINE CANCER

The overall five-year survival rate for women with endometrial cancer is 73 percent.

Endometrial carcinoma, cancer of the lining of the uterus, is the fourth most common malignancy in women in the United States, behind BREAST CANCER, bowel cancer (COLORECTAL CANCER), and LUNG CANCER. Overall, about two to three percent of women will develop endometrial cancer.

CAUSES

There are several risk factors for the development of endometrial cancer including

- A history of infertility and MENSTRUAL IRREGULARITIES
- Late natural menopause
- OBESITY
- Estrogen replacement therapy without progestins
- DIABETES

SYMPTOMS

Approximately 90 percent of women with endometrial carcinoma will have VAGINAL BLEEDING as their only symptom. Fortunately, most women recognize the importance of this symptom and seek medical consultation within three months.

DIAGNOSIS

PHYSICAL EXAMINATION seldom reveals any evidence of endometrial carcinoma, although OBESITY and HYPERTENSION are commonly associated constitutional factors. Endometrial BIOPSY is the accepted first step in evaluating a woman with abnormal uterine bleeding (VAGINAL BLEEDING; MENSTRUAL IRREGULARITIES) or suspected endometrial problems.

A PAP SMEAR is an unreliable diagnostic test in the evaluation of uterine cancer, since only 30 percent to 50 percent of women with endometrial cancer will have an abnormal PAP SMEAR. (Its main role is detecting CERVICAL CANCER.)

Hysteroscopy (a form of ENDOSCOPY) and DILATION AND CURETTAGE should be reserved for situations in which an office endometrial BIOPSY cannot be performed, bleeding recurs after a negative BIOPSY, or the specimen obtained is inadequate to explain the bleeding.

Transvaginal ULTRASOUND may be a useful adjunct to endometrial BIOPSY for evaluating abnormal uterine bleeding (VAGINAL BLEEDING; MENSTRUAL IRREGULARITIES) and for selecting women for additional testing.

COMPLICATIONS

Some women, experience pelvic pressure or discomfort indicative of uterine enlargement or disease spread. Bleeding may not have occurred because of cervical stenosis (in which the cervix blocks the blood from passing out of the uterus), and may be associated with the collection of blood within the uterine cavity, and a worse prognosis.

TREATMENT

SELF TREATMENT:

None.

MEDICAL TREATMENT:

Medical therapy is secondary to surgical treatment. Postoperative radiation therapy may result in improved survival. Women with metastatic (spread) disease may benefit from hormonal therapy or chemotherapy.

SURGICAL TREATMENT:

The surgical procedure would minimally include

- Sampling of peritoneal fluid for evaluation (CYTOLOGY)
- Exploration of the abdomen and pelvis with BIOPSY or excision of any suspicious lesions
- Total HYSTERECTOMY
- Removal of both fallopian tubes and ovaries
- Sampling of lymph nodes in the pelvis and alongside the abdominal aorta

PREVENTION

Screening for endometrial cancer should currently not be undertaken because of the lack of an appropriate, cost-effective, and acceptable test that reduces mortality. Abnormal perimenopausal and postmenopausal uterine bleeding (VAGINAL BLEEDING; MENSTRUAL IRREGULARITIES) should always be taken seriously and properly investigated,

VAGINITIS

Vaginitis is an inflammation of the vagina that can cause bothersome symptoms. Vaginitis is a common problem that, although annoying, does not pose major health problems.

Vaginitis is an inflammation that can usually be treated with antibiotics or vaginal creams.

CAUSES

Vaginitis is usually a result of some infectious agent, although other irritants can cause inflammation as well. Frequent causes of vaginitis include

- *Candida* organisms (a yeast infection)
- *Trichomonas* organisms
- Bacterial vaginosis
- Lack of estrogen in postmenopausal women
- A foreign body, such as a lost tampon in the vagina

SYMPTOMS

The symptoms of vaginitis include

- Vaginal ITCHING and burning
- VAGINAL DISCHARGE
- Foul odor

DIAGNOSIS

The symptoms themselves can usually point to the diagnosis of vaginitis. Important information for the physician to know in the patient's MEDICAL HISTORY includes

- The character of the VAGINAL DISCHARGE, especially whether it is itchy or odorous
- Any new sexual partners, since some causes of vaginitis are sexually transmitted
- Use of douches, since they can cause a chemical reaction
- Recent treatment with antibiotics
- Any new medications, such as oral contraceptives
- Any medical problems, such as DIABETES

To diagnose the cause of vaginitis, a PHYSICAL EXAMINATION of the vulva, or entrance to the vagina, and the vagina will be done. A sample of the VAGINAL DISCHARGE is obtained and examined under a microscope.

If the cause of the vaginitis is sexually transmitted, CULTURES for CHLAMYDIA and gonorrhea and a BLOOD TEST for syphilis and human immunodeficiency virus (HIV) are sometimes warranted.

COMPLICATIONS

Infections need to be treated promptly to avoid progression. Unattended vaginitis could potentially progress to wider infection, PELVIC INFLAMMATORY DISEASE, and infertility.

TREATMENT

SELF TREATMENT:

If the patient has had documented yeast infections in the past and experiences the classic recurrent symptoms (ITCHING and thick white, odorous VAGINAL DISCHARGE), self treatment with over-the-counter clotrimazole may be appropriate.

MEDICAL TREATMENT:

- For vaginitis caused by candidal organisms, treatment is usually a vaginal cream or suppository. An oral medication (FLUCONAZOLE) is also available.
- For a trichomonal vaginitis, an oral antibiotic (METRONIDAZOLE) is prescribed. It is important that both sexual partners receive treatment simultaneously, or the infection can recur.
- For bacterial vaginosis, treatment is usually an oral antibiotic (METRONIDAZOLE) or vaginal cream. Sometimes this infection can be sexually transmitted and the partner or partners needs treatment also.

SURGICAL TREATMENT:

None.

PREVENTION

Strategies to help prevention of vaginitis include

- Taking showers rather than baths
- Wearing cotton panties or pantyhose with a cotton crotch rather than nylon
- Wiping from front to back after urination or bowel movements
- Avoiding frequent douching
- Limiting sweets and increasing yogurt intake
- Maintaining a healthy body weight
- Limiting the number of sexual partners and employing safe-sex techniques

VARICOSE VEINS

Varicose veins are dilated curving veins usually on the legs. Veins return blood to the heart and lungs to be reoxygenated and then to be recirculated to the rest of the body via the arteries.

The pressure in veins is much lower than in the arteries, so blood's return trip via the veins is more difficult, especially since it's uphill most of the time from the legs when standing or sitting. The veins normally have one-way valves that help blood flow back toward the heart, but in varicose veins, the valves often fail, allowing blood to pool and contributing to the swelling problem.

Varicose veins are not dangerous and in most cases improve with self-treatment.

CAUSES

Although hereditary factors play a major role for many people, other causes include

- Prolonged standing or sitting
- OBESITY
- Lack of exercise
- Age
- Pregnancy
- Anything that causes long-term obstructions of the veins

Women are more often affected than men.

SYMPTOMS

The symptoms are

- Swollen, knotted, visible veins
- Swelling in the legs (ANKLE SWELLING)
- In long-standing cases, SKIN CHANGES such as discoloration, ITCHING, skin ulcers, and other skin breakdown problems

DIAGNOSIS

The diagnosis is apparent from seeing the veins on the legs. Blood flow studies (ULTRASOUND) may be used to document problems in the deeper veins under the muscles of the legs that are not visible on the surface.

COMPLICATIONS

- The skin breakdown (SKIN CHANGES) can lead to infections and ulceration.
- A clot may form in the vein and cause a tender swollen lump (a superficial thrombophlebitis). This is not dangerous.

TREATMENT

SELF TREATMENT:

- Tight belts or stockings that constrict the legs at the top should be avoided; they can make the obstruction to the vein flow worse.
- Elastic stockings specifically made for leg swelling should be worn. Care should be taken if the skin becomes dry or begins to break down.
- Elevation of the legs whenever possible during the day and at night helps, especially if the legs are raised a few inches above the level of the heart.

MEDICAL TREATMENT:

Diuretics such as HYDROCHLOROTHIAZIDE may be used if necessary for severe swelling, but the self-treatment measures are preferred.

SURGICAL TREATMENT:

Sclerotherapy (injection of chemicals that shrink the vein) and surgical removal (VARICOSE VEIN REMOVAL) are reserved for the most bothersome cases.

PREVENTION

Persons with varicose veins should avoid OBESITY and prolonged standing or sitting, and should adhere to a regimen of regular exercise.

TESTS & SURGERIES

ABORTION

Abortions can be performed for a number of reasons, such as because the woman's physical or emotional health is in danger or because the woman chooses to terminate the pregnancy.

An abortion is a procedure to effect the expulsion or removal of a developing fetus from a woman's uterus before the time when the fetus is expected to live on its own outside the uterus.

For abortions in the first trimester, the procedure can be done as an outpatient, usually in a doctor's office or a clinic. Later abortions often require a hospital setting.

PREOPERATIVE PREPARATION

A BLOOD TEST or urine test is performed to confirm the existence of the pregnancy.

Before any abortion procedure, the woman should explore her feelings regarding the pregnancy. Sometimes women are very sure in their decisions, other times they need help from friends, family, or independent counselors to help them arrive at the right decision for them regarding their pregnancy. Although decisions are often difficult, making the decision earlier in the pregnancy increases the safety and the ease of the procedure.

ANESTHESIA

Usually, a local anesthetic is used. The patient may also receive intravenous medications for pain relief during the procedure. A sedative may be added for abortions in the second trimester, because the procedure is more involved and can take longer. General anesthesia is rarely necessary since the procedure is generally short and general anesthesia increases the risk of complications.

PROCEDURE

In the first trimester, abortions are performed by suction curettage and take about 15 minutes. For this procedure

- The woman assumes the normal position for a gynecologic examination with her feet in stirrups.
- The cervix is cleansed with an antiseptic solution and then a local anesthetic is administered.
- The cervix is grasped with a holder and dilators gradually enlarge the opening of the womb.
- A curette is inserted into the uterus.
- The curette is attached to suction or a vacuum pump and the pregnancy is suctioned out.

In the second trimester, a suction curettage procedure called a dilation and evacuation, or D & E, may still be performed. In this procedure, the cervix is pretreated with Laminaria to dilate the cervix. (Laminaria are thin rods which absorb moisture from the body and swell, causing a gradual dilation of the uterine cervix.) Instruments other than just a suction curette are necessary, and the abortion procedure is usually longer in duration.

For later abortions, the pregnancy may be terminated by inducing labor with drugs. These medications can be administered vaginally, into the uterine cavity, or through an intravenous line. This procedure to terminate a pregnancy is usually performed in a hospital setting. Depending upon the medication used, labor may take as few as 12 hours to more than 24 hours to terminate the pregnancy. Because the placenta may not deliver intact, forceps or a dilation and curettage may be necessary to ensure that the uterus is empty.

HOSPITAL RECOVERY

In later-term induced-labor abortions, an overnight stay may be required.

AT-HOME RECOVERY

Antibiotics may be prescribed to decrease the risk of postoperative infection.

The woman should have a follow-up examination in two to six weeks. A normal menstrual period can be expected four to six weeks after a pregnancy termination.

COMPLICATIONS AND RISKS

After an abortion, uterine cramps and bleeding much like a period are to be expected. However, infection and excessive bleeding are serious complications.

WARNING SIGNS:

- Heavy VAGINAL BLEEDING, soaking a pad in a half hour
- FEVER higher than 101°F
- Foul smelling VAGINAL DISCHARGE
- Severe ABDOMINAL PAIN

ALLERGY TESTING

Allergy testing is used by a wide variety of doctors including allergists, otolaryngologists (ear, nose, and throat specialists), and dermatologists.

When patients have symptoms that may be a result of an allergic reaction, allergy testing can help identify the item that triggered the reaction (the item is called an *allergen*). However, because people can have positive reactions to allergy tests but not experience noticeable symptoms when exposed to the substance, the results of such testing must be interpreted carefully.

Allergy tests are most helpful for evaluating symptoms of hay fever. They play a smaller role in investigating causes of reactions such as ASTHMA and hives. Their use in evaluating food allergies is more uncertain, and they are probably unwarranted in the general evaluation of nonspecific symptoms such as FATIGUE.

There are a number of ways to test for allergies. The most certain way is to challenge and rechallenge a person to the item to which they are supposed to be allergic. That is, expose the person, look for a reaction, and repeat the same procedure again later to be certain. However, given the time and confounding factors, this approach is not always practical. The two most common methods for allergy testing are

- Skin tests in which the skin's reaction to a potential allergen is monitored
- Radioallergosorbent tests (RAST) or other BLOOD TESTS in which the laboratory searches for specific immunologic substances in the blood

PREPARATION

Because they modify the body's reaction to allergens, antihistamines and PREDNISONE should be discontinued before various types of skin tests.

ANESTHESIA

None.

PROCEDURE

For skin testing

- A drop of purified allergen is placed on the skin.
- A small prick with a needle is made at the site to allow the allergen to come in contact with the immune system.

- If a hive forms within minutes, the test is positive and complete, but if the result is negative or unclear, a small amount of the allergen may be injected directly into the skin with a needle to be sure the test is not positive.

When skin testing some types of allergens, especially metals such as nickel, the material may be taped against the skin for a few days rather than injected.

For RAST and other BLOOD TESTS, blood is drawn from a vein and analyzed in special laboratories for specific antibodies to certain allergens. This method is particularly useful when investigating certain rare occupational exposures that cause lung symptoms and for fungal reactions. RAST is easy and widely available, but it is expensive and fraught with false-positive results.

HOSPITAL RECOVERY

Patients are observed for at least 15 minutes after skin testing so that any generalized reaction (see below) can be treated promptly.

AT-HOME RECOVERY

None.

COMPLICATIONS AND RISKS

In rare cases, skin tests may cause more than a local reaction on the skin. Examples of more drastic reactions include

- Wheezing
- Low blood pressure
- Diffuse hives (RASH)
- BREATHING DIFFICULTY or SWALLOWING DIFFICULTIES from swelling of the throat

Severe local reactions can be treated with topical HYDROCORTISONE.

For RAST, the main "risks" are incurring the expense of further testing due to false-positive results.

AMPUTATION

Amputation is usually a procedure of last resort. Although often life-saving, it can be very traumatic for the patient and his or her family.

An amputation is an operation on a damaged or nonfunctional extremity that involves removal of the limb or portion of the limb. The need for an amputation may arise in cases of traumatic damage, infection, or loss of blood supply due to vascular problems (GANGRENE). Amputations in the upper extremity are usually done by an orthopedic surgeon; amputations in the legs may be done by an orthopedic, general, or vascular surgeon.

ALTERNATIVE TREATMENTS

Amputation procedures are generally done after all nonsurgical treatments have been attempted; some new, minimally invasive procedures such as ANGIOPLASTY, which is done to improve blood flow to limbs suffering from an inadequate blood supply, may help save the limb or change the level at which amputation must be done.

PREOPERATIVE PREPARATION

Amputations are generally done on an urgent basis for patients who are already ill with other underlying problems; laboratory tests and other diagnostic tests, such as ELECTROCARDIOGRAPHY, chest X-ray (RADIOGRAPHY), and BLOOD TESTS will be done to evaluate general health. Other tests may be done to maximize treatment of underlying or associated conditions before surgery.

Overnight fasting is required with general anesthesia.

ANESTHESIA

Although both general anesthesia and regional anesthesia (nerve blocks of arm or leg) may be used, the associated medical conditions of the patient may dictate the anesthesia.

PROCEDURE

The specific amputation type is dictated by the location of the part being removed. Removal of digits on the hand or feet require only small incisions; amputation at various levels of the arm and leg are carefully planned to remove nonviable muscle, bone, and soft tissue at a level where healing will take place. During the operation, blood vessels are tied off and bone is sawed through if necessary.

For appropriate patients, the level is planned to allow fitting with a prosthetic limb that may provide for some levels of function.

HOSPITAL RECOVERY

The length of the hospital stay may be dictated by the underlying medical condition that necessitated the amputation. Medical treatment in the hosptial may be required for associated conditions, even though treatment of the amputation could continue on an outpatient basis.

Because of infections or infected limbs, patients may require intravenous antibiotic treatment either by vein or through a more permanent catheter implanted under the skin. Initially, intravenous or intramuscular pain medicine such as MORPHINE or MEPERIDINE may be required; many patients may be able to switch to oral medication such as an ACETAMINOPHEN AND CODEINE COMBINATION after several days.

AT-HOME RECOVERY

Rehabilitation will continue at home. This is generally the stage at which prosthetic (artificial limb) fitting takes place, and physical therapy is directed towards improved residual limb usage. Oral pain medication such as an ACETAMINOPHEN AND CODEINE COMBINATION may be needed for several weeks or months after the amputation.

If there was an underlying condition, such as ATHEROSCLEROSIS or DIABETES, that caused the limb problem, these conditions must be carefully monitored to decrease the risk of further problems.

COMPLICATIONS AND RISKS

As with any surgery, there is a risk of surgical wound infection. Patients in whom an underlying infection made the amputation necessary should be especially aware of potential problems; symptoms include increased redness, swelling, pain, and drainage from the surgery site. Patients may note FEVER, chills, or sweats if they have an infection.

After recovery, those patients who have been fitted with a prosthesis should monitor skin conditions at the amputation, as skin breakdown may point out a prosthetic fit problem.

ANEURYSM, REMOVAL OF

Aneurysms can be life threatening, and if they rupture, the results are often catastrophic. Prompt repair of unstable aneurysms is crucial.

An ANEURYSM is a bulging out or ballooning of a blood vessel. There are two main dangers associated with an ANEURYSM: 1) Within the ballooned out area, clots can form; and 2) the weakness of the wall can cause the vessel to rupture.

ANEURYSMS most often develop in the aorta, the body's largest blood vessel, in the chest portion leading from the heart or in the abdominal portion before the aorta divides into branches that provide blood to the legs. When an aortic ANEURYSM is threatening to rupture and the risk of surgery is warranted, a thoracic or vascular surgeon will repair or remove it. In some cases an interventional radiologist may also be able to repair an ANEURYSM using special devices passed through the blood vessels.

Cerebral ANEURYSMS of the brain blood vessels are usually repaired by a neurosurgeon. An ANEURYSM can also occur in the heart muscle and require repair.

ALTERNATIVE TREATMENTS

Not all ANEURYSMS need to be operated on. If the ANEURYSM is relatively small and not causing any problems, it can be monitored for expansion over a period of years using ULTRASOUND. Some blood pressure–lowering medicines, such as METOPROLOL and PROPRANOLOL, can help slow or stabilize progressive expansion.

PREOPERATIVE PREPARATION

COMPUTED TOMOGRAPHY, ULTRASOUND, and angiograms (RADIOGRAPHY) are all used to define the extent and size of the ANEURYSM. Because the surgery is more stressful to the heart than most other operations and most people with ANEURYSMS have some degree of heart disease, special tests of the heart, such as a CARDIAC STRESS TEST, are also often performed.

Overnight fasting is required with general anesthesia.

ANESTHESIA

General anesthesia is necessary, and a heart-lung machine may also be needed.

Newer techniques that involve placement of special devices called *stents* inside an ANEURYSM can be performed under local anesthesia.

PROCEDURE

For aortic ANEURYSMS in the chest or abdomen

- An incision is made in the chest or abdomen along the midline.
- The ANEURYSM is located and the vessel is clamped off above and below the ANEURYSM site.
- The diseased section is removed and replaced with a synthetic pipe that is sized and sewn into place.
- The incision is then closed with sutures.

For some patients, a new technique may be possible using special grafts (stents) that can be placed inside the ANEURYSM and secured into place using plastic tubes (catheters) guided through the blood vessels and manipulated with the help of X rays (RADIOGRAPHY).

HOSPITAL RECOVERY

- The hospital stay is usually about seven to ten days, often with the first day in the intensive care unit.
- If the chest cavity was opened for surgery, chest tubes (drainage tubes that run under the rib cage to collection containers) are usually needed.
- A catheter in the bladder to drain urine for a day or two is common.

AT-HOME RECOVERY

- Activity can be gradually increased with full recovery in about four to six weeks.
- Synthetic grafts can get infected, so prophylactic antibiotics may be recommended before any subsequent procedures.

COMPLICATIONS AND RISKS

- Excessive bleeding
- Loss of blood flow to nearby branch arteries leading to damage of the areas they feed—for example, the spinal nerves (causing paralysis), the intestines (causing GANGRENE of the bowel), kidneys (causing kidney damage or KIDNEY FAILURE)
- Infection of the wound or graft

TESTS & SURGERIES

ANGIOPLASTY

Angioplasty, a relatively new technique in the treatment of vascular diseases, is now one of the most frequently performed cardiovascular procedures in the United States.

Angioplasty is used to shape the inside of a blood vessel to improve blood flow past blockages (see ATHEROSCLEROSIS). Various techniques to open up blockages in arteries using devices on long plastic tubes have been developed, but the most commonly used device is a narrow, inflatable, one- to two-inch-long balloon attached to a long plastic tube called a catheter.

The long plastic tube is usually inserted through a hole punctured through the skin into the arteries in the groin, and is then passed up to the target vessel until the balloon is placed alongside a blockage. It is then inflated to force an increase in the interior space of the vessel.

Besides balloons, other related devices include rotating small blades, drill-like devices, and lasers. The target vessels are usually partially occluded arteries to the heart (causing ANGINA) or large vessels in the leg (causing claudication—pain in the legs during activity that is relieved by rest).

ALTERNATIVE TREATMENTS

Angioplasty is best used when surgery (such as CORONARY ARTERY BYPASS GRAFT SURGERY) is otherwise necessary and when medications are not enough. Medications for ANGINA (one indication for angioplasty) include NITROGLYCERIN, calcium channel blockers (DILTIAZEM), and beta-blockers (METOPROLOL, ATENOLOL). Medications for claudication usually provide a modest benefit.

PREOPERATIVE PREPARATION

A CARDIAC STRESS TEST and angiogram X ray (RADIOGRAPHY) are helpful in selecting the right patients for angioplasty and planning the procedure.

ANESTHESIA

Local anesthesia is all that is needed, but a surgical team and general anesthesia are usually available on standby.

PROCEDURE

- The balloon catheter is inserted into an artery in the thigh or occasionally in the upper arm.

- The catheter is guided with the help of RADIOGRAPHY to the site of the blockage.
- The balloon is inflated and deflated repeatedly to expand the opening of the blocked artery.
- X rays (RADIOGRAPHY), pressure readings, and ULTRASOUND images may be used to evaluate the vessel before and after the procedure.
- The catheter is withdrawn and the opening to the entry artery compressed or repaired.

HOSPITAL RECOVERY

- One to two days in the hospital may be required to allow the insertion site to start healing safely.
- The heart is monitored closely for the first 24 hours with continuous ELECTROCARDIOGRAPHY.
- Intravenous blood thinners, such as HEPARIN and ASPIRIN, may be used to reduce the chance of a clot forming where the lining of the artery is disrupted.

AT-HOME RECOVERY

For the first week or two, patients should generally avoid vigorous exercise involving bending at the insertion site.

COMPLICATIONS AND RISKS

Bleeding at the insertion site after the catheter is removed is the most common complication. The bleeding can be under the skin and may show up as an enlarging lump or as increasing pain in the area.

More serious but rare complications include

- Allergic reactions to the X ray contrast material, or dye, that is used to make the artery more visible during the procedure (see RADIOGRAPHY)
- Tearing, perforating, or completely occluding the target artery, possibly leading to HEART ATTACK and even death (very rare)

A few percent of patients may need emergency bypass surgery to help deal with these complications. (See CORONARY ARTERY BYPASS GRAFT SURGERY.)

BIOPSY

Because biopsy is usually the definitive test for certain diseases and because many different tests can be run on a biopsy sample, the test is extremely helpful in diagnosis.

A biopsy is a procedure in which a small sample of tissue is taken from a particular part of the body so that it can be prepared and examined under a microscope. More advanced tests may also be done on this tissue sample, such as CULTURES for viruses or other germs. Often biopsies are used to check for cancer, but many other uses exist.

PREPARATION

Most biopsies don't require any preparation. If a sample is to be taken from the linings of the lungs or the gastrointestinal tract, fasting can minimize any risk of vomiting.

ANESTHESIA

Almost all biopsies are done with local anesthesia. Rarely, general anesthesia might be necessary if the biopsy is to be taken from a difficult area (for example, a brain biopsy).

PROCEDURE

The exact procedure varies with each biopsy location. Special scopes through which small samples can be removed are commonly used for biopsies of the gastrointestinal tract and lung (see ENDOSCOPY). Special catheters passed through the veins or arteries can be used in a biopsy of the heart (CARDIAC CATHETERIZATION). COMPUTED TOMOGRAPHY or ULTRASOUND can guide certain biopsies of internal organs using special needles passed through the skin directly to the organ.

RECOVERY

In most cases, biopsies are performed on an outpatient basis, and patients are released the same day. Observation can range from a few minutes for skin biopsy to hours or overnight for biopsy of an internal organ.

COMPLICATIONS AND RISKS

A biopsy is a relatively simple and safe procedure. Bleeding or infection are always a possibility but are rare. Some organs can be perforated during a biopsy and may require surgery; this complication is also rare.

BLADDER REMOVAL

Surgical removal of the bladder involves removing the bladder and creating a so-called urinary diversion, in which a segment of bowel is used to connect the ureters to a stoma—an opening to the outside of the abdomen. This urinary diversion allows urine to drain out into a collecting pouch on the outside of the body.

The surgery is performed by a urologist or general surgeon in a hospital setting.

Surgical removal of the bladder is usually performed only in the case of invasive bladder cancer.

ALTERNATIVE TREATMENTS

In some patients, a combination of radiation therapy and chemotherapy can replace surgery.

PREOPERATIVE PREPARATION

Cystoscopy (a form of ENDOSCOPY) and a BIOPSY of the tumor are usually necessary to confirm the diagnosis and determine the extent of the cancer.

The surgery requires a complete bowel preparation involving antibiotics and enemas to clean out the colon and decrease the chance of infection after surgery.

Overnight fasting is required with general anesthesia.

ANESTHESIA

General anesthesia.

PROCEDURE

- An incision is made in the lower portion of the abdomen over the bladder.
- The ureters from the kidneys to the bladder are identified and cut.
- The bladder is removed. Frequently, the prostate (in men) or uterus and ovaries (in women) are removed during this same procedure, as well.
- A conduit is fashioned from a section of the small intestine.
- The conduit is connected to the ureters on one end and the skin on the other.

- A stoma, or opening in the skin, is created for the collecting device, which can be fitted tightly with an appliance to hold it in place.
- The incision is closed with sutures.

HOSPITAL RECOVERY

- The hospital stay is usually about 10 to 14 days, often with the first day spent in the intensive care unit.
- An intravenous line remains in place for about seven days until bowel function returns.

AT-HOME RECOVERY

- Strenuous activity must be restricted for about six weeks.
- A nurse may visit the patient in the home or while he or she is still in the hospital to teach the patient self-care techniques for the stoma site.
- Minor postoperative pain may require oral pain medication such as ACETAMINOPHEN AND CODEINE COMBINATION.

COMPLICATIONS AND RISKS

- Delayed return of bowel function, signaled by an inability to eat and keep down food
- Leakage from one of the urine connections, signaled by FEVER and excessive drainage from the surgical wound

BLOOD COUNT

Red blood cells carry oxygen to all parts of the body using the protein hemoglobin. White blood cells help fight infections. Smaller bits of tissue called platelets help seal leaks in blood vessels and aid in the formation of blood clots. Blood counts are the measurement of all three of these items in the blood.

One of the most common laboratory blood tests, a blood count can help make the diagnosis of anemia or assess the body's response to an infection or its ability to fight one.

Preparation

No special preparation is required for a blood count. Fasting, for example, is not required for a blood count like it is for some other BLOOD TESTS.

Procedure

Blood is usually drawn from a vein in the middle of the arm, but other sites can be used in special circumstances. The procedure is usually as follows:

- A tourniquet is applied to the upper arm for a short period to enlarge the vein, making it easier to see and get blood from.
- The vein site is swabbed with alcohol or iodine to prevent infection.
- A sterile needle punctures the vein (a procedure called *venipuncture*) and suction draws out the required amount of blood.
- A dressing (bandage) is then applied. It can usually be removed in a few hours.

Complications and Risks

A bruise at the site of the venipuncture is the most common complication. An infection at the site is possible but extremely rare.

BLOOD PRESSURE TEST

Most people can learn to take their own blood pressure measurements, but it is necessary to do it carefully to get the most accurate results.

Blood pressure is one of the "vital signs." Chronic high blood pressure (HYPERTENSION) can contribute to many diseases, and because it causes no symptoms, monitoring it with this test is crucial.

Preparation

The patient should be sitting quietly for a few minutes, comfortably resting the arm to be measured at chest height.

Procedure

- A blood pressure cuff is wrapped around the upper arm.
- The pressure is raised in the cuff with a pump until it is well above the patient's blood pressure, so that no flow is getting under the cuff.
- Very slowly, the pressure is released, and using a stethoscope, the person performing the test listens for the sound of blood flowing through the artery.
- When the pulse can be heard, the pressure of the cuff is recorded. This first number (the *systolic* pressure) is the peak pressure of the blood with each heartbeat.
- The pressure in the cuff continues to go down until the sound of the pulse momentarily disappears again, and the pressure of the cuff is recorded again. This is the second number (the *diastolic* pressure). It represents the lowest the blood pressure gets between heartbeats.
- The two measurements are normally written together: for example, *120/80*.

Recovery

The only recovery consists of waiting the minute or two for the blood flow in the arm to return to normal. (It is not uncommon for the lower arm and hand to have the sensation of "pins and needles" for a few moments.)

Complications and Risks

None.

BLOOD TESTS

Much can be learned from the chemistry of the blood, and there are many different laboratory tests that can be performed on a single sample. With the exception of different amounts of blood needed for different tests, the procedure for blood tests varies little as far as the patient is concerned.

Common tests include liver and kidney function, blood mineral balance, blood cholesterol levels, and blood sugar levels.

Screening tests for blood cholesterol and blood sugar levels are often performed on certain age groups and populations identified as being at risk for certain diseases (such as ATHEROSCLEROSIS or DIABETES) and are a reasonable and effective way to prevent some health problems.

Blood tests can be performed for many reasons. They can be used to screen for disease in apparently healthy people, to help make a diagnosis, or to monitor the progress of a disease or treatment.

Preparation

Fasting for three or more hours may be necessary for some specific blood tests. Ask your doctor beforehand.

Procedure

Blood is usually drawn from a vein in the middle of the arm, but other sites can be used in special circumstances. The procedure is usually as follows:

- A tourniquet is applied to the upper arm for a short period to enlarge the vein, making it easier to see and get blood from.
- The vein site is swabbed with alcohol or iodine to prevent infection.
- A sterile needle punctures the vein (a procedure called *venipuncture*) and suction draws out the required amount of blood.
- A dressing (bandage) is then applied. It can usually be removed in a few hours.

Complications and Risks

A bruise at the site is the most common complication. An infection at the site is possible but extremely rare.

False alarm test results can also be considered a common "complication" of using blood tests to screen healthy people. Approximately 50 percent of healthy people who have a 20-item blood panel performed will have at least one false-positive test result.

BONE MINERAL DENSITY

Most patients don't need this test since almost all women should be taking steps to prevent osteoporosis anyway, and others may show signs of it by simpler less expensive methods.

Bone mineral density testing, or densitometry, is used to measure the concentration of calcified material in the bones and help assess OSTEOPOROSIS or rickets. In this test a radiation beam is passed through the bone and analyzed.

PREPARATION

None.

ANESTHESIA

None.

PROCEDURE

Usually, the vertebral spine, a wrist bone, or the hip bone is tested. It is placed in the beam and a percent of normal bone concentration is reported (for example, 70 percent of normal density).

RECOVERY

None.

COMPLICATIONS AND RISKS

None. An insignificant amount of radiation is used and poses no danger to the patient. Although not exactly a complication or risk, the major drawback of the test is its cost; it is an expensive test that has little clinical value. It can be of value, however, to the woman who is otherwise ambivalent about hormone replacement therapy for postmenopausal OSTEOPOROSIS.

CARDIAC CATHETERIZATION

A catheter is a long plastic tube that can be inserted into a vein or artery and can be manipulated with the help of RADIOGRAPHY. In a cardiac catheterization, catheters are passed up to the heart. Dye can be injected into the coronary arteries, and into heart chambers in order to film the blood flow into and out of the chambers with RADIOGRAPHY.

Pressure measurements can also be made that help check heart valve function (see HEART VALVE DISEASE). The X-ray films of the arteries help identify any blockages that could interfere with blood flow to the heart muscle (as a result of ATHEROSCLEROSIS, for example).

The definitive test for atherosclerosis of the heart is cardiac catheterization with coronary angiography. It is used to plan most heart surgeries.

PREPARATION

For individuals with a known allergy to the contrast dye, special preparation with medicines are useful in reducing allergic reactions. A cardiac catheterization is performed in patients who have fasted at least four to six hours, unless it's an emergency.

ANESTHESIA

Local anesthetic is used at the sight where the catheter is inserted.

PROCEDURE

- A vein, artery, or one of each in the arm or leg is chosen as the entry point.
- The vessel is penetrated with a needle, or a small surgical incision is performed (a "cut down") to isolate the vessel.
- Guide wires are used to thread catheters up to the heart and to change to differently shaped catheters for different tasks.
- Pressure readings are recorded.
- A blood thinner such as HEPARIN is given to minimize the chance of blood clots forming on or in the catheters.
- Dye may be injected by hand with a syringe, or a higher-volume pump may be used for certain pictures.

- When the procedure is done, the catheters are removed and pressure is carefully applied to allow the entrance site to seal. If a "cut down" was necessary, the artery or vein is sewn and the skin sutured closed.

HOSPITAL RECOVERY

- Usually, patients may walk cautiously after six hours if the leg was the entry point, although overnight bed rest is common.
- An intravenous line with fluids is maintained initially.
- Patients may be released the next day, although some hospitals may let patients go home in the evening after a morning procedure.

AT-HOME RECOVERY

Avoidance of stressful activity that could affect the puncture site is reasonable for a few days.

COMPLICATIONS AND RISKS

- An allergic reaction to the dye is one of the most common complications, occurring in a few percent of patients.
- Less common but even more severe complications include blood clots forming on the catheters and breaking off and going downstream possibly leading to a STROKE, HEART ATTACK, or GANGRENE depending on where the clot travels.
- Heart rhythm abnormalities (ARRHYTHMIAS) may be seen when catheters touch the inside of the heart or during dye injections.
- The artery that serves as the entry site may be damaged and need additional special repair.
- Approximately 1 in 1000 patients could have a life-threatening complication progressing to death.

CARDIAC STRESS TEST

Many types of stress testing are available nowadays to check blood flow to the heart and overall circulatory function.

This test, sometimes called a treadmill test, involves monitoring the subject's heart as it is put through the paces of moderate to strenuous exercise. In some cases, when strenuous exercise cannot be performed, the state of exertion can be simulated by using certain drugs.

Usually, a physician with some additional training in the area or a specially trained nurse or exercise physiologist performs a cardiac stress test. Advanced cardiac life-support equipment and a physician trained in its use need to be nearby in case any cardiac problems arise because of the extreme exertion.

PREPARATION

Depending on the type of stress test, certain medications may be suspended before the test. THEOPHYLLINE and caffeine are avoided for stress tests where certain drugs are used to affect the heart. Beta-blockers such as ATENOLOL or METOPROLOL may be suspended before other types of stress tests because of their affect on the circulatory system.

The patient should avoid a large meal prior to the test. Baseline ELECTROCARDIOGRAPHY is checked before the stress is started so that the tester has a point of comparision with which to judge later readings.

PROCEDURE

There are two major categories of cardiac stress tests. The oldest and usually the best method is to use exercise to stress the heart while ELECTROCARDIOGRAPHY and BLOOD PRESSURE TESTING are monitored for changes. The exercise is usually on a treadmill, although stationary bicycles are sometimes used. NUCLEAR MEDICINE or ULTRASOUND techniques may be used during the procedure to assess other aspects of the heart's function.

The second approach uses drugs instead of exercise to stimulate the heart. The patient usually lays down quietly for this type of "stress," and it is most helpful in patients who cannot otherwise achieve the adequate cardiac stress levels through exercise. (This technique is useful for patients with disabilities, for example.)

RECOVERY

After the stress, the patient is monitored for a minimum of five to six minutes or until the physician feels it is safe to stop. For some NUCLEAR MEDICINE techniques, the patient may have to be scanned for 20 to 30 minutes and return late in the day for a repeat scan. (This technique is useful for patients with disabilities, for example.)

COMPLICATIONS AND RISKS

Generally, the risks associated with this test are low, and if a patient is so vulnerable to exercise-related stress that a complication does occur, it's better that it happens during the test in a monitored setting with health professionals rather than out on the street or at home during some other stressful activities.

Complications include

- Changes in heart rhythm (ARRHYTHMIA)
- Low blood pressure
- FAINTING OR FAINTNESS
- HEART ATTACK (rare)
- Cardiac arrest (extremely rare)

The overall risk of life-threatening complication is near 1 in 10,000. However, some patients should have their cardiac stress deferred. Such patients include those with

- HEART VALVE DISEASE
- Uncontrolled ANGINA
- Uncontrolled high blood pressure (HYPERTENSION)
- Uncontrolled CONGESTIVE HEART FAILURE

CAROTID ENDARTECTOMY

The carotid arteries run through the neck on either side of the Adam's apple up to the brain and are the major source of blood flow to the brain. ATHEROSCLEROSIS can cause enough plaque build-up to interfere with blood flow to the brain or to serve as a site for clot formation, which can lead to either transient ischemic attack or STROKE. In carotid endartectomy, a vascular-, cardiothoracic-, or neurosurgeon opens the carotid artery and cleans out the plaque material in the area that is most problematic.

Carotid endartectomy is a procedure performed only on patients at high-risk for stroke and transient ischemic attack.

PREOPERATIVE PREPARATION

ASPIRIN, which is commonly used to treat transient ischemic attack, may be withheld temporarily before surgery to avoid bleeding complications.

Because approximately 70 percent of the people with ATHEROSCLEROSIS of their carotid artery also have it in their heart, some type of cardiac evaluation, such as ELECTROCARDIOGRAPHY, CARDIAC STRESS TESTING, or CARDIAC CATHETERIZATION, may be warranted depending on the patient's other risk factors.

ULTRASOUND of the carotid artery and cerebral angiography (RADIOGRAPHY) are usually performed before the surgery is even considered to identify the problem and select the best candidate to benefit from surgical correction.

Overnight fasting is required with general anesthesia.

ANESTHESIA

General anesthesia is the most common, but local anesthesia with an intravenous sedative is an option in some cases.

PROCEDURE

- An incision is made along the neck under the jaw to identify the area of the carotid artery to be opened.
- Clamps are placed on the artery above and below the area of plaque build-up.
- Care is taken to not dislodge any plaque that could travel downstream and cause a STROKE.
- The artery is opened.
- The atherosclerotic debris is carefully removed.
- The artery is sewn closed, and the clamps are removed.
- The skin is sutured closed.

Monitoring by ELECTROENCEPHALOGRAPHY is sometimes done during the procedure in order to detect any complications during the time the patient is under general anesthesia.

HOSPITAL RECOVERY

Patients are usually kept in the hospital for three or four days. ASPIRIN or other blood thinners such as HEPARIN may be used to decrease the risk of complications and improve blood flow.

AT-HOME RECOVERY

Patients can generally return to work in a few weeks. Wound care, such as cautious cleaning and inspection for signs of infection, is appropriate.

COMPLICATIONS AND RISKS

Carotid endartectomy and the preoperative angiography (RADIOGRAPHY) both carry a significant risk of STROKE. Complication rates vary from one to ten percent or more depending on the hospital and the surgeon. (Generally, hospitals that perform many carotid endartectomies have lower complication rates.)

Because of this significant risk, patients are very carefully selected so that the benefits clearly outweigh the risks. In recent years, the surgery has been reserved for patients who experience significant transient ischemic attacks associated with tight blockages in the carotid arteries. However, it may also modestly benefit patients with tight blockages not causing symptoms if performed at a hospital with a low complication rate.

Besides the risk of stroke, possible complications include excessive bleeding and infection at the wound sight.

CARPAL TUNNEL RELEASE

Surgical carpal tunnel release is recommended for patients who have not obtained relief of symptoms with conservative treatment.

Carpal tunnel release is a surgical procedure to relieve continuous or episodic pressure on the median nerve. Entrapment or compression of the median nerve and its blood supply cause CARPAL TUNNEL SYNDROME.

ALTERNATIVE TREATMENTS

Anti-inflammatory medication, such as IBUPROFEN or NAPROXEN, given orally or steroids given by injection directly into the area may be helpful. A splint to keep the wrist in neutral position, worn either full time or at night, may also relieve the symptoms.

PREOPERATIVE PREPARATION

In general, routine diagnostic tests such as ELECTROCARDIOGRAPHY and BLOOD TESTS may be done to make an assessment of general health. Specific preparation will depend on what type of setting (hospital, surgical center, or office surgery) the procedure will take place.

Overnight fasting is required for general anesthesia.

ANESTHESIA

Adequate anesthesia for a carpal tunnel release can be provided by general anesthesia, regional anesthesia (a nerve block of the arm only), or local anesthesia (a nerve block in the area of the carpal tunnel only).

PROCEDURE

Carpal tunnel release can be done either as an open procedure through a small incision overlying the underside of the wrist, or as an endoscopic procedure through small stab incisions to allow access for instruments and a lighted magnifying endoscope (see ENDOSCOPY).

Regardless of the method employed, the goal of the operation is to release the pressure from the transverse carpal ligament that constricts the space where the median nerve runs next to the tendons of the wrist and finger flexor muscles.

- In the open procedure, the incision is made and the transverse carpal ligament is exposed; in the endoscopic procedure, the instruments are put in place through small stab incisions.
- The ligament is carefully divided, releasing the pressure on the median nerve.
- The incisions in the skin are closed, leaving the cut ligament to heal on its own in the released position.

HOSPITAL RECOVERY

Carpal tunnel release is generally done as an outpatient procedure, so no hospital stay is necessary beyond the time it takes for anesthesia to wear off.

AT-HOME RECOVERY

- The affected arm and hand should remain elevated for 24 to 48 hours after the surgery to decrease swelling.
- The wrist may be placed in a splint or brace to limit the motion of the wrist joint.
- Oral pain medicine, such as an ACETAMINOPHEN AND CODEINE COMBINATION, is generally adequate for pain relief, and may be needed for 10 to 14 days after the operation.
- A period of restricted activity should be expected, and patients are generally advised to limit lifting, carrying, and other wrist movement activities for several weeks.

COMPLICATIONS AND RISKS

As with any surgery, there is a low risk of surgical wound infection; this would be noticed as increased redness, pain, swelling, and drainage from the wound and possibly a low-grade FEVER.

The operation itself may cause some irritation of the median nerve or flexor tendons; increasing NUMBNESS, tingling, or weakness should be evaluated by a physician.

CATARACT REMOVAL

In most cases today, cataract surgery includes removal of the cataract and replacement with a new plastic lens implant. The implanted lens corrects most of the need for glasses after surgery, but glasses may still be needed for reading or far vision.

A CATARACT is an opacity in the clear lens of the eye. The lens is positioned directly behind the colored portion of the eye known as the iris and is important for focusing a clear image on the back of the eye. When a CATARACT forms, visual function may be impaired. If the patient and eye surgeon (the ophthalmologist) agree that cataract surgery is necessary, plans for the operation can be made. The procedure is usually done on an outpatient basis and the results are extremely successful in the vast majority of cases.

ALTERNATIVE TREATMENTS

Some CATARACTS can change the need for glasses due to a change in the optical properties of the lens. In these cases, adjusting the glasses by increasing the nearsighted correction or reducing the farsighted correction can improve visual function.

Some CATARACTS are small and affect visual function because of their central location. In this case, self-administered pupil-dilating eyedrops can allow a patient to see around the cataract and improve eyesight.

If these measures are inadequate to control the problem, cataract surgery may be required.

PREOPERATIVE PREPARATION

Before the operation the surgeon or a technician will measure the patient for the appropriate implant power. Everyone requires an implant power specific to his or her own eye. The goal is to avoid large differences in spectacle requirements between the two eyes. The power can be adjusted to reduce or eliminate any near- or farsightedness that may have been present before.

Other preoperative tests can include BLOOD TESTS, ELECTROCARDIOGRAPHY (if over 40 years of age), and more sophisticated tests if the patient has complex medical problems.

In general, patients are asked not to eat or drink after midnight the night before surgery if the operation is planned for the morning. A light breakfast may be allowed if the surgery is to be performed in the afternoon. If a patient is on blood pressure or other heart medicine, this should be taken as usual on the morning of surgery. The patient should consult with the eye surgeon and medical doctor about adjusting anti-coagulants, or blood thinning, medication such as

HEPARIN, WARFARIN, and ASPIRIN. Patients with DIABETES may be instructed to modify their medication on the day of surgery when the diet is being altered.

ANESTHESIA

In most cases, local anesthesia is used for the surgery. The patient is sedated with medication administered through an intravenous line. The eye surgeon or anesthesiologist then injects local anesthetic around the eye, which blocks movement of the eye and lid, numbs the pain fibers, and blurs the vision in the eye. If the patient is unable to lie still for the operation, general anesthesia may be necessary. Some patients may be deemed good candidates for topical anesthesia, in which the surgery is performed with anesthetic eyedrops only and without sedation or general anesthesia.

PROCEDURE

Although there are several techniques available for removing a cataract, the most common today is a procedure called *phacoemulsification*, which takes only 30 to 45 minutes.

- The pupil is dilated widely with eyedrops before the patient is brought to the operating room.
- After anesthetic administration, the skin around the eye is cleansed with special soap and drapes are positioned so that only the eye to be treated is exposed.
- A device is inserted to separate the eyelids and hold the eye open.
- A small incision (approximately ⅛ inch) is made in the upper portion of the eye at the edge of the iris.
- The phacoemulsification unit (a device the size of a marking pen with a small tapered tip) is introduced through the incision.
- The device breaks up and sucks out the clouded interior of the lens.
- The implant is placed inside the "skin" of the old lens in the space where the cataract was.
- The incision is closed with one stitch, or it may be self-sealing and require no stitches.

Antibiotics and cortisone-like medication may then be administered by injection or by placing a special drug-soaked dissolvable contact lens over the eye.

HOSPITAL RECOVERY

The surgery is done as an outpatient, which means that following the operation and some relaxation time, the patient, accompanied by a friend or relative, is allowed to go home.

AT-HOME RECOVERY

Postoperative discomfort is usually minimal. The patient will be examined by the surgeon the next day and will be given instructions on the use of eyedrop medications. The next follow-up visit occurs within one week of the surgery and later appointments occur at longer intervals.

Because of the small incision technique, recovery time is rapid and restrictions are minimal. Activities of daily living are all permissible. Care should be taken to avoid falling, injury to the eye, or exposure to irritating materials around the eye. Swimming with the head under water should be avoided for approximately two weeks.

COMPLICATIONS AND RISKS

Problems occur only rarely, with the worst complications being the most rare. Complications include

- Loss of vision in the eye due to infection or bleeding
- Retinal detachment
- Reversible swelling of the retina
- GLAUCOMA
- Swelling of the front of the eye (the cornea)

In some cases the tissue behind the implant may become hazy and require laser treatment to restore clarity. Finally, the best prediction of implant power may, on rare occasion, be poorly suited to the patient when actually implanted, requiring lens implant exchange or a contact lens.

WARNING SIGNS:

- Severe pain and redness that seem to be worsening
- Decrease in vision after the first postoperative day
- Pus discharge from the eye

These problems should prompt a call to and examination by the surgeon.

COLOSTOMY

Having a colostomy can be traumatic, and a patient can require a period of adjustment, but the operation should not prevent a person from leading a normal life.

A colostomy involves the creation of an opening between the abdominal wall and large bowel. The patient has bowel movements through the opening (or stoma) and must wear an appliance that holds an impermeable plastic bag in place to collect the fecal material.

Colostomy is required for patients who have their rectum removed or who need to have the fecal stream diverted from the distal large intestine. The operation can be necessary to decompress the colon when there is an INTESTINAL OBSTRUCTION. It can be a temporary situation or, when the rectum is removed on account of a disease such as COLORECTAL CANCER, permanent.

ALTERNATIVE TREATMENTS

None.

PREOPERATIVE PREPARATION

A colostomy is sometimes performed during another procedure, usually removal of the rectum or an emergency operation on the colon for infection (see DIVERTICULAR DISEASE) when sewing the colon back together right away is too dangerous.

If scheduled ahead of time, the patient is taught preoperatively about the care and maintenance of the colostomy and a point on the abdominal wall suitable for the colostomy is marked before the operation so that it will be located in the optimal position.

Except when performed in an emergency, colostomy requires the usual preparation. BLOOD TESTS and ELECTROCARDIOGRAPHY, for example, are standard before almost any surgery.

Overnight fasting is required with general anesthesia.

ANESTHESIA

General anesthesia.

PROCEDURE

- An opening in the abdominal wall, usually in the left lower abdomen, is made.

- When the colon is obstructed on the left side, the colostomy is made from a loop of colon in the right upper abdomen.
- The end (or sometimes a loop) of large intestine is brought out through the opening and sewn to the edges of the skin.
- The opening is covered with an appliance and a bag to collect the fecal contents.

HOSPITAL RECOVERY

Recovery depends on the primary operation—whether the colostomy was performed during a more extensive procedure such as removal of the rectum. Generally, the procedure requires three to seven days in the hospital.

AT-HOME RECOVERY

Recovery depends on the primary operation. Activity should be restricted for approximately three to six weeks.

COMPLICATIONS AND RISKS

- The end of the bowel may retract into the abdominal wall causing difficulty with fitting the appliance.
- Infections can occur along the side of the stoma.
- A HERNIA—the protrusion of internal structures through the opening—may occur alongside the stoma.
- An abnormally long portion of colon may protrude, or prolapse, through the opening.
- If the appliance does not fit adequately, leakage of fecal material can damage the skin around the stoma.

COMPUTED TOMOGRAPHY

Computed tomography allows physicians to visualize areas of the body that formerly could only be examined through open surgery.

Computed tomography, or CT, is an X-ray procedure that uses computer technology to make a series of X-ray images, or scans, of a body part—much like slices of bread—that can then be reconstructed by the computer and viewed from different angles.

A technician may run the machine, but a radiologist administers the contrast, if any, and interprets the results.

PREPARATION

Special preparation depends on the part of the body studied and whether contrast material, a type of dye that allows better visualization of the area studied, is to be administered. For patients allergic to contrast material, special preparation with medication such as DIPHENHYDRAMINE and PREDNISONE may be required. If the bowel or kidneys are scanned, fasting may be required for three to four hours before the procedure.

PROCEDURE

- The patient lies on a table.
- If contrast material is needed, an intravenous line may be started to administer the material.
- The area of the body to be imaged is passed into the scanning area.

The procedure may take 15 minutes or as long as an hour, depending on the size of the area studied, whether X rays are obtained both before and after injection of contrast material, and the ability of the patient to cooperate by lying still.

RECOVERY

Computed tomography is generally performed on an outpatient basis, and patients need no recovery time.

COMPLICATIONS AND RISKS

There is essentially little risk to undergoing CT. The amount of radiation from most scans is comparable to the amount of radiation one is exposed to during a day at the beach.

Individuals allergic to contrast material can experience serious reactions, including hives, and loss of blood pressure.

CORONARY ARTERY BYPASS GRAFT SURGERY

When ATHEROSCLEROSIS interferes with the blood flow to the heart muscle because of blockages in the coronary arteries, one of the ways to improve blood flow to the heart is coronary artery bypass graft surgery. A vein, usually from the leg, or an artery from along the breast bone is used to reroute the blood and bypass the blockages.

The selection of patients for bypass surgery has been studied a great deal, yet there remains some controversial areas. In properly selected patients, bypass surgery may increase the likelihood of a patient being alive five years later by 10 percent to 30 percent or more. It may also relieve disabling angina when medications are not enough.

ALTERNATIVE TREATMENTS

Medications such as NITROGLYCERIN, ATENOLOL, and DILTIAZEM can relieve symptoms and, in some cases, even prolong life. ANGIOPLASTY may also be an option for some patients facing bypass surgery.

PREOPERATIVE PREPARATION

A CARDIAC STRESS TEST can be very helpful in selecting which patients may benefit the most from bypass surgery. A coronary angiogram (RADIOGRAPHY) and CARDIAC CATHETERIZATION is also critical in selecting patients and planning the actual bypass operation. The patient may need to avoid ASPIRIN for approximately one week before surgery. Other tests routinely done before the operation include

- BLOOD TESTS of various kinds
- ELECTROCARDIOGRAPHY
- Chest X ray (RADIOGRAPHY)

Overnight fasting is required for general anesthesia.

ANESTHESIA

General anesthesia is administered and an artificial heart-lung bypass machine is used to sustain life during parts of surgery in which the bypass grafts are being sewn.

PROCEDURE

- The chest is opened by some of the surgical team while veins in the leg, or occasionally the arm, are removed carefully to be used for the "bypass." In addition, one or two arteries along each side of the breastbone (the internal mammary arteries) may be isolated for bypass use.
- The heart is stopped while the heart-lung machine sustains life.

- The one end of the bypass vessel is sewn carefully to the aorta and the other end is sewn to the coronary artery beyond the blocked area. This may be repeated, if necessary, for other blockages.
- The heart is restarted and the chest is closed in multiple steps.

HOSPITAL RECOVERY

In some hospitals, uncomplicated bypass surgery now only requires three days in the hospital with close home-care follow-up. Most hospitals, though, keep patients five to ten days, depending on the progress of recovery. Monitoring in the intensive care unit for one to two days is commonly followed by monitoring with ELECTROCARDIOGRAPHY for a few additional days. Gradually chest tubes, intravenous lines, and other support systems are removed.

AT-HOME RECOVERY

Patients are usually allowed to drive after six weeks. Before that, they may return to work full or part-time depending on their doctor's recommendation. Even during the first few days home, patients should get dressed and go out for progressively longer walks.

COMPLICATIONS AND RISKS

Mild complications can include

- A suppressed appetite and mild depression can be common shortly after bypass surgery, so getting back to routine activities as soon as possible is helpful.
- The most common problems are tenderness at incision sites (legs and breastbone); less often, infection at these sites can be an issue.

More serious complications—including STROKE, HEART ATTACK, need for emergency reoperation, and even death—are quite uncommon but vary with age and the individual. For middle-aged men, the risk of death may be less than one percent. For older patients, mortality can be five to ten percent in some higher-risk patients.

CULTURE

A culture is a test in which a sample from a patient's body is taken and tested for any germs that can be grown from it. When they are grown, or cultured, the bacteria, viruses, or other microorganisms can then be identified. The most appropriate antibiotic treatment can also be suggested by testing various ones against the germ grown from a culture.

A culture is a common test used to confirm the presence and identity of any infectious agents.

PREPARATION

Cultures are best done before someone is treated with antibiotics, since the drugs may inhibit the growth of bacteria and lead to false-negative results.

To prevent contamination with the normal bacteria that are always on the skin and in the mouth, rigorous skin preparation with antibacterial swabs precedes the sample taking.

ANESTHESIA

None, unless the culture is part of a BIOPSY procedure.

PROCEDURE

There are various ways to sample for germs:

- A throat swab takes a small sample from the back of the throat to test for streptococcal bacteria, the cause of strep throat.
- Blood samples can be drawn (see BLOOD TEST) to look for PNEUMONIA and BLOOD POISONING.
- Bone samples may be needed to document infection and select antibiotics in cases of osteomyelitis.
- Fluid accumulations around lungs, heart, joint spaces, or abdomen may be aspirated by needle.
- Urine, sputum, or stool may be cultured.

RECOVERY

Depending on the technique, little recovery time is needed.

COMPLICATIONS AND RISKS

If a needle is used for the sample, there is a remote possibility of excessive bleeding or infection. False-positive results are also a "risk" that can lead to unnecessary treatment.

Cytology is a test closely related to a biopsy, but cytology requires fewer cells, and therefore, less tissue needs to be collected.

CYTOLOGY

Cytology uses a small sample of cells spread on a microscope slide to look for changes that can be clues to cancer or infections. The samples are somewhat easier to obtain than a BIOPSY but may also be collected with needles and special scopes just like a BIOPSY. Some common examples of cytologic tests are the PAP SMEAR to look for cancer of the cervix and the sputum cytology to look for lung cancer or certain infections such as *Pneumocystis carinii* PNEUMONIA.

PREPARATION

For samples taken from the stomach or lungs, fasting for a few hours may be required to minimize the risk of vomiting.

ANESTHESIA

Usually, no anesthesia is required, but local anesthesia can be used, depending on how the sample is collected.

PROCEDURE

The exact procedure varies with the sample to be taken. To collect a PAP SMEAR, a wooden spatula is used. Special scopes with brushes are commonly used for samples collected from the lungs or gastrointestinal tract.

Needles may be used to aspirate cells from some organs such as the thyroid gland or suspected tumors in the lung, breast, or abdomen. Sometimes accumulations of fluid around the heart, lungs, or in the abdomen will be drained off and searched for cells to be studied.

RECOVERY

Taking a cytology specimen usually requires little or no observation. When a needle is used, a period of observation of up to 24 hours may be necessary.

COMPLICATIONS AND RISKS

Bleeding and infection at the site from which the sample was taken are possible, but rare, complications.

DILATION AND CURETTAGE

Dilation and curettage (D & C) is used for both diagnostic and therapeutic reasons. Some of the more common reasons include

- Diagnosis of endometrial abnormalities (such as UTERINE CANCER or hyperplasia), incomplete or missed abortion, or molar pregnancy (the presence of a degenerated ovum, or egg)
- Evaluation of the endometrial lining in cases of infertility
- The control or treatment of dysfunctional uterine bleeding

The procedure is usually performed in an outpatient surgery center or an operating room of a hospital by a gynecologist.

Dilation and curettage is the second most common gynecologic procedure and is used to diagnose cancer and other serious diseases as well as to treat dysfunctional uterine bleeding.

ALTERNATIVE TREATMENTS

Depending on the reason for the D & C, options may include hormonal therapy, hysteroscopy (a form of ENDOSCOPY), or endometrial sampling.

PREOPERATIVE PREPARATION

Depending on the type of anesthetic being used, overnight fasting may be required.

ANESTHESIA

A variety of anesthetic techniques can be used for a D & C, including local anesthetic such as a paracervical block, intravenous sedation, spinal or epidural anesthetic, or general anesthetic.

PROCEDURE

- The patient is positioned in stirrups similar to that for an office pelvic examination.
- A speculum is placed in the vagina and the cervix is located.
- A clamp is placed on the cervix after the vagina has been cleansed.
- The cervix is dilated to the appropriate size for viewing and instruments.

- Either a suction curettage (scraping) or sharp curettage is performed to clean out the uterine contents.
- If the procedure is being performed for diagnostic reasons, the material obtained is sent to pathology for a definitive diagnosis.

HOSPITAL RECOVERY

The D & C is an outpatient procedure and postoperative recovery may range from 15 minutes to a few hours, depending on the type of anesthetic used and how long it takes the patient to come out of it.

AT-HOME RECOVERY

Recovery at home is minimal. Patients should expect some minimal vaginal spotting for a few days after the procedure. Patients also need to refrain from intercourse for one to two weeks and avoid any vigorous activity immediately after the procedure.

COMPLICATIONS AND RISKS

At home, patients should look for any signs of infection developing. These may include

- Lower ABDOMINAL PAIN and tenderness (although cramping is normal)
- Temperature higher than 100.4°F
- Any foul-smelling VAGINAL DISCHARGE

ELECTROCARDIOGRAPHY

Electrocardiography is a very common test used to evaluate the health of the heart.

Commonly referred to as an EKG or ECG, electrocardiography uses a machine to measure and record (on paper or computer screen) the electrical activity of the heart. With each heartbeat, the heart has an electrical discharge spike that can be recorded using electrodes on the surface of the body. The shape and pattern of the spikes can help diagnose a wide variety of heart problems, including myocardial infarction (HEART ATTACK) and problems with the electrical system of the heart.

Preparation

The skin may be shaved where the electrode recording patches are placed on the chest, arms, and legs. Otherwise, the procedure requires no preparation.

Anesthesia

None.

Procedure

- The patient lies down quietly.
- The recording electrodes are placed on specific sites on the chest wall, arms, and legs.
- The machine is started and a sample (usually three to four seconds) from each electrode site is recorded.

The EKG may be monitored continuously during some procedures and surgeries.

In an attempt to diagnose certain heart rhythm problems (ARRHYTHMIAS), portable EKG monitors (called *Holter monitors*) may be worn for 24 hours or more to give an extended picture of the heart's rhythm.

Recovery

None.

Complications and Risks

Occasionally, the adhesive or gel used at the electrode sites can cause some local skin irritation.

ELECTROENCEPHALOGRAPHY

Electroencephalography is done to help evaluate patients with a variety of brain disorders, from headaches to mental changes to seizures.

Electroencephalography (EEG) is a test of brain function that records the electrical activity of the brain. This test is used to aid in the evaluation of patients with a variety of problems. A change in brain function, seizures, or a loss of consciousness are the most common reasons for this test, but it may be used for patients with HEADACHE, mental changes, weakness, or changes in sensation. The test is performed by a technologist and typically requires one to two hours.

PREPARATION

No extensive preparation is needed and patients should continue to take their medications unless specifically instructed otherwise. Because electrodes will be placed on the scalp, the hair should be clean, hair dressings should not be used, and hair pieces should not be worn on the day of the EEG. Because it is frequently desirable for the patient to sleep during a portion of the test, coffee or other caffeine-containing beverages should be avoided on the day of the test.

PROCEDURE

- The technologist asks some questions about the problem for which the test is being performed.
- Electrodes are attached all over the head with a special paste or glue.
- The patient is asked to lie quietly with the eyes closed.
- The technologist may ask the patient to hyperventilate for a few minutes and look at a flashing light or do some other simple stimulative activities.
- The electrodes are removed.
- The completed recording is reviewed by a physician, usually as a neurologist, and a report is sent to the doctor who requested the test.

RECOVERY

If a sedative is used to help obtain sleep during the test, the patient may be slightly drowsy following the test.

COMPLICATIONS AND RISKS

None.

ENDOSCOPY

Using a tube to look inside the body has been done for years. However, the wide variety of areas that can now be seen and the equipment used to do it has changed rapidly over the past two decades, making endoscopy one of the most versatile diagnostic tools.

Endoscopy is the use of a lighted tube inserted into the body to see internal structures. The tube may be rigid—for direct vision—or flexible with fiber-optic equipment—for transmitting images and even videotaping.

The physician who performs the endoscopy varies depending on which part of the body is to be inspected. Most procedures are done on an outpatient basis.

Examples of endoscopy that use the available openings in the body include

- Gastroscopy (stomach)
- Colonoscopy and sigmoidoscopy (colon)
- Bronchoscopy (lungs)
- Cystoscopy (bladder)
- Hysteroscopy (uterus)

In other cases, the skin may be opened to allow a scope to penetrate into an area. Among these procedures are

- Arthroscopy to look into a joint
- Laparoscopy to look in the abdomen

Besides helping to make a diagnosis, endoscopy can be used to treat certain conditions. RECTAL- OR COLON POLYP REMOVAL, transurethral resection of the prostate (see PROSTATE GLAND REMOVAL), joint surgery and a rapidly expanding area of endoscopic surgery for GALLBLADDER REMOVAL are just a few of the surgical applications for endoscopy.

PREOPERATIVE PREPARATION

- In most cases, some degree of fasting is best. This may be several hours or even overnight.
- For patients with HEART VALVE DISEASE, prophylactic antibiotics, such as AMPICILLIN and gentamicin, may be needed.

ANESTHESIA

Anesthesia choice depends on the body part being viewed.

- No anesthesia may be necessary for sigmoidoscopy of the rectum and lower colon.
- Local anesthesia, using topical sprays to numb an area, may be used for bronchoscopy of the lungs.
- General or spinal anesthetic may be appropriate for laparoscopy of the abdomen or pelvis.

PROCEDURE

- The patient may be sedated with an intravenous injection before the procedure.
- The scope is passed carefully into the opening.
- All the areas passed are inspected and possibly photographed or even videotaped if necessary.
- BIOPSY may be performed, repairs made, and even diseased parts removed.
- The scope is removed.
- If an incision was necessary, it is closed and dressed.

HOSPITAL RECOVERY

Most endoscopy only requires a brief (less than an hour) observation period after the procedure. If sedation is used, the patient may be kept longer (up to one or two hours). For laparoscopic surgery, overnight stays may be necessary.

Mild analgesics like an ACETAMINOPHEN AND CODEINE COMBINATION may be needed for more involved procedures.

AT-HOME RECOVERY

When an incision in the skin was needed, keeping the wound clean and limiting activity for a few days may be required.

COMPLICATIONS AND RISKS

- Perforation of a body part—such as the colon, esophagus, or lung—with the scope is rare. Perforation may require surgery to repair and can be a serious complication. The problem would be apparent within minutes to hours of the procedure.
- Local bleeding can usually be dealt with without difficulty, but in rare circumstances, it can be excessive or life threatening.
- Infection is rare and can develop only if the skin is cut for the procedure or if the patient has other unusual risks such as HEART VALVE DISEASE.

FIBROID TUMOR REMOVAL

The removal of FIBROID TUMORS of the uterus without removing the uterus itself is called *myomectomy*. It is performed when fibroids are large, cause pain, or cause abnormal bleeding *and* when the woman wants to bear children in the future. The operation can give a woman sufficient time to have children before fibroids cause a HYSTERECTOMY to be necessary.

In the majority of women who undergo myomectomy, fibroids grow back and become problematic again.

ALTERNATIVE TREATMENTS

Small fibroids or fibroids that cause no symptoms may be observed rather than removed. Nonsteroidal anti-inflammatory drugs such as IBUPROFEN may decrease pain and bleeding from fibroids.

Women who have problems with fibroids and do not desire children may elect to undergo HYSTERECTOMY. There is no permanent cure for symptomatic fibroids other than removal.

PREOPERATIVE PREPARATION

An ULTRASOUND is the most common test performed during the preparation for surgery.

Leuprolide (a synthetic form of the gonadotropin-releasing hormone) given in monthly injections for three to six months may decrease the size of fibroids thereby allowing for easier surgery with less blood loss.

Prior to scheduled surgery, a woman will undergo preoperative BLOOD TESTS to assess her BLOOD COUNT, kidney function, and liver functions. Chest X ray (RADIOGRAPHY) and ELECTROCARDIOGRAPHY may be performed depending on a woman's age and hospital center.

The night before surgery, the woman usually has some sort of bowel cleansing, such as an enema, and must refrain from eating for 8 to 12 hours before surgery.

ANESTHESIA

General anesthesia or regional anesthesia, such as epidural or spinal block, may be used. With regional anesthesia, a sedative may be administered so that the patient is awake but not anxious.

PROCEDURE

- A six to eight inch incision is made in the abdomen.
- The uterus is raised out of the abdomen and a superficial incision is made over an accessible fibroid.
- The fibroid is shelled out and removed in one piece.
- If possible, all of the fibroids are removed through the same incision.
- The holes left by the fibroids in the uterus are then sewn tightly with thread that disappears over time.
- The abdomen is sewn closed in many layers.

Myomectomy is most commonly done as described; however, in certain cases, the procedure may be done vaginally or through hysteroscopy (a form of ENDOSCOPY).

HOSPITAL RECOVERY

Immediately after surgery, a woman has a catheter inserted in her bladder to remove urine and an intravenous tube inserted to deliver fluids and pain medicines. On the first postoperative day, she can and should be encouraged to walk. She is also allowed to drink fluids. Usually she can eat regular food once she has passed gas through her rectum. The length of the hospital stay is three to four days.

AT-HOME RECOVERY

The main instructions for recovery are rest and plenty of fluids. Pain medication, such as an ACETAMINOPHEN AND CODEINE COMBINATION, may be needed. The patient should refrain from using tampons or douches and from having sexual intercourse for the first month after surgery. Stairs must be taken slowly and activity gradually increased as tolerated. Most women are healthy and return to work in six weeks.

Women who desire immediate pregnancy are advised to wait three months before attempting conception. If the inside of the uterine cavity was entered, the uterine wall may be weak and cesarean section may be the only delivery option.

COMPLICATIONS AND RISKS

Infection, although rare, is a risk in any surgery.

GALLBLADDER REMOVAL

The gallbladder is not absolutely necessary, and most patients have no problems after their gallbladders are removed.

The gallbladder can be removed in a procedure called *cholecystectomy* for any of three reasons

- Gallstones that cause symptoms
- Complications of gallstones (see CHOLECYSTITIS AND CHOLANGITIS)
- Benign or malignant tumors (occasionally)

ALTERNATIVE TREATMENTS

The orally administered bile salts, ursodeoxycholate or chenodeoxycholate, dissolve cholesterol GALLSTONES in selected patients. Unfortunately, most patients have stones that are not amenable to this treatment. Dissolution requires from 12 to 24 months, the treatments are expensive, and stones recur in the majority of patients.

GALLSTONES have also been fragmented with sound waves (ULTRASONIC LITHOTRIPSY). The fragments are passed from the gallbladder and dissolved with bile salts. Again, this has only been effective in a select minority of patients and recurrence rates are high.

PREOPERATIVE PREPARATION

Diagnostic tests to confirm the presence of stones include ULTRASOUND and sometimes X rays (RADIOGRAPHY) enhanced with different contrast agents depending on the nature of the problem suspected.

BLOOD TESTS and ELECTROCARDIOGRAPHY are standard before almost any surgery.

Overnight fasting is required with general anesthesia.

ANESTHESIA

General anesthesia.

PROCEDURE

For open cholecystectomy

- A standard incision is made in the upper middle of the abdomen or just below the ribs.
- The duct emptying the gallbladder into the common bile duct (the main duct connecting the liver to the

intestines) is identified, tied off with sutures or clips, and divided.

- The artery to the gallbladder is likewise identified, tied off, and divided.
- The gallbladder is then dissected from the liver and minor bleeding is controlled by electrocoagulation of small blood vessels.
- The surgeon may then perform an X ray (RADIOGRAPHY) called an *intraoperative cholangiogram* before removing the gallbladder. (In this procedure, radiologic dye is injected into the gallbladder duct while the X ray is taken. The X ray shows the entire bile duct system and any stones that have passed into the common bile duct can be seen. It also excludes injury to major bile ducts.)
- The abdominal wound is closed in layers with sutures and the skin is closed with sutures or clips.

For laparoscopic cholecystectomy (Laparoscopy is a form of ENDOSCOPY.)

- A puncture wound is made near the navel.
- A camera is placed into the abdomen. (The surgeon and assistants can then watch the operation on a video monitor.)
- Three additional puncture wounds are made in the abdomen along the rib cage for other instruments to be inserted.
- The gallbladder is removed through one of the puncture wounds.
- Puncture wounds are closed with sutures or clips.

Laparoscopic cholecystectomy is possible in 95 percent of patients.

HOSPITAL RECOVERY

Patients requiring open cholecystectomy require three to five days to regain normal bowel function. Intravenous fluids and medications are required until liquid is tolerated orally. Activity is encouraged despite pain.

Patients undergoing laparoscopic cholecystectomy have less pain and take liquids within hours of the operation. They usually spend only one day in the hospital.

AT-HOME RECOVERY

Recovery from open cholecystectomy requires from two to four weeks. Patients require pain medications such as an ACETAMINOPHEN AND CODEINE COMBINATION for one or two weeks, but are usually able to resume daily activities after one week. Strenuous activity and lifting of weight greater than about 20 pounds should be avoided for six to eight weeks.

Recovery time is markedly reduced with laparoscopic cholecystectomy. Most patients require pain medications for only several days and return to full activity after one or two weeks.

Patients may drive a car when they no longer have pain and when they are not taking pain medications that cause drowsiness.

COMPLICATIONS AND RISKS

- Leakage of bile from the gallbladder bed can cause a collection of bile beneath the liver. This prolongs upper right ABDOMINAL PAIN and delays recovery from the operation. The collection of bile may have to be drained.
- Bile duct injury causes a leak of a large amount of bile. This causes the patient to develop jaundice and abscesses in the abdomen, especially near the liver. Bile may leak through the wound. This complication will require another operation for correction and can be quite serious.
- PNEUMONIA may result because postoperative incisional pain may make deep breathing and coughing difficult.
- Wound infection is a possibility, but can be treated with antibiotics and with drainage of pus from the wound.

HEART VALVE REPLACEMENT

The implantation of new valves is performed to relieve symptoms of congestive heart failure, fainting, or angina caused by a damaged valve.

When a heart valve malfunctions enough to severely impair heart function (see HEART VALVE DISEASE), it may need to be replaced or repaired. During open heart surgery, cardiothoracic surgeons often decide to repair some heart valves, but sometimes only replacement with an artificial valve will suffice. Replacement valves are either categorized as mechanical valves, which are metallic or made of related alloys, or tissue valves, which are made from cow or pig tissue that has been specially processed.

ALTERNATIVE TREATMENTS

Special catheter treatments using balloons (valvuloplasty—a cousin of ANGIOPLASTY) can be useful in certain situations to delay the need for open heart surgery and replacement.

PREOPERATIVE PREPARATION

Echocardiograms (ULTRASOUND), CARDIAC CATHETERIZATION, and special exercise tests (CARDIAC STRESS TESTS) may be used to help decide the proper timing of valve replacement. This is often a difficult and unclear area. The physician does not want to put in an artificial valve too soon if the damaged one can be tolerated for additional months or years. Yet if one waits too long, sudden death or irreversible heart damage may occur.

ANESTHESIA

General anesthesia and a heart-lung machine are required for open heart surgery.

PROCEDURE

- The chest is opened and the ribs spread to allow access to the heart.
- The appropriate heart chamber is opened and the valve is inspected.
- If the valve can be repaired, it is (this option is often preferable).
- If the valve cannot be repaired, it is removed. Newer techniques attempt to preserve as much of the tissue supporting the old valve as possible.

- The appropriate artificial valve is sewn into place and the incisions are closed.

A heart-lung machine circulates and oxygenates enough blood to sustain life during the main portions of the operation.

HOSPITAL RECOVERY

Open heart surgery usually requires a five- to ten-day hospital stay. Anticoagulants such as HEPARIN and WARFARIN may be needed to discourage clot formations. Chest tubes and continuous ELECTROCARDIOGRAPHY will be in place for the first few days, which are spent in a surgical intensive care unit.

AT-HOME RECOVERY

- Working and other activities are gradually increased.
- Driving can usually be resumed after six weeks.
- Wound care to avoid infections is necessary until healing occurs.
- Prophylactic administration of antibiotics such as AMPICILLIN or gentamicin is helpful in preventing serious infections in patients with heart valve replacements. These drugs are given before certain procedures like dental work, bowel surgery, or vaginal surgery.

COMPLICATIONS AND RISKS

Valve replacement surgery can have mortality rates as high as five to ten percent so it is done only when the risk of leaving the original valve in place is significantly greater than that of replacement.

Infection of the wound or valve and valve malfunction can occur at any time.

Clots may form on artificial valves and cause malfunction or even travel to the brain or limbs causing STROKE or GANGRENE. This occurs rarely and can be minimized with anticoagulants such as HEPARIN or WARFARIN.

HEMORRHOID BANDING

Banding is particularly useful for patients with large or prolapsed internal hemorrhoids, but it is not effective with external hemorrhoids because application of a rubber band in this area is too painful.

Hemorrhoid banding is a method for destroying and thus eliminating internal HEMORRHOIDS. The rubber band that is applied causes the tissue to die and slough off while controlling the vein so that it doesn't bleed. The procedure is most often performed by a general or a colorectal surgeon in an outpatient setting.

Alternative treatments

Patients may obtain temporary relief with warm baths (sitz baths), which soothe and cleanse the perianal area. Anal suppositories with or without cortisone may also ameliorate symptoms.

Other surgical treatments include HEMORRHOID REMOVAL and infrared or electrocoagulation of HEMORRHOIDS.

The development and progression of HEMORRHOIDS can be avoided or impeded by avoiding CONSTIPATION and straining with bowel movements. A high-fiber diet is best for long-term control of bowel habits, but many patients require fiber supplements such as psyllium or methylcellulose to control the consistency of bowel movements. Regular exercise may also be beneficial in the prevention of HEMORRHOIDS.

Preoperative preparation

Patients should evacuate their rectum before the procedure. This usually requires an enema given on the day of the procedure.

Anesthesia

None.

Procedure

- Anoscopy (see ENDOSCOPY) is performed to locate the hemorrhoid to be banded.
- The area at the base of the hemorrhoid is grasped and tested to be sure that it is in an area where there are no pain fibers.

- The hemorrhoid is grasped and pulled into a special instrument, and an elastic band is then released to contract around the base of the hemorrhoid.
- The band is left in place, and the instruments are withdrawn.

HOSPITAL RECOVERY

The procedure is usually performed in the office and requires no specific monitoring. Patients may feel pressure or mild discomfort in the rectum and are usually observed until that feeling subsides.

AT-HOME RECOVERY

Very little, if any, pain medication, such as an ACETAMINOPHEN AND CODEINE COMBINATION, is required. Diet should be altered and fiber supplements or stool softeners given to control bowel movements.

The patient may note minor RECTAL BLEEDING with bowel movements, especially as hemorrhoidal tissue sloughs.

COMPLICATIONS AND RISKS

- Excessive pain may result if the skin in the anal canal is included in the rubber band. It should be treated by removing the rubber band.
- Significant RECTAL BLEEDING can occur infrequently when the hemorrhoidal tissue sloughs, usually one to three days after treatment, and the patient should see his or her doctor at that time.
- Patients, especially elderly men, may have difficulty passing their urine due to a reflex caused by the discomfort.
- Infection at the site of the treatment may occur but is rare.

HEMORRHOID REMOVAL

Hemorrhoid removal is the most thorough method of removing symptomatic hemorrhoids, but recurrence is not uncommon.

HEMORRHOIDS that cause persistent symptoms, especially bleeding, despite medical treatment, and that are not amenable to less invasive treatments, require formal surgery to remove them. This operation is performed by a general or colorectal surgeon in a hospital setting.

ALTERNATIVE TREATMENTS

Patients can sometimes obtain relief from symptoms with warm baths (sitz baths), which soothe and cleanse the perianal area, thus avoiding all medical treatment. However, this is not a cure for HEMORRHOIDS, and severe cases need more aggressive therapy.

Dietary changes and fiber supplements can be instituted to control bowel habits. Anal suppositories with or without cortisone may ameliorate symptoms.

HEMORRHOID BANDING is a possible treatment in select patients with internal HEMORRHOIDS. Infrared or electrocoagulation of HEMORRHOIDS may also be an option.

PREOPERATIVE PREPARATION

It is helpful to control CONSTIPATION and bowel habits preoperatively with a high-fiber diet, fiber supplements, and stool softeners. The rectum should be evacuated with enemas on the night before and morning of surgery. Overnight fasting is required for general anesthesia.

ANESTHESIA

Local anesthesia with sedation, regional anesthesia (spinal block), or general anesthesia may be used for this surgery.

PROCEDURE

- The patient is placed in either a prone position with the buttocks taped apart or supine with the legs in stirrups.
- The anus is examined and the groups of hemorrhoids to be removed are identified.
- The hemorrhoid is tied off with a suture.
- The hemorrhoid is cut from the anal muscles and removed.

- The wound in the rectum is closed with a running suture, but the external skin wound is left open. (If the anal skin is closed, there may be increased postoperative pain and a higher incidence of infection and stricture of the anus.)

HOSPITAL RECOVERY

Many patients can be discharged the same day of the operation. Those with pain that is not well controlled with oral pain medications, difficulty passing urine, and with concomitant medical problems may require observation in the hospital for one to two days.

AT-HOME RECOVERY

Patients require pain medication such as an ACETAMINOPHEN AND CODEINE COMBINATION for several days until pain subsides. Pain may be worse after bowel movements and medication may be required intermittently for one to two weeks. Bowel movements should be controlled with a high-fiber diet, fiber supplements, and stool softeners.

Sitz baths (soaking the anal area in warm water) are begun the day after surgery and are performed two to three times per day to soothe and cleanse the surgical sites. Activity is encouraged but limited by pain. Patients normally have a small amount of bleeding that ceases immediately after bowel movements.

COMPLICATIONS AND RISKS

- Infection is rare, but can be serious, causing FEVER and severe, worsening pain.
- In rare cases, significant postoperative RECTAL BLEEDING can occur; this complication requires prompt attention.
- Stricture, or stenosis, of the anal canal can occur as wounds heal, but is rare. In this complication, the patient has difficulty and pain passing bowel movements, and stool caliber is decreased.

HERNIA REPAIR

Hernia repair is usually a low-risk operation, but a large, complex hernia, especially those arising in abdominal scars, may require a more involved, riskier procedure.

HERNIA is a common condition and hernia repair is a commonly performed operation for general surgeons. A HERNIA in the groin or abdominal wall is repaired to ameliorate symptoms and to avoid future enlargement and any subsequent complications.

Patients should be able to return to full activity after recovery from the repair, but the HERNIA can recur in as many as ten percent of patients over their lifetime.

ALTERNATIVE TREATMENTS

There is no medical treatment for a HERNIA. In very ill patients, for whom surgery would be risky, a HERNIA may be observed and the operation reserved for complications, should they develop.

PREOPERATIVE PREPARATION

There are no specific tests required for hernia repair. Patients should be evaluated and prepared as appropriate for their medical problems and for the type of anesthesia they will require. BLOOD TESTS and ELECTROCARDIOGRAPHY are not uncommon; overnight fasting is required for general anesthesia.

A bowel preparation involving the removal of fecal contents and the administration of antibiotics (see SMALL BOWEL RESECTION) may be performed before repair of a complex incisional HERNIA.

ANESTHESIA

Simple hernia repairs can be performed under local anesthetic with intravenous sedation. A more complex operation will require a general anesthesia. Laparoscopic repair (see below) always requires a general anesthetic.

PROCEDURE

For open repair

- An incision is made directly over the area.
- The incision is carried through the skin, subcuta-

neous tissues, and the strong connective tissue that gives the abdominal wall its strength (called the superficial fascia).

- The hernia is located and the sac of herniated tissue is opened.
- Abdominal contents are reinserted.
- The base of the sac is closed with sutures and the excess sac is removed.
- One of several repairs is then performed: 1) A section of deep fascia is sutured over the defect; or 2) if the fascia is weak, as it often is with a recurrent hernia, a piece of woven mesh material is used to close the defect or reinforce the repair.
- The incision is sutured closed in successive layers.

For laparoscopic repair

- The abdominal cavity or the space between the abdominal cavity and the hernia is filled with carbon dioxide gas through a puncture wound near the navel to give the surgeons room to work.
- A laparoscope is inserted through a small incision and placed into the space, allowing the surgeon and surgical assistants to watch the procedure on a video monitor.
- Instruments are placed through two other puncture wounds.
- The hernia is reduced from the inside and the edges of the defect and fascia important for its repair are cut free.
- A piece of mesh material is put over the defect and stapled in placed.
- The puncture wounds are closed with sutures.

An incisional HERNIA is repaired by reopening the abdominal wound. The edges of the defect are defined and cut back to normal muscle and fascia. The wound is reclosed using sutures. If the defect is large, a piece of mesh may be required to bridge the defect or to reinforce the repair.

HOSPITAL RECOVERY

Patients most often undergo hernia repair as an outpatient; that is, they leave the hospital as soon as they recover from the anesthetic and are able to walk. Some patients may require admission to the hospital to observe and treat coexisting medical problems.

Patients who require incisional hernia repair are hospitalized for several days since they essentially undergo abdominal surgery when their wound is reopened and reclosed. They may develop decreased bowel motility and may not be able to eat. Therefore, they often require intravenous fluids until they can tolerate food.

AT-HOME RECOVERY

- Normal activity is encouraged, but patients will require pain medication such as an ACETAMINOPHEN AND CODEINE COMBINATION.
- Strenuous activity including lifting of weight greater than 10 to 20 pounds is restricted for six to eight weeks.
- Patients may drive a car when they no longer have pain and when they are not taking pain medications that make them drowsy.

Many surgeons are more liberal after laparoscopic repair and allow patients to return to full unrestricted activity as soon as their pain subsides.

COMPLICATIONS AND RISKS

Wound infection causes redness and swelling, FEVER, increasing pain, and, possibly, drainage from the incision. It is treated with antibiotics and with drainage of pus from the wound.

Ecchymosis refers to a small amount of bleeding under the skin causing a large amount of black and blue in the area around the wound. In the groin, ecchymosis can extend into scrotum and penis. This can be quite alarming to the patient, but has no significance. Ecchymosis disappears spontaneously over 10 to 14 days.

Hematoma is a collection of blood below the wound manifested by a firm swelling. It may be associated with ecchymosis. If large, a hematoma may cause discomfort and should be evaluated by the surgeon.

Recurrent HERNIA is not uncommon and requires repair, usually with prosthetic mesh material.

HIP ARTHROPLASTY

The goal of a hip arthroplasty (total hip replacement) is to replace the hip joint surfaces that are painful and degenerated from OSTEOARTHRITIS or RHEUMATOID ARTHRITIS with an artificial ball and socket joint made of advanced metal, plastic, and ceramic materials. The operation, performed by an orthopedic surgeon, promises improved function and decreased pain.

Total hip replacement is usually a very successful operation; it has a satisfaction rate greater than 90 percent.

ALTERNATIVE TREATMENTS

The decision to have a hip arthroplasty is based on how the symptoms of the hip arthritis interfere with everyday life activities. No medications or noninvasive techniques for improving the quality of worn or damaged hip joint surfaces are currently available.

PREOPERATIVE PREPARATION

General laboratory BLOOD TESTS and other diagnostic tests such as ELECTROCARDIOGRAPHY are usually done to evaluate general health status. RADIOGRAPHY may be used to help plan the operation.

ANESTHESIA

General anesthesia or regional anesthesia (spinal or epidural block) is used. A sedative may be given with regional anesthesia so that the patient is awake but not anxious.

PROCEDURE

- A variety of surgical incisions are made on the side of the upper thigh.
- The muscles are moved to the side to expose the hip (ball and socket) joint area.
- Using power instruments, the upper end of the femur (the ball) and the acetabulum (the socket) are cut and reamed to remove worn cartilage.
- Implants sized to fit the patient are then either press fitted or cemented onto the femur and into the acetabulum to create a new, low-friction ball and socket joint.
- Muscles involved in movements of the hip are then reattached to their normal positions.

HOSPITAL RECOVERY

Most patients will be in the hospital for about five to ten days after the operation. Intravenous or intramuscular pain medicine is generally used for the first several days after surgery; patients can usually be changed to oral pain medicine such as an ACETAMINOPHEN AND CODEINE COMBINATION after that time.

Physical therapy is initiated in the hospital to educate patients about restrictions, and to start exercises for range of motion and strengthening. Depending on the type of hip arthroplasty, patients will start with limited weight bearing with an assistive device (crutches or walker).

AT-HOME RECOVERY

Patients continue the rehabilitation process at home with an emphasis on improving range of motion and hip muscle strength. Restrictions on weight bearing decrease as the hip heals and muscle strength returns. There may be some restrictions on certain sitting positions, and stooping and bending until soft tissues around the hip are healed.

Therapists provide some assistive devices to aid in everyday activities that stress the hip (special aids for the bath and shower, and grabbers for picking up objects from the floor, for example).

Oral pain medications such as an ACETAMINOPHEN AND CODEINE COMBINATION may be required for two to four weeks after the patient comes home.

COMPLICATIONS AND RISKS

- As with any surgical procedure, there is a small risk of surgical wound infection.
- Dislocation of the hip joint before the soft tissues heal may occur if patients are not careful about positioning restrictions.
- Deep vein THROMBOSIS is a serious but rare occurrence.

HIP NAILING

A hip nailing, or hip pinning, operation is done to fix a fracture of the femur bone around the hip joint.

Hip nailing stabilizes a BONE FRACTURE of the femur, or thigh bone, near the hip in the best position for bone healing and the best position for normal hip function. This is necessary to stabilize the joint for walking and standing. An orthopedic surgeon performs the operation and can use a variety of implants, ranging from pins and screws to larger metallic implants. The results of the procedure are generally associated with the severity of the fracture being repaired.

ALTERNATIVE TREATMENTS

Fractures of the femur around the hip joint are difficult to treat without surgery. The forces and motion that go through the fracture area impair healing of the bone.

PREOPERATIVE PREPARATION

General diagnostic tests include BLOOD TESTS, ELECTROCARDIOGRAPHY, chest X rays (RADIOGRAPHY), and other tests to determine general health. Most fractures can be evaluated with plain X rays (RADIOGRAPHY), but occasionally, other more specialized studies, such as a bone scan (see NUCLEAR MEDICINE) or COMPUTED TOMOGRAPHY, may be needed to provide information about more complex fractures.

ANESTHESIA

- General anesthesia for more complex procedures
- Regional anesthesia, such as spinal or epidural block, for less complex procedures

PROCEDURE

- The patient is positioned on a special table to allow for the application of traction (to help with the fracture alignment).
- Special X-ray (RADIOGRAPHY) equipment is positioned so the surgeon can see the fracture during the operation.
- A surgical incision is made on the outside part of the upper thigh.

- The surgeon aligns the fracture pieces and fixes them in place with the appropriate fixation device (pin, screw, or nail).
- The incision is then closed with sutures.

HOSPITAL RECOVERY

Patients may be hospitalized after their hip procedure anywhere from three to seven days, depending on the severity of the injury and the extent of the operation. Postoperatively, intravenous or intramuscular pain medicines such as MORPHINE and MEPERIDINE are used to decrease discomfort. Most patients will be able to switch to oral pain medicine such as an ACETAMINOPHEN AND CODEINE COMBINATION after several days. Physical therapy is initiated in the hospital to teach patients limited weight bearing with crutches or a walker.

AT-HOME RECOVERY

Most BONE FRACTURES around the hip require three to six months to heal fully, although patients will be able to increase their activity level as healing progresses. A home physical therapy program or outpatient physical therapy is continued to increase the range of motion and the strength of the area.

COMPLICATIONS AND RISKS

As with any surgery, there is the slight risk of postoperative wound infection. This would be associated with increased pain, redness, swelling, and drainage from the area of the surgical incision.

Although the healing rate is generally very good, occasionally a fracture may not heal and may require further surgical treatment. In cases where the bone is not supporting the fixation devices, they may loosen or break, requiring another operation.

Patients will notice some loss of range of motion of the hip joint and some decreased strength; these are the result of the injury, and a return to fully normal function after the fracture should not be expected.

Some patients may see an increase in RHEUMATOID ARTHRITIS and arthritic changes with time after a hip fracture, regardless of the type of repair.

HYSTERECTOMY

A *total* hysterectomy is the operation to remove the uterus and cervix (which is the bottom part of the uterus). A *partial* hysterectomy, removal of the uterus without the cervix, is performed very rarely. Hysterectomy does not include removal of the fallopian tubes and ovaries, although this is often done at the same time.

Hysterectomies may be performed by one of two routes depending upon the indication. Abdominal hysterectomy—removal of the uterus through an incision in the abdomen—is used when there are very large FIBROID TUMORS, UTERINE CANCER, OVARIAN CANCER, or scarring from previous abdominal surgery or infection such as PELVIC INFLAMMATORY DISEASE.

In *vaginal* hysterectomy the uterus is removed through an incision in the vagina. Although recuperation is much easier from this type of surgery, it is only practical when the uterus is not greatly enlarged. Indications for vaginal hysterectomy include symptomatic small to moderate FIBROID TUMORS, persistent abnormal VAGINAL BLEEDING, certain precancerous conditions of the uterus, and when the uterus is falling (prolapsing) into the vagina. A vaginal hysterectomy can also be performed with the aid of laparoscopy (a form of ENDOSCOPY), which makes the procedure more versatile.

The exact indications for hysterectomy have been the focus of much controversy lately, but there is no doubt that the operation is useful and even life-saving in certain circumstances.

ALTERNATIVE TREATMENTS

Alternative treatments depend on the indication for the surgery. Small or asymptomatic fibroids may be observed rather than removed. Abnormal uterine bleeding may be controlled by hormones—estrogen, progesterone, or a combination of the two. In certain cases abnormal uterine bleeding may be prevented by ablation, or charring, of the interior lining.

PREOPERATIVE PREPARATION

During the workup before a hysterectomy, women most frequently have a pelvic ULTRASOUND to assess the uterus and ovaries. In cases of abnormal bleeding a BIOPSY of the inside lining of the uterus (endometrium) may be performed to rule out cancer such as UTERINE CANCER.

Preoperative BLOOD TESTS may include BLOOD COUNTS, liver and kidney assessments, and a sampling of blood to be kept in the blood bank in case the need for transfusion arises. A chest X ray (RADIOGRAPHY) and ELECTROCARDIOGRAPHY may be performed depending on the woman's age and hospital center.

The night before surgery the woman usually has some kind of bowel cleansing such as an enema and does not eat for eight to twelve hours prior to surgery.

ANESTHESIA

General anesthesia and regional anesthesia (spinal or epidural block) are both options. A sedative may be given with regional anesthesia so that the patient is awake but not anxious.

PROCEDURE

For abdominal hysterectomy

- An incision is made in the abdomen.
- The blood vessels to the uterus and the surrounding tissue are cut and tied off.
- The uterus is removed through the abdominal incision.
- The abdomen is then sewn closed in many layers with thread that disappears over time.
- The skin is closed with thread or staples.

For vaginal hysterectomy

- An incision is made at the top of the vagina.
- The blood vessels and surrounding tissue are cut and tied off.
- The organs are removed through the vaginal incision.

To perform a laparoscopically assisted vaginal hysterectomy, small incisions are made near the navel and at two other sites in the lower abdomen to allow a laparoscope (see ENDOSCOPY) to pass into the abdominal cavity. The surgery is performed with the aid of images obtained through the scope.

Hospital recovery

Immediately after surgery, a woman has a catheter placed in her bladder for urination and an intravenous catheter inserted to deliver fluids and pain medications. On the first postoperative day a woman should be encouraged to walk as much as possible. Depending on the type of surgery, she may be able to drink fluids and consume a general diet on the first day. After an abdominal hysterectomy a patient drinks clear fluids and consumes regular food only after having passed gas through her rectum. Diet may be advanced more quickly after vaginal surgery.

The hospital stay is usually three to four days for an abdominal hysterectomy and two to three days for a vaginal hysterectomy.

At-home recovery

The main instructions for recovery are rest and plenty of fluids. Pain medication, such as an ACETAMINOPHEN AND CODEINE COMBINATION, may be needed. The patient should refrain from using tampons or douches and from having sexual intercourse for the first month after surgery. Stairs must be taken slowly and activity gradually increased as tolerated. Most women are healthy and feel capable of returning to a normal routine in six weeks.

Complications and risks

All types of hysterectomy, like all other surgery, carry risks of infection. Blood loss, anesthesia problems, and injury to other organs, such as the intestines and bladder, are remote possibilities.

An ileostomy can be temporary if the bowels are to be reattached at some point, or it can be permanent when the large intestine has been removed.

ILEOSTOMY

An ileostomy is an opening created between the abdominal wall and the portion of the small intestines called the *ileum*. The patient has bowel movements through the opening, called a *stoma*, and must wear an appliance that holds an impermeable plastic bag in place to collect the wastes. Ileostomy is required for patients who have their large intestine removed on account of disease such as COLORECTAL CANCER or who need to have the fecal stream diverted from the large intestine as in some cases of ULCERATIVE COLITIS.

ALTERNATIVE TREATMENTS

None.

PREOPERATIVE PREPARATION

An ileostomy is performed during another procedure, usually removal of part or all of the colon. If the procedure is scheduled in advance, the patient is taught about the ileostomy and a point on the abdominal wall suitable for the ileostomy is marked before the operation so that it will be located in the optimal position.

BLOOD TESTS, ELECTROCARDIOGRAPHY, and other tests to evaluate general health status are standard before almost any surgery.

Overnight fasting is required with general anesthesia.

ANESTHESIA

General anesthesia.

PROCEDURE

Ileostomy is usually performed in conjunction with another operation, which means an abdominal incision has already been made.

- After the other procedure, such as SIGMOID COLON REMOVAL, an opening is made in the abdominal wall, usually in the right lower abdomen.

- The end, or sometimes a loop, of small intestine is brought out through the opening and sewn to the skin edges to create an opening in the bowel for bowel movements.
- The opening is covered with an ileostomy appliance and a bag.

HOSPITAL RECOVERY

It depends on the primary operation, but generally, ileostomy requires a hospital stay of three to seven days. Liquids and soft foods are introduced after a few days.

AT-HOME RECOVERY

It depends on the primary operation, but activity should generally be restricted for three to six weeks. Pain medication, such as an ACETAMINOPHEN AND CODEINE COMBINATION, may be prescribed if necessary.

COMPLICATIONS AND RISKS

- The end of the bowel may retract into the abdominal wall causing difficulty with fitting the appliance.
- Infections can occur alongside the stoma.
- If the appliance does not fit adequately, leakage of fecal material can damage the skin around the ileostomy.
- DIARRHEA may occur since absorption of water by the colon is no longer possible and patients are more susceptible to DIARRHEA during gastrointestinal illnesses.

KIDNEY REMOVAL

Because the body is equipped with two kidneys, one can be removed without severely compromising the body's ability to eliminate wastes through the urine.

Kidney removal, also called *nephrectomy*, is necessary in several circumstances. Severely infected or cancerous kidneys are candidates for removal. A nonfunctioning kidney (KIDNEY FAILURE) may need to be removed to make room for a KIDNEY TRANSPLANT. A functioning kidney from a living donor is also removed in this manner.

PREOPERATIVE PREPARATIONS

Intravenous pyelogram (RADIOGRAPHY) and COMPUTED TOMOGRAPHY, are usually necessary. BLOOD TESTS and ELECTROCARDIOGRAPHY are also standard before almost any surgery. Overnight fasting is required with general anesthesia.

ANESTHESIA

General anesthesia.

PROCEDURE

- A generous incision is made along the flank.
- The renal vein, renal artery, and the ureter are tied off and cut and the organ is removed.
- The kidney's attachments to the surrounding structures are cut and the organ is removed.
- Internal muscles are repaired and vessels tied off.
- The external incision is closed with sutures.

HOSPITAL RECOVERY

Hospital stay is usually five to seven days. Fluids are administered intravenously for several days until the patient can eat.

AT-HOME RECOVERY

Activity should be limited for approximately six weeks.

COMPLICATIONS AND RISKS

- Excessive bleeding (hemorrhage) is a danger with this procedure and may require transfusion.
- Because the incision in the flank is so large and so near the bottom of the lung, pneumothorax (collapsed lung) is a possible complication.

KIDNEY TRANSPLANT

In this procedure, a kidney from a living related donor or from a compatible organ donor is transplanted into a person with KIDNEY FAILURE. The operation is performed in the hospital setting by either a transplant specialist or a urologist.

With current methods to control rejection, the likelihood that kidney transplantation will be a success is very good provided a suitable donor can be found.

ALTERNATIVE TREATMENTS

Although dialysis can offset many of the problems associated with failing kidneys, quality of life may often be better with transplantation.

PREOPERATIVE PREPARATION

The donated organ and the recipient patient must be precisely cross-matched to minimize the risk of rejection. Cross-matching usually entails BLOOD TESTS.

As with other major sugery, overnight fasting and preoperative tests, such as BLOOD TESTS and ELECTROCARDIOGRAPHY, are usually required.

ANESTHESIA

General anesthesia.

PROCEDURE

The diseased kidney can be removed from the transplant recipient (KIDNEY REMOVAL) well before the transplant operation—up to several weeks in advance—with kidney functions being performed through dialysis. The donor kidney, however, cannot be removed any sooner than about 12 hours before transplantation. Once the donor kidney is available, the procedure can begin:

- An incision is made along the flank.
- The vein and artery that will be connected to the graft kidney are identified.
- The graft kidney is placed in the selected site.
- The graft kidney's artery and vein are attached to the patient's own vessels.
- The graft kidney's ureter is connected to the patient's bladder.
- The surgical incision is closed with sutures.

HOSPITAL RECOVERY

The length of time the patient must stay at the hospital is extremely variable and depends on the occurrence of complications; three weeks is common. Occasionally, part of the postoperative stay is in the intensive care unit, and some dialysis treatments may still be required. Part of the treatment immediately after includes immunosuppressive medication, such as CYCLOSPORINE, AZATHIOPRINE, and PREDNISONE, which can cause significant side effects.

Sutures stay in place for about one week, and the intravenous line remains for a few days.

AT-HOME RECOVERY

Recovery at home takes a minimum of six weeks—often longer, depending on any complications. Recovery entails significant restrictions on activities and close monitoring of health status.

COMPLICATIONS AND RISKS

- Poor graft function can be a temporary or long-term problem. Poor urine output can signal diminished function.
- Graft rejection is the most feared of the complications. In rejection, the host's body treats the new kidney as an invader and the immune system attacks it (hence the use of immunosuppressant medication after surgery). Pain in the area of the transplant and FEVER are warning signs of rejection.
- Opportunistic infections are a danger because the artificially weakened immune system makes the recipient unable to fight off otherwise simple bacterial and viral invaders.

KNEE ARTHROPLASTY

The goal of knee arthroplasty is to replace worn and arthritic knee cartilage with metal, plastic, or ceramic surfaces to improve function and decrease pain. This operation is done by an orthopedic surgeon.

More than 90 percent of patients with advanced knee arthritis have decreased pain and improved function after knee arthroplasty.

ALTERNATIVE TREATMENTS

Degenerative conditions of the knee such as OSTEOARTHRITIS and RHEUMATOID ARTHRITIS are treated initially with anti-inflammatory or pain medicines, such as IBUPROFEN and acetaminophen, and with decreased activity. Physical therapy may be helpful.

No medications or noninvasive techniques for improving or restoring degenerative knee cartilage surfaces are currently available.

PREOPERATIVE PREPARATION

Laboratory tests, such as BLOOD COUNT and other BLOOD TESTS, and other diagnostic tests, such as ELECTROCARDIOGRAPHY and chest X ray (RADIOGRAPHY), are done to evaluate general health.

Overnight fasting is required for general anesthesia.

ANESTHESIA

General anesthesia and regional anesthesia (spinal or epidural block) are both options. A sedative may be given with regional anesthesia so that the patient is awake but not anxious.

PROCEDURE

- An incision is made on the front part of the knee.
- By moving the patella (knee cap) and its associated tendons out of the way, the worn surfaces of the knee joint (femur and tibia) are exposed.
- Using power instruments and special surgical guides to align the cut surfaces, the worn surfaces are removed.

- The removed material is replaced by metal and plastic implants that are sized to the individual patient and are then press fitted or cemented into place.
- The patella mechanism is then allowed to return to its normal position.
- The incision is closed with sutures.

HOSPITAL RECOVERY

Most patients undergoing knee arthroplasty will be in the hospital between five and ten days. Intravenous or intramuscular pain medications may be administered for the first several days; patients can usually switch to oral pain medicine, such as an ACETAMINOPHEN AND CODEINE COMBINATION, at that time.

Physical therapy to regain range of motion and improve strength is initiated in the hospital. Patients are generally limited to restricted weight bearing with an assistive device (crutches or walker).

AT-HOME RECOVERY

Patients continue the rehabilitation process at home—either with at-home physical therapy or as an outpatient. Exercises are continued to improve range of motion and strength. Restrictions on activity and weight bearing are progressively relaxed as the knee heals.

Patients may continue to use oral pain medicine, such as an ACETAMINOPHEN AND CODEINE COMBINATION, for two to four weeks after they come home.

COMPLICATIONS AND RISKS

- As with any operation, there is a small risk of surgical wound infection.
- On rare occasions, blood clots in the legs (deep vein THROMBOSIS) can be a dangerous complication.

LUMBAR DISK REMOVAL

The objective of a disk removal surgery, called *diskectomy*, is to decompress nerve roots that are irritated by a portion of the intervertebral disk (see HERNIATED DISK). Disk removal surgery is done by surgeons with specialized training in spine surgery, usually orthopedic surgeons or neurosurgeons.

Although most of the time the surgery is done in a hospital setting, some types of diskectomies may be done as outpatient surgery.

Lumbar disk removal is helpful for about 80 percent of the patients who experience no improvement with conservative treatment.

ALTERNATIVE TREATMENTS

Almost all patients with disk problems should initially undergo conservative treatment with rest, anti-inflammatory medication, such as IBUPROFEN, and possibly physical therapy to allow for recovery without surgery.

PREOPERATIVE PREPARATION

An evaluation of the patient's general health can include routine BLOOD TESTS and more specialized tests such as ELECTROCARDIOGRAPHY and chest X rays (RADIOGRAPHY) as needed.

Overnight fasting is required for general anesthesia.

ANESTHESIA

Anesthesia is usually general, but occasionally, regional anesthetic (anesthesia of the lower back and legs) or local anesthetic (anesthesia of the surgery site only) may be used with or without a sedative.

PROCEDURE

The goal of the diskectomy is to free affected nerve roots that are compressed or stretched by HERNIATED DISK material. This may be done through an open incision with the aid of magnifying glasses or a microscope, or by an endoscopic approach (see ENDOSCOPY).

For the open, or microdiskectomy

- An incision is centered over the affected disk space.
- The overlying soft tissues are carefully cut to reveal the nerve root.
- The nerve is carefully moved to the side, and the offending disk material is removed.

- The wound is closed with sutures in layers.

In the endoscopic approach

- A small tube that allows passage of small instruments and an endoscope is passed through the muscle along the spine and placed in the center of the disk.
- Disk material is then removed in front of the bulging material to decompress the nerve root indirectly.

HOSPITAL RECOVERY

Depending on the setting of the procedure, some patients may be able to go home the same day or the day after the procedure. Patients can generally walk unassisted after the operation on that same day.

Oral pain medicine such as an ACETAMINOPHEN AND CODEINE COMBINATION is usually adequate to control discomfort; some patients may require some intravenous or intramuscular pain medicine right after the procedure, though.

AT-HOME RECOVERY

Most patients require a period of convalescence and reduced activity after surgery. Patients should avoid repeated stooping, bending, lifting, and prolonged sitting for several weeks. Some patients with less demanding jobs may be able to return to limited work as soon as two to three weeks after the operation.

Oral pain medicine (ACETAMINOPHEN AND CODEINE COMBINATION) is generally needed for several weeks after the operation.

COMPLICATIONS AND RISKS

As with any surgery, there is a small risk of surgical wound infection, but it is rare.

Surgery around the irritated nerve root may cause some additional pain, NUMBNESS, or tingling similar to the original symptoms of a HERNIATED DISK with nerve root entrapment, and should be evaluated by a physician.

LUMBAR PUNCTURE

During the lumbar puncture, or spinal tap, a small needle is put into the fluid-filled space that surrounds the brain and spinal cord to remove fluid for laboratory tests. The needle is inserted between the bones of the spine in the lower back below the end of the spinal cord. This test is performed to diagnose infections, such as meningitis, and bleeding into this space (subarachnoid hemorrhage), and to obtain fluid to test for other diseases such as MULTIPLE SCLEROSIS.

A lumbar puncture is performed to test for such diseases as multiple sclerosis or meningitis, and to inject drugs in the spinal cord area to treat some conditions.

PREPARATION

There is no specific preparation for this test.

ANESTHESIA

A local anesthetic is used.

PROCEDURE

Usually the patient is asked to curl up on his or her side, although sometimes the patient is asked to sit and bend forward. Sometimes the test is done in an X-ray (RADIOGRAPHY) room where a fluoroscope can be used to aid the procedure.

- The skin is cleaned with an antiseptic and a local anesthetic is injected.
- A needle is inserted into the spinal canal.
- Once the needle is in the spinal fluid, the pressure may be measured and fluid collected.
- Once the spinal fluid has been collected, the needle is removed.

RECOVERY

The patient is usually kept flat in bed for about an hour following the test and then may resume normal activity but should avoid lifting or straining for 24 hours. There may be soreness in the lower back for a few days.

COMPLICATIONS AND RISKS

In extremely rare cases in which there is an unsuspected increase in the pressure in the brain, a lumbar puncture can cause a worsening of neurologic symptoms.

LUNG RESECTION

Lung resection is the surgical removal of a portion of the lung.

Lung resection can be used to remove suspicious nodules, or "spots," in the lung or, in a relatively new procedure, to reduce lung volume in patients with EMPHYSEMA.

Removal of suspicious lesions is often needed for diagnosis and attempted cure (see LUNG CANCER).

Volume reduction surgery removes lung tissue damaged by EMPHYSEMA, decreasing lung volume and allowing the rib cage and diaphragm to assume a more normal position. Removing damaged lung also allows the more normal lung tissue to function better.

Specific criteria must be met before patients are deemed candidates for this surgery. In general, patients must have severe EMPHYSEMA with significant lung overinflation. Patients are not candidates if they are active smokers, are severely obese (OBESITY), or have another severe illness.

ALTERNATIVE TREATMENTS

For emphysema patients, optimal medical therapy should be attempted before surgery.

PREOPERATIVE PREPARATION

For lung resection of suspected LUNG CANCERS, an evaluation for any possible spread of the cancer is performed. COMPUTED TOMOGRAPHY is often used for this purpose.

Other tests used before lung surgery may include

- BLOOD TESTS, including BLOOD COUNT
- ELECTROCARDIOGRAPHY
- PULMONARY FUNCTION TESTING
- Chest X ray (RADIOGRAPHY)

Overnight fasting is required for general anesthesia.

ANESTHESIA

General anesthesia.

PROCEDURE

There are two major approaches: open surgery or surgery using thoracoscopy (a form of ENDOSCOPY). For open surgery

- An incision is made in the center of the chest.
- The sternum (breastbone) separated.

- The suspicious nodule or the portion of the emphysematous lung is removed with a stapling device that cuts and seals lung tissue with staples.
- A strip of bovine (cow) heart tissue may be used to strengthen the incision.
- The incision is closed in layers with sutures.

For the thoracoscopic approach

- Three small holes are made on one side of the chest.
- The thoracoscope and other instruments are inserted through the holes.
- Surgical removal is performed as above except through the thoracoscope.
- The instruments are removed and the puncture wounds closed.

HOSPITAL RECOVERY

Chest tubes and intravenous fluids are usually required for two to three days after the surgery. Mechanical ventilation (a breathing machine) may also be needed initially. The total hospital stay is usually between five to seven days.

AT-HOME RECOVERY

Over three to six weeks, activity may be gradually increased. Pain medication, such as an ACETAMINOPHEN AND CODEINE COMBINATION, may be prescribed. Driving is usually deferred for six weeks if the breast bone was cut during surgery. Some wound care is necessary.

COMPLICATIONS AND RISKS

Wound infection, excessive bleeding, PNEUMONIA, and other complications of major surgery are a possibility. Also, the quantity of remaining lung tissue has to be enough to sustain the patient. Preoperative tests are used to predict postoperative lung function, but patients are sometimes left with an inadequate amount of functional lung tissue after resection. Very rarely, patients require prolonged use of mechanical ventilation (a breathing machine).

MAGNETIC RESONANCE IMAGING

Although relatively new, magnetic resonance imaging is now a frequently used diagnostic technique that has a wide variety of applications.

Magnetic resonance imaging (sometimes called MR or MRI) is a form of radiologic testing that allows physicians to distinguish fine details of internal structures. Unlike RADIOGRAPHY and COMPUTED TOMOGRAPHY, magnetic resonance imaging does not use X-ray radiation.

The technology used is very complex: Using an extremely powerful magnetic field, some portion of the body's atoms are lined up parallel to each other like rows of magnets. A pulse of radio waves transiently shifts the atom particles and they emit a detectable radio signal as they shift back into line. The signals are assembled with the help of a computer to build an image of the body area.

PREPARATION

Patients with heart pacemakers, hearing aids, or any other metal parts in the body may not be able to have the test and need to tell their doctors before an exam. Otherwise no special preparation is necessary.

ANESTHESIA

None is needed, but in rare instances, patients who are claustrophobic may need sedation before the procedure.

PROCEDURE

- The patient lays down and is moved into the large cylinder that houses the magnets.
- Sometimes a special dye or contrast medium is used to enhance the images and this is injected by vein into the body.
- The test may take 30 to 90 minutes, during which time the patient must remain very still.

RECOVERY

None.

COMPLICATIONS AND RISKS

There are no known risks associated with this procedure.

MALIGNANT MELANOMA REMOVAL

A malignant melanoma is a pigmented form of SKIN CANCER. It begins as a result of an abnormal proliferation of the pigment-producing cells in the skin called *melanocytes*.

Melanoma is associated with recurrent severe sunburns during childhood, adolescence, or early adulthood.

ALTERNATIVE TREATMENTS

Malignant melanoma requires surgical removal.

PREOPERATIVE PREPARATION

Overnight fasting may be required for general anesthesia.

ANESTHESIA

General anesthesia or regional anesthesia may be used.

PROCEDURE

For superficial tumors

- The surgeon numbs the skin with a local anesthetic.
- The surgeon uses a scalpel to cut around the tumor.
- Adequate margins of normal skin are also removed.
- The two sides are then stitched together.
- The removed tissue is examined to make sure all of the tumor has been removed .

When the tumor is deeper and when the skin area of the tumor drains to a defined set of lymph nodes, the lymph nodes may need to be surgically removed also and examined for any melanoma cells that may have spread from the skin to the bundle of lymph nodes. If cells are found in the lymph nodes, medicines that kill cancer cells (chemotherapy) may be given to treat melanoma cells that may have spread to other sites besides the skin and lymph nodes. The patient will also undergo a variety of X-ray (RADIOGRAPHY) methods to search for signs of tumor in other sites.

RECOVERY

No hospital stay is usually required.

COMPLICATIONS AND RISKS

Infection and excessive bleeding are possible but rare.

MASTECTOMY, MODIFIED RADICAL

In most cases, radiation treatments are not required if a modified radical mastectomy is performed, but depending on the stage of disease, patients may require chemotherapy.

The modified radical mastectomy, or total mastectomy, is a time-honored treatment for BREAST CANCER. It involves the removal of the entire breast and contents of the armpit area. The operation is most commonly performed in the hospital by a general surgeon or a surgical oncologist.

ALTERNATIVE TREATMENTS

Lumpectomy (MASTECTOMY, PARTIAL) and radiation treatments may be appropriate for some tumors of the breast.

PREOPERATIVE PREPARATION

The patient undergoing modified radical mastectomy requires mammography (RADIOGRAPHY) to assess the health of the opposite breast. Patients should have a chest X ray (RADIOGRAPHY) and a battery of tests that include serum liver function tests to exclude tumor in the liver (see BLOOD TESTS).

Some patients with large cancers should have a bone scan (see NUCLEAR MEDICINE) and tests to examine the liver, such as COMPUTED TOMOGRAPHY or liver scan (see NUCLEAR MEDICINE), to exclude the possibility that the tumor has spread to the bones or to the liver.

Overnight fasting is required for general anesthesia.

ANESTHESIA

General anesthesia.

PROCEDURE

- The patient is placed on the operating room table on her back.
- An incision is made over the breast and skin flaps are created to close the wound by cutting between the skin and the breast tissue.
- The breast is then removed from the chest wall by removing the fascia (the lining of the chest wall muscles).
- The muscles of the chest wall are preserved. (Previously the operation—called the radical mastectomy—removed these muscles and caused significant chest wall deformity. This is no longer felt to be necessary.)

- The blood vessels and important nerves in the armpit area are identified through the same incision and preserved.
- The contents of the armpit including the lymph nodes are removed and sent for pathologic examination (see BIOPSY).
- The skin is closed with sutures or clips.

Some women choose to have breast reconstruction, either immediately or later after they have recovered from their operation and treatment. This is performed by a plastic surgeon.

HOSPITAL RECOVERY

Since lymph fluid may collect in the wound, a drainage tube is sometimes placed in the armpit and under the skin flaps. The surgery requires a short one- to three-day hospital stay. Patients require oral pain medications such as an ACETAMINOPHEN AND CODEINE COMBINATION. They are encouraged to resume normal activity, to perform exercises and use their arms as soon as possible after the operation.

AT-HOME RECOVERY

Patients may continue to require pain medications such as an ACETAMINOPHEN AND CODEINE COMBINATION at home. They should increase their activity and their exercises. Many patients go home with drains in their armpits and must care and empty the drains until they are ready to be removed. Chemotherapy, if needed, is begun when the wounds are healed and drains are removed.

COMPLICATIONS AND RISKS

- Hematoma is a collection of blood in the wound. It usually resolves spontaneously, but if large, it may have to be evacuated surgically.
- Seroma is a collection of lymph fluid in the armpit. It can occur despite the use of drains. It may resolve on its own, but if uncomfortable may need to be aspirated with a needle.
- Wound infection is a possibility with all surgery, but it is rare.

MASTECTOMY, PARTIAL

For most types of breast cancer, lumpectomy is followed by sampling of lymph nodes from the armpit area, radiation treatments, and depending on the stage of the disease, chemotherapy.

A partial mastectomy is the removal of part of the breast to treat benign and malignant tumors of the breast (see BREAST CANCER). Removal of a cancer of the breast with an adequate margin of tissue is called *lumpectomy*. Sometimes an entire quadrant of the breast is required to remove a cancer. The operation is most commonly performed in a hospital by a general surgeon or a surgical oncologist.

ALTERNATIVE TREATMENTS

Modified radical mastectomy is another more involved operation to treat tumors of the breast (see MASTECTOMY, MODIFIED RADICAL).

PREOPERATIVE PREPARATION

The patient undergoing breast BIOPSY (removal of a lump for diagnosis) usually requires mammography (RADIOGRAPHY) to assess the characteristics of the lump and to be sure there are no other lesions in the same or opposite breast.

Patients with BREAST CANCER should have a chest X ray (RADIOGRAPHY) and a battery of tests including serum liver function tests (see BLOOD TESTS) to exclude tumor in the liver. Some patients with large cancers should have a bone scan (see NUCLEAR MEDICINE) and tests to examine the liver, such as COMPUTED TOMOGRAPHY or a liver scan (see NUCLEAR MEDICINE), to exclude spread of the cancer.

Overnight fasting is required for general anesthesia.

ANESTHESIA

Breast BIOPSY and lumpectomy may be performed under local anesthesia. Many patients require general anesthetic when BIOPSY of the armpit lymph nodes or a larger resection is required.

PROCEDURE

- The patient is placed on the operating room table on her back.
- An incision is made over the lump.
- The lump and an appropriate amount of surrounding tissue are removed.

- The lump is sent for pathologic examination (BIOPSY).
- If the contents of the armpit need to be removed or sampled, another incision is made in the armpit.
- Wounds are closed with sutures or clips.

HOSPITAL RECOVERY

Breast BIOPSY is usually performed as an outpatient, but more extensive operations, such as lumpectomy or quadrantectomy, require a short one- to two-day hospital stay. Since lymph fluid may collect in the wound, a drainage tube is sometimes placed in the armpit area and left in place to collect fluid until drainage ceases. Patients require oral pain medications such as an ACETAMINOPHEN AND CODEINE COMBINATION. Patients are encouraged to resume normal activity, perform exercises, and use their arms as soon as possible after the operation.

AT-HOME RECOVERY

Patients may continue to require pain medications at home. They should increase their activity and their exercises gradually. Many patients go home with wound drains in place and must care for and empty the drains until they are ready to be removed.

Radiation and chemotherapy can begin when wounds are healed and drains are removed.

COMPLICATIONS AND RISKS

- Hematoma is a collection of blood in the wound. It usually resolves spontaneously, but if large, it may have to be evacuated surgically.
- Seroma is a collection of lymph fluid in the armpit. It can occur despite the use of drains. It may resolve on its own, but if uncomfortable may need to be aspirated with a needle.
- Wound infection is a possibility with all surgery, but it is rare.
- Recurrence of tumor may occur in some patients. Total mastectomy (MASTECTOMY, MODIFIED RADICAL) may be required at that time to eliminate the disease.

MEDICAL HISTORY

In approximately 70 percent of cases, all a physician really needs to make a diagnosis and address a problem is the information a patient can tell him or her.

PHYSICAL EXAMINATION and diagnostic tests contribute only a small portion of the information required to make a diagnosis. A medical history involves the communication of information about a patient's symptoms, past illnesses, health habits, family history, and other pertinent topics.

PREPARATION

To get the most for yourself from a medical history, it helps to organize and even write down information to give to the doctor or to refer to during the history. For example, dates of prior hospitalizations, immunizations, and surgeries are important pieces of information. It's also helpful to record any adverse or allergic reactions you had to a specific medication.

Some aspects of the family history are very helpful and worth asking a relative about. For example, the patient should know about any family history of

- Unexpected deaths at a young age
- BREAST CANCER
- COLORECTAL CANCER
- Thyroid cancer
- Premature heart disease such as a HEART ATTACK
- DIABETES

If the visit to the doctor is to evaluate a specific symptom, it can be helpful to read the appropriate section in this book, note what things make the problem more or less suspicious, the timing and duration of the symptom, and any other clues.

PROCEDURE

The key aspects of a medical history are

- The chief complaint—the main reason a patient is seeking medical advice
- History of the present illness
- Past medical history
- Family medical history
- Social history including occupation, hobbies, smoking and alcohol use, sexual orientation
- General review of body systems

Depending on the setting a doctor may focus on a limited number of topics or cover most of this list.

It is very important to be as open as possible about answers even if they are embarrassing; a physician is in a better position to help if he or she knows the whole story.

NUCLEAR MEDICINE

Nuclear medicine is the use of radioactive chemicals for a medical purpose. Some type of scan or imaging of the body is the most common use. The radioactive substance is injected into the body and its radio signal is then detectable from the outside. Common scans using nuclear techniques include bone scans, heart muscle scans, thyroid scans, and lung scans.

Radioactive iodine to treat HYPERTHYROIDISM is an example of the therapy side of nuclear medicine. A radiopharmacist may prepare the material, a radiologist or cardiologist certified in nuclear medicine usually performs the test or treatment.

Nuclear medicine encompasses a wide variety of tests and therapies. It can be used to obtain images useful in diagnosis, and it can actually treat certain disorders.

PREPARATION

This varies widely with the specific test. Preparation mainly consists of communicating the appropriate information to the physician conducting the test. The physician must know about

- Any medications the patient is taking because they may need to be avoided for a day or so before the test (THEOPHYLLINE, for example, must be discontinued before certain heart scans.)
- Any chance that the patient is pregnant (Nuclear medicine can adversely affect a developing fetus.)

PROCEDURE

Almost all nuclear scans require ingesting a radioactive material into the bloodstream. Then special cameras record the radiation coming from the organ being studied.

Scans commonly take 20 to 60 minutes, and patience is required because of the time it takes to get a useful picture.

RECOVERY

For hyperthyroidism treatment with radioactive iodine, patients may be kept in a hospital room for a day or so.

COMPLICATIONS AND RISKS

The radiation dose is generally quite small, and for the average patient, the cumulative exposure is insignificant.

OCCULT BLOOD TESTING

Approximately half of all colorectal cancers bleed at some time, and this bleeding is not always enough to be noticed. A laboratory test for this occult (hidden) blood is often necessary.

Occult blood testing of stool is an attempt to detect the small amounts of blood emitted by COLORECTAL CANCERS that are not otherwise visible. The test also detects blood from sources other than cancers—from meat or benign gastrointestinal problems—leading to false alarms. Despite the frequent false-positive results, the test is useful. One recent study documented the benefit, albeit modest, of a yearly occult blood test: The mortality from colon cancer over a 13-year period in people aged 50 to 80 dropped from 8 deaths per 1000 people to 5 deaths per 1000 people in those who had an occult blood screening yearly. The use of flexible sigmoidoscopy (a form of ENDOSCOPY) may be an alternative to occult blood screening.

PREPARATION

One should follow the directions included with each testing kit, but in general, to minimize the chances of a false-positive result, one should avoid red meat and ASPIRIN or other anti-inflammatory drugs such as IBUPROFEN for a few days before the test.

PROCEDURE

The test is performed by the subject at home with a special kit. Because different kit manufacturers have slightly different procedures, it is important to follow the directions on the particular package. Generally, stool is sampled over a period of three days.

COMPLICATIONS AND RISKS

There is nothing dangerous about this test, but false positive results do generate additional tests and costs (for example, ENDOSCOPY and RADIOGRAPHY).

OVARIAN CYST REMOVAL

Persistent ovarian cysts may need to be removed. Ruptured or twisted cysts may need emergency surgery. There are several techniques available for the procedure including traditional open surgery and removal with laparoscopy (a form of ENDOSCOPY).

Advances in surgical techniques have made ovarian cyst removal much less difficult in recent years.

PREOPERATIVE PREPARATION

BLOOD TESTS and possibly an ULTRASOUND may be necessary. Overnight fasting is required with general anesthesia.

ANESTHESIA

General or spinal anesthesia are the norm, but local anesthesia with sedation may be possible with laparoscopy.

PROCEDURE

For open surgery
- An incision is made in the abdomen.
- The blood vessel to the ovary is clamped.
- If the cyst is malignant, the ovary is removed.
- The incision is sewn shut in layers with sutures.

For surgery using laparoscopy (ENDOSCOPY), the procedure is performed through small puncture wounds in the abdomen.

HOSPITAL RECOVERY

An abdominal incision may require three to seven days in the hospital, less with a laparoscopy.

AT-HOME RECOVERY

Patients should limit vigorous activity for about six weeks. Sexual activity may be resumed when the doctor feels the wounds have healed.

COMPLICATIONS AND RISKS

- Infection at the site of entry through the skin
- Persistent bleeding, but this occurs rarely

PACEMAKER INSERTION

Pacemaker insertion is done to help regulate the heart rhythm, and especially to keep the heart from going too slow and causing faintness.

A pacemaker is an electronic device that helps regulate the heart rhythm and correct ARRHYTHMIAS. There are many types of pacemakers today. They all have a battery, one or more electrode wires that go to the heart, and a control center. Standard pacemakers keep the heart from going too slow in order to avoid FAINTING OR FAINTNESS or cardiac arrest. Newer types of pacemakers have features that can speed up the heart during exercise.

Related devices, such as implantable defibrillators and antitachycardia pacemakers, can deliver electrical shocks to abort abnormal rhythms automatically.

A cardiologist or cardiothoracic surgeon usually performs the procedure.

ALTERNATIVE TREATMENTS

For abnormally slow heart rhythms causing symptoms of FAINTING OR FAINTNESS, a pacemaker is the most appropriate treatment. There are some drug therapies for certain ARRHYTHMIAS, however. Some abnormally fast rhythms (called *tachycardias*) may respond to the selective use of medicaitons such as

- PROCAINAMIDE
- Quinidine
- Sotalol
- Amiodarone

PREOPERATIVE PREPARATION

ELECTROCARDIOGRAPHY and special pacing studies of the heart may be required. BLOOD TESTS to assess general health may also be performed.

ANESTHESIA

Local anesthesia is used under the collarbone near the vein where the electrode wire is passed.

PROCEDURE

- The pacemaker battery and control center are placed under the skin.

- The electrode wire is passed via one of the large veins nearby into the heart's inside wall.
- X rays (RADIOGRAPHY) are used to confirm or adjust the location of the electrode.
- The pacemaker's performance is tested and adjusted, and the incision is closed.

HOSPITAL RECOVERY

Pacemaker insertions are now done as outpatient surgery or with very brief hospital stays of one to two days. The heart is monitored with ELECTROCARDIOGRAPHY and the arm on the side of the incision is restricted in its motion for a short time.

AT-HOME RECOVERY

Vigorous activity with the arm should be avoided for a few weeks so that the electrode gets a chance to settle into the heart muscle and continue to make good electrical contact with the tissue.

Especially in the early weeks after a pacemaker insertion, antibiotics may be recommended to avoid infection in patients undergoing procedures, such as dental work, in which bacteria could be released into the blood stream.

COMPLICATIONS AND RISKS

A wound infection, purulent drainage, or FEVER can occur early after the surgery, as can excessive bleeding.

The pacemaker signal wire can dislodge or even, rarely, perforate the heart wall, although this can be adjusted again in most cases.

Pacemaker electrodes or batteries can malfunction, leading to loss of function and causing FAINTING OR FAINTNESS.

A pacemaker can be a lifesaving procedure and is well worth the risks when inserted in appropriately selected patients.

PAP SMEAR

Pap smear is short for the *Papanicolaou* smear named for the Greek physician who developed the test.

The Pap smear tests for cancer or precancerous changes in the uterine cervix (see CERVICAL CANCER). The Pap smear is performed in the office by a primary care physician or an obstetrician-gynecologist. This is a painless, though possibly uncomfortable, part of a routine pelvic examination.

Women who are sexually active or who have reached 18 years of age should have routine pelvic examinations and Pap smears.

PREPARATION

None.

PROCEDURE

- A speculum is inserted to open the vagina.
- Cells shed from the cervix are collected by means of scraping the inside of the cervix with a small wooden spatula.
- The cells collected are spread on a slide and sent to the laboratory to be examined (see CYTOLOGY).

If an abnormality is detected, further testing may be required, including

- A procedure called colposcopy (a form of ENDOSCOPY and BIOPSY)
- Another pelvic examination with insertion of a speculum to visualize the cervix
- BIOPSY of the cervix

RECOVERY

This is an outpatient procedure and is usually performed in a doctor's office.

COMPLICATIONS

Occasionally, there may be troublesome VAGINAL BLEEDING, requiring sutures to be placed. This rarely happens with the new office procedures. Other possible complications include local or systemic infections requiring antibiotic therapy. Patients should call the doctor if there is any bleeding that is heavier than a normal menstrual period (MENSTRUAL IRREGULARITIES), DIZZINESS, FEVER, or increasing pain unresponsive to mild pain medication, such as IBUPROFEN or NAPROXEN.

PENILE IMPLANT

A penile implant is a procedure in which an inflatable prosthesis is inserted into the penis. The procedure is intended as a remedy for IMPOTENCE that is otherwise untreatable.

These devices work very well and provide a reliable means of obtaining an erection suitable for intercourse.

ALTERNATIVE TREATMENTS

Self-injection of an agent that stimulates erection or a special vacuum pump can be used in some cases.

PREOPERATIVE PREPARATION

The groin area is usually shaved in the areas of the incision. Overnight fasting is required for general anesthesia.

ANESTHESIA

General anesthesia.

PROCEDURE

- An incision is made at the base of the penis.
- Incisions are made in the corporal bodies of the penis on either side of the urethra.
- The corporal bodies are dilated, or stretched, to allow the placement of the implant.
- The proper size of implant is selected and inserted along with the reservoir of fluid for inflation.
- The incision is closed with sutures.

HOSPITAL RECOVERY

The patient usually has to spend another two days in the hospital. Pain medication is prescribed as needed.

AT-HOME RECOVERY

Activity needs to be moderately restricted for several weeks after the surgery. Abstinence from sexual intercourse is required for six weeks.

COMPLICATIONS AND RISKS

Infection of the surgical wound or the area around the prosthesis is the only real danger.

PEPTIC ULCER SURGERY

Although becoming less common with the advent of new therapies for ulcers, peptic ulcer surgery is still useful and highly effective in certain circumstances.

Operations for peptic ulcer disease and ULCERS of the stomach and duodenum are performed for bleeding, obstruction of the stomach, perforation of an ulcer, malignancy (STOMACH CANCER), and failure of medical treatments to control symptoms. The operations are designed to decrease the amount of acid secreted by the stomach and to stop bleeding when it is present.

Three procedures are commonly performed for peptic ulcer disease, depending on the patient's circumstances: highly selective vagotomy, vagotomy and pyloroplasty, or vagotomy and antrectomy.

ALTERNATIVE TREATMENTS

Medical treatments for ulcers include antacids or medicines designed to decrease gastric acid secretion. Medications include CIMETIDINE, RANITIDINE, and OMEPRAZOLE.

Most cases of bleeding from ulcers spontaneously resolve and don't require surgery.

PREOPERATIVE PREPARATION

Ulcers are diagnosed preoperatively by esophagastroscopy (a form of ENDOSCOPY) or upper gastrointestinal series (see RADIOGRAPHY). Gastric ulcers should undergo BIOPSY to exclude a malignant ulcer.

A bowel preparation involving cathartics and enemas is performed, and antibiotics such as AMPICILLIN and METRONIDAZOLE are given prophylactically to avoid postoperative infectious complications.

Overnight fasting is required with general anesthesia.

ANESTHESIA

General anesthesia.

PROCEDURE

- An incision is made in the upper abdomen.
- For highly selective vagotomy, all of the branches of the vagus nerves to the stomach are cut but branches to the lower stomach, which is important for gastric emptying, and branches to other organs are spared.

- With vagotomy and pyloroplasty, the main trunks of the vagus nerves are cut, interrupting innervation to all of the abdominal organs. Gastric emptying is impaired and the opening of the stomach to the intestine is cut and resewn to allow it to empty.
- With vagotomy and antrectomy, the main vagus nerves are cut and the lower portion of the stomach is removed. The remaining stomach is then sewn to the duodenum or to the small bowel below.
- The incision is closed with sutures.

Highly selective vagotomy can be performed with laparoscopy (a form of ENDOSCOPY) through several puncture wounds in the abdominal wall.

HOSPITAL RECOVERY

Patients require pain medications such as MORPHINE and MEPERIDINE postoperatively and are not able to eat until healing has occurred. They require intravenous fluids. Recovery is quickest for patients who have had highly selective vagotomy or vagotomy and pyloroplasty. Healing after vagotomy and antrectomy is longer since part of the stomach is removed. The hospital stay generally ranges from four to seven days.

AT-HOME RECOVERY

Recovery at home requires another six to eight weeks. Patients are encouraged to return to normal activity, but should avoid lifting and strenuous activities for two months.

COMPLICATIONS AND RISKS

- DIARRHEA may occur after vagotomy. It usually improves in several weeks.
- Dumping syndrome is a complex of symptoms caused by a stomach that empties too rapidly and includes nausea, DIARRHEA, and DIZZINESS.
- Ulcers may recur.
- Anastomotic leak leads to leakage of intestinal contents from the area where the stomach was sewn to the intestine. This, in turn, leads to abscess formation or to sepsis (BLOOD POISONING).
- PNEUMONIA may result because postoperative pain may make deep breathing and coughing difficult.
- Wound infection is an unlikely possibility.

PERIODONTAL SURGERY

Nearly all periodontal surgery is preventable with good oral hygiene.

A component of preventive dental care, periodontal surgery manipulates soft (gingiva) and hard (bone) tissues supporting the teeth to correct various problems, which left uncorrected, could result in tooth loss.

ALTERNATIVE TREATMENTS

Treatment alternatives may include more frequent dental hygiene visits for nonsurgical periodontal procedures such as scaling and root planing.

PREOPERATIVE PREPARATION

Diagnostic casts to examine the occlusion as well as X rays (RADIOGRAPHY) and measurements of gingival pocket depths are used to determine the need for surgical treatment.

ANESTHESIA

Local anesthetic.

PROCEDURE

Periodontal surgery aims at reducing or eliminating gum pockets around the teeth by removing infected gingival tissue, encouraging reattachment of healthy gingival tissue, or grafting of gum tissue and bone.

Synthetic membrane barriers are used to help guide regeneration of bone. These fibers are placed into the gum lining, and synthetic bone grafts may be used.

RECOVERY

Postoperative management is performed routinely one week after treatment to see if the graft has taken. Consistent dental hygiene visits are necessary to maintain the health of the gum tissues.

COMPLICATIONS AND RISKS

On occasion, exposure of the root surface and sensitivity may be present initially after surgical treatment. Additional complications may arise if the grafted material does not function properly.

PHYSICAL EXAMINATION

Along with medical history, the physical examination is the most basic and the oldest of diagnostic explorations.

The physical examination consists of careful looking (inspection), tapping with the fingers (percussion), feeling with the fingers (palpation), and listening with a stethoscope (auscultation). Depending on the body part examined, a doctor may use all of these methods (as during an examination of the heart, lungs, or abdomen) or just one or two (during an examination of the skin). Occasionally even smell is useful; for example, ketoacidosis—a condition in DIABETES—produces a characteristic odor to the breath, and wounds that are infected can smell.

A primary care physician has a broader repertoire of physical examination techniques to choose from. A specialist may examine a patient in greater depth, but the examination is usually limited to one organ system.

PREPARATION

None.

ANESTHESIA

None.

PROCEDURE

An examination may focus on one or two body parts or be more general, depending on the patient's need, the problem, and the available time.

An almost endless number of individual steps can be performed during a physical examination. For example, hundreds of techniques can be used to test the nervous system alone.

Although it's not possible to perform a truly "complete" physical examination, a general physical exam usually consists of the basics, including

- Vital signs, including body temperature, blood pressure (see BLOOD PRESSURE TEST), pulse, respiratory rate, and general characteristics such as weight and height
- Head, eyes, ears, nose, and throat (often using special scopes)

- Neck, including the glands, the arteries that carry blood to the head, and thyroid
- Chest, including heart and lungs
- Abdomen
- Pelvic examination in women
- Scrotal examination in men
- Rectal exam both
- Legs, arms, spine, and other joints
- Skin
- Nervous system, including reflexes, muscle strength, coordination, and mental function

In recent years the belief has become more accepted that certain parts of a general screening examination are much more important than others. For example, depending on the patient's age, sex, and individual risk factors, a doctor may be much more effective spending more time on a skin or breast examination than a nervous system or joint examination.

HOSPITAL RECOVERY

None.

AT-HOME RECOVERY

None.

COMPLICATIONS AND RISKS

None. A physical examination is extremely safe.

PROSTATE GLAND REMOVAL

Removal of the prostate is an operation performed for PROSTATE CANCER that is confined to the prostate. The procedure is also used to treat advanced cases of enlarged prostate that cannot be managed by other means (see PROSTATE, ENLARGED).

The surgery is performed in the hospital and usually by a urologist. There is more than one technique in use for this surgery: the *retropubic* approach and the *perineal* approach.

For patients with cancer confined to the prostate, prostate gland removal provides an excellent chance of cure.

ALTERNATIVE TREATMENTS

Radiation therapy and hormonal (palliative) therapy are alternatives for select patients.

PREOPERATIVE PREPARATION

- A needle BIOPSY is usually needed to confirm the diagnosis.
- A bone scan is performed to look for evidence that the cancer has spread. (see NUCLEAR MEDICINE).
- The patient should have no food or drink after midnight the night before surgery.

ANESTHESIA

General anesthesia.

PROCEDURE

- In the retropubic approach, the incision is made in the lower abdomen. In the perineal approach, the incision is made in the area between the scrotum and the anus.
- The lymph nodes in the area are removed (retropubic approach only).
- The prostate gland is cut away from the urethra and the bladder.
- The gland is removed.
- The bladder and the urethra are connected to each other again.
- The external incision is closed with sutures.

HOSPITAL RECOVERY

- The patient usually has to spend another three to five days in the hospital.
- Pain medication such as ACETAMINOPHEN AND CODEINE COMBINATION is prescribed as needed.
- An intravenous line is usually left in place for two days.
- Solid food is resumed after one to two days.

AT-HOME RECOVERY

- A Foley catheter that runs from the bladder down the urethra and out the penis is left in place for two to three weeks to drain urine.
- Activity must be restricted for approximately six weeks.

COMPLICATIONS AND RISKS

The two biggest complications associated with prostate gland removal are

- INCONTINENCE—Most patients leak urine after the catheter is removed. This condition generally improves with time; after about six months, approximately 90 percent of men have no leakage problems or leak only a small amount when they are straining or lifting.
- IMPOTENCE—Despite techniques to spare the nerves responsible for achieving erection, IMPOTENCE is still common after prostatectomy.

PULMONARY FUNCTION TESTS

Pulmonary function tests measure lung size or volume and the ability to exhale air forcefully, which helps to identify lung disease.

A number of physiologic tests can be performed in a pulmonary function laboratory for the purpose of establishing lung function. These measurements often include

- The total lung volume
- The ability to exhale forcefully
- The total amount of air exhaled in a full breath
- The diffusing capacity of the lung (how quickly and evenly a gas distributes in the lung)

These tests are often used in the diagnosis of diseases such as ASTHMA, EMPHYSEMA, and chronic bronchitis (BRONCHITIS, CHRONIC).

PREPARATION

None.

PROCEDURE

To test lung volume, either the helium-dilution technique or body plethysmography are used. The helium-dilution technique involves inhaling a known volume and concentration of helium for several minutes. The concentration of helium decreases as it enters the lung. By measuring the decrease in helium concentrations caused by its larger volume of distribution, lung volume can be estimated. Body plethysmography requires patients to sit inside an air-tight box and breathe through a mouthpiece. Lung volume is determined by measuring the change in box volume and pressure.

To test the ability to exhale, patients are asked to take in a full breath and then forcefully exhale as long and hard as they can. The volume of the air exhaled in the first second of trying, called the FEV_1, can help demonstrate when airflow obstruction is present. The total amount of air exhaled from a full exhalation (called the *forced vital capacity*, or *FVC*) is also helpful in diagnosis.

Another commonly performed pulmonary function test is the diffusing capacity for carbon monoxide. In this test, patients are asked to inhale minute quantities of carbon monoxide to test the diffusion of this gas into pulmonary blood vessels.

COMPLICATIONS AND RISKS

None.

RADIAL KERATOTOMY

Radial keratotomy is a surgical procedure designed to correct nearsightedness in patients who cannot tolerate glasses or contact lenses.

In this surgery, performed on the front surface of the eye (the cornea), several spoke-like incisions are made outside the line of sight. This causes a subtle bulge of the sides of the cornea, flattening the center and reducing the degree of myopia. The operation works best in patients with a low degree of nearsightedness.

The amount of correction possible depends on the age of the patient. The older the patient, the more effect is possible with the same amount of surgery. The operation is performed by an ophthalmologist with special training in this type of corneal surgery.

ALTERNATIVE TREATMENTS

Alternative treatments include the use of glasses or contact lenses. In patients with a visually significant CATARACT, CATARACT REMOVAL with lens implant insertion will greatly reduce the preoperative nearsightedness.

PREOPERATIVE PREPARATION

Contact lenses can alter the measurements taken during the examination. Hard contact lenses should therefore be left out at least two weeks before the examination. Soft lenses should be removed at least three days before.

ANESTHESIA

The surgery is performed with anesthetic eyedrops only. The patient is sedated with a drug such as DIAZEPAM.

PROCEDURE

- The skin around the eye is cleansed and a light drape is placed over the face.
- A device is gently inserted under the lids to keep the eye open.
- The eye is numbed with a series of anesthetic drops and the corneal thickness is measured.
- The diamond-tipped instrument is then set for the depth of the individual cornea.
- The line of sight is lightly marked with a circular marker. The incisions in the periphery of the cornea will extend up to the edge of this circle.

- The cornea is lightly marked with either four or eight incisions, depending on the degree of nearsightedness, more myopia requiring more incisions.
- Marks are also made if astigmatism is to be corrected.
- Once the necessary marks have been made, the diamond blade is used to make the necessary incisions.

When the surgery is completed, an antibiotic-cortisone combination eye drop is instilled along with another eye drop that reduces postoperative pain. The patient is allowed to return home with the help of a friend or relative.

When two eyes are to be done, they are done one week apart. In this way the knowledge about the response in the first eye can be used to modify the proposed procedure on the other eye.

HOSPITAL RECOVERY

Radial keratotomy is an outpatient procedure. Except for a few moments of observation, no hospital stay is required.

AT-HOME RECOVERY

Drops are used in the eye for one week. The patient should not swim with the head under water for two weeks after surgery. Until the vision has stabilized and the eyes are comfortable, it is unwise to operate dangerous machinery.

COMPLICATIONS AND RISKS

Scratchy discomfort is usually present for up to a week after radial keratotomy. Glare, light sensitivity, and fluctuation of vision are common after surgery and subside by about six weeks. Patients may observe a slight ghost image around objects and may feel it takes a second for images to focus clearly. This symptom also seems to subside with time. Undercorrection and overcorrection may occur with this procedure. Complications such as infection, perforation, postoperative wound rupture, CATARACT, and retinal detachment are very rare. There is ample evidence to suggest that the effect in moderate to higher degrees of nearsighted surgical correction may not be stable after one year.

RADIOGRAPHY

When diseases or abnormalities are suspected, radiography is used to view internal parts of the body.

Using X rays to take pictures of parts of the body not easily seen is called *radiography*. X rays can identify broken or diseased bones, chest abnormalities, or signs of perforated organs in the abdomen. Special X-ray techniques can detect foreign bodies such as glass under the skin; they can also be used to detect signs of BREAST CANCER (a test called *mammography*).

Primary care physicians, emergency medicine physicians, surgeons, and other specialists all use X rays for one reason or another.

Some X rays require injection of special dye, or contrast material, to make certain structures better visible on the X-ray film. The contrast material may be injected into a vein in the arm or via a catheter directly into blood vessels near the body part being studied; for example, in an angiogram, the dye is injected into the blood vessels that are under examination. Other X rays require drinking a liquid with barium in it (the upper gastrointestinal, or GI, series) or running barium into the colon (the lower GI series) to enhance X-ray images of the esophagus, stomach, and intestines.

PREPARATION

Individuals who are allergic to the contrast material used for some X rays may need special preparation with antihistamines or other drugs to suppress adverse reactions. Such drugs include PREDNISONE and DIPHENHYDRAMINE.

If there is any chance of pregnancy, the patient should discuss it with her doctor, because X rays may cause abnormalities in the early development of a fetus.

Some examinations require fasting.

ANESTHESIA

None.

PROCEDURE

- Contrast material, if any is needed, is administered, orally or by injection.
- The patient is positioned in front of the source of the X rays.

- A special film is placed behind the patient to receive the X-ray image.
- A lead apron can be placed over areas not in the picture.
- The technician usually steps out of the room, and the picture is taken.

RECOVERY

None, except that angiograms or delayed films (if needed) may require a few hours.

COMPLICATIONS AND RISKS

- The risk of X rays is generally insignificant except to a fetus early in development. However, some X rays involve more radiation than others, and excessive repeat examinations over a period of years could increase a person's risk for certain cancers or LEUKEMIA. Therefore, doctors try to order X rays only when necessary.
- The radiation from a chest X ray is said to be comparable to the amount one would get from a day on the beach.
- Allergic reactions to contrast materials can range from mild flushing to wheezing, low blood pressure, or even death. Serious reactions are extremely rare and can be treated promptly with DIPHENHYDRAMINE, fluids, and epinephrine.
- There is an extremely small risk of perforation of the colon with a lower GI series.

RECTAL- OR COLON POLYP REMOVAL

Some types of rectal or colon polyps should be removed because they are either cancerous or have the potential to become malignant.

A COLON POLYP or rectal polyp is an abnormal growth in the colon or rectum. It may be benign, but many benign polyps have the potential to become malignant (to become COLORECTAL CANCER) and should be removed. Many polyps contain cancer already and have to be removed. Polyps may be removed without surgery using colonoscopy (a form of ENDOSCOPY). Other polyps are too large or too broad based for colposcopy and require more traditional surgical removal in a hospital setting.

ALTERNATIVE TREATMENTS

A polyp that is small (less than four millimeters in diameter) can be observed with regular ENDOSCOPY, but usually it is easier to remove it.

PREOPERATIVE PREPARATION

Patients who are to undergo polyp removal receive a mechanical bowel preparation. This consists of the removal of fecal contents by beginning a liquid diet one to two days before the operation. Later, a large volume of nonabsorbable liquid is ingested or laxatives are given to clear the intestine of feces. Some patients also require enemas.

Patients undergoing surgical removal are also given oral nonabsorbable antibiotics to kill bacteria in the bowel and, therefore, lessen any chance of postoperative infection. The patient is not allowed any food or water after midnight on the night preceding polyp removal.

ANESTHESIA

Endoscopic polypectomy can be performed with sedation alone. Surgical removal of polyps requires a general anesthetic.

PROCEDURE

Endoscopic polypectomy:

- A flexible scope is passed through the rectum and colon.

- The polyp is located and the feasibility of resection is assessed.
- A wire snare is passed through the scope and looped around the base of the polyp.
- The loop is tightened and electrocautery is used to cut the base of the polyp and coagulate any blood.
- When free, the polyp is grasped, taken out through the anus, and sent to the laboratory for pathologic examination.

Surgical removal of a polyp:

- An abdominal incision is made.
- Although the growth can be removed by opening the colon and removing the polyp, it is more often removed with a whole segment of colon because the patient will then be properly treated if cancer is later found in the polyp (see SIGMOID COLON REMOVAL).

HOSPITAL RECOVERY

Endoscopic polyp removal can be performed as an outpatient procedure or with a short hospital stay. Surgical removal requires more extensive recovery (see SIGMOID COLON REMOVAL).

AT-HOME RECOVERY

Endoscopic polyp removal requires no special at-home recovery. Recovery from open surgical removal may require several weeks (see SIGMOID COLON REMOVAL).

COMPLICATIONS AND RISKS

- Perforation of the bowel may occur with endoscopic polyp removal.
- RECTAL BLEEDING may occur after endoscopic polyp removal.
- See SIGMOID COLON REMOVAL for complications of surgical polyp removal.

Sigmoid colon removal is performed if there are benign or malignant tumors or other diseases present in the area.

SIGMOID COLON REMOVAL

The sigmoid colon is removed most frequently for benign and malignant tumors (COLORECTAL CANCER) and for diverticulitis (DIVERTICULAR DISEASE). It is occasionally removed if the colon twists on itself (a condition called *volvulus*), for inflammatory disease of the colon such as CROHN DISEASE, and for ENDOMETRIOSIS. The operation is performed by general or colorectal surgeons.

ALTERNATIVE TREATMENTS

Endoscopic polyp removal (see RECTAL- OR COLON POLYP REMOVAL) may be an option for smaller tumors.

PREOPERATIVE PREPARATION

Patients receive a mechanical and antibiotic bowel preparation. This consists of the removal of fecal contents by beginning a liquid diet one to two days before surgery. Later, a large volume of nonabsorbable liquid is ingested or laxatives are given by mouth to clear the intestine of feces. Some patients also require enemas. Finally, oral nonabsorbable antibiotics are given to kill bacteria in the bowel. Overnight fasting is required for general anesthesia.

ANESTHESIA

General anesthesia.

PROCEDURE

- An abdominal incision is usually made vertically down the middle.
- The blood supply to the sigmoid colon and the fatty tissue in which it runs (mesocolon) is divided between clamps and tied with sutures.
- The bowel is clamped and divided above and below the diseased area.
- The affected segment is removed.
- Colonic continuity is restored either by suturing the ends together or by stapling them with a specially designed colonic stapling device.
- If a COLOSTOMY is required, the colon is brought out through the abdominal wall.
- The abdominal wall is closed in layers with sutures.

HOSPITAL RECOVERY

Intestinal motility decreases after the operation, and patients do not tolerate oral nutrition or fluid until bowel function returns. Bowel function, manifest by return of bowel sounds and passing of flatus and feces, returns in about three to five days. Intravenous fluids and pain medications such as MORPHINE and MEPERIDINE are required until that time. Once bowel function resumes, a liquid diet is begun and patients are advanced to a regular diet as tolerated. Intravenous fluids are stopped and oral medications such as an ACETAMINOPHEN AND CODEINE COMBINATION begun.

The patient is encouraged to get out of bed and walk as soon as possible and to cough and deep breathe to avoid respiratory complications.

Patients are discharged from the hospital as soon as they are on a regular diet. This usually requires seven to ten days.

AT-HOME RECOVERY

Recovery at home requires another several weeks. Patients gradually increase their activity as pain subsides. Bowel habits usually return to normal as the patient resumes normal dietary habits and daily routines.

Patients may drive a car when their pain has subsided and they are not taking pain medications that cause drowsiness.

COMPLICATIONS AND RISKS

- Postoperative ileus is prolonged loss of motility after abdominal surgery. Eating causes ABDOMINAL SWELLING and VOMITING. The patient may require parenteral nutrition (nutrition not delivered orally). Prolonged ileus usually resolves spontaneously, but it does prolong hospitalization.
- Postoperative INTESTINAL OBSTRUCTION can be caused by scars from the operation or problems at the area where the bowel was sewn together.
- Anastomotic leak is a failure of the intestine to heal, causing leaking of intestinal contents, an abscess, or soiling of the abdominal cavity.
- PNEUMONIA may result because postoperative pain may make deep breathing and coughing difficult.
- Wound infection is an unlikely possibility.

SPLEEN REMOVAL

Spleen removal is performed to remove and evaluate the extent of tumors, to treat abscesses, and to remove the organ when it is trapping and sequestering blood cells or platelets.

The spleen is an organ in the upper left abdomen, which is part of the immune system. It also clears old and damaged blood components from the circulation. The spleen can be involved with malignant tumors (especially lymphoma [see LYMPHOMA, NON-HODGKIN]), can develop abscesses, and may enlarge considerably in response to other systemic illnesses. Spleen removal (splenectomy) may be necessary to remove and evaluate the extent of tumors, to treat abscesses, or to remove the organ when it is trapping and sequestering blood cells. Finally, the spleen is susceptible to injury during trauma to the chest, flank, and abdomen. Removal of the spleen may be necessary to stop bleeding.

Splenectomy is performed by a trauma or general surgeon.

ALTERNATIVE TREATMENTS

Most disorders of the spleen are treated initially with medications such as PREDNISONE for autoimmune diseases. Removal of the spleen is performed when medical treatment is not effective.

Techniques have been developed to remove the spleen using laparoscopy (a form of ENDOSCOPY), which decreases postoperative pain and time to complete recovery.

PREOPERATIVE PREPARATION

Patients undergoing elective removal of the spleen receive pneumococcal vaccine several weeks before operation. BLOOD TESTS and ELECTROCARDIOGRAPHY are sometimes performed to assess general health before the operation. Overnight fasting is required with general anesthesia.

ANESTHESIA

General anesthesia.

PROCEDURE

For surgical removal

- An incision is made in the middle of the upper abdomen or below the left rib cage.
- The spleen's attachments to other organs are cut.
- The splenic artery and vein (the main blood supply) are then tied with sutures and divided.

- The spleen is removed.
- The abdominal wound is closed in layers with sutures and the skin is closed with sutures or clips.

For laparoscopic removal

- Five or six puncture wounds are made.
- A video camera is inserted through one of these wounds and instruments through the others.
- The surgeon and assistants remove the spleen while watching the surgery on a video monitor.
- The surgery is similar to the open procedure described above.
- The spleen is divided into smaller pieces and is removed through one of the puncture wounds.
- The puncture wounds are closed with sutures.

HOSPITAL RECOVERY

Patients undergoing open splenectomy remain in the hospital for three to ten days, depending on the reason for removal of their spleen. They are not able to take liquids or foods early after the surgery and need intravenous fluids and medications such as MORPHINE and MEPERIDINE.

Patients who undergo laparoscopic removal of the spleen remain in the hospital for one to five days.

AT-HOME RECOVERY

Postoperative convalescence at home is variable and ranges from two to eight weeks for open operation and from one to three weeks for laparoscopic surgery. Patients may require oral pain medication such as an ACETAMINOPHEN AND CODEINE COMBINATION.

Patients may drive a car when their pain has subsided and they are not taking pain medications that cause drowsiness.

COMPLICATIONS AND RISKS

- Postoperative bleeding may occur.
- An intra-abdominal abscess causes FEVER, ABDOMINAL PAIN, and prolonged recovery.
- PNEUMONIA may result because postoperative incisional pain may make deep breathing and coughing difficult.
- Wound infection is an unlikely possibility.

THYROIDECTOMY

The thyroid gland is located in the neck. Its hormone is vital to proper metabolic functioning. A number of conditions related to the thyroid gland may require surgical treatment.

A surgeon treats three groups of patients with thyroid disease: those with an overactive gland (HYPERTHYROIDISM), those with an underactive gland (HYPOTHYROIDISM), and those with suspicious masses (tumors, cysts, or nodules) in the gland. Removal of all or part of the thyroid may be required in each of these situations. The operation is performed by a general surgeon, an endocrine surgeon, or an otolaryngologist (an ear, nose, and throat specialist).

Surgery is also performed for goiter—a benign enlargement of the gland—when the goiter causes symptoms.

Alternative treatments

HYPERTHYROIDISM may be treated with antithyroid drugs and radioactive iodine. The type of treatment is based on many factors, including the patients age, other medical conditions, and the severity and progression of the disease.

HYPOTHYROIDISM can be treated with replacement of thyroid hormone.

Nodules in the thyroid gland consist of masses that function and those that do not (cysts and solid) growths. Cysts may be treated with thyroid hormone if they show no signs of cancer on aspiration. Functioning nodules may be observed if the patient does not have HYPERTHYROIDISM.

Preoperative preparation

Patients should have thyroid function tests (see BLOOD TESTS) and a thyroid scan (see NUCLEAR MEDICINE). Patients with nodules should also undergo BIOPSY to distinguish among cysts, benign nodules, and cancer.

Patients with HYPERTHYROIDISM who are candidates for surgery require suppression of the gland with iodine alone or with a combination of iodine and propylthiouracil. Some patients are also given PROPRANOLOL to block the effects of thyroid hormone on other organs.

BLOOD TESTS and ELECTROCARDIOGRAPHY, among other tests of general health, are standard before almost any surgery. Overnight fasting is required with general anesthesia.

Anesthesia

General anesthesia.

PROCEDURE

- An incision is made across the lower neck and skin flaps are made above and below the incision.
- The muscles covering the thyroid gland are retracted or divided and the gland is exposed. The vein to the middle of the gland and the arteries to the top and the bottom are identified, tied off, and cut.
- The lobe is removed from the windpipe with the isthmus (the portion that connects the two lobes).
- If the entire gland is to be removed, the opposite lobe is removed in a similar manner.
- The wounds are closed with sutures or clips.

HOSPITAL RECOVERY

Hospital stay is usually one to two days. Patients usually experience postoperative pain and require pain medications such as ACETAMINOPHEN AND CODEINE COMBINATION.

Sutures may be removed in three to five days.

AT-HOME RECOVERY

Patients who have had a total thyroidectomy require lifetime replacement of thyroid hormone.

COMPLICATIONS

- Thyroid storm refers to a severe case of HYPERTHYROIDISM that may occur in patients who have not been prepared adequately preoperatively with antithyroid medications.
- A hematoma is a collection of blood beneath the wound. If large, it can press on the windpipe and interfere with breathing.
- Injury to the recurrent laryngeal nerve causes paralysis of the vocal cord and a hoarse voice.
- HYPOTHYROIDISM will occur when all or most of the thyroid gland is removed. It is treated by giving thyroid hormone replacement.

TRACHEOSTOMY

Tracheostomy is often performed as an emergency procedure when airway obstruction is acute.

A tracheostomy is a procedure that establishes an alternative pathway for the passage of air while breathing. An opening is made in the neck into the trachea (the windpipe) to allow passage of air if the upper airway is obstructed or if long-term ventilation of the lungs is required.

Indications for tracheostomy fall into three major categories, including

- Upper airway obstruction resulting from tumors such as LARYNGEAL CANCER, trauma, infection, neuromuscular disorders, or malformations
- Diseases of the lungs such as EMPHYSEMA or severe PNEUMONIA that require prolonged ventilator support
- The inability of the patient to manage secretions from either the mouth or the lungs

Surgeons and emergency medicine physicians are trained in this procedure.

ALTERNATIVE TREATMENTS

When an emergency airway is required there are several options. Often ventilation can be achieved using an oxygen mask over the nose and mouth. An endotracheal tube can be passed through the mouth and larynx and into the trachea if this is medically safe and possible.

PREOPERATIVE PREPARATION

In an emergency setting, there is often little time for preoperative preparation.

When the tracheostomy is elective, routine preoperative tests such as BLOOD COUNT and other BLOOD TESTS are performed.

Overnight fasting is required with general anesthesia.

ANESTHESIA

Anesthesia may be either general or local. Local anesthesia is often combined with sedation.

PROCEDURE

- An incision is made in the front of the neck over the trachea.

- The midline of the muscles of the trachea is identified and the muscles are gently separated.
- Retraction is used to hold the muscles to the sides, exposing the area of the trachea and the thyroid.
- An opening is made in the front wall of the trachea and secretions are immediately suctioned out.
- A tube is placed through the opening into the trachea, sutured to the skin, and secured around the neck with a cloth band.

HOSPITAL RECOVERY

Recovery usually includes a one night stay in the intensive care unit followed by one week in the hospital. During this time, the patient and caregivers learn proper care and cleaning of the tracheostomy tube.

AT-HOME RECOVERY

Recovery at home is centered on proper care of the tracheostomy tube. Since the normal airflow is diverted from the nose, the functions of air humidification and clearance of secretions are altered. Initially the patient will require humidified air. Suctioning of secretions from the lungs with a catheter is necessary.

A tracheostomy can be temporary. When the tube is removed, the opening will slowing close by contracture of scarring. A few patients will need an operation to completely close the opening.

COMPLICATIONS AND RISKS

A blockage of the tube may occur if the tube is not cleaned frequently enough to keep it clear. Mucus or dried secretions may plug the trachea or deeper bronchi in the lungs if proper humidification and suctioning are not observed.

The tracheostomy tube may become dislodged from the trachea if the cloth ties securing it around the neck are not kept snug.

Finally, in rare cases, there may be bleeding from the tube. Bleeding from the trachea is potentially a very serious sign of erosion of the tracheostomy tube into an artery.

TUBAL LIGATION

Tubal ligation is a highly effective, permanent contraceptive procedure that only women who do not desire any more children should undergo.

Tubal ligation is a permanent form of contraception. This procedure should be considered only by women who have completed childbearing or by women who do not desire to bear children. Tubal ligation is highly effective: Less than 0.5 percent of patients undergoing the procedure become pregnant. However, if the procedure fails, approximately 50 percent of pregnancies will be ectopic. Therefore, if a woman misses a period following tubal ligation, a pregnancy test is mandatory. Should the test be positive, the woman must seek immediate medical care.

Alternative treatments

Alternatives to tubal ligation include VASECTOMY for the woman's partner and injectable or implantable hormonal contraceptives. These methods are as effective as tubal ligation. However, the latter two are reversible. Other birth control methods such as intrauterine devices (IUDs) and barrier methods are available, but are not as consistently effective as surgical sterilization.

Preoperative preparation

In order to reduce the risk of pregnancy at the time of the surgery, tubal ligation should be performed within the first ten days of the menstrual cycle. A BLOOD COUNT and pregnancy test are done upon admission. Overnight fasting is required for general anesthesia.

Anesthesia

The majority of tubal ligations are performed under general anesthesia, although spinal anesthesia is an alternative.

Procedure

For tubal ligation performed by laparoscopy (a form of ENDOSCOPY)

- Two incisions, a half inch in size, are made at the belly button and pubic area.
- A laparoscope is inserted through the lower incision.
- Gas is used to distend the abdomen.

- The pelvis is examined.
- A segment of the fallopian tube is destroyed, which prohibits the passage of the egg and sperm so that fertilization of the egg does not occur.
- The laparoscope is then removed, the gas allowed to escape, and the incisions at the belly button and pubic area are closed with sutures.

Vaginal and postpartum tubal ligations entail a different approach, but most tubal ligations are performed laparoscopically.

HOSPITAL RECOVERY

A tubal ligation is an outpatient procedure. After the surgery, a nurse monitors vital signs and observes the patient for surgical or anesthetic complications. Pain medicine such as an ACETAMINOPHEN AND CODEINE COMBINATION may be administered, and most patients will get drowsy.

If no problems arise, the patient will be given liquids, and when able, will be assisted to the rest room. Most patients remain in the recovery room for approximately two hours after the procedure. Rarely, patients will experience nausea and VOMITING severe enough to require an overnight stay.

AT-HOME RECOVERY

Upon arrival home, the patient should rest. Fluids and a bland diet are best the day of surgery. IBUPROFEN is effective for relief of cramping. Driving is not recommended for 24 hours following surgery, but within three days of surgery, the patient should be able to resume normal activities. Intercourse and use of tampons are restricted for two weeks after tubal ligation.

COMPLICATIONS AND RISKS

Major complications of tubal ligation are rare (less than one percent). They include internal bleeding and intra-abdominal infection. A laparotomy (incision of the abdomen) may be needed to correct these complications. Death occurs in 1 in 30,000 procedures.

ULTRASONIC LITHOTRIPSY

Ultrasonic lithotripsy is a procedure in which kidney stones or gallstones are broken into fragments, using shock waves.

An ultrasonic lithotripter is a device designed to fragment KIDNEY STONES and GALLSTONES without surgery. After fragmentation, the pieces of the stone either pass spontaneously in urine or bile, are dissolved, or must be removed using ENDOSCOPY or surgical techniques.

ALTERNATIVE TREATMENTS

See KIDNEY STONES and GALLSTONES.

PREOPERATIVE PREPARATION

Stones must be identified before the procedure with X rays (RADIOGRAPHY) for KIDNEY STONES, and ULTRASOUND for GALLSTONES. Overnight fasting is required for general anesthesia.

ANESTHESIA

Intravenous sedation or general anesthesia is used.

PROCEDURE

- The patient is placed into a water bath or in contact with a gel-filled flexible membrane.
- Shock waves are sent through the water or gel.
- X rays (RADIOGRAPHY) for KIDNEY STONES, or ULTRASOUND for GALLSTONES are used to locate the stones.
- Shock waves are generated by the lithotripter and focused precisely on the stone.
- Fragmentation requires multiple shock waves.

HOSPITAL RECOVERY

Patients are discharged the same or the next day.

AT-HOME RECOVERY

Patients may require pain medication such as an ACETAMINOPHEN AND CODEINE COMBINATION after treatment.

COMPLICATIONS AND RISKS

- Shock waves can damage tissues near the stone.
- Patients can experience bleeding in the urine or bile.

ULTRASOUND

Ultrasound uses sound waves like sonar to bounce off a body part under the skin. The reflection can be used to give a picture of the shape and consistency of the internal organs. Ultrasound has a wide variety of uses including looking for GALLSTONES, clots in blood vessels, or ATHEROSCLEROSIS. When used for studying the heart valves and heart muscle, it is called *echocardiography*.

Unlike other radiologic imaging techniques, ultrasound uses no radiation and no iodonated contrast materials or dyes.

PREPARATION

There may be minor preparation, such as drinking lots of fluids to fill the bladder, before certain pelvic ultrasounds.

PROCEDURE

- When the test is to be performed entirely externally, a special gel is put on the skin to help the ultrasound probe make optimal contact with the skin.
- The transducer—the device that generates and collects the sound waves—is placed in direct contact with the skin and passed over the area to be viewed.
- The pictures can be seen in real time on a video monitor or as still images.

There are also special ultrasound probes that are passed into the body. Examples of these include a rectal probe to look at the prostate, a vaginal probe to look at the pelvic organs, a probe on an endoscope (see ENDOSCOPY) to go down the esophagus to look at the heart and aorta (transesophageal echocardiography), and even special ultrasound probes that can pass through the skin into an artery.

RECOVERY

Usually, no observation is required for an ultrasound. In the case of passing an ultrasound catheter into an artery, an overnight stay may be necessary. If a sedative is used, then observation for an hour or so may be needed.

COMPLICATIONS AND RISKS

Routine ultrasound tests are without any significant side effects. If an artery is penetrated to study it from the inside, there is a small chance of bleeding and other risks.

URINALYSIS

A urinalysis helps in the diagnosis of many conditions affecting the kidneys, urinary tract, liver, and other metabolic functions.

Urine is the liquid produced by the continuous filtration of blood by the kidneys. The kidneys are very efficient, so urine should not contain any blood sugar or blood cells, and only minimal amounts of protein.

Urine is a "window" to the kidneys and can serve as an important clue to kidney function, urinary tract infections, and even liver and other metabolic diagnoses. Urine can also be analyzed for additional chemicals and special proteins. In some cases, a 24-hour collection is needed.

PREPARATION

When looking for infection, caution must be used in the collecting of a urine specimen to minimize contamination with skin near the urethra, the passageway and body opening where urine comes out. Prolonged standing can affect the amount of protein lost in the urine in some individuals, so specific instructions may be given if this is suspected.

PROCEDURE

- The opening of the urethra to the outside of the body is cleansed with a sterile pad.
- The middle portion of the urine stream (after the first few seconds) is the portion that is caught in a sterile cup.
- The sample is sent to the lab for analysis.

RECOVERY

None.

COMPLICATIONS AND RISKS

None.

VARICOSE VEIN REMOVAL

VARICOSE VEINS, found usually in the legs, result when the valves of the veins break and are unable to keep blood from backing up. Blood has a tendency to stagnate in the dilated veins. Because the pressure inside VARICOSE VEINS is greater than that of normal veins, the veins are engorged and visible on the surface of the skin.

A tendency to develop VARICOSE VEINS seems to run in families. Other predisposing factors include previous clots or inflammations of the leg veins, called thrombophlebitis, or any condition that obstructs the normal outflow of the venous blood from the legs, such as pregnancy, tight garments, or OBESITY.

Because there is no evidence that proves the removal of superficial leg veins will truly alter the course of disease due to varicose veins, removal of the superficial veins is considered a cosmetic procedure.

ALTERNATIVE TREATMENTS

The first approach to VARICOSE VEINS should be the use of support stockings with pressure capacities between 30 and 50 mm Hg. Elevating the legs, avoiding prolonged standing, and removing any potential outlet obstruction of the legs are important first steps. However, once the valves in the veins are broken, or collapsed, there is no way to repair them. In rare severe cases, deep vein replacement surgery can be attempted.

There are no strictly medical therapies that eliminate VARICOSE VEINS.

For very small, thin VARICOSE VEINS, or small dilated surface blood vessels, another technique is available. The surgeon can introduce a small needle into the vessel and inject salty water or a chemical that causes the vessel to contract and become occluded (closed off). This procedure is called *sclerotherapy.* After the procedure, the patient usually wears a compression bandage or garment to keep the treated, sclerosed veins occluded and allow scar formation to make the occlusion permanent.

Newer technology consists of machines that emit laser light. One wavelength of laser light is very well absorbed by the pigment inside the blood vessels but not by skin tissues. Therefore, the laser light can obliterate vessels containing red blood cells and not injure the other skin tissues. This technology is starting to be used to treat small superficial vessels in the skin of the legs that patients wish to have removed for cosmetic reasons.

PREOPERATIVE PREPARATION

None.

ANESTHESIA

Usually none is needed for sclerotherapy. For vein removal, a local anesthetic is used.

PROCEDURE

- The surgeon makes an incision in the skin above the vein.
- The varicose vein is then cut through and tied off at both ends of the cut with a suture.
- The surgeon performs the same procedure at another part of the same vein some distance away.
- The surgeon can then remove the tied-off vein through the skin. (The patient is left with two small scars at each end of the site where the vein was removed.)

Again, whether this procedure prevents the occurrence of conditions resulting from VARICOSE VEINS is controversial, but it definitely removes the unsightly vein.

HOSPITAL RECOVERY

The procedure is usually performed on an outpatient basis and requires no hospital stay.

AT-HOME RECOVERY

Wound care is necessary for the first few weeks.

COMPLICATIONS AND RISKS

Excessive bleeding and local wound infection are possibilities but are rare.

VASECTOMY

Vasectomy is a minor surgical procedure to cut the tubes that carry sperm from the testes to the urethra. The elective procedure is done for sterilization only. Usually performed by a urologist, vasectomy takes place in an outpatient setting.

Vasectomy is probably the most effective form of birth control. The procedure is simple and very safe.

ALTERNATIVE TREATMENTS

There are no other options as far as male sterilization is concerned. Other methods of birth control are available, of course.

PREOPERATIVE PREPARATION

The scrotum is usually shaved in the areas of the incision. Otherwise, there are no special preparations.

ANESTHESIA

Local anesthesia.

PROCEDURE

- A small incision is made in the skin of the scrotum.
- The vas deferens (the duct that runs from each testicle) is identified and cut; the ends are then tied off.
- The incision is sewn up.
- The procedure is then repeated on the opposite side.

A postoperative semen analysis is sometimes performed to ensure the absence of sperm. Other birth control is necessary until the laboratory studies confirm the sterility.

RECOVERY

Activity should be restricted for one or two days. Oral pain medication such as an ACETAMINOPHEN AND CODEINE COMBINATION may be prescribed if necessary. It can be helpful to wear underwear with good scrotal support (briefs, for example) for a few weeks after surgery.

COMPLICATIONS

Complications are very uncommon. The only dangers are the remote possibility of infection at the wound sight and excessive bleeding.

A visual acuity test is given to determine the level of visual function and to help provide a prescription for correction if vision is not normal.

VISUAL ACUITY

Measurement of visual acuity is one way to determine a patient's level of visual function. The most common method employs the Snellen visual acuity chart. This chart is comprised of a series of letters or optotypes, larger at the top and smaller at the bottom. A person with normal vision should be able to see a series of smaller letters at a distance of 20 feet. If these are the smallest letters the patient can see, the visual acuity is reported as 20/20. If an individual can see letters that are even smaller, the visual acuity, depending on the line accurately read, may be 20/15 or 20/10. This would mean that a person with normal vision would be required to move closer than 20 feet to see letters designed to be read at 15 or even 10 feet. If a person can only see larger letters, e.g., the 20/50 line, this would mean that he or she could see the letters at 20 feet, while a person with normal eyesight could stand 50 feet away and still see the letters. Legal blindness can be defined as a visual acuity of 20/200 or less in the better-seeing eye.

PROCEDURE

The test is administered in either a dim or moderately illuminated room with the target 20 feet from the subject. Sometimes mirrors are used to simulate a 20-foot distance in a room that is not that long. The test may be administered with or without glasses.

- One eye is covered, and the fellow eye is tested.
- The ophthalmologist places different lenses in front of the open eye in an effort to determine which combination of lenses results in the best possible performance on the visual acuity test.
- The second eye is tested in the same manner, while the fellow eye is covered.
- Both eyes are tested simultaneously to determine the best combination of lenses for visual acuity.

COMPLICATIONS AND RISKS

None.

PART III: PRESCRIPTION DRUGS

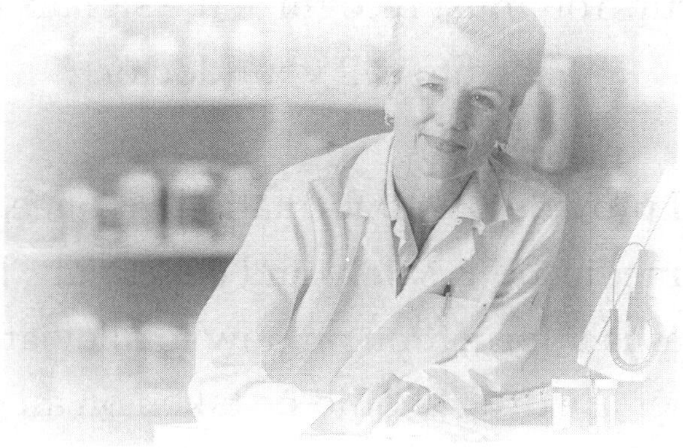

The right drug for the right patient in the right dose at the right time. This rule sums up the decisions made when your doctor gives you a prescription. You've helped make those decisions by giving your doctor your complete medical history, which should include any previous allergic reactions you've suffered, any other drugs you may be taking, and any chronic health problems you may have. Once you leave your doctor's office with your prescription in hand, however, you have still more to do as a responsible patient and a smart consumer.

Drug therapy is an important component of health care. Once you receive a prescription, you must know how and when to properly administer your medication. You must understand and comply with your dosage schedule. You must know what to do to prevent certain side effects and how to handle any side effects that might occur. You must recognize the signals that indicate the need to call your doctor.

Part III provides the information you need to take prescription medications safely and effectively. Included in the drug profiles is information on how to alleviate certain side effects, whether the drug should be taken on an empty stomach or with meals, whether it is likely to affect your ability to drive, and whether generic equivalents are available for a prescribed trade-name medication. You will discover which side effects are common to some medications and which side effects constitute danger signals that require immediate attention from your physician.

Of course, your doctor and pharmacist are your best sources of information about the medications prescribed to you, but it doesn't hurt to be as informed as you can be about the treatments affecting your body.

acetaminophen and codeine combination

BRAND NAMES (Manufacturers)
acetaminophen with codeine (various manufacturers)
Aceta with Codeine (Century)
Capital with Codeine (Carnrick)
Phenaphen-650 with Codeine (Robins)
Phenaphen with Codeine (Robins)
Tylenol with Codeine (McNeil)
Ty-tabs (Major)

TYPE OF DRUG
Analgesic combination

INGREDIENTS
acetaminophen and codeine

DOSAGE FORMS
Tablets (300 mg acetaminophen with 7.5 mg, 15 mg, 30 mg, or 60 mg codeine; 325 mg acetaminophen with 30 mg or 60 mg codeine; 650 mg acetaminophen with 30 mg codeine)
Capsules (325 mg acetaminophen with 15 mg, 30 mg, or 60 mg codeine)
Oral elixir (120 mg acetaminophen and 12 mg codeine per 5-ml spoonful, with 7% alcohol)
On the label of the vial of tablets or capsules, the name of this drug may be followed by a number that refers to the amount of codeine present (#1 has 7.5 mg codeine, #2 has 15 mg codeine, #3 has 30 mg codeine, and #4 has 60 mg codeine).

STORAGE
This medication should be stored at room temperature. It should never be frozen.

USES

Acetaminophen and codeine combination is used to relieve mild to severe pain (formulations of this medication with higher codeine contents are used to relieve more severe pain). Codeine is a narcotic analgesic that acts upon on the central nervous system (brain and spinal cord) to relieve pain.

TREATMENT

In order to avoid stomach upset, you can take this medication with food or milk.

This medication works most effectively if you take it at the onset of pain, rather than waiting until the pain becomes intense.

Measure the dose of the liquid form of this medication carefully with a specially designed 5-ml measuring spoon. An ordinary kitchen teaspoon is not accurate enough for measuring the dosage.

If you are taking this medication on a regular schedule and you miss a dose, take the missed dose as soon as possible, unless it is almost time for the next dose. In that case, don't take the missed dose at all; return to your regular dosing schedule. Do not double the next dose.

SIDE EFFECTS

Minor. Constipation, dizziness, drowsiness, dry mouth, false sense of well-being, flushing, light-headedness, loss of appetite, nausea, painful or difficult urination, or sweating. These side effects should disappear as your body adjusts to the medication.

If you are constipated, increase the amount of fiber in your diet (fresh fruits and vegetables, salads, bran, and whole-grain breads), exercise, and drink more water (unless your doctor directs you to do otherwise).

To reduce mouth dryness, chew sugarless gum or suck on ice chips or hard candy.

If you feel dizzy or light-headed, sit or lie down for a while; get up slowly from a sitting or reclining position; and be careful on stairs.

Major. Tell your doctor about any side effects that are persistent or particularly bothersome. IT IS ESPECIALLY IMPORTANT TO TELL YOUR DOCTOR about anxiety, difficulty in breathing, excitation, fatigue, palpitations, rash, restlessness, sore throat and fever, tremors, unusual bleeding or bruising, weakness, or yellowing of the eyes or skin.

INTERACTIONS

This medication interacts with several other types of drugs:

1. Concurrent use with other central nervous system depressants (such as alcohol, antihistamines, barbiturates, benzodiazepine tranquilizers, muscle relaxants, and phenothiazine tranquilizers) or with tricyclic antidepressants can cause extreme drowsiness.

2. A monoamine oxidase (MAO) inhibitor taken within 14 days of this medication can lead to unpredictable and severe side effects.

3. Long-term use and high doses of the acetaminophen portion of this medication can increase the effects of oral anticoagulants (blood thinners, such as warfarin); this combination may lead to bleeding complications.

4. Anticonvulsants (antiseizure medications), barbiturates, and alcohol can increase the liver toxicity caused by large doses of the acetaminophen portion of this medication.

BE SURE TO TELL YOUR DOCTOR about any medications you are currently taking, especially any listed above.

WARNINGS

• Tell your doctor about unusual or allergic reactions you have had to any medications, especially to acetaminophen, codeine, or other narcotic analgesics (such as hydrocodone, hydromorphone, meperidine, methadone, morphine, oxycodone, and propoxyphene).

• Tell your doctor if you now have or if you have ever had an acute abdominal condition, asthma, a blood disorder, brain disease, colitis, epilepsy, gallstones or gallbladder disease, head injuries, heart disease, kidney disease, liver disease, lung disease, mental illness, prostate disease, thyroid disease, or urethral strictures.

• If this drug makes you dizzy or drowsy, do not take part in any activity that requires alertness, such as driving a car or operating potentially dangerous equipment.

• Before having surgery or any other medical or dental treatment, be sure to tell your doctor or dentist that you are taking this medication.

• Because this product contains codeine, it has the potential for abuse and must be used with caution. Usually, it should not be taken on a regular schedule for longer than ten days at a time. Tolerance develops quickly; do not increase the dosage or stop taking the drug abruptly unless you first consult your doctor. If you have been taking large amounts of this medication for long periods, you may experience a withdrawal reaction (diarrhea, excessive yawning, gooseflesh, irritability, muscle aches, nausea, runny nose, shivering, sleep disorders, stomach cramps, sweating, trembling, vomiting, or weakness). Your doctor may, therefore, want to reduce the dosage gradually.

• Because this product contains acetaminophen, additional drugs that contain acetaminophen should not be taken without first getting your doctor's approval. Be sure to check the labels on over-the-counter pain, sinus, allergy, asthma, diet, cough, and cold products before you use them in order to see if they also contain acetaminophen.

• Be sure to tell your doctor if you are pregnant. The effects of this medication during pregnancy have not been thoroughly studied in humans. Codeine used regularly in large doses during pregnancy can result in addiction of the fetus, leading to withdrawal symptoms (diarrhea, excessive crying, excessive yawning, irritability, fever, sneezing, tremors, or vomiting) at birth. Also, tell your doctor if you are breast-feeding an infant. Small amounts of this drug may pass into breast milk and cause drowsiness in the nursing infant.

---

albuterol

BRAND NAMES (Manufacturers)

Albuterol Sulfate (Copley)
Proventil (Schering)
Ventolin (Glaxo)

TYPE OF DRUG

Bronchodilator

INGREDIENT

albuterol

DOSAGE FORMS

Tablets (2 mg and 4 mg)
Inhalation aerosol (each spray delivers 90 mcg)
Inhalation solution (0.5% and 0.083%)
Oral syrup (2 mg per 5-ml spoonful)
Capsule for inhalation (200 mcg)

STORAGE

Albuterol tablets and oral syrup should be stored at room temperature in a tightly closed, light-resistant container. The inhalation aerosol should be stored away from excessive heat—the contents are pressurized and can explode if heated.

USES

Albuterol is used to relieve wheezing and shortness of breath caused by lung diseases such as asthma, bronchitis, and emphysema. This drug acts directly on the muscles of the bronchi (breathing tubes) to relieve bronchospasms (muscle contractions of the bronchi), which allows air to move more freely to and from the lungs.

TREATMENT

To lessen stomach upset, take albuterol tablets and oral syrup with food (unless your doctor directs you to do otherwise).

Each dose of oral syrup should be measured carefully with a 5-ml measuring spoon designed for that purpose. Ordinary kitchen teaspoons are not accurate enough.

The inhalation aerosol form of this medication is usually packaged with an instruction sheet. Read the directions carefully before using this medication. You may wish to consult your doctor or pharmacist about the proper administration of this drug. The container should be shaken well just before each use. The contents tend to settle on the bottom, so it is necessary to shake the bottle in order to distribute the ingredients evenly inside and equalize the doses.

If more than one inhalation is necessary, wait at least one full minute between doses, in order to receive the full benefit of the first dose.

If you miss a dose of this medication and remember within an hour, take the missed dose immediately; then follow your regular dosing schedule for the next dose. If you miss the dose by more than an hour, just wait until the next scheduled dose. Do not double the dose.

SIDE EFFECTS

Minor. Anxiety, dizziness, flushing, headache, insomnia, irritability, loss of appetite, muscle cramps, nausea, nervousness, restlessness, sweating, tremors, vomiting, weakness, or dryness or irritation of the mouth or throat (from the inhalation aerosol). These side effects should disappear as your body adjusts to the medication.

To help prevent dryness or irritation of the mouth or throat, rinse your mouth with water after each dose of the inhalation aerosol.

In order to avoid difficulty in falling asleep, check with your doctor to see if you can take the last dose of this medication several hours before bedtime each day.

If you feel dizzy, sit or lie down for a while; get up from a sitting or reclining position slowly; and be careful on stairs.

Major. Tell your doctor about any side effects that are persistent or particularly bothersome. IT IS ESPECIALLY IMPORTANT TO TELL YOUR DOCTOR about chest pain, difficult or painful urination, itching, palpitations, or rash.

INTERACTIONS

Albuterol interacts with several other types of drugs:

1. The beta blockers (acebutolol, atenolol, labetalol, metoprolol, nadolol, pindolol, propranolol, timolol) antagonize (act against) this medication, decreasing its effectiveness.

2. Monoamine oxidase (MAO) inhibitors, tricyclic antidepressants, antihistamines, levothyroxine, and over-the-counter (nonprescription) cough, cold, asthma, allergy, diet, and sinus medications may increase the side effects of this medication.

3. There may be a change in the dosage requirements of insulin or oral antidiabetic medications when albuterol is started.

4. The blood-pressure-lowering effects of guanethidine may be decreased by this medication.
5. The use of albuterol with other bronchodilator drugs (either oral or inhalant drugs) can have additive side effects. Discuss this with your doctor.

BE SURE TO TELL YOUR DOCTOR about any other medications that you are taking, especially any listed above.

WARNINGS

• Tell your doctor about unusual or allergic reactions you have had to medications, especially to albuterol or any related drug (metaproterenol, terbutaline, amphetamines, ephedrine, epinephrine, isoproterenol, norepinephrine, phenylephrine, phenylpropanolamine, pseudoephedrine).
• Tell your doctor if you now have or if you have ever had diabetes mellitus, an enlarged prostate gland, epilepsy, glaucoma, heart disease, high blood pressure, or thyroid disease.
• This medication can cause dizziness. Your ability to perform tasks that require alertness, such as driving a car or operating potentially dangerous equipment, may be decreased. Appropriate caution should, therefore, be taken.
• Before having surgery or any other medical or dental treatment, be sure to tell the doctor or dentist that you are taking this medication.
• Do not exceed the recommended dosage of this medication; excessive use may lead to an increase in side effects or a loss of effectiveness.
• Avoid contact of the aerosol inhalation with your eyes.
• Do not puncture, break, or burn the aerosol container. The contents are under pressure and may explode.
• Contact your doctor if you do not respond to the usual dose of this medication. It may be an indication that your asthma is getting worse, which may require additional therapy.
• Be sure to tell your doctor if you are pregnant. The effects of this medication during pregnancy have not been thoroughly studied in humans, but it has caused side effects in the offspring of animals that received large doses during pregnancy. Also, tell your doctor if you are breast-feeding an infant. It is not known if albuterol passes into breast milk.

---

allopurinol

BRAND NAMES (Manufacturers)

allopurinol (various manufacturers)
Lopurin (Boots)
Zyloprim (Burroughs Wellcome)

TYPE OF DRUG

Antigout

INGREDIENT

allopurinol

DOSAGE FORM

Tablets (100 mg and 300 mg)

STORAGE

Allopurinol tablets should be stored at room temperature in a tightly closed container.

USES

This medication is used to treat chronic gout and to lower blood uric acid levels. Allopurinol blocks the body's production of uric acid. Allopurinol should not be used to treat acute gout attacks.

TREATMENT

In order to avoid stomach irritation, you can take allopurinol with food or with a full glass of water or milk. It may take one to three weeks before the full effects of this medication are observed.

Drink at least 10 to 12 glasses (eight ounces each) of fluids per day while taking this medication in order to prevent the formation of kidney stones.

If you miss a dose of this medication, take the missed dose as soon as possible, unless it is almost time for the next dose. In that case, do not take the missed dose at all; just return to your regular dosing schedule. Do not double the next dose.

Take this drug for the full duration of prescribed therapy, as the full benefit of allopurinol may be delayed for several weeks.

SIDE EFFECTS

Minor. Diarrhea, drowsiness, nausea, stomach upset, or vomiting. These side effects should disappear as your body adjusts to the medication.
Major. Tell your doctor about any side effects that are persistent or particularly bothersome that may be the result of this medication. IT IS ESPECIALLY IMPORTANT TO TELL YOUR DOCTOR about blurred vision, chills, difficult or painful urination, fatigue, fever, loss of hair, muscle aches, numbness or tingling sensations, paleness, rash, sore throat, unusual bleeding or bruising, or yellowing of the eyes or skin.

INTERACTIONS

Allopurinol interacts with several other types of drugs:
1. Alcohol, diuretics (water pills), and pyrazinamide can increase blood uric acid levels, thus decreasing the effectiveness of allopurinol.
2. Allopurinol can increase the body's store of iron salts, which can lead to iron toxicity.
3. When combined with allopurinol, ampicillin can increase the chance of skin rash; thiazide diuretics and captopril can increase the chance of allergic reactions; and cyclophosphamide can increase the chance of blood disorders. Allopurinol can also increase the blood levels and side effects of drugs such as mercaptopurine, azathioprine, oral anticoagulants (blood thinners) and theophylline.
4. Vitamin C can make the urine acidic, which can increase the risk of kidney stone formation with this medication.

Before starting to take allopurinol, BE SURE TO TELL YOUR DOCTOR about any medications you are currently taking, especially any of those listed above.

WARNINGS

• Tell your doctor about unusual or allergic reactions you have had to any medications, especially to allopurinol.
• Tell your doctor if you now have or if you have ever had blood disorders, kidney disease, or liver disease. Also, tell your doctor if you have a relative with idiopathic hemochromatosis (a disorder of iron metabolism).
• This drug may cause dizziness or drowsiness. Do not take part in any activity that requires alertness, such as driving a car or operating dangerous equipment.
• Be sure to tell your doctor if you are pregnant. Although this drug appears to be safe in animals, studies in pregnant women have not been conducted. Also, tell your doctor if you are breast-feeding an infant. It is not known whether allopurinol passes into breast milk.

---

alprazolam

BRAND NAME (Manufacturer)
Xanax (Upjohn)
TYPE OF DRUG
Benzodiazepine sedative/hypnotic
INGREDIENT
alprazolam
DOSAGE FORM
Tablets (0.25 mg, 0.5 mg, 1 mg, and 2 mg)
STORAGE
This medication should be stored at room temperature in a tightly closed, light-resistant container.

USES

Alprazolam is prescribed to treat symptoms of anxiety and anxiety associated with depression. It may work by acting as a depressant of the central nervous system. This drug is currently used to relieve nervousness and panic disorder. Alprazolam is effective for this purpose for short periods, but it is important to try to remove the cause of the anxiety as well.

TREATMENT

This drug should be taken exactly as directed by your doctor. It can be taken with food or a full glass of water if stomach upset occurs.

If you are taking this medication regularly and you miss a dose, take the missed dose immediately if you remember within an hour of the scheduled dose. If more than an hour has passed, skip the dose you missed and wait for the next scheduled dose. Do not double the dose.

SIDE EFFECTS

Minor. Bitter taste in mouth, constipation, diarrhea, dizziness, drowsiness (after a night's sleep), dry mouth, excessive salivation, fatigue, flushing, headache, heartburn, loss of appetite, nausea, nervousness, sweating, or vomiting. As you adjust to the drug, these effects should disappear.

To relieve constipation, increase the amount of fiber in your diet (fresh fruits and vegetables, salads, bran, and whole-grain breads), try to get regular exercise, and drink more water (unless your doctor directs you to do otherwise).

Dry mouth can be relieved by chewing sugarless gum or by sucking on ice chips.

If you feel dizzy, sit or lie down for a while; get up slowly from a sitting or reclining position; and be careful on stairs.

Major. Tell your doctor about any side effects that are persistent or particularly bothersome. IT IS ESPECIALLY IMPORTANT TO TELL YOUR DOCTOR about blurred or double vision, chest pain, severe depression, difficulty in urinating, fainting, falling, fever, hallucinations, joint pain, mouth sores, nightmares, palpitations, rash, shortness of breath, slurred speech, sore throat, uncoordinated movements, unusual excitement, unusual tiredness, or yellowing of the eyes or skin.

INTERACTIONS

Alprazolam interacts with several other types of drugs:
1. To prevent oversedation, this drug should not be taken with alcohol, other sedative drugs, central nervous system depressants (such as antihistamines, barbiturates, muscle relaxants, pain medications, narcotics, medicines for seizures, and phenothiazine tranquilizers), or antidepressant medications.
2. This medication may decrease the effectiveness of carbamazepine, levodopa, and oral anticoagulants (blood thinners).
3. Disulfiram, oral contraceptives (birth control pills), isoniazid, and cimetidine can increase the blood levels of alprazolam, which can lead to toxic effects.
4. Concurrent use of rifampin may decrease the effectiveness of alprazolam.

Before starting to take alprazolam, BE SURE TO TELL YOUR DOCTOR about any medications you are currently taking, especially any of those listed above.

WARNINGS

• Tell your doctor about unusual or allergic reactions you have had to any medications, especially to alprazolam or other benzodiazepine tranquilizers (such as chlordiazepoxide, clorazepate, diazepam, flurazepam, halazepam, lorazepam, oxazepam, prazepam, temazepam, or triazolam).
• Tell your doctor if you now have or if you have ever had liver disease, kidney disease, epilepsy, lung disease, myasthenia gravis, narrow-angle glaucoma, porphyria, mental depression, mental illness, or sleep apnea.
• This medicine can cause drowsiness. Avoid tasks that require mental alertness, such as driving a car or using potentially dangerous equipment.
• This medication has the potential for abuse and must be used with caution. Tolerance may develop quickly; do not increase the dosage of the drug without first consulting your doctor. It is also important not to stop this drug suddenly if you have been taking it in large amounts or if you have used it for several months. Your doctor will want to reduce the dosage gradually.
• This is a safe drug when used properly. When it is combined with other sedative drugs or alcohol, however, serious side effects can develop.

• Be sure to tell your doctor if you are pregnant. This medicine may increase the chance of birth defects if it is taken during the first three months of pregnancy. In addition, too much use of this medicine during the last six months of pregnancy may result in addiction of the fetus—leading to withdrawal side effects in the newborn. Also, use of this medicine during the last weeks of pregnancy may cause drowsiness, slowed heartbeat, and breathing difficulties in the infant. Also, tell your doctor if you are breast-feeding an infant. This medicine can pass into breast milk and cause excessive drowsiness, slowed heartbeat, and breathing difficulties in nursing infants.

---

amantadine

BRAND NAMES (Manufacturers)
amantadine hydrochloride (various manufacturers)
Symadine (Reid-Rowell)
Symmetrel (DuPont)
TYPE OF DRUG
Antiparkinsonism agent and antiviral
INGREDIENT
amantadine
DOSAGE FORMS
Capsules (100 mg)
Oral syrup (50 mg per 5-ml spoonful)
STORAGE
Amantadine should be stored at room temperature in a tightly closed container. This medication should never be frozen.

USES

Amantadine is used to treat the symptoms of Parkinson's disease and to prevent or treat respiratory tract infections caused by influenza A virus. It is thought to relieve the symptoms of Parkinson's by increasing the levels of dopamine, an important chemical in the brain, which is lacking in these patients. Amantadine is also an antiviral agent that slows the growth of the influenza virus.

TREATMENT

Amantadine can be taken on an empty stomach or with food or milk.

Each dose of the oral syrup should be measured carefully with a specially designed 5-ml measuring spoon. If you are taking amantadine to treat a viral infection, you should start taking it as soon as possible after exposure to the infection. Continue to take this medication for the entire time prescribed by your doctor (usually seven to 14 days), even if the symptoms of infection disappear before the end of that period. If you stop taking the drug too soon, the virus is given a chance to continue growing and the infection could recur.

Amantadine works best when the level of medicine in your bloodstream is kept constant. Therefore, take the doses at evenly spaced intervals day and night. For example, if you are to take two doses a day, the doses should be spaced 12 hours apart.

If you are taking amantadine to treat Parkinson's disease, you should know that the full effects of this medication may not become apparent for several weeks.

If you miss a dose of this medication, take the missed dose as soon as possible, unless it is almost time for the next dose. In that case, don't take the missed dose at all; just return to your regular dosing schedule. Do not double the next dose.

SIDE EFFECTS

Minor. Constipation, dizziness, dry mouth, fatigue, headache, insomnia, loss of appetite, nausea, or vomiting. These side effects should gradually disappear.

To relieve constipation, increase the amount of fiber in your diet (fresh fruits and vegetables, salads, bran, and whole-grain breads), exercise, and drink more water (unless your doctor directs you to do otherwise).

If you feel dizzy, sit or lie down for a while; get up slowly from a sitting or reclining position.

To relieve mouth dryness, chew sugarless gum or suck on ice chips or hard candy.

Major. Tell your doctor about any side effects that are persistent or particularly bothersome. IT IS ESPECIALLY IMPORTANT TO TELL YOUR DOCTOR about anxiety, confusion, convulsions, depression, difficulty urinating, fluid retention, hallucinations, purplish-red spots on the skin, shortness of breath, skin rash, slurred speech, or visual disturbances.

INTERACTIONS

Amantadine interacts with several other types of drugs:
1. Concurrent use of amantadine and alcohol can lead to dizziness, fainting, and confusion.
2. Phenothiazine tranquilizers and tricyclic antidepressants in combination with amantadine can lead to confusion, hallucinations, and nightmares.

BE SURE TO TELL YOUR DOCTOR about any medications you are currently taking, especially any of those listed above.

WARNINGS

• Tell your doctor about unusual or allergic reactions you have had to any medications, especially to amantadine.
• Before starting to take amantadine, tell your doctor if you now have or if you have ever had epilepsy, heart or blood vessel disease, kidney disease, liver disease, mental disorders, or stomach ulcers.
• If this drug makes you dizzy, avoid taking part in any activity that requires alertness, such as driving a car or operating potentially dangerous equipment.
• If you are taking amantadine to treat Parkinson's disease, do not stop taking the medication unless you first consult your doctor. Stopping the drug abruptly may lead to a worsening of the disease. Your doctor may, therefore, want to reduce your dosage gradually to prevent this from occurring. In addition, tolerance to the benefits of amantadine can develop in several months. If you notice a loss of effectiveness, BE SURE TO CONTACT YOUR DOCTOR.
• Be sure to tell your doctor if you are pregnant. Although amantadine appears to be safe in humans, birth defects

have been reported in the offspring of animals that received large doses during pregnancy. Also, tell your doctor if you are breast-feeding an infant. Small amounts of amantadine pass into breast milk and can cause side effects in the nursing infant.

---

amitriptyline

BRAND NAMES (Manufacturers)
Amitril (Parke-Davis)
amitriptyline hydrochloride (various manufacturers)
Elavil (Stuart)
Endep (Roche)
Enovil (Hauck)

TYPE OF DRUG
Tricyclic antidepressant

INGREDIENT
amitriptyline

DOSAGE FORM
Tablets (10 mg, 25 mg, 50 mg, 75 mg, 100 mg, and 150 mg)

STORAGE
Store at room temperature in a tightly closed container.

USES

Amitriptyline is used to relieve the symptoms of mental depression. This medication belongs to a group of drugs referred to as the tricyclic antidepressants. These medicines are thought to relieve depression by increasing the concentration of certain chemicals necessary for nerve transmission in the brain.

TREATMENT

This medication should be taken exactly as your doctor prescribes. It can be taken with water or with food to lessen the chance of stomach irritation, unless your doctor tells you to do otherwise.

The effects of therapy with this medication may not become apparent for two or three weeks.

If you miss a dose of this medication, take the missed dose as soon as possible, and then return to your regular dosing schedule. However, if the dose you missed was a once-a-day bedtime dose, do not take that dose in the morning; check with your doctor instead. If the dose is taken in the morning, it may cause some unwanted side effects. Never double the dose.

SIDE EFFECTS

Minor. Constipation, cramps, diarrhea, dizziness, drowsiness, dry mouth, fatigue, heartburn, loss of appetite, nausea, peculiar tastes in the mouth, restlessness, sweating, vomiting, weakness, or weight gain or loss. As your body adjusts to the medication, these side effects should disappear.

This medication may cause increased sensitivity to sunlight. You should, therefore, avoid prolonged exposure to sunlight and sunlamps. Wear protective clothing and use an effective sunscreen.

Amitriptyline may cause your urine to turn blue-green; this effect is harmless.

Dry mouth can be relieved by chewing sugarless gum or by sucking on ice chips or hard candy.

To relieve constipation, increase the amount of fiber in your diet (fresh fruits and vegetables, salads, bran, and whole-grain breads), exercise, and drink more water (unless your doctor directs you to do otherwise).

To avoid dizziness when you stand, contract and relax the muscles of your legs for a few moments before rising. Do this by alternately pushing one foot against the floor while raising the other foot slightly, so that you are "pumping" your legs in a pedaling motion.

Major. Tell your doctor about any side effects that are persistent or particularly bothersome. IT IS ESPECIALLY IMPORTANT TO TELL YOUR DOCTOR about agitation, anxiety, blurred vision, chest pain, confusion, convulsions, difficulty in urinating, enlarged or painful breasts (in both sexes), fainting, fever, fluid retention, hair loss, hallucinations, headaches, impotence, mood changes, mouth sores, nervousness, nightmares, numbness in the fingers or toes, palpitations, ringing in the ears, seizures, skin rash, sleep disorders, sore throat, tremors, uncoordinated movements or balance problems, unusual bleeding or bruising, or yellowing of the eyes or skin.

INTERACTIONS

Amitriptyline interacts with a number of other types of medications:

1. Extreme drowsiness can occur when this medicine is taken with central nervous system depressants (such as alcohol, antihistamines, barbiturates, benzodiazepine tranquilizers, muscle relaxants, narcotics, pain medications, phenothiazine tranquilizers, and sleeping medications) or with other antidepressants.

2. Amitriptyline may decrease the effectiveness of antiseizure medications and may block the blood-pressure-lowering effects of clonidine and guanethidine.

3. Oral contraceptives (birth control pills) or estrogen-containing drugs can increase the side effects and reduce the effectiveness of the tricyclic antidepressants (including amitriptyline).

4. Cimetidine can decrease the elimination of amitriptyline from the body, thus increasing the possibility of side effects.

5. Tricyclic antidepressants may increase the side effects of thyroid medication and of over-the-counter (nonprescription) cough, cold, allergy, asthma, sinus, and weight-control medications.

6. The concurrent use of tricyclic antidepressants and monoamine oxidase (MAO) inhibitors should be avoided because the combination may result in fever, convulsions, or high blood pressure. At least 14 days should separate the use of amitriptyline and the use of an MAO inhibitor.

Before starting to take amitriptyline, BE SURE TO TELL YOUR DOCTOR about any medications you are currently taking, especially any of those listed above.

WARNINGS

• Tell your doctor if you have had unusual or allergic reactions to medications, especially to amitriptyline or any of the other tricyclic antidepressants (imipramine, doxepin, trimipramine, amoxapine, protriptyline, desipramine, maprotiline, nortriptyline).

• Tell your doctor if you have a history of alcoholism, or if you have ever had asthma, diabetes, high blood pressure, liver or kidney disease, heart disease, a heart attack, circulatory disease, stomach problems, intestinal problems, difficulty in urinating, enlarged prostate gland, epilepsy, glaucoma, thyroid disease, mental illness, or electroshock therapy.

• If this drug makes you dizzy or drowsy, do not take part in any activity that requires alertness, such as driving a car or operating potentially dangerous equipment.

• Before having surgery or other medical or dental treatment, tell your doctor or dentist you are taking this drug.

• Do not stop taking this drug suddenly. Abruptly stopping it can cause nausea, headache, stomach upset, fatigue, or a worsening of your condition. Your doctor may want to reduce the dosage gradually.

• The effects of this medication may last as long as seven days after you have stopped taking it, so continue to observe all precautions during that period.

• Be sure to tell your doctor if you are pregnant. Studies have not been done in humans; however, studies in animals have shown that this type of medication can cause side effects to the fetus when given to the mother in large doses during pregnancy. Also, tell your doctor if you are breast-feeding an infant. Small amounts of this drug can pass into breast milk and may cause irritability or sleeping problems, in nursing infants.

---

amlodipine

BRAND NAME (Manufacturer)
Norvasc (Pfizer)
TYPE OF DRUG
Antianginal and antihypertensive
INGREDIENT
amlodipine
DOSAGE FORM
Tablets (2.5 mg, 5 mg, and 10 mg)
STORAGE
This medication should be stored at room temperature in a tightly closed container away from heat and direct sunlight.

USES

Amlodipine belongs to a group of drugs known as calcium channel blockers and is used to prevent the symptoms of angina (chest pain). It can also be used to treat high blood pressure. Amlodipine dilates the blood vessels of the heart and increases the amount of oxygen that reaches the heart muscle, though it is unclear exactly how it operates.

TREATMENT

This medication should be taken exactly as prescribed by your doctor. Amlodipine can be taken with meals or with a full glass of water if stomach upset occurs. Try to develop a set schedule for taking it.

Amlodipine does not relieve chest pain once it has begun; it is only used to prevent angina attacks.

If you miss a dose and remember within four hours, take the missed dose and resume your regular schedule. If more than four hours have passed, skip the dose you missed and then take your next dose as scheduled. Do not double the dose.

This medication does not cure angina but can help to control the condition as long as you continue to take the medicine.

SIDE EFFECTS

Minor. Constipation, diarrhea, dizziness, drowsiness, headache, insomnia, light-headedness, nausea, nervousness, stomach pain, or vomiting.

To relieve constipation, increase the amount of fiber in your diet (fresh fruits and vegetables, salads, bran and whole-grain breads), exercise, and drink more water (unless your doctor directs you to do otherwise).

Major. Tell your doctor about any side effects that are persistent or particularly bothersome. IT IS ESPECIALLY IMPORTANT TO TELL YOUR DOCTOR about confusion, depression, eye pain, or visual changes, fatigue, fluid retention, flushing, palpitations, skin rash.

INTERACTIONS

At this time, amlodipine does not appear to interact with other drugs when used according to directions.

WARNINGS

• Tell you doctor about unusual or allergic reactions you have had to any medications, especially amlodipine.

• Tell your doctor if you have ever had liver disease, obstructive coronary artery disease, or heart failure.

• If this drug makes you drowsy or dizzy, avoid taking part in any activity that requires alertness, such as driving a car or operating potentially dangerous equipment.

• Be sure to tell your doctor if you are pregnant. Extensive studies in pregnant women have not been conducted, but side effects have been reported in the offspring of animals that received large doses of amlodipine during pregnancy. Also, be sure to tell your doctor if you are breast-feeding an infant. It is not known if amlodipine passes into breast milk.

---

amoxicillin

BRAND NAMES (Manufacturers)
amoxicillin (various manufacturers)
Amoxil (SmithKline Beecham)
Polymox (Bristol)
Trimox (Squibb)
Utimox (Parke-Davis)
Wymox (Wyeth-Ayerst)
TYPE OF DRUG
Antibiotic

INGREDIENT

amoxicillin

DOSAGE FORMS

Capsules (250 mg and 500 mg)
Chewable tablets (125 mg and 250 mg)
Oral suspension (125 mg and 250 mg per 5-ml spoonful)
Oral suspension drops (50 mg per ml)

STORAGE

Amoxicillin tablets and capsules should be stored at room temperature in tightly closed containers. The oral suspension should be stored in the refrigerator in a tightly closed container. Any unused portion of the suspension should be discarded after 14 days because the drug loses its potency after that time. This medication should never be frozen.

USES

Amoxicillin antibiotic is used to treat a wide variety of bacterial infections, including infections in the middle ear, skin, upper and lower respiratory tracts, and urinary tract. Amoxicillin acts by severely injuring the cell walls of the infecting bacteria, thereby preventing them from growing and multiplying.

Amoxicillin kills susceptible bacteria but is not effective against viruses, parasites, or fungi.

TREATMENT

Amoxicillin can be taken either on an empty stomach or along with food or milk (in order to prevent stomach upset).

The suspension form of this medication should be shaken well just before measuring each dose. The contents tend to settle on the bottom of the bottle, so it is necessary to shake the container to distribute the ingredients evenly and equalize the doses. Each dose should then be measured carefully with a specially designed 5-ml measuring spoon or the 1-ml dropper provided, as directed by your doctor or pharmacist. An ordinary kitchen teaspoon is not accurate enough.

It is important to continue to take this medication for the entire time prescribed by your doctor (usually seven to 14 days), even if the symptoms of infection disappear before the end of that period. If you stop taking the drug too soon, resistant bacteria are given the chance to continue growing, and the infection could recur.

Amoxicillin works best when the level of medicine in your bloodstream is kept constant. It is best, therefore, to take the doses at evenly spaced intervals day and night. For example, if you are to take three doses a day, the doses should be spaced eight hours apart.

If you miss a dose of this drug, take the missed dose immediately. However, if you don't remember to take the missed dose until it is almost time for your next dose, take it; space the next dose about halfway through the regular interval between doses; then return to your regular schedule. Do not skip any doses.

SIDE EFFECTS

Minor. Diarrhea, heartburn, nausea, or vomiting. These side effects should disappear as your body adjusts to the drug.

Major. Tell your doctor about any side effects that are persistent or particularly bothersome. IT IS ESPECIALLY IMPORTANT TO TELL YOUR DOCTOR about bloating, chills, cough, darkened tongue, difficulty in breathing, fever, irritation of the mouth, muscle aches, rash, rectal or vaginal itching, severe or bloody diarrhea, or sore throat. Also, if your symptoms of infection seem to be getting worse rather than improving, contact your doctor.

INTERACTIONS

Amoxicillin interacts with other types of medications:

1. Probenecid can increase the blood concentration of this medication.

2. Amoxicillin may decrease the effectiveness of oral contraceptives (birth control pills), and pregnancy could result. You should, therefore, use a different or additional (barrier) form of birth control while taking this medication. Discuss this with your doctor.

3. The concurrent use of amoxicillin and allopurinol can increase the risk of developing a rash.

BE SURE TO TELL YOUR DOCTOR about any medications you are currently taking.

WARNINGS

- Tell your doctor about unusual or allergic reactions you have had to any medications, especially to amoxicillin, ampicillin, or penicillin or to cephalosporin antibiotics, penicillamine, or griseofulvin.
- Tell your doctor if you now have or if you have ever had kidney disease, asthma, or allergies.
- This medication has been prescribed for your current infection only. Another infection later on, or one that someone else has, may require a different medicine. You should not give your medicine to other people or use it for other infections, unless your doctor specifically directs you to do so.
- Diabetics taking amoxicillin should know that this drug may cause a false-positive sugar reaction with a Clinitest urine glucose test. To avoid this problem while taking amoxicillin, you should switch to Clinistix or Tes-Tape to test your urine for sugar.
- Be sure to tell your doctor if you are pregnant. Although amoxicillin appears to be safe during pregnancy, extensive studies in humans have not been conducted. Also, tell your doctor if you are breast-feeding an infant. Small amounts of this medication pass into breast milk and may temporarily alter the bacterial balance in the intestinal tract of the nursing infant, resulting in diarrhea.

---

ampicillin

BRAND NAMES (Manufacturers)

ampicillin (various manufacturers)
D-Amp (Dunhall)
Omnipen (Wyeth-Ayerst)
Polycillin (Apothecon)
Principen (Apothecon)
Totacillin (SmithKline Beecham)

TYPE OF DRUG
Antibiotic
INGREDIENT
ampicillin
DOSAGE FORMS
Capsules (250 mg and 500 mg)
Oral suspension (125 mg and 250 mg per 5-ml spoonful)
Oral suspension drops (100 mg per ml)
STORAGE
Ampicillin capsules should be stored at room temperature; ampicillin liquid suspension and drops should be refrigerated but should never be frozen. Do not keep any of these medications beyond the expiration date. All containers should be closed tightly to keep out moisture.

USES

Ampicillin is used to treat a wide variety of bacterial infections, including middle ear infections in children and infections of the respiratory, urinary, and gastrointestinal tracts. This type of antibiotic acts by severely injuring the cell walls of the infecting bacteria, thereby preventing them from growing and multiplying. Ampicillin kills susceptible bacteria but is not effective against viruses, parasites, or fungi.

TREATMENT

It is best to take ampicillin on an empty stomach (one hour before or two hours after a meal) with a full glass of water (not juice or soda pop). Always follow your doctor's directions.

If you have been prescribed the liquid suspension form of this drug, be sure to shake the bottle well before taking this medication. The contents tend to settle on the bottom of the bottle, so it is necessary to shake the container to distribute the ingredients evenly and equalize the doses. Be sure to use specially marked droppers or spoons in order to accurately measure the correct amount of liquid. Household teaspoons vary in size and may not give you the correct dosage.

Ampicillin works best when the level of medicine in your bloodstream is kept constant. It is, therefore, best to take the doses at evenly spaced intervals day and night. For example, if you are to take four doses a day, the doses should be spaced six hours apart.

If you miss a dose, take it as soon as possible. If it is already time for the next dose, take it; space the next two doses at half the normal time interval (for example, if you were supposed to take one capsule every six hours, take your next two doses every three hours); then resume your normal dosing schedule.

Please remember that it is very important that you continue to take this medication for the entire duration prescribed to you by your doctor (usually seven to 14 days), even if the symptoms are no longer apparent before the end of that period. If you stop taking this medication too soon, resistant bacteria are given a chance to continue growing, and the infection could recur.

SIDE EFFECTS

Minor. Diarrhea, nausea, or vomiting. These side effects should disappear as your body adjusts to the medication.

Major. Tell your doctor about any side effects that are persistent or particularly bothersome. IT IS ESPECIALLY IMPORTANT TO TELL YOUR DOCTOR about darkened tongue, difficulty in breathing, fever, joint pain, mouth sores, rash, rectal or vaginal itching, severe or bloody diarrhea, or sore throat. Also, if your symptoms of infection seem to be getting worse rather than improving, you should contact your doctor.

INTERACTIONS

This drug interacts with other types of medications:
1. Ampicillin interacts with allopurinol, chloramphenicol, erythromycin, paromomycin, tetracycline, and troleandomycin.
2. Ampicillin may decrease the effectiveness of oral contraceptives (birth control pills), and pregnancy could result. You should, therefore, use a different or additional (barrier) form of birth control while taking the antibiotic ampicillin.

BE SURE TO TELL YOUR DOCTOR about any medications you are taking, especially any of those listed above.

WARNINGS

- Tell your doctor about unusual or allergic reactions you have had to any medications, especially to penicillin, ampicillin, amoxicillin, cephalosporin antibiotics, penicillamine, or griseofulvin.
- Tell your doctor if you have or have ever had liver or kidney disease, asthma, hay fever, or other allergies.
- This medication has been prescribed for your current infection only. Another infection later on, or one that someone else has, may require a different medicine. Do not give your medicine to other people or use it for other infections, unless your doctor directs you to do so.
- Diabetics taking ampicillin should know that this drug may cause a false-positive sugar reaction with a Clinitest urine glucose test. To avoid this problem while taking ampicillin, you should switch to Clinistix or Tes-Tape to test your urine for sugar.
- Be sure to tell your doctor if you are pregnant. Although ampicillin appears to be safe during pregnancy, extensive studies in humans have not been conducted. Also, tell your doctor if you are breast-feeding an infant. Small amounts of this medication pass into breast milk and may temporarily alter the bacterial balance in the intestinal tract of the nursing infant, resulting in diarrhea.

---

aspirin

BRAND NAMES (Manufacturers)
A.S.A. Enseals* (Lilly)
aspirin* (various manufacturers)
Bayer* (Glenbrook)
Bayer Children's* (Glenbrook)
Easprin (Parke-Davis)
Ecotrin* (SmithKline Beecham)
Empirin* (Burroughs Wellcome)

Measurin* (Winthrop Pharmaceuticals)
ZORprin (Boots)
*Available over-the-counter (without a prescription)

TYPE OF DRUG

Analgesic and anti-inflammatory

INGREDIENT

aspirin

DOSAGE FORMS

Tablets (65 mg, 81 mg, 325 mg, and 500 mg)
Chewable tablets (75 mg and 81 mg)
Chewing gum (227 mg)
Enteric-coated tablets (165 mg, 325 mg, 500 mg, 650 mg, and 975 mg)
Sustained-release tablets (650 mg and 800 mg)
Caplets (325 mg and 500 mg)
Suppositories (60 mg, 65 mg, 120 mg, 125 mg, 130 mg, 195 mg, 200 mg, 300 mg, 325 mg, 600 mg, 650 mg, and 1.2 g)

STORAGE

Store at room temperature in a tightly closed container. Moisture causes aspirin to decompose. Discard the medicine if it has a vinegary odor.

USES

Aspirin is used to treat mild to moderate pain, fever, and inflammatory conditions, such as rheumatic fever, rheumatoid arthritis, and osteoarthritis. Because it prevents the formation of blood clots, aspirin has also been shown to be effective in reducing the risk of transient ischemic attacks (small strokes) and to have a protective effect against certain heart attacks in men with angina (chest pain).

Aspirin is a useful medication that is utilized in the treatment of a wide variety of diseases. Because it is so common and so readily available, you may not think of it as "real medicine." This is a common misconception; aspirin certainly is "real medicine." If your doctor prescribes or recommends aspirin for your condition, it is for a good reason. FOLLOW YOUR DOCTOR'S DIRECTIONS CAREFULLY!

TREATMENT

To avoid stomach irritation, you should take aspirin with food or with a full glass of water or milk.

Chewable aspirin tablets may be chewed, dissolved in fluid, or swallowed whole.

Swallow the sustained-release or enteric-coated tablets whole. Crushing, chewing, or breaking these tablets destroys their sustained-release activity and increases side effects.

To use the suppository, remove the foil wrapper and moisten the suppository with water (if it is too soft to insert, refrigerate the suppository for half an hour or run cold water over it before you remove the wrapper). Lie on your left side with your right knee bent. Push the suppository into the rectum, pointed end first. Lie still for a few minutes. Avoid having a bowel movement for at least an hour in order to give the drug time to be absorbed into your system.

If you are using aspirin to treat an inflammatory condition, it may take two or three weeks until the full benefits are observed.

If you are taking aspirin on a regular schedule and you miss a dose, take the missed dose as soon as possible, unless it is almost time for the next dose. In that case, do not take the missed dose at all; just return to your regular dosing schedule. Do not double the next dose.

SIDE EFFECTS

Minor. Heartburn, nausea, or vomiting. These side effects should disappear as your body adjusts to the medication.

Major. Tell your doctor about any side effects that are persistent or particularly bothersome. IT IS ESPECIALLY IMPORTANT TO TELL YOUR DOCTOR about any loss of hearing or ringing in the ears; bloody or black, tarry stools; confusion; difficult or painful urination; difficulty in breathing; dizziness; severe stomach pain; skin rash; or unusual weakness.

INTERACTIONS

Aspirin interacts with a number of other types of medications:

1. Aspirin can increase the effects of anticoagulants (blood thinners), such as warfarin, leading to bleeding complications.

2. The antigout effects of probenecid and sulfinpyrazone may be blocked by aspirin.

3. Aspirin can increase the gastrointestinal side effects of nonsteroidal anti-inflammatory drugs, alcohol, phenylbutazone, and adrenocorticosteroids (cortisonelike medicines).

4. Ammonium chloride, methionine, and furosemide can increase the side effects of aspirin.

5. Acetazolamide, methazolamide, antacids, and phenobarbital can decrease the effectiveness of aspirin.

6. Aspirin can increase the side effects of methotrexate, penicillin, thyroid hormone, phenytoin, sulfinpyrazone, naproxen, valproic acid, insulin, and oral antidiabetic medications.

7. Aspirin can decrease the effects of spironolactone.

Before starting to take aspirin, BE SURE TO TELL YOUR DOCTOR about any medications you are currently taking, especially any of those listed above.

WARNINGS

- Tell your doctor about unusual or allergic reactions you have had to any medications, especially to aspirin, methyl salicylate (oil of wintergreen), tartrazine, diclofenac, diflunisal, flurbiprofen, fenoprofen, ibuprofen, indomethacin, ketoprofen, meclofenamate, mefenamic acid, naproxen, piroxicam, sulindac, tolmetin, or etodolac.
- Before starting to take aspirin, be sure to tell your doctor if you now have or if you have ever had asthma, bleeding disorders, congestive heart failure, diabetes, glucose-6-phosphate dehydrogenase deficiency, gout, hemophilia, high blood pressure, kidney disease, liver disease, nasal polyps, peptic ulcers, or thyroid disease.
- Before having surgery or any other medical or dental treatment, be sure to tell your doctor or dentist that you are taking aspirin. Aspirin is usually discontinued five to seven days before surgery, in order to prevent bleeding complications.

• The use of aspirin in children (about 16 years of age or less) with the flu or chicken pox has been associated with a rare, life-threatening condition called Reye's syndrome. Aspirin should, therefore, not be given to children with signs of an infection.
• Large doses of aspirin (greater than eight 325-mg tablets per day) can cause erroneous urine glucose test results. People with diabetes should, therefore, check with their doctor before changing insulin doses while taking this medication.
• Additional medications that contain aspirin should not be taken without your doctor's approval. Be sure to check the labels on over-the-counter (nonprescription) pain, sinus, allergy, asthma, cough, and cold preparations to see if they contain aspirin.
• Be sure to tell your doctor if you are pregnant. Aspirin has been shown to cause birth defects in the offspring of animals that received large doses during pregnancy. Large doses of aspirin given to a pregnant woman close to term can prolong labor and cause bleeding complications in the mother and heart problems in the infant. Also, tell your doctor if you are breast-feeding an infant. Small amounts of aspirin pass into breast milk.

---

atenolol

BRAND NAMES (Manufacturers)
atenolol (various manufacturers)
Tenormin (ICI Pharma)
TYPE OF DRUG
Beta-adrenergic blocking agent
INGREDIENT
atenolol
DOSAGE FORM
Tablets (25 mg, 50 mg, and 100 mg)
STORAGE
Atenolol should be stored at room temperature in a tightly closed, light-resistant container.

USES

Atenolol is used to treat high blood pressure and angina (chest pain). It belongs to a group of medicines known as beta-adrenergic blocking agents or, more commonly, beta blockers. These drugs work by controlling impulses along certain nerve pathways. The result is a decreased workload for the heart.

TREATMENT

Atenolol can be taken with a glass of water, with meals, immediately following meals, or on an empty stomach, depending on your doctor's instructions. Try to take the medication at the same time(s) each day.

Try not to miss any doses of this medication. If you do miss a dose, take the missed dose as soon as possible. However, if the next scheduled dose is within eight hours (if you are taking this medicine only once a day) or within four hours (if you are taking this medicine more than once a day), do not take the missed dose at all; just return to your regular dosing schedule. Do not double the next dose.

It is important to remember that atenolol does not cure high blood pressure, but it will help to control the condition as long as you continue to take it.

SIDE EFFECTS

Minor. Anxiety; constipation; decreased sexual ability; diarrhea; difficulty in sleeping; drowsiness; dryness of the eyes, mouth, and skin; headache; nausea; nervousness; stomach discomfort; tiredness; or weakness. These side effects should disappear as your body adjusts to the medicine.

If you are extra-sensitive to the cold, be sure to dress warmly during cold weather.

To relieve constipation, increase the amount of fiber in your diet (fresh fruits and vegetables, salads, bran, and whole-grain breads), and drink more water (unless your doctor directs you to do otherwise).

Plain, nonmedicated eye drops (artificial tears) may help to relieve eye dryness.

Sucking on ice chips or chewing sugarless gum helps relieve mouth or throat dryness.

Major. Tell your doctor about any side effects that are persistent or particularly bothersome. IT IS ESPECIALLY IMPORTANT TO TELL YOUR DOCTOR about breathing difficulty or wheezing; cold hands or feet (due to decreased blood circulation to skin, fingers, and toes); confusion; dizziness; fever and sore throat; hair loss; hallucinations; light-headedness; mental depression; nightmares; reduced alertness; skin rash; swelling of the ankles, feet, or lower legs; or unusual or unexplained bleeding or bruising.

INTERACTIONS

Atenolol interacts with a number of other medications:
1. Indomethacin has been shown to decrease the blood-pressure-lowering effects of the beta blockers. This negative effect may also happen with aspirin or other salicylates.
2. Concurrent use of beta blockers and calcium channel blockers (diltiazem, nifedipine, and verapamil) or disopyramide can lead to heart failure or very low blood pressure.
3. Cimetidine and oral contraceptives (birth control pills) can often increase the side effects of beta-adrenergic blocking agents.
4. Side effects may also be increased when beta blockers are taken with clonidine, digoxin, epinephrine, phenylephrine, phenylpropanolamine, phenothiazine tranquilizers, prazosin, or monoamine oxidase (MAO) inhibitors. At least 14 days should separate the use of a beta blocker and the use of an MAO inhibitor.
5. Alcohol, barbiturates, and rifampin can decrease the effectiveness of atenolol.
6. Beta blockers may antagonize (work against) the effects of theophylline, aminophylline, albuterol, isoproterenol, metaproterenol, and terbutaline.
7. Beta blockers can also interact with insulin or oral antidiabetic agents—raising or lowering blood-sugar levels or masking the symptoms of low blood sugar.

8. The action of beta blockers may be increased if they are used with chlorpromazine, furosemide, or hydralazine, which may have a negative effect.
9. In patients who have congestive heart failure treated with digitalis glycosides (for example, digoxin or digitoxin), caution should be used as both atenolol and digitalis products may slow heart conduction.

BE SURE TO TELL YOUR DOCTOR about any medications you are currently taking, especially any of those listed above.

WARNINGS

• Before starting to take this medication, it is important to tell your doctor if you have ever had unusual or allergic reactions to any beta blocker (acebutolol, atenolol, betaxolol, bisoprolol, carteolol, esmolol, labetalol, metoprolol, nadolol, penbutolol, pindolol, propranolol, and timolol).

• Tell your doctor if you now have or if you have ever had allergies, asthma, hay fever, eczema, slow heartbeat, bronchitis, diabetes mellitus, emphysema, heart or blood vessel disease, kidney disease, liver disease, thyroid disease, or poor circulation in the fingers or toes.

• In diabetics, atenolol may block some of the warning signs of low blood sugar (hypoglycemia), such as rapid pulse rate, but not others, such as dizziness or sweating.

• You may want to check your pulse while taking this medication. If your pulse is much slower than your usual rate (or if it is less than 50 beats per minute), check with your doctor. A pulse rate that is too slow may cause circulation problems.

• Atenolol may affect your body's response to exercise. Make sure you discuss with your doctor a safe amount of exercise for your medical condition.

• It is important that you do not stop taking this medicine without first checking with your doctor. Some conditions may become worse when the medicine is stopped suddenly, and the danger of a heart attack is increased in some patients. Your doctor may want you to gradually reduce the amount of medicine you take before stopping completely. Make sure that you have enough medicine on hand to last through vacations and holidays.

• Before having surgery or any other medical or dental treatment, tell the physician or dentist that you are taking this medicine. Often, this medication will be discontinued 48 hours prior to any major surgery.

• This medicine can cause dizziness, drowsiness, lightheadedness, or decreased alertness. Therefore, exercise caution while driving or using dangerous equipment.

• While taking this medicine, do not use any over-the-counter (nonprescription) asthma, allergy, cough, cold, sinus, or diet preparations unless you first check with your pharmacist or doctor. Some of these medicines can cause high blood pressure when taken at the same time as a beta blocker.

• Be sure to tell your doctor if you are pregnant. Animal studies have shown that some beta blockers can cause problems in pregnancy when used at very high doses. Adequate studies have not been done in humans, but there has been some association between beta blockers used during pregnancy and low birth weight, as well as breathing problems and slow heart rate in the newborn infants. However, other reports have shown no effects on newborn infants. Also, tell your doctor if you are breast-feeding an infant. Small amounts of atenolol may pass into breast milk.

---

azathioprine

BRAND NAME (Manufacturer)
Imuran (Burroughs Wellcome)
TYPE OF DRUG
Immunosuppressant
INGREDIENT
azathioprine
DOSAGE FORM
Tablets (50 mg)
STORAGE
Azathioprine should be stored at room temperature in a tightly closed, light-resistant container. This medication should not be refrigerated.

USES

This medication is used to prevent rejection of kidney transplants and to control the symptoms of severe rheumatoid arthritis. It is not clear how azathioprine works therapeutically for either condition, but it is known to act on the body's immune system.

TREATMENT

In order to prevent nausea and vomiting, you can take azathioprine with food or after a meal (unless your doctor directs you to do otherwise).

Try not to miss any doses of this medication. If you do miss a dose, take the missed dose as soon as possible, unless it is almost time for the next scheduled dose. In that case, do not take the missed dose at all; just return to your regular dosing schedule. Do not double the next dose. If you miss more than one dose, CHECK WITH YOUR DOCTOR.

SIDE EFFECTS

Minor. Diarrhea, nausea, or vomiting. These side effects should disappear over time and as your body adjusts to the medication.
Major. Tell your doctor about any side effects that are persistent or particularly bothersome. IT IS ESPECIALLY IMPORTANT TO TELL YOUR DOCTOR about darkened urine, fever, hair loss, joint pains, mouth sores, muscle aches, skin rash, sore throat, unusual bleeding or bruising, or yellowing of the eyes or skin.

INTERACTIONS

BE SURE TO TELL YOUR DOCTOR if you are already taking allopurinol. This medication can possibly increase the blood levels of azathioprine, which can lead to serious side effects.

WARNINGS

• Be sure to tell your doctor about any unusual or allergic reactions that you have had to any medications, especially to those you may have experienced after taking azathioprine.

• Before starting to take this medication, be sure to tell your doctor if you now have or if you have ever had gout, kidney disease, liver disease, pancreatitis, or recurrent infections.

• Azathioprine is potent medicine. Your doctor will want to monitor your therapy carefully with blood tests, so that you take the least amount of this medication that you possibly can.

• Do not stop taking this medication unless you first check with your doctor. Stopping therapy with this drug abruptly may lead to a worsening of your condition. Your doctor may, therefore, want to start you on another drug before therapy with azathioprine is stopped.

• There is a chance that azathioprine may cause unwanted effects months or years later. These delayed effects may include certain types of cancer. Be sure to discuss these possible effects with your doctor.

• Azathioprine can increase your susceptibility to infections. It is, therefore, important to contact your doctor at the first sign of infection. Your dose of azathioprine may need to be adjusted.

• Be sure to tell your doctor if you are pregnant. Birth defects have been reported in the offspring of animals that received large doses of azathioprine during pregnancy. This drug also has the potential for producing birth defects in human offspring. Use of this drug is not recommended during pregnancy. Birth defects may occur in the offspring if either the male or female is using this drug at the time of conception. Use of birth control is recommended while taking this drug. Also, tell your doctor if you are breast-feeding an infant. It is not known whether azathioprine passes into breast milk.

---

azithromycin

BRAND NAME (Manufacturer)
Zithromax (Pfizer)
TYPE OF DRUG
Antibiotic
INGREDIENT
azithromycin
DOSAGE FORM
Capsules (250 mg)
STORAGE
This product should be stored at room temperature in a closed, light-resistant container.

USES

Azithromycin is used to treat a wide variety of bacterial infections, including those of the upper and lower respiratory tracts and skin and certain sexually transmitted diseases. This medicine acts by preventing bacteria from manufacturing protein and thereby preventing their growth. Azithromycin kills certain bacteria but is not effective against viruses, parasites, or fungi.

TREATMENT

It is best to take azithromycin on an empty stomach (one hour before and two hours after a meal). Azithromycin works best when the level of medicine in your bloodstream is kept constant. Therefore, it is best to take the doses at the same time every day.

If you miss a dose, take it immediately. However, if you don't remember to take your scheduled dose until the next day, skip the missed dose and go back to your regular dosing schedule. Do not double the next dose.

It is important to continue to take this medicine for the entire time period prescribed by the doctor (usually five days), even if the symptoms disappear before the end of that period. If you stop taking this drug too soon, resistant bacteria (bacteria that will not be killed by the antibiotic) are given a chance to continue to grow and infection could recur.

SIDE EFFECTS

Minor. Diarrhea, nausea, vomiting, headache, dizziness, abdominal pain. These effects should disappear as your body adjusts to the medication.

This medication can cause increased sensitivity to sunlight. It is important to avoid prolonged exposure to sunlight and sunlamps. Wear protective clothing and use an effective sunscreen.

If you feel dizzy or light-headed, sit or lie down for a while; get up slowly from a sitting or reclining position; and be careful on stairs.

Major. Tell your doctor about any side effects that are persistent or particularly bothersome. IT IS ESPECIALLY IMPORTANT TO TELL YOUR DOCTOR about fever, palpitations, rash, shortness of breath, swelling of the face or neck, sore throat, rectal or vaginal itching, unusual bruising or bleeding, or yellowing of the eyes or skin. Also, if your symptoms of infection seem to be getting worse rather than improving, you should contact your doctor.

INTERACTIONS

Azithromycin interacts with several medications:

1. Azithromycin potentially can increase blood levels of aminophylline, theophylline, carbamazepine, cyclosporin, phenytoin, digoxin, triazolam, phenobarbital, ergotamine, dihydroergotamine, or oral anticoagulants (blood thinners, such as warfarin); this may lead to serious side effects.

2. Antacids containing aluminum and magnesium will decrease the efficacy of azithromycin. Take antacids one hour before, or two hours after your dose of azithromycin.

3. Terfenadine, astemizole, and loratidine may cause irregular heart rate when taken with azithromycin.

BE SURE TO TELL YOUR DOCTOR about any medications you are currently taking, especially any listed above.

WARNINGS

• Tell your doctor about any unusual reactions you have to any medications, especially to azithromycin, erythromycin, or clarithromycin.

• Tell you doctor if you have or ever had kidney disease, liver disease, or heart disease.

• This medication has been prescribed for your current infection only. Another infection later on, or one that someone else has, may require a different medicine. You should not give your medication to other people or use it for other infections, unless your doctor specifically directs you to do so.
• Before having surgery or any other medical or dental treatment, be sure to tell your doctor or dentist you are taking azithromycin.
• Be sure to tell your doctor if you are pregnant. The effects of this medicine during pregnancy have not been thoroughly studied in humans. Also, tell your doctor if you are breast-feeding an infant. It is not known if azithromycin passes into breast milk.

---

bromocriptine

BRAND NAME (Manufacturer)
Parlodel (Sandoz)
TYPE OF DRUG
Dopamine agonist and antiparkinsonism agent
INGREDIENT
bromocriptine
DOSAGE FORMS
Tablets (2.5 mg)
Capsules (5 mg)
STORAGE
Bromocriptine should be stored at room temperature in a tightly closed, light-resistant container.

USES

This medication is used to treat the symptoms of Parkinson's disease and to decrease milk production in women who choose not to breast-feed their infants. Bromocriptine relieves the symptoms of Parkinson's disease by replacing a chemical (dopamine) that is diminished in the brains of these patients. Bromocriptine prevents milk production by blocking the action of the responsible hormone (prolactin). Bromocriptine is also used to treat acromegaly (a growth disorder).

TREATMENT

In order to avoid stomach irritation, you can take the medication with food or with a full glass of water or milk.

If you miss a dose of this medication and remember within four hours, take the missed dose immediately. If more than four hours have passed, do not take the missed dose at all; just return to your regular dosing schedule. Do not double the next dose.

SIDE EFFECTS

Minor. Abdominal pain, constipation, diarrhea, dizziness, drowsiness, fatigue, headache, insomnia, light-headedness, loss of appetite, nasal congestion, nausea, or vomiting. These should disappear as your body adjusts to the drug.

Dizziness or fainting may occur, especially following the first dose. It is best, therefore, to take the first dose while lying down. If you feel dizzy or light-headed with later doses, sit or lie down; get up slowly.

To relieve constipation, increase the amount of fiber in your diet (fresh fruits and vegetables, salads, bran, and whole-grain breads). You can also increase your exercise and drink more water (unless your doctor directs you to do otherwise).

Major. Tell your doctor about any side effects that are persistent or particularly bothersome. IT IS ESPECIALLY IMPORTANT TO REPORT about abnormal, involuntary movements; anxiety; confusion; convulsions; depression; difficulty in swallowing; fainting; fluid retention; hallucinations; nervousness; nightmares; skin rash; shortness of breath; tingling in the hands or feet; or visual disturbances.

INTERACTIONS

Bromocriptine interacts with several medications:
1. Phenothiazine tranquilizers, methyldopa, haloperidol, metoclopramide, reserpine, and monoamine oxidase (MAO) inhibitors decrease the beneficial effects of bromocriptine.
2. Dosages of any antihypertensive medications may require adjustment when bromocriptine is started.

Before starting to take bromocriptine, BE SURE TO TELL YOUR DOCTOR about any medications you are currently taking, especially if you are taking any of those medications listed above.

WARNINGS

• Tell your doctor about unusual or allergic reactions you have had to any medications, especially to bromocriptine or ergotamine.
• Before starting treatment with this medication, be sure to tell your doctor if you now have or have ever had heart or blood-vessel disease, kidney disease, liver disease, or mental disorders.
• Alcohol should be avoided with this medication.
• If this drug makes you dizzy or drowsy, avoid tasks that require alertness, such as driving a car.
• Do not stop taking bromocriptine unless you first check with your doctor. Stopping the drug abruptly may lead to a worsening of your condition. Your doctor may want to reduce your dosage gradually to prevent this from occurring.
• Be sure to tell your doctor if you are pregnant. It is generally recommended that bromocriptine not be used during pregnancy because there have been reports of birth defects in both animals and humans whose mothers received the drug during pregnancy. Also, be sure to tell your doctor if you are breast-feeding an infant. Bromocriptine blocks milk production.

---

captopril

BRAND NAME (Manufacturer)
Capoten (Squibb)
TYPE OF DRUG
Antihypertensive

INGREDIENT
captopril
DOSAGE FORM
Tablets (12.5 mg, 25 mg, 50 mg, and 100 mg)
STORAGE
Captopril should be stored at room temperature in a tightly closed container.

USES

Captopril is used to treat high blood pressure and congestive heart failure. It is a vasodilator (it dilates the blood vessels) that acts by blocking the production of chemicals that may be responsible for constricting or narrowing blood vessels.

TREATMENT

To obtain maximum benefit from captopril, you should take it on an empty stomach one hour before meals. In order to become accustomed to taking this medication, try to take it at the same time(s) every day.

It may be several weeks before you notice the full effects of this medication.

If you miss a dose of this medication, take the missed dose as soon as possible, unless it is almost time for the next dose. In that case, do not take the missed dose at all; just wait until the next scheduled dose. Do not double the dose.

Captopril does not cure high blood pressure, but it will help control the condition as long as you continue to take this drug.

SIDE EFFECTS

Minor. Abdominal pain, constipation, cough, diarrhea, dizziness, dry mouth, fatigue, flushing, headache, insomnia, loss of appetite, loss of taste, nausea, or vomiting. These side effects should disappear as your body adjusts to the medication.

This medication can increase your sensitivity to sunlight. It is, therefore, important to avoid prolonged exposure to sunlight and sunlamps. Always wear protective clothing and sunglasses when out of doors, and use an effective sunscreen.

To relieve constipation, increase the amount of fiber in your diet (fresh fruits and vegetables, salads, bran, and whole-grain breads). You can also increase your level of exercise and drink more water (unless your doctor directs you to do otherwise).

To relieve mouth dryness, suck on ice chips or a piece of hard candy or chew sugarless gum.

To avoid dizziness or light-headedness when you stand, contract and relax the muscles of your legs for a few moments before rising. Do this by pushing one foot against the floor while raising the other foot slightly, alternating feet so that you are "pumping" your legs.

Major. Tell your doctor about any side effects that are persistent or particularly bothersome. IT IS ESPECIALLY IMPORTANT TO TELL YOUR DOCTOR about chest pain; chills; difficult or painful urination; fever; itching; mouth sores; palpitations; prolonged vomiting or diarrhea; rash; sore throat; swelling of the face, hands, or feet; tingling in the fingers or toes; unusual bleeding or bruising; or yellowing of the eyes or skin.

INTERACTIONS

Captopril interacts with several other types of medications:

1. Diuretics (water pills) and other antihypertensive medications can cause an excessive drop in blood pressure when combined with captopril (especially with the first dose).
2. The combination of captopril with spironolactone, triamterene, amiloride, potassium supplements, or salt substitutes can lead to hyperkalemia (dangerously high levels of potassium in the bloodstream).
3. Antineoplastic agents (anticancer drugs) or chloramphenicol can increase the bone marrow side effects of captopril.
4. Concurrent use of captopril and allopurinol can increase the risk of developing an allergic reaction to the medication.
5. Indomethacin can decrease the blood-pressure-lowering effects of captopril.
6. Captopril can delay the body's elimination of lithium. Concurrent use of captopril and lithium may cause lithium toxicity.

Before starting captopril, BE SURE TO TELL YOUR DOCTOR about any drugs you are taking, especially any of those listed above.

WARNINGS

• Tell your doctor about any unusual or allergic reactions you have or have had to medications, especially to captopril or enalapril.
• Tell your doctor if you now have or if you have ever had aortic stenosis, blood disorders, kidney disease, kidney transplant, liver disease, systemic lupus erythematosus, or a heart attack or stroke.
• Be careful—excessive perspiration, dehydration, or prolonged vomiting or diarrhea can lead to an excessive drop in blood pressure while you are taking this medication. Contact your doctor if you have any of these symptoms.
• Before having surgery or other medical or dental treatment, tell your doctor you are taking this drug.
• The first few doses of this drug may cause dizziness. Try to avoid any sudden changes in posture which can lead to light-headedness.
• If you have high blood pressure, do not take any over-the-counter (nonprescription) medications for weight control, or for allergy, asthma, sinus, cough, or cold problems unless you first check with your doctor.
• Do not stop taking this medication unless you first consult your doctor. Stopping this drug abruptly may lead to a rise in blood pressure.
• Be sure to tell your doctor if you are pregnant. Captopril has been found to cause birth defects in the fetus if taken during the second or third trimester of pregnancy. Also tell your doctor if you are breast-feeding an infant. Captopril passes into breast milk. The effects of this drug on the infant have not been determined.

carbamazepine

BRAND NAMES (Manufacturers)
carbamazepine (various manufacturers)
Epitol (Lemmon)
Tegretol (Geigy)
Tegretol Chewable (Geigy)
TYPE OF DRUG
Anticonvulsant
INGREDIENT
carbamazepine
DOSAGE FORMS
Tablets (200 mg)
Chewable tablets (100 mg)
Oral suspension (100 mg per 5-ml spoonful)
STORAGE
Carbamazepine tablets and oral suspension should be stored at room temperature in tightly closed containers.

USES

This medication is used for the treatment of seizure disorders, for relief of neuralgia (nerve pain), and for a wide variety of mental disorders. The mechanism of carbamazepine's antiseizure activity is unknown, but it is not related to other anticonvulsants. Carbamazepine is not an ordinary pain reliever—it should not be used for minor aches or pains.

TREATMENT

Carbamazepine can be taken with food if stomach upset occurs, unless your doctor directs otherwise.

Carbamazepine works best when the level of medicine in your bloodstream is kept constant. It is best, therefore, to take it at evenly spaced intervals day and night. For example, if you are to take four doses a day, the doses should be spaced six hours apart.

Try not to miss any doses of this medication. If you do miss a dose, take the missed dose as soon as possible, unless it is almost time for the next dose. In that case, do not take the missed dose at all; just return to your regular dosing schedule. Do not double the next dose unless your doctor directs you to do so. If you are taking carbamazepine for a seizure disorder and you miss two or more doses, be sure to contact your doctor.

SIDE EFFECTS

Minor. Agitation; blurred vision; confusion; constipation; diarrhea; dizziness; drowsiness; dry mouth; headache; loss of appetite; muscle or joint pain; nausea; restlessness; sweating; vomiting; or weakness. These side effects should disappear over time and as your body adjusts to the medication.

This medication can increase your sensitivity to sunlight. It is important to avoid prolonged exposure to sunlight and sunlamps. Always wear protective clothing and sunglasses when out of doors, and use sunscreen.

To relieve constipation, increase the amount of fiber in your diet (fresh fruits and vegetables, salads, bran, and whole-grain breads), exercise, and drink more water (unless your doctor directs you to do otherwise).

To relieve mouth dryness, suck on ice chips or a piece of hard candy or chew sugarless gum.

If you feel dizzy or light-headed, sit or lie down for a while; get up slowly from a sitting or reclining position; and be careful on stairs.

Major. Be sure to tell your doctor about any side effects that are persistent or particularly bothersome. IT IS ESPECIALLY IMPORTANT FOR YOU TO TELL YOUR DOCTOR about abdominal pain, chills, depression, difficulty in breathing, difficulty in urinating, eye discomfort, fainting, fever, hair loss, hallucinations, impotence, loss of balance, mouth sores, nightmares, numbness or tingling sensations, palpitations, ringing in the ears, skin rash, sore throat, swelling of the hands and feet, twitching, unusual bleeding or bruising, or yellowing of the eyes or skin.

INTERACTIONS

Carbamazepine interacts with other types of medications:

1. Concurrent use of it with central nervous system depressants (such as alcohol, antihistamines, barbiturates, benzodiazepine tranquilizers, muscle relaxants, narcotics, pain medications, and phenothiazine tranquilizers) or with tricyclic antidepressants can cause extreme drowsiness.

2. Phenobarbital, phenytoin, and primidone can decrease blood levels and effectiveness of carbamazepine.

3. Isoniazid, propoxyphene, verapamil, cimetidine, troleandomycin, and erythromycin can increase the blood levels of carbamazepine, which can also increase side effects.

4. The combination of lithium and carbamazepine can lead to central nervous system side effects.

5. Carbamazepine can decrease the effectiveness of phenytoin, oral anticoagulants (blood thinners, such as warfarin), doxycycline, oral contraceptives (birth control pills), ethosuximide, valproic acid, aminophylline, and theophylline.

6. The use of carbamazepine within 14 days of the use of a monoamine oxidase (MAO) inhibitor can lead to serious side effects.

Before you start to take carbamazepine, BE SURE TO TELL YOUR DOCTOR about any medications you are currently taking, especially any of those listed above.

WARNINGS

• Tell your doctor about unusual or allergic reactions you have had to any medications, especially to carbamazepine or to tricyclic antidepressants (such as amitriptyline, desipramine, doxepin, imipramine, protriptyline, or nortriptyline).

• Tell your doctor if you now have or if you have ever had bone marrow depression, blood disorders, difficulty urinating, glaucoma, heart or blood vessel disease, kidney disease, or liver disease.

• Before having surgery or any other medical or dental treatment, be sure to tell your doctor or dentist that you are taking this medication.

• If this medication makes you dizzy or drowsy, do not take part in any activity that requires alertness, such as driving a car or operating potentially dangerous equipment.

• If you are taking this medication to control any type of seizure disorder, do not stop taking it suddenly. If you stop abruptly, you may experience uncontrollable seizures.
• Be sure to tell your doctor if you are pregnant. Birth defects have been reported more often in infants whose mothers have seizure disorders. It is unclear if the increased risk of birth defects is associated with the disorder or with the anticonvulsant medications, such as carbamazepine, that are used to treat the condition. The risks and benefits of treatment should be discussed with your doctor. Also, tell your doctor if you are breast-feeding an infant. Small amounts of carbamazepine pass into breast milk.

---

cefaclor

BRAND NAME (Manufacturer)
Ceclor (Lilly)
TYPE OF DRUG
Cephalosporin antibiotic
INGREDIENT
cefaclor
DOSAGE FORMS
Capsules (250 mg and 500 mg)
Oral suspension (125 mg, 187 mg, 250 mg, and 375 mg per 5-ml spoonful)
STORAGE
Cefaclor capsules should be stored at room temperature in a tightly closed container. The oral suspension form of this drug should be stored in the refrigerator in a tightly closed container. Any unused portion of the oral suspension should be discarded after 14 days because the drug loses its potency after that time. This medication should never be frozen.

USES

This medication is used to treat a wide variety of bacterial infections, including those of the middle ear, skin, upper and lower respiratory tract, and urinary tract. This drug acts by severely injuring the cell walls of the infecting bacteria, thereby preventing them from growing and multiplying. Cefaclor kills susceptible bacteria, but it is not effective against viruses, parasites, or fungi.

TREATMENT

Cefaclor can be taken either on an empty stomach or with food or a glass of milk (to avoid an upset stomach).

The contents of the suspension form of cefaclor tend to settle on the bottom of the bottle, so it is necessary to shake the container well to distribute the ingredients evenly and equalize the doses. Each dose should then be measured carefully with a specially designed 5-ml measuring spoon or with the dropper provided. An ordinary kitchen teaspoon is not accurate enough.

Cephalosporin antibiotics work best when the level of medicine in your bloodstream is kept at a constant level. It is best, therefore, to take the doses at evenly spaced intervals day and night. For example, if you are to take three doses a day, the doses should be spaced eight hours apart.

If you miss a dose of this medication, take the missed dose immediately. If you do not remember to take the missed dose until it is almost time for your next dose, take it; space the following dose halfway through the regular interval between doses; then return to your regular dosing schedule. Try not to skip any doses.

It is important to continue to take this medication for the entire time prescribed by your doctor (usually seven to 14 days), even if the symptoms disappear before the end of that period. If you stop taking this drug too soon, resistant bacteria are given a chance to continue growing, and the infection could recur.

SIDE EFFECTS

Minor. Abdominal pain, diarrhea, dizziness, fatigue, headache, heartburn, loss of appetite, nausea, or vomiting. These minor side effects can be expected to disappear in time as your body becomes accustomed to the medication.

If you feel dizzy, sit or lie down for a while; get up slowly from a sitting or reclining position.

Major. Tell your doctor about any side effects that are persistent or particularly bothersome. IT IS ESPECIALLY IMPORTANT TO TELL YOUR DOCTOR about darkened tongue, difficulty in breathing, fever, itching, joint pain, rash, rectal or vaginal itching, severe diarrhea (which can be watery or can contain pus or blood), sore mouth, stomach cramps, tingling in the hands or feet, or unusual bleeding or bruising. Also, if symptoms of infection seem to be getting worse rather than improving, contact your doctor.

INTERACTIONS

Cefaclor interacts with several other types of medications:
1. Probenecid can increase the blood concentrations and side effects of this medication.
2. The side effects, especially effects on the kidneys, of furosemide, bumetanide, ethacrynic acid, colistin, vancomycin, polymyxin B, and aminoglycoside antibiotics can be increased by cefaclor.

BE SURE TO TELL YOUR DOCTOR about any medications you are currently taking, especially any listed above.

WARNINGS

• Be sure to tell your doctor about any unusual or allergic reactions you have or have ever had to any medication, especially to cefaclor or other cephalosporin antibiotics (such as cefamandole, cephalexin, cephradine, cefadroxil, cefazolin, cefixime, cefoperazone, cefotaxime, cefpodoxime, cefprozil, ceftizoxime, cephalothin, cephapirin, cefuroxime, and moxalactam) or to penicillin antibiotics.
• Tell your doctor if you now have or if you have ever had kidney disease.
• This medication has been prescribed for your current infection only. Another infection later on, or one that someone else has, may require a different medicine. You should not give your medication to other people or use it for other infections.
• Diabetics who are taking cefaclor should know that this medication can cause a false-positive sugar reaction with a Clinitest urine glucose test. To avoid this problem while taking cefaclor, you should switch to Clinistix or Tes-Tape to test your urine sugar content.

• Be sure to tell your doctor if you are pregnant. Although the cephalosporin antibiotics appear to be safe when administered during pregnancy, extensive and conclusive studies in human subjects have not been conducted. Also, be sure that you tell your doctor if you are breast-feeding an infant. Small amounts of this medication can pass into breast milk and may temporarily alter the bacterial balance in the intestinal tract of the nursing infant, resulting in gastrointestinal problems in the infant.

---

chlordiazepoxide

BRAND NAMES (Manufacturers)
chlordiazepoxide hydrochloride (various manufacturers)
Libritabs (Roche)
Librium (Roche)
Mitran (Hauck)
TYPE OF DRUG
Benzodiazepine sedative/hypnotic
INGREDIENT
chlordiazepoxide
DOSAGE FORMS
Capsules (5 mg, 10 mg, and 25 mg)
Tablets (5 mg, 10 mg, and 25 mg)
STORAGE
This medication should be stored at room temperature in tightly closed, light-resistant containers.

USES

Chlordiazepoxide is prescribed to treat the symptoms of anxiety and alcohol withdrawal. It is not clear exactly how this medicine works, but it may relieve anxiety by acting as a depressant of the central nervous system. This drug is used to relieve nervousness. It is effective for this purpose, but it is important to remove the cause of the anxiety as well.

TREATMENT

This medication should be taken exactly as directed by your doctor. It can be taken with food or a full glass of water if stomach upset occurs. Do not take this medication with a dose of antacids, since they may retard its absorption.

If you are taking this medication regularly and you miss a dose, take the missed dose immediately. If more than an hour has passed, however, skip the dose you missed and wait for the next scheduled dose. Do not double the dose.

SIDE EFFECTS

Minor. Bitter taste in the mouth, constipation, depression, diarrhea, dizziness, drowsiness (after a night's sleep), dry mouth, excessive salivation, fatigue, flushing, headache, heartburn, loss of appetite, nausea, nervousness, sweating, or vomiting. As your body adjusts to the medicine, these side effects should disappear.

To relieve constipation, increase the fiber in your diet (fresh fruits and vegetables, salads, bran, and whole-grain breads), exercise, and drink more water (unless your doctor instructs you to do otherwise).

Dry mouth can be relieved by chewing sugarless gum or by sucking on ice chips.

If you feel dizzy, sit or lie down for a while; get up slowly from a sitting or reclining position; and be careful on stairs.

Major. Tell your doctor about any side effects that are persistent or particularly bothersome. IT IS ESPECIALLY IMPORTANT TO TELL YOUR DOCTOR about blurred or double vision, chest pain, difficulty in urinating, fainting, falling, fever, hallucinations, joint pain, mouth sores, nightmares, palpitations, rash, severe depression, shortness of breath, slurred speech, sore throat, uncoordinated movements, unusual excitement, unusual tiredness, or yellowing of the eyes or skin.

INTERACTIONS

Chlordiazepoxide interacts with several other drugs:

1. To prevent oversedation, this drug should not be taken with alcohol, other sedative drugs, central nervous system depressants (such as antihistamines, barbiturates, muscle relaxants, pain medicines, narcotics, medicines for seizures, and phenothiazine tranquilizers), or with antidepressants.

2. This medication may decrease the effectiveness of carbamazepine, levodopa, and oral anticoagulants (blood thinners) and may increase the effects of phenytoin.

3. Disulfiram, oral contraceptives (birth control pills), isoniazid, and cimetidine can increase the blood levels of chlordiazepoxide, which can lead to toxic effects.

4. Concurrent use of rifampin may decrease the effectiveness of chlordiazepoxide.

BE SURE TO TELL YOUR DOCTOR about any medications you are currently taking, especially any of the medications that are listed above.

WARNINGS

• Tell your doctor about unusual or allergic reactions you have had to any medications, especially to chlordiazepoxide or other benzodiazepine tranquilizers (such as alprazolam, clorazepate, diazepam, flurazepam, halazepam, lorazepam, oxazepam, prazepam, temazepam, and triazolam).

• Tell your doctor if you now have or if you have ever had liver disease, kidney disease, epilepsy, lung disease, myasthenia gravis, porphyria, sleep apnea, mental depression, or mental illness.

• This medicine can cause drowsiness. Avoid tasks that require alertness, such as driving a car or operating potentially dangerous machinery.

• Before having surgery or any other medical or dental treatment, tell your doctor or dentist that you are taking this drug.

• This medication has the potential for abuse and must be used with caution. Tolerance may develop quickly; do not increase the dosage of the drug without first consulting your doctor. It is also important not to stop this drug suddenly if you have been taking it in large amounts or if you have used it for several weeks. Your doctor may want to reduce your dosage of this medication gradually to avoid complications.

• This is a safe drug when used properly. When it is combined with other sedative drugs or alcohol, however, serious side effects may develop.
• Be sure to tell your doctor if you are pregnant. This medicine may increase the chance of birth defects if it is taken during the first three months of pregnancy. In addition, too much use of this medicine during the last six months of pregnancy may lead to addiction of the fetus, resulting in withdrawal side effects in the newborn. Also, use of this medicine during the last weeks of pregnancy may cause excessive drowsiness, slowed heartbeat, and breathing difficulties in the infant. Tell your doctor if you are breast-feeding an infant. This medicine can pass into breast milk and cause excessive drowsiness, slowed heartbeat, and breathing difficulties in the nursing infant.

chlorpromazine

BRAND NAMES (Manufacturers)
chlorpromazine hydrochloride (various manufacturers)
Ormazine (Hauck)
Sonazine (Cord)
Thorazine (SmithKline Beecham)
Thorazine Spansules (SmithKline Beecham)
Thor-Prom (Major)
TYPE OF DRUG
Phenothiazine tranquilizer
INGREDIENT
chlorpromazine hydrochloride
DOSAGE FORMS
Tablets (10 mg, 25 mg, 50 mg, 100 mg, and 200 mg)
Sustained-release capsules (30 mg, 75 mg, 150 mg, 200 mg, and 300 mg)
Oral concentrate (30 mg per ml and 100 mg per ml)
Oral syrup (10 mg per 5-ml spoonful)
Suppositories (25 mg and 100 mg)
STORAGE
The tablet and capsule forms of this drug should be stored at room temperature in tightly closed, light-resistant containers. The oral syrup and suppository forms of this drug should be stored in the refrigerator in tightly closed, light-resistant containers. If the oral concentrate or syrup turns to a slight yellow color, the medicine is still effective and can be used. However, if it changes color markedly or has particles floating in it, it should not be used. Chlorpromazine should never be frozen.

USES

Chlorpromazine is prescribed to treat the symptoms of certain types of mental illness, such as emotional symptoms of psychosis, the manic phase of manic-depressive illness, and severe behavioral problems in children. This medication is thought to relieve the symptoms of mental illness by blocking certain chemicals involved with nerve transmission in the brain.

Chlorpromazine may also be used to treat tetanus, porphyria, uncontrollable hiccups, anxiety before surgery, and nausea and vomiting.

TREATMENT

To avoid stomach irritation, take the tablet or capsule forms of this medication with a meal or with a glass of water or milk (unless your doctor directs you to do otherwise). The sustained-release capsules should be taken whole; do not crush, break, or open them prior to swallowing. Breaking the capsule would result in releasing the medication all at once—defeating the purpose of the extended-release capsules.

Measure the oral syrup carefully with a specially designed 5-ml measuring spoon. An ordinary kitchen teaspoon is not accurate enough.

The oral-concentrate form of this medication should be measured carefully with the dropper provided, then added to four ounces (one-half cup) or more of water, milk, a carbonated beverage, or to applesauce or pudding immediately prior to administration. Be careful that the serving size is not more than the patient is willing or able to drink or eat; otherwise, the full dose may not be consumed. To prevent possible loss of effectiveness, the medication should not be diluted in tea, coffee, or apple juice.

To use the suppository form of this medication, remove the foil wrapper and moisten the suppository with water (if the suppository is too soft to insert, refrigerate it for half an hour or run cold water over it before removing the wrapper). Lie on your left side with your right knee bent. Push the suppository into the rectum, pointed end first. Lie still for a few minutes. Try to avoid having a bowel movement for at least an hour.

If you miss a dose of this medication, take the missed dose as soon as possible, then return to your regular schedule. If it is almost time for the next dose, however, skip the one you missed and return to your regular schedule. Do not double the dose (unless your doctor directs you to do so).

Antacids and antidiarrheal medicines may decrease the absorption of this medication from the gastrointestinal tract. Therefore, at least one hour should separate doses of one of these medicines and chlorpromazine.

The full effects of this medication for the control of emotional or mental symptoms may not become apparent for two weeks after you start to take it.

SIDE EFFECTS

Minor. Blurred vision, constipation, decreased sweating, diarrhea, dizziness, drooling, drowsiness, dry mouth, fatigue, jitteriness, menstrual irregularities, nasal congestion, restlessness, tremors, vomiting, or weight gain. As your body adjusts to the medication, these side effects should disappear.

This medication can cause increased sensitivity to sunlight. It is, therefore, important to avoid prolonged exposure to sunlight or sunlamps. Wear protective clothing and use an effective sunscreen.

Chlorpromazine can also cause discoloration of the urine to red, pink, or red-brown. This is a harmless effect.

If you are constipated, increase the amount of fiber in your diet (fresh fruits and vegetables, salads, bran, and whole-grain breads), exercise, and drink more water (unless your doctor directs you to do otherwise).

Chew sugarless gum or suck on ice chips or a piece of hard candy to reduce mouth dryness.

To avoid dizziness or light-headedness when you stand, contract and relax the muscles of your legs for a few moments before rising to move the blood. Do this by pushing one foot against the floor while raising the other foot slightly, alternating feet so that you are "pumping" your legs in a pedaling motion.

Major. Tell your doctor about any side effects that are persistent or particularly bothersome. IT IS ESPECIALLY IMPORTANT TO TELL YOUR DOCTOR about breast enlargement (in both sexes); chest pain; convulsions; darkened skin; difficulty in swallowing or breathing; fainting; fever; impotence; involuntary movements of the face, mouth, jaw, or tongue; palpitations; rash; sleep disorders; sore throat; uncoordinated movements; unusual bleeding or bruising; visual disturbances; or yellowing of the eyes or skin.

INTERACTIONS

Chlorpromazine will interact with several types of medications:

1. It can cause extreme drowsiness when combined with alcohol or other central nervous system depressants (such as barbiturates, benzodiazepine tranquilizers, muscle relaxants, narcotics, and pain medications) or with tricyclic antidepressants.

2. Chlorpromazine can decrease the effectiveness of amphetamines, guanethidine, anticonvulsants, and levodopa.

3. The side effects of cyclophosphamide, epinephrine, monoamine oxidase (MAO) inhibitors, phenytoin, and tricyclic antidepressants may be increased by this medication.

4. Chlorpromazine can increase the absorption of propranolol, which can increase the risks of side effects.

5. Lithium may increase the side effects and decrease the effectiveness of this medication.

Before starting to take chlorpromazine, BE SURE TO TELL YOUR DOCTOR about any medications that you are currently taking, especially any of those drugs listed above.

WARNINGS

- Tell your doctor about unusual or allergic reactions you have had to any medications, especially to chlorpromazine or any other phenothiazine tranquilizers (such as fluphenazine, mesoridazine, perphenazine, prochlorperazine, promazine, thioridazine, and trifluoperazine) or to loxapine.
- Tell your doctor if you have a history of alcoholism, or if you now have or ever had blood disease, bone marrow disease, brain disease, breast cancer, blockage in the urinary or digestive tract, drug-induced depression, epilepsy, high or low blood pressure, diabetes mellitus, glaucoma, heart or circulatory disease, liver disease, lung disease, Parkinson's disease, peptic ulcers, or an enlarged prostate gland.
- Tell your doctor about any recent exposure to a pesticide or an insecticide. Chlorpromazine may increase the side effects from the exposure.
- To prevent oversedation, avoid drinking alcoholic beverages while taking this medication.
- If this drug makes you dizzy or drowsy, avoid any activity that requires alertness. Be careful on stairs, and avoid getting up suddenly from a lying or sitting position.
- Before having surgery or any other medical or dental treatment, be sure to tell your doctor or dentist that you are taking this medication.
- Some of the side effects caused by this drug can be prevented by taking an antiparkinsonism drug. Discuss this with your doctor.
- This medication can decrease sweating and heat release from the body. You should, therefore, avoid becoming overheated by strenuous exercise in hot weather and should avoid taking hot baths, showers, and saunas.
- Do not stop taking this medication suddenly. If the drug is stopped abruptly, you may experience nausea, vomiting, stomach upset, headache, increased heart rate, insomnia, tremors, or a worsening of your condition. Your doctor may want to reduce the dosage gradually.
- If you are planning to have a myelogram or any other procedure in which dye will be injected into your spinal cord, tell your doctor that you are taking this medication.
- Avoid spilling the oral concentrate or oral syrup forms of this medication on your skin or clothing; it may cause redness and irritation of the skin.
- While you are being treated with this medication, do not take any over-the-counter (nonprescription) medications for weight control or for cough, cold, allergy, asthma, or sinus problems without first checking with your doctor. The combination of these medications with chlorpromazine may cause high blood pressure.
- Be sure to tell your doctor if you are pregnant. Small amounts of this medication cross the placenta. Although there are reports of safe use of this drug during pregnancy, there are also reports of liver disease and tremors in newborn infants whose mothers received this medication close to term. Also, tell your doctor if you are breast-feeding an infant. Small amounts of this medication pass into breast milk and may affect the nursing infant.

---

chlorpropamide

BRAND NAMES (Manufacturers)

chlorpropamide (various manufacturers)
Diabinese (Pfizer)

TYPE OF DRUG

Oral antidiabetic

INGREDIENT

chlorpropamide

DOSAGE FORM

Tablets (100 mg and 250 mg)

STORAGE

Store at room temperature in a tightly closed container. This medication should not be refrigerated.

USES

Chlorpropamide is used for the treatment of diabetes mellitus that appears in adulthood and cannot be managed by control of diet alone. This type of diabetes is known as non-insulin-dependent diabetes (sometimes called maturity-onset or Type II diabetes). Chlorpropamide lowers blood sugar by increasing the release of insulin from the pancreas.

TREATMENT

In order for this medication to work correctly, it must be taken as your doctor has directed. It is best to take this medicine at the same time each day in order to maintain a constant blood-sugar level. It is important, therefore, to try not to miss any doses of this medication. If you do miss a dose, take it as soon as possible, unless it is almost time for the next dose. In that case, do not take the missed dose at all; just return to your regular dosing schedule. Do not double the next dose. Tell your doctor if you feel any side effects from missing a dose.

Diabetics who are taking oral antidiabetic medication may need to be switched to insulin if they develop diabetic coma, have a severe infection, are scheduled for major surgery, or become pregnant.

SIDE EFFECTS

Minor. Diarrhea, headache, heartburn, loss of appetite, nausea, stomach discomfort, stomach pain, or vomiting. These side effects usually disappear during treatment, as your body adjusts to the medication.

Chlorpropamide may increase your sensitivity to sunlight. Use caution during exposure to the sun. You may want to wear protective clothing and sunglasses. Use an effective sunscreen and avoid exposure to sunlamps.

Major. If any side effects are persistent or particularly bothersome, it is important to notify your doctor. IT IS ESPECIALLY IMPORTANT TO TELL YOUR DOCTOR about dark urine, fatigue, itching of the skin, light-colored stools, sore throat and fever, unusual bleeding or bruising, or yellowing of the eyes or skin.

Chlorpropamide can also cause retention of body water, which in turn can lead to drowsiness; muscle cramps; seizures; swelling or puffiness of the face, hands, or ankles; and tiredness or weakness. IT IS IMPORTANT TO TELL YOUR DOCTOR if you notice the appearance of any of these side effects.

INTERACTIONS

Chlorpropamide will interact with several other types of medications:

1. Chloramphenicol, fenfluramine, guanethidine, insulin, miconazole, monoamine oxidase (MAO) inhibitors, oxyphenbutazone, oxytetracycline, phenylbutazone, probenecid, aspirin or other salicylates, sulfinpyrazone, or sulfonamide antibiotics, when combined with chlorpropamide, can lower blood-sugar levels—sometimes to dangerously low levels.

2. Thyroid hormones, dextrothyroxine, epinephrine, phenytoin, thiazide diuretics (water pills), or cortisone-like medications (such as dexamethasone, hydrocortisone, and prednisone), when combined with chlorpropamide, can actually increase blood-sugar levels.

3. Rifampin can decrease the blood levels of chlorpropamide, which can lead to a decrease in its effectiveness.

4. Antidiabetic medications can increase the effects of anticoagulants (blood thinners, such as warfarin), which can lead to bleeding complications.

5. Beta-blocking medications (acebutolol, atenolol, betaxolol, bisoprolol, carteolol, esmolol, labetalol, metoprolol, nadolol, penbutolol, pindolol, propranolol, and timolol), combined with chlorpropamide, can result in either high or low blood-sugar levels. Beta blockers can also mask the symptoms of low blood sugar, which can be dangerous.

6. Avoid drinking alcoholic beverages while taking this medication (unless otherwise directed by your doctor). Some patients who take this medicine suffer nausea, vomiting, dizziness, stomach pain, pounding headache, sweating, or redness of the face and skin when they drink alcohol. Also, large amounts of alcohol can lower blood sugar to dangerously low levels.

BE SURE TO TELL YOUR DOCTOR about any medications you are currently taking, especially any of those listed above.

WARNINGS

• It is important to tell your doctor if you have ever had unusual or allergic reactions to this medicine or to any sulfa medication (sulfonamide antibiotics, acetazolamide, diuretics [water pills], or other oral antidiabetics).

• Tell your doctor if you now have or if you have ever had kidney disease, liver disease, severe infection, or thyroid disease.

• Be sure to follow the special diet that your doctor gave you. This is an essential part of controlling your blood sugar and is necessary in order for this medicine to work properly.

• Before having surgery or any other medical or dental treatment, be sure to tell your doctor or dentist that you are taking this medicine.

• Have tests conducted for sugar in your blood or urine, as directed by your doctor. It is a convenient way to determine whether or not your diabetes is being controlled by this medicine.

• Eat or drink something containing sugar right away if you experience any symptoms of low blood sugar (such as anxiety, chills, cold sweats, cool or pale skin, drowsiness, excessive hunger, headache, nausea, nervousness, rapid heartbeat, shakiness, or unusual tiredness or weakness). It is important that your family and friends know the symptoms of low blood sugar and what to do if they observe any of these symptoms in you.

• Even if the symptoms of low blood sugar are corrected by eating or drinking sugar, it is important to contact your doctor as soon as possible after experiencing them. The blood-sugar-lowering effects of this medicine can last for hours, and the symptoms may return during this period. Good sources of sugar are orange juice, corn syrup, honey, sugar cubes, and table sugar. You are at greatest risk of developing low blood sugar if you skip or delay meals, exercise more than usual, cannot eat because of nausea or vomiting, or drink large amounts of alcoholic beverages.

• Be sure to tell your doctor if you are pregnant. Since extensive studies have not yet been conducted, it is not known whether this medication can cause problems when administered to a pregnant woman. Cautious use of this medication is thus warranted.

It is also important to tell your doctor if you are currently breast-feeding an infant. It has been determined that this medicine can pass from the mother's blood into breast milk. For this reason this medication is not recommended for use by any woman who is breast-feeding.

---

cholestyramine

BRAND NAMES (Manufacturers)
Cholybar (Parke-Davis)
Questran (Bristol Labs)
Questran Light (Bristol Labs)

TYPE OF DRUG
Antihyperlipidemic (lipid-lowering drug)

INGREDIENT
cholestyramine

DOSAGE FORMS
Oral powder (4 g of cholestyramine per 9 g of powder or 4 g of cholestyramine per 5 g of powder)
Bar (4 g of cholestyramine per bar)

STORAGE
Cholestyramine should be stored at room temperature in a tightly closed container. This medication should not be refrigerated.

USES

This medication is used to lower blood cholesterol and to treat itching associated with liver disease. Cholestyramine chemically binds to bile salts in the gastrointestinal tract and prevents the body from producing cholesterol.

TREATMENT

Cholestyramine is usually taken before meals. Each dose should be measured carefully and then added to 2 to 6 ounces of water, milk, fruit juice, or another noncarbonated drink. To avoid swallowing of air, this mixture should be taken slowly. The powder can also be mixed with soup, applesauce, or crushed pineapple. You should never take cholestyramine dry; you might accidentally inhale the powder, which could irritate your throat and lungs. For the bar form of the drug, chew thoroughly. As with the powder, this should be followed with plenty of fluids.

If you miss a dose of this medication, take it as soon as possible, unless it is almost time for the next dose. In that case, do not take the missed dose at all; just return to your regular dosing schedule. Do not double the next dose.

Cholestyramine does not cure hypercholesterolemia (high blood-cholesterol levels), but it will help to control the condition as long as you continue to take it.

SIDE EFFECTS

Minor. Anxiety, belching, constipation, diarrhea, dizziness, drowsiness, fatigue, gas, headache, hiccups, loss of appetite, nausea, stomach pain, vomiting, or weight loss or gain. These side effects should disappear as your body adjusts to the medication.

To relieve constipation, increase the amount of fiber in your diet (fresh fruits and vegetables, salads, bran, and whole-grain breads), exercise, and drink more water (unless your doctor directs you to do otherwise).

If you feel dizzy, sit or lie down for a while; get up slowly from a sitting or reclining position; and be careful on stairs.

Major. Tell your doctor about any side effects you experience that are persistent or particularly bothersome. IT IS ESPECIALLY IMPORTANT TO TELL YOUR DOCTOR about backaches; bloody or black, tarry stools; difficult or painful urination; fluid retention; muscle or joint pains; rash or irritation of the skin, tongue, or rectal area; ringing in the ears; swollen glands; tingling sensations; unusual bleeding or bruising; or unusual weakness.

INTERACTIONS

Cholestyramine interferes with the absorption of a number of other drugs, including phenylbutazone, warfarin (a blood thinner), thiazide diuretics (water pills), digoxin, penicillins, tetracycline, phenobarbital, folic acid, iron, thyroid hormones, cephalexin, clindamycin, trimethoprim, and fat-soluble vitamins (A, D, E, and K). The effectiveness of these medications will be decreased by cholestyramine. To avoid this interaction, take the other medications one hour before or four to six hours after a dose of cholestyramine.

BE SURE TO TELL YOUR DOCTOR about any medications you are currently taking, especially those listed above.

WARNINGS

• Tell your doctor about unusual or allergic reactions you have had to any medications, especially to cholestyramine.

• Tell your doctor if you now have or if you have ever had bleeding disorders, biliary obstruction, heart disease, hemorrhoids, gallstones or gallbladder disease, kidney disease, malabsorption, stomach ulcers, or an obstructed intestine.

• Cholestyramine should be used only in conjunction with diet, weight reduction, or correction of other conditions that could be causing elevated levels of blood cholesterol.

• This product contains the color additive FD&C Yellow No. 5 (tartrazine), which can cause allergic-type reactions (fainting, rash, shortness of breath) in certain susceptible individuals.

• The color of cholestyramine powder may vary from batch to batch. This does not change the effectiveness of the medication.

• Be sure to tell your doctor if you are pregnant. Although cholestyramine appears to be safe (because very little is absorbed into the bloodstream), extensive studies in humans during pregnancy have not been conducted. Also, tell your doctor if you are breast-feeding an infant. It is not known whether cholestyramine passes into breast milk. However, cholestyramine can decrease the absorption of some vitamins in the mother, which could result in decreased vitamins to the nursing infant.

---

cimetidine

BRAND NAMES (Manufacturers)
cimetidine (various manufacturers)
Tagamet (SmithKline Beecham)
TYPE OF DRUG
Gastric-acid-secretion inhibitor (decreases stomach acid)
INGREDIENT
cimetidine
DOSAGE FORMS
Tablets (200 mg, 300 mg, 400 mg, and 800 mg)
Oral liquid (300 mg per 5-ml spoonful, with 2.8% alcohol)
STORAGE
Cimetidine tablets and oral liquid should be stored at room temperature in tightly closed, light-resistant containers. This medication should never be frozen. If cimetidine is not properly stored (especially if it is exposed to light or heat) it may develop a strong, unpleasant odor.

USES

Cimetidine is used to treat duodenal and gastric ulcers. It is also used in the long-term treatment of excessive stomach acid secretion and in the prevention of recurrent ulcers. It is also used to treat gastro-esophagal reflux (backflow of stomach contents into the esophagus), which can cause heartburn. Cimetidine works by blocking the effects of histamine in the stomach, which reduces stomach acid secretion.

TREATMENT

Take cimetidine with, or shortly after, meals and again at bedtime (unless your doctor directs otherwise).

The tablets should not be crushed or chewed, because cimetidine has a bitter taste and an unpleasant odor.

The oral liquid should be measured carefully with a specially designed 5-ml measuring spoon. An ordinary kitchen teaspoon is not accurate enough.

Antacids can block the absorption of cimetidine. If you are taking antacids as well as cimetidine, at least one hour should separate doses of the two medications.

If you miss a dose of cimetidine, take the missed dose as soon as possible, unless it is almost time for the next dose. In that case, do not take the missed dose at all; just return to your regular dosing schedule. Do not double the next dose.

SIDE EFFECTS

Minor. Diarrhea, dizziness, drowsiness, headache, or muscle pain. These side effects should disappear as your body adjusts to the medication.

If you feel dizzy, sit or lie down for a while; stand up slowly; and be careful on stairs.

Major. Tell your doctor about any side effects that are persistent or particularly bothersome. IT IS ESPECIALLY IMPORTANT TO TELL YOUR DOCTOR about confusion, fever, hair loss, enlarged or painful breasts (in both sexes), hallucinations, impotence, palpitations, rash, sore throat, unusual bleeding or bruising, weakness, or yellowing of the eyes or skin.

INTERACTIONS

Cimetidine interacts with other types of medications:
1. It can decrease the elimination, and thus increase the side effects, of theophylline, aminophylline, oxtriphylline, phenytoin, carbamazepine, beta blockers, benzodiazepine tranquilizers (such as clorazepate, chlordiazepoxide, diazepam, flurazepam, halazepam, and prazepam), tricyclic antidepressants, oral anticoagulants (blood thinners, such as warfarin), lidocaine, verapamil, quinidine, nifedipine, metronidazole, codeine, and morphine.
2. The combination of cimetidine and anticancer drugs may increase the risk of blood disorders.
3. The absorption of ketoconazole is decreased by cimetidine; at least two hours should separate doses of these two drugs.
4. Cimetidine may decrease the blood levels and effectiveness of digoxin.

BE SURE TO TELL YOUR DOCTOR about any medications you are currently taking, especially any of those listed above.

WARNINGS

• Tell your doctor about any unusual or allergic reactions you have had to medications, especially to cimetidine, famotidine, nizatidine, or ranitidine.
• Tell your doctor if you now have or if you have ever had arthritis, kidney disease, liver disease, or organic brain syndrome.
• Cimetidine can decrease the elimination of alcohol from the body, which can prolong its intoxicating effects.
• Cimetidine should be taken continuously for as long as your doctor prescribes. Stopping therapy early may be a cause of ineffective treatment.
• Cigarette smoking may block the beneficial effects of therapy with cimetidine.
• If this drug makes you dizzy or drowsy, do not take part in any activity that requires alertness, such as driving a car or operating potentially dangerous equipment.
• Be sure to tell your doctor if you are pregnant. Cimetidine appears to be safe during pregnancy; however, extensive testing has not been conducted. Also, tell your doctor if you are breast-feeding an infant. Small amounts of cimetidine pass into breast milk.

---

ciprofloxacin

BRAND NAME (Manufacturer)
Cipro (Miles)
TYPE OF DRUG
Antibiotic

INGREDIENT
ciprofloxacin
DOSAGE FORM
Tablets (250 mg, 500 mg, and 750 mg)
STORAGE
Ciprofloxacin tablets should be stored at room temperature in tightly closed containers away from direct light.

USES

Ciprofloxacin is an antibiotic that is used to treat a wide variety of bacterial infections. It chemically attaches to the bacteria and prevents their growth and multiplication. Ciprofloxacin is not effective against viruses, parasites, or fungi.

TREATMENT

Ciprofloxacin is best taken two hours after a meal with a full glass (8 ounces) of water, however, it can be taken with or without meals. You should drink several additional glasses of water or other fluid every day, unless your doctor directs you to do otherwise. Drinking extra water will help to prevent some of the unwanted side effects of ciprofloxacin.

Ciprofloxacin works best when the level of medicine in your bloodstream is kept constant. It is best, therefore, to take the doses at evenly spaced intervals day and night. For example, if you are to take two doses a day, the doses should be spaced 12 hours apart.

It is very important that you do not miss any doses of this medication. If you do miss a dose, take it as soon as you remember. However, if you do not remember to take the missed dose until it is almost time for your next dose, skip the missed dose and go back to your regular dosing schedule. Do not double the next dose.

Ciprofloxacin therapy may be required for four to six weeks or longer. It is important to continue to take this drug for the entire time prescribed, even if the symptoms of infection disappear before the end of that period. If you stop taking the drug too soon, resistant bacteria are given a chance to continue growing, and your infection could recur.

SIDE EFFECTS

Minor. Diarrhea, headache, light-headedness, nausea, stomach irritation, or vomiting. These side effects should disappear as your body adjusts to the medication.

Major. Tell your doctor about any side effects that are persistent or particularly bothersome. IT IS ESPECIALLY IMPORTANT TO TELL YOUR DOCTOR about blood in your urine, change in your vision, confusion, convulsions (seizures), agitation, dizziness, hallucinations, lower back pain, muscle or joint pain, pain or difficulty in urinating, restlessness, skin rash, tremor, unpleasant taste, unusual bleeding or bruising, or yellowing of the eyes or skin. Also, if the symptoms of your infection do not improve in several days, contact your doctor.

INTERACTIONS

Ciprofloxacin interacts with several other drugs:

1. Use of antacids with ciprofloxacin can decrease the absorption of this medicine. Do not take antacids within two hours of taking this medicine.

2. Use of sucralfate with ciprofloxacin can decrease the absorption of ciprofloxacin. Do not take a dose of sucralfate within two hours of a dose of ciprofloxacin unless directed to do so by your doctor.

3. Use of medicine containing theophylline along with ciprofloxacin can lead to increased bloodstream levels of theophylline and therefore to an increased chance of theophylline-related side effects.

4. Regular consumption of large quantities of caffeine-containing products (coffee, tea, or caffeine-containing soft drinks) with ciprofloxacin may lead to exaggerated or prolonged effects of caffeine. Therefore, your doctor may wish for you to restrict intake of caffeine during treatment.

5. Use of probenecid with ciprofloxacin can increase the bloodstream levels of ciprofloxacin and thus increase the risk of ciprofloxacin-related side effects.

Before starting to take ciprofloxacin, BE SURE TO TELL YOUR DOCTOR about any other medications you are currently taking, especially any of those medications listed above.

WARNINGS

• Tell your doctor about unusual or allergic reactions you have had to any medications, especially to ciprofloxacin, enoxacin, ofloxacin, norfloxacin, cinoxacin, or nalidixic acid.

• Before starting to take this medication, be sure to tell your doctor if you now have or if you have ever had brain or spinal cord disease, epilepsy, kidney disease, or liver disease.

• To decrease the potential for harmful effects on your kidneys, you should increase your intake of fluids (nonalcoholic) unless your doctor directs you to do otherwise.

• Ciprofloxacin can cause dizziness or light-headedness, so patients taking this medicine should know how they react to this medicine before they operate an automobile or machinery, or engage in activities requiring alertness or coordination.

• This medicine can make your skin more sensitive to the sun. When you first begin taking this drug, avoid too much sun and do not use a sunlamp until you see how your skin responds to short periods of sun exposure. This is especially important if you tend to sunburn easily. Wear protective clothing and use an effective sunscreen when out of doors.

• Ciprofloxacin has been prescribed for your current infection only. Another infection later on, or one that someone else has, may require a different medicine. You should not give your medicine to other people or use it for other infections, unless your doctor specifically directs you to do so.

• Be sure to call your doctor if you experience a rash, swelling of the face, or difficulty breathing after taking ciprofloxacin.

• Be sure to tell your doctor if you are pregnant. This drug is not recommended for use in pregnant women because it can result in serious adverse effects in the developing fetus. Also, tell your doctor if you are breastfeeding an infant. It is not known whether ciprofloxacin passes into breast milk.

clarithromycin

BRAND NAME (Manufacturer)
Biaxin (Abbott)
TYPE OF DRUG
Antibiotic
INGREDIENT
clarithromycin
DOSAGE FORM
Tablets (250 mg and 500 mg)
STORAGE
Clarithromycin tablets should be stored at room temperature in a tightly closed, light resistant container.

USES

Clarithromycin is used to treat a wide variety of bacterial infections including infections of the upper and lower respiratory tracts and skin. It acts by preventing the bacteria from manufacturing protein, which prevents their growth. Clarithromycin kills susceptible bacteria, but it is not effective against viruses, parasites, or fungi.

TREATMENT

Clarithromycin may be taken without regard to meals. If stomach upset should occur, clarithromycin may be taken with food or milk, unless your doctor tells you otherwise. The coated tablets should be swallowed whole; do not crush or chew these tablets.

Clarithromycin works best when the level of medicine in your bloodstream is kept constant. It is best, therefore, to take the doses at evenly spaced intervals, day and night. If you are to take two doses a day, the doses should be spaced 12 hours apart.

It is very important that you do not miss any doses of this medication. If you do miss a dose, take it as soon as you remember. However, if you do not remember to take the missed dose until it is almost time for your next dose, skip the missed dose and go back to you regular dosing schedule. Do not double the dose.

It is important to continue to take this medication for the entire time prescribed by your doctor (usually seven to 14 days), even if the symptoms disappear before the end of that period. If you stop taking the drug too soon, resistant bacteria are given a chance to continue growing and the infection could recur.

SIDE EFFECTS

Minor. Abdominal pain/discomfort, abnormal taste, diarrhea, dyspepsia, headache, nausea. These side effects should disappear as your body adjusts to the medication.
Major. Tell your doctor about any side effects that are persistent or particularly bothersome. IT IS ESPECIALLY IMPORTANT TO TELL YOUR DOCTOR about fever, hearing loss, rash, rectal or vaginal itching, yellowing of the eyes or skin, or persistent diarrhea. Also, if your symptoms of infection seem to be getting worse rather than improving, you should contact your doctor.

INTERACTIONS

Clarithromycin can decrease the elimination of carbamazepine, aminophylline, theophylline, and oxtriphylline from the body, which can lead to serious side effects. Blood levels of digoxin and oral anticoagulants (blood thinners, such as warfarin) may also be increased by clarithromycin. Clarithromycin can increase the possibililty of irregular heart rate when taken with certain antihistamine drugs (terfenadine, loratidine, astemizole).

BE SURE TO TELL YOUR DOCTOR about any medications you are currently taking, especially any of those listed above.

WARNINGS

• Tell your doctor about any unusual or allergic reactions you have had to any medications, especially to clarithromycin, erythromycin, or azithromycin.
• Tell your doctor if you have now or have ever had kidney disease or liver disease.
• This medication has been prescribed for your current infection only. Another infection later on, or one that someone else has, may require a different medication. You should not give your medicine to other people or use it for another infection, unless your doctor specifically directs you to do so.
• Before having surgery or any other medical or dental treatment, be sure to tell your doctor or dentist that you are taking clarithromycin.
• Be sure to tell your doctor if you are pregnant. The effects of this medication during pregnancy have not been thoroughly studied in humans. Also, tell your doctor if you are breast-feeding an infant. It is not known whether clarithromycin passes into breast milk.
• Tell your doctor about any heart problems or irregular heart rate before taking clarithromycin.

clindamycin

BRAND NAMES (Manufacturers)
Cleocin HCl (Upjohn)
Cleocin Pediatric (Upjohn)
clindamycin (various manufacturers)
TYPE OF DRUG
Antibiotic
INGREDIENT
clindamycin palmitate hydrochloride
DOSAGE FORMS
Capsules (75 mg, 150 mg, and 300 mg)
Oral suspension (75 mg per 5-ml spoonful)
Vaginal cream (2%)
STORAGE
Clindamycin capsules and oral suspension should be stored at room temperature in tightly closed containers. The oral suspension should not be refrigerated or frozen; when chilled, it thickens and becomes difficult to pour. The suspension form of this medication should be discarded after 14 days because it loses potency.

USES

Clindamycin is an antibiotic that is used orally or vaginally to treat a wide variety of bacterial infections. It chemically attaches to the bacteria and prevents their growth and multiplication. Clindamycin kills susceptible bacteria, but it is not effective against viruses, parasites, or fungi.

TREATMENT

In order to prevent irritation to your esophagus (swallowing tube) or stomach, you should take clindamycin with food or a full glass of water or milk (unless your doctor directs you to do otherwise).

The suspension form of this medication should be shaken well just before measuring each dose. The contents tend to settle on the bottom of the bottle, so it is necessary to shake the container to distribute the ingredients evenly and equalize the doses. Each dose should then be measured carefully with a specially designed 5-ml measuring spoon. An ordinary kitchen teaspoon is not accurate enough.

Clindamycin works best when the level of medicine in your bloodstream is kept constant. It is best, therefore, to take the doses at evenly spaced intervals day and night.

Try not to miss any doses of this medication. If you do miss a dose, take it as soon as you remember. However, if you do not remember to take the missed dose until it is almost time for your next dose, take the missed dose immediately; space the following dose about halfway through the regular interval between doses; then continue with your regular dosing schedule.

It is important to continue to take this medication for the entire time prescribed by your doctor (usually seven to 14 days), even if your symptoms of infection disappear before the end of that period. If you stop taking the drug too soon, resistant bacteria are given a chance to continue growing, and your infection could recur.

SIDE EFFECTS

Minor. Diarrhea, loss of appetite, nausea, stomach or throat irritation, or vomiting. These side effects should disappear as your body adjusts to the medication. If the diarrhea becomes prolonged, CONTACT YOUR DOCTOR. Do not take antidiarrheal medicine.

Major. Tell your doctor about any side effects that are persistent or particularly bothersome. IT IS ESPECIALLY IMPORTANT TO TELL YOUR DOCTOR about bloody or pus-containing diarrhea, hives, itching, muscle or joint pain, skin rash, unusual bleeding or bruising, or yellowing of the eyes or skin. Also, if the symptoms of your infection do not improve in several days, contact your doctor. This medication may not be effective for your particular infection.

INTERACTIONS

Clindamycin should not interact with other medications if it is used according to directions.

WARNINGS

- Tell your doctor about unusual or allergic reactions you have had to any medications, especially to clindamycin or lincomycin.
- Before starting to take this medication, be sure to tell your doctor if you now have or if you have ever had colitis, kidney disease, or liver disease.
- Before having surgery or any other medical or dental treatment, be sure to tell your doctor or dentist that you are taking clindamycin.
- The 75 mg and 150 mg capsules of this medication contain the color additive FD&C Yellow No. 5 (tartrazine), which can cause allergic-type symptoms (fainting, shortness of breath, rash) in certain susceptible individuals.
- Clindamycin has been prescribed for your current infection only. Another infection later on, may require a different medicine. You should not give your medicine to other people or use it for other infections, unless your doctor specifically directs you to do so.
- Your doctor may tell you to avoid vaginal sexual intercourse when using the vaginal cream. This cream contains mineral oil, which will make condoms and vaginal diaphrams less effective and increase the likelihood of pregnancy.
- Be sure to tell your doctor if you are pregnant. Although clindamycin appears to be safe during pregnancy, extensive studies in humans have not been conducted. Also, tell your doctor if you are breast-feeding an infant. Small amounts of clindamycin pass into breast milk and can be transmitted to a nursing infant.

---

clonazepam

BRAND NAME (Manufacturer)
Klonopin (Roche)
TYPE OF DRUG
Benzodiazepine anticonvulsant
INGREDIENT
clonazepam
DOSAGE FORM
Tablets (0.5 mg, 1 mg, and 2 mg)
STORAGE
Clonazepam should be stored at room temperature in a tightly closed, light-resistant container.

USES

This medication is used to treat certain seizure disorders and other mental disorders. It is unclear exactly how clonazepam works to treat convulsions, but it appears that this drug prevents the spread of seizures to all parts of the brain.

TREATMENT

This medication can be ingested either on an empty stomach or with food or milk. However, take it only as directed by your doctor.

Clonazepam works best when the level of medicine in your bloodstream is kept constant. It is best, therefore, to take the doses at evenly spaced intervals over the course of the day and night. For example, if you are to take three doses a day, the doses should be spaced eight hours apart.

Try not to miss any doses of this medication. If you do miss a dose and remember within an hour, take the dose immediately. If more than an hour has passed, do not take the missed dose at all; just return to your regular dosing schedule. Do not double the next dose. If you miss two or more doses, CONTACT YOUR DOCTOR.

SIDE EFFECTS

Minor. Constipation, diarrhea, drowsiness, dry mouth, headache, increased appetite, insomnia, loss of appetite, nausea, runny nose, or weight loss or gain. These side effects should disappear as your body adjusts to the medication.

In order to relieve constipation, increase the amount of fiber in your diet (fresh fruits and vegetables, salads, bran, and whole-grain breads), exercise, and drink more water (unless your doctor directs you to do otherwise).

To relieve mouth dryness, chew sugarless gum or suck on ice chips or a piece of hard candy.

Major. Tell your doctor about any side effects that are persistent or particularly bothersome. IT IS ESPECIALLY IMPORTANT TO TELL YOUR DOCTOR about behavioral problems, confusion, depression, fever, fluid retention, hair loss, hallucinations, hysteria, increased or decreased urination, muscle weakness, palpitations, skin rash, slurred speech, sore gums, tremors, unusual bleeding or bruising, unusual body movements, or yellowing of the eyes or skin.

Clonazepam can also produce an increase in salivation, so it should be used cautiously by people who have swallowing difficulties. Contact your doctor if salivation becomes a problem.

INTERACTIONS

Clonazepam interacts with several other types of drugs:

1. Concurrent use of it with other central nervous system depressants (such as alcohol, antihistamines, barbiturates, benzodiazepine tranquilizers, muscle relaxants, narcotics, pain medications, phenothiazine tranquilizers, and sleeping medications) or with tricyclic antidepressants can cause extreme drowsiness.

2. Phenobarbital and phenytoin can decrease the blood levels and effectiveness of clonazepam.

3. Concurrent use of clonazepam and valproic acid can lead to increased seizure activity.

Before starting to take this medication, BE SURE TO TELL YOUR DOCTOR about any medications you are currently taking, especially any of those listed above.

WARNINGS

• Tell your doctor about unusual or allergic reactions you have had to any medications, especially to clonazepam or to other benzodiazepine tranquilizers (such as alprazolam, chlordiazepoxide, clorazepate, diazepam, flurazepam, halazepam, lorazepam, oxazepam, prazepam, temazepam, and triazolam).

• Tell your doctor if you now have or if you have ever had glaucoma, kidney disease, liver disease, or lung disease.

• If this drug makes you dizzy or drowsy, do not take part in any activity that requires alertness, such as driving a car or operating potentially dangerous equipment. Children should be careful while playing.

• Do not stop taking this medication unless you first check with your doctor. If you have been taking this medication for several months or longer, stopping the drug abruptly could lead to a withdrawal reaction and a worsening of your condition. Your doctor may, therefore, want to reduce your dosage of this medication gradually.

• Be sure to tell your doctor if you are pregnant. Although no harmful effects have been reported during pregnancy, extensive studies have not been conducted. The risks and benefits of clonazepam therapy during pregnancy should be discussed with your doctor. Also, tell your doctor if you are breast-feeding an infant. Small amounts of clonazepam pass into breast milk and may cause excessive drowsiness in nursing infants.

---

codeine

BRAND NAMES (Manufacturers)
Codeine Phosphate (various manufacturers)
Codeine Sulfate (various manufacturers)
TYPE OF DRUG
Analgesic and cough suppressant
INGREDIENT
codeine
DOSAGE FORMS
Tablets (15 mg, 30 mg, and 60 mg)
Oral solution (15 mg per 5-ml measuring spoon)
STORAGE
Codine tablets and oral solution should be stored at room temperature in a tightly closed, light-resistant container.

USES

Codeine is a narcotic analgesic that acts directly on the central nervous system (brain and spinal cord). It is used to relieve mild to moderate pain or in order to suppress coughing.

TREATMENT

In order to avoid stomach upset, you can take codeine with food or milk.

This drug works best if you take it at the onset of pain, rather than waiting until the pain has already beome intense.

If you are taking this medication on a regular schedule and you miss a dose, take the missed dose as soon as possible, unless it is almost time for your next dose. In that case, do not take the missed dose at all; just return to your regular dosing schedule. Do not double the next dose.

SIDE EFFECTS

Minor. Constipation, dizziness, drowsiness, dry mouth, false sense of well-being, flushing, light-headedness, loss of appetite, nausea, painful or difficult urination, or sweating. These side effects should disappear as your body adjusts to the medication.

If you are constipated, increase the amount of fiber in your diet (fresh fruits and vegetables, salads, bran, and whole-grain breads), exercise, and drink more water (unless your doctor directs you to do otherwise).

Chew sugarless gum or suck on ice chips or a piece of hard candy to reduce mouth dryness.

If you feel dizzy, light-headed, or nauseated, sit or lie down for a while; get up from a sitting or lying position slowly; and be careful on stairs.

Major. Tell your doctor about any side effects that are persistent or particularly bothersome. IT IS ESPECIALLY IMPORTANT TO TELL YOUR DOCTOR about anxiety, breathing difficulties, excitation, fatigue, palpitations, rash, restlessness, sore throat and fever, tremors, or weakness.

INTERACTIONS

Codeine interacts with several other types of medications:

1. Concurrent use of this medication with other central nervous system depressants (such as alcohol, antihistamines, barbiturates, benzodiazepine tranquilizers, muscle relaxants, and phenothiazine tranquilizers) or with tricyclic antidepressants can cause extreme drowsiness.

2. A monoamine oxidase (MAO) inhibitor taken within 14 days of this medication can lead to unpredictable and severe side effects.

3. Cimetidine, combined with this medication, can cause confusion, disorientation, and shortness of breath.

BE SURE TO TELL YOUR DOCTOR about any medications you are currently taking.

WARNINGS

• Tell your doctor about unusual or allergic reactions you have had to medications, especially to codeine or to any other narcotic analgesics (such as hydrocodone, hydromorphone, meperidine, methadone, morphine, oxycodone, and propoxyphene).

• Tell your doctor if you now have or if you have ever had acute abdominal conditions, asthma, brain disease, colitis, epilepsy, gallstones or gallbladder disease, head injuries, heart disease, kidney disease, liver disease, lung disease, mental illness, emotional disorders, prostate disease, thyroid disease, or urethral stricture.

• If this drug makes you dizzy or drowsy, do not take part in any activity that requires alertness, such as driving an automobile or operating potentially dangerous equipment or machinery.

• Before having surgery or other medical or dental treatment, tell your doctor or dentist you are taking this drug.

• Because this product contains codeine, it has the potential for abuse and must be used with caution. Usually, it should not be taken on a regular schedule for longer than ten days (unless your doctor directs you to do so). Tolerance develops quickly; do not increase the dosage or stop taking the drug abruptly unless you first consult your doctor. If you have been taking large amounts of this medication for long periods, you may experience a withdrawal reaction (muscle aches, diarrhea, gooseflesh, runny nose, nausea, vomiting, shivering, trembling, stomach cramps, sleep disorders, irritability, weakness, excessive yawning, or sweating) when you stop taking it. Your doctor may, therefore, want to reduce the dosage gradually.

• Be sure to tell your doctor if you are pregnant. The effects of this medication during the early stages of pregnancy have not been thoroughly studied in humans. However, codeine, used regularly in large doses during the later stages of pregnancy, can result in addiction of the fetus, leading to withdrawal symptoms (irritability, excessive crying, tremors, fever, vomiting, diarrhea, sneezing, or excessive yawning) at birth. Also, tell your doctor if you are breast-feeding an infant. Small amounts of this medication may pass into breast milk and cause excessive drowsiness in the nursing infant.

---

colchicine

BRAND NAMES (Manufacturers)
colchicine (various manufacturers)
Colchicine (Abbott)
TYPE OF DRUG
Antigout
INGREDIENT
colchicine
DOSAGE FORM
Tablets (0.5 mg, 0.6 mg, and 0.65 mg)
STORAGE
Colchicine should be stored at room temperature in a tightly closed, light-resistant container.

USES

Colchicine is used to relieve the symptoms of a gout attack and to prevent further attacks. Colchicine prevents the movement of uric acid crystals, which are responsible for the pain in the joints that occurs during an attack of gout.

TREATMENT

Colchicine can be taken on an empty stomach or with food or a full glass of water or milk (as directed by your doctor).

If you are taking colchicine to control a gout attack, it is important that you understand how to take it and when it should be stopped. CHECK WITH YOUR DOCTOR.

If you miss a dose of this medication, take the missed dose as soon as possible, unless it is almost time for the next dose. In that case, do not take the missed dose at all; just return to your regular dosing schedule. Do not double the next dose.

SIDE EFFECTS

Minor. Abdominal pain, diarrhea, nausea, or vomiting. These side effects should disappear as your body adjusts to the medication.

Major. Tell your doctor about any side effects that are persistent or particularly bothersome. IT IS ESPECIALLY IMPORTANT TO TELL YOUR DOCTOR about difficult or painful urination, fever, loss of hair, muscle pain, persistent diarrhea, skin rash, sore throat, tingling in the hands or feet, or unusual bleeding or bruising.

INTERACTIONS

Colchicine interacts with several types of medications:
1. It can decrease absorption of vitamin B_{12}.
2. The action of colchicine can be blocked by vitamin C and can be enhanced by sodium bicarbonate or ammonium chloride.
3. Colchicine can increase the drowsiness caused by central nervous system depressants.

BE SURE TO TELL YOUR DOCTOR about any medications you are currently taking.

WARNINGS

• Tell your doctor about unusual or allergic reactions you have had to any medications.
• Tell your doctor if you now have or if you have ever had blood disorders, gastrointestinal disorders, heart disease, kidney disease, or liver disease.
• Large amounts of alcohol can increase the blood levels of uric acid, which can decrease the effectiveness of colchicine.
• Colchicine is not an analgesic (pain reliever) and does not relieve pain other than that of gout.
• Be sure to tell your doctor if you are pregnant. Colchicine is not recommended for use during pregnancy because it has been reported to cause birth defects in both animals and humans. Also, tell your doctor if you are breast-feeding an infant. It is not known whether colchicine passes into breast milk.

---

cyclophosphamide

BRAND NAME (Manufacturer)
Cytoxan (Bristol-Myers Oncology)
TYPE OF DRUG
Antineoplastic (anticancer drug)
INGREDIENT
cyclophosphamide
DOSAGE FORM
Tablets (25 mg and 50 mg)
STORAGE
Cyclophosphamide should be stored at room temperature in a tightly closed container.

USES

Cyclophosphamide belongs to a group of drugs known as alkylating agents or nitrogen mustards. It is used to treat a variety of cancers. Cyclophosphamide works by binding to the rapidly growing cancer cells, preventing their multiplication and growth. Cyclophosphamide has also been used as an immunosuppressant in order to treat severe rheumatoid arthritis and other diseases.

TREATMENT

In order to obtain maximum benefit, you should take cyclophosphamide on an empty stomach. However, if stomach upset occurs, you can take it with food or milk (unless your doctor directs you to do otherwise).

The timing of the doses of this medication is important. Be sure you completely understand your doctor's instructions on how and when this medication should be taken. Try not to miss any doses.

If you miss a dose of this medication, do not take the missed dose at all; just return to your regular dosing schedule. Do not double the next dose.

SIDE EFFECTS

Minor. Diarrhea, loss of appetite, nausea, or vomiting. These side effects may disappear as your body adjusts to the medication. However, it is important to continue taking this medication despite the nausea and vomiting that may occur. Cyclophosphamide also causes hair loss, which is reversible when the medication is stopped.
Major. Tell your doctor about any side effects that are persistent or particularly bothersome. IT IS ESPECIALLY IMPORTANT TO TELL YOUR DOCTOR about blood in the urine, chills, cough, darkening of the skin or fingernails, difficult or painful urination, fever, menstrual irregularities, mouth sores, sore throat, unusual bleeding or bruising, or yellowing of the eyes or skin.

INTERACTIONS

This drug interacts with several other types of drugs:
1. It can decrease the absorption of digoxin from the gastrointestinal tract.
2. Phenobarbital can increase the side effects of cyclophosphamide.
3. Concurrent use of allopurinol, chloramphenicol, chlorpromazine, or thiazide diuretics (water pills) with cyclophosphamide can lead to bone-marrow suppression.
4. Cyclophosphamide can increase the effect of warfarin (blood thinner).

Before starting to take this medication, BE SURE TO TELL YOUR DOCTOR about any medications you are currently taking, especially any of those listed above.

WARNINGS

• Tell your doctor about unusual or allergic reactions you have had to any medications, especially to cyclophosphamide.
• Before starting to take this medication, be sure to tell your doctor if you have ever had blood disorders, chronic or recurrent infections, gout, kidney disease, or liver disease.
• Before having surgery or any other medical or dental treatment, tell your doctor or dentist you are taking this drug.
• Cyclophosphamide tablets contain the color additive FD&C Yellow No. 5 (tartrazine), which can cause allergic-type reactions (fainting, shortness of breath, rash) in certain susceptible individuals.
• You should not receive any immunizations or vaccinations while taking this medication. Cyclophosphamide decreases the effectiveness of the vaccine and may result in an infection if a live-virus vaccine is administered.
• It is important to drink plenty of fluids (three quarts each day) while taking this medication. If the drug is allowed to concentrate in the bladder, it can cause bloody urine and can damage the kidneys or bladder.

• This medication can lower your platelet count, which can decrease your body's ability to form blood clots. You should, therefore, be especially careful while brushing your teeth, flossing, or using toothpicks, razors, or fingernail scissors. Try to avoid falls and other injuries.
• This drug can decrease fertility in both men and women.
• Be sure to tell your doctor if you are pregnant. Birth defects have been reported in both animals and humans whose mothers received cyclophosphamide during pregnancy. The risks should be discussed with your doctor. Also, tell your doctor if you are breast-feeding an infant. Since the drug passes into breast milk, a woman should stop breast-feeding before starting cyclophosphamide therapy.

Women of childbearing potential who are not already pregnant when treatment with cyclophosphamide is begun need to use some sort of birth control to prevent pregnancy from occurring. However, oral contraceptives (birth control pills) may not be recommended by your doctor since they may interfere with this medication. Consult with your physician about alternative methods of birth control.

cyclosporine

BRAND NAME (Manufacturer)
Sandimmune (Sandoz)
TYPE OF DRUG
Immunosuppressant
INGREDIENT
cyclosporine
DOSAGE FORMS
Oral solution (100 mg per ml, with 12.5% alcohol)
Soft gelatin capsules (25 mg and 100 mg)
STORAGE
Cyclosporine oral solution and capsules should be stored in the original container at room temperature. This medication should never be refrigerated or frozen. Once the solution has been opened, it should be used within two months.

USES

Cyclosporine is used to prevent organ rejection after kidney, liver, and heart transplants. It is not clearly understood how cyclosporine works, but it appears to prevent the body's rejection of foreign tissue. Cyclosporine is also used to treat severe psoriasis.

TREATMENT

To make it more palatable, the solution should be diluted with milk, chocolate milk, or orange juice (preferably at room temperature). The dose should be measured carefully with the dropper provided and placed in one of the fluids listed above. Use a glass container (cyclosporine chemically binds to wax-lined and plastic surfaces). Stir well and drink at once—do not allow the mixture to stand before drinking. Refill the glass with the same beverage and drink this solution to ensure that the whole dose is taken. The dropper should be wiped with a clean towel after use and stored in its container. If the dropper has been cleaned, make sure it is completely dry before using it again.

It is important not to miss any doses of this medication. If you do miss a dose, take the missed dose as soon as possible, unless it is almost time for the next dose. In that case, do not take the missed dose at all; just return to your regular dosing schedule. Do not double the next dose.

SIDE EFFECTS

Minor. Abdominal discomfort, diarrhea, flushing, headache, hiccups, leg cramps, loss of appetite, nausea, or vomiting. These side effects should disappear as your body adjusts to the medication.
Major. Tell your doctor about any side effects that are persistent or particularly bothersome. IT IS ESPECIALLY IMPORTANT TO TELL YOUR DOCTOR about acne; bleeding, tender, or enlarged gums; convulsions; difficult or painful urination; enlarged and painful breasts (in both sexes); fever; hair growth; hearing loss; muscle pain; rapid weight gain (three to five pounds within a week); sore throat; tingling of the hands or feet; tremors; unusual bleeding or bruising; or yellowing of the eyes or skin.

INTERACTIONS

Cyclosporine interacts with several other types of drugs:
1. Carbamazepine, isoniazid, rifampin, phenytoin, phenobarbital, and trimethoprim/sulfamethoxazole can decrease the blood levels of cyclosporine, decreasing its effectiveness.
2. Cimetidine, diltiazem, erythromycin, ketoconazole, oral contraceptives, danazol, and amphotericin B can increase the blood levels of cyclosporine, which can lead to an increase in side effects.
3. Tell your doctor if you are currently taking corticosteroids, verapamil, or nonsteroidal anti-inflammatory drugs.

BE SURE TO TELL YOUR DOCTOR about any medications you are currently taking.

WARNINGS

• Tell your doctor about unusual or allergic reactions you have had to any medications, especially to cyclosporine or to polyoxyethylated castor oil.
• Before starting to take this medication, be sure to tell your doctor if you now have or if you have ever had hypertension (high blood pressure) or gastrointestinal disorders.
• Repeated laboratory tests are necessary while you are taking cyclosporine to ensure that you are receiving the correct dosage and to avoid liver and kidney damage.
• Certain cancers have occurred in patients receiving cyclosporine and other immunosuppressant drugs after transplantation. No causal effect has been established, however.
• Do not stop taking this medication without first consulting your doctor. If the drug is stopped abruptly, organ rejection may occur. Your doctor may, therefore, want to reduce your dosage gradually or start you on another drug if treatment with this drug is to be discontinued.

• Be sure to tell your doctor if you are pregnant. Although extensive studies in humans have not been conducted, cyclosporine has caused fetal damage when administered to pregnant animals. Also, tell your doctor if you are breast-feeding, because cyclosporine passes into breast milk.

---

diazepam

BRAND NAMES (Manufacturers)
diazepam (various manufacturers)
Diazepam Intensol (Roxene)
Valium (Roche)
Valrelease (Roche)
Vazepam (Major)
TYPE OF DRUG
Sedative/hypnotic
INGREDIENT
diazepam
DOSAGE FORMS
Oral solution (5 mg per 5-ml spoonful)
Oral intensol solution (5 mg per ml)
Tablets (2 mg, 5 mg, and 10 mg)
Sustained-release capsules (15 mg)
STORAGE
This medication should be stored at room temperature in a tightly closed, light-resistant container.

USES

Diazepam is prescribed to treat symptoms of anxiety and sometimes to treat muscle spasms, convulsions, seizures, or alcohol withdrawal. It is not clear exactly how this medicine works, but it may relieve anxiety by acting as a depressant of the central nervous system (brain and spinal cord). Diazepam is currently used by many people to relieve nervousness. It is effective for this purpose for short periods, but it is important to try to remove the cause of the anxiety as well.

TREATMENT

The oral intensol solution should be mixed with a nonalcoholic liquid or semi-solid food such as water, juice, soda or sodalike beverages, applesauce, or pudding. Use only the calibrated dropper provided. Stir the liquid or food gently for a few seconds after adding the oral intensol solution. The entire amount of the mixture should be consumed immediately. Do not store prepared mixtures for future use.

The tablet or capsule form of this medication should be taken exactly as directed by your doctor. It can be taken with food or a full glass of water if stomach upset occurs. Do not take this medication with a dose of antacids, since they may retard its absorption.

If you are taking this medication regularly and you miss a dose and remember within an hour, take the missed dose immediately. If more than an hour has passed, skip the dose you missed and wait for the next scheduled dose. Do not double the next dose.

SIDE EFFECTS

Minor. Bitter taste in the mouth, constipation, depression, diarrhea, dizziness, drowsiness (after a night's sleep), dry mouth, excessive salivation, fatigue, flushing, headache, heartburn, loss of appetite, nausea, nervousness, sweating, or vomiting. These side effects should disappear once your body gets accustomed to the medication.

To relieve constipation, increase the amount of fiber in your diet (fresh fruits and vegetables, salads, bran, and whole-grain breads), exercise, and drink more water (unless your doctor directs you to do otherwise).

Dry mouth can be relieved by chewing sugarless gum or by sucking on ice chips or hard candy.

If you feel dizzy, sit or lie down for a while; get up slowly from a sitting or reclining position; and be careful on stairs.

Major. Tell your doctor about any side effects that are persistent or particularly bothersome. IT IS ESPECIALLY IMPORTANT TO TELL YOUR DOCTOR about blurred or double vision, chest pain, difficulty in urinating, fainting, falling, fever, joint pain, hallucinations, mouth sores, nightmares, palpitations, rash, severe depression, shortness of breath, slurred speech, sore throat, uncoordinated movements, unusual excitement, unusual tiredness, or yellowing of the eyes or skin.

INTERACTIONS

This medication interacts with several other types of medications:

1. To prevent oversedation, this drug should not be taken with alcohol, other sedative drugs, or central nervous system depressants (such as antihistamines, barbiturates, muscle relaxants, pain medicines, narcotics, medicines for seizures, and tranquilizers), or with antidepressants.

2. This medication may decrease the effectiveness of carbamazepine, levodopa, and oral anticoagulants (blood thinners) and may increase the effects of phenytoin.

3. Disulfiram, oral contraceptives (birth control pills), isoniazid, fluoxetine, valproic acid, propranolol, metoprolol, ketoconazole, and cimetidine can increase the blood levels of diazepam, which can lead to toxic effects.

4. Concurrent use of rifampin may decrease the effectiveness of diazepam.

BE SURE TO TELL YOUR DOCTOR about any medications you are currently taking, especially any of those listed above.

WARNINGS

• Tell your doctor about unusual or allergic reactions you have had to any medications, especially to diazepam or other benzodiazepine tranquilizers (such as alprazolam, flurazepam, halazepam, lorazepam, oxazepam, prazepam, temazepam, and triazolam).

• Be sure to tell your doctor if you now have or if you have ever had liver disease, kidney disease, epilepsy, lung disease, myasthenia gravis, porphyria, mental depression, or mental illness.

• This medicine can cause drowsiness. Avoid tasks that require alertness, such as driving a car or operating potentially dangerous machinery.

• This medication has the potential for abuse and must be used with caution. Tolerance may develop quickly;

do not increase your dosage of the drug without first consulting your doctor. It is also important not to stop taking this drug suddenly if you have been taking it in large amounts or if you have used it for several weeks. Your doctor may want to reduce your dosage gradually.

• This is a safe drug when used properly. When it is combined with other sedative drugs or alcohol, however, serious side effects can develop.

• Be sure to tell your doctor if you are pregnant. This medicine may increase the chance of birth defects if it is taken during the first three months of pregnancy. In addition, too much use of this medicine during the last six months of pregnancy may cause the baby to become dependent on it, resulting in withdrawal side effects in the newborn. Use of diazepam during the last weeks of pregnancy may cause excessive drowsiness, slowed heartbeat, and breathing difficulties in the infant. Be sure to tell your doctor if you are breast-feeding an infant. This medication can pass into breast milk and cause excessive drowsiness, slowed heartbeat, and breathing difficulties in nursing infants.

---

dicloxacillin

BRAND NAMES (Manufacturers)
dicloxacillin sodium (various manufacturers)
Dycill (SmithKline Beecham)
Dynapen (Apothecon)
Pathocil (Wyeth-Ayerst)

TYPE OF DRUG
Penicillin antibiotic

INGREDIENT
dicloxacillin

DOSAGE FORMS
Capsules (125 mg, 250 mg, and 500 mg)
Oral suspension (62.5 mg per 5-ml spoonful)

STORAGE
Dicloxacillin capsules should be stored at room temperature in a tightly closed container. The oral suspension should be stored in the refrigerator in a tightly closed container. Any unused portion of the suspension should be discarded after 14 days because the drug loses its potency after that time. This medication should never be frozen.

USES

Dicloxacillin is used to treat a wide variety of bacterial infections, especially those caused by *Staphylococcus* bacteria. It acts by severely injuring the cell membranes of the infecting bacteria, thereby preventing them from growing and multiplying. Dicloxacillin kills susceptible bacteria, but it is not effective against viruses, parasites, or fungi.

TREATMENT

Dicloxacillin should be taken on an empty stomach or with a glass of water, one hour before or two hours after a meal. This medication should never be taken with fruit juices or carbonated beverages because the acidity of these drinks destroys the drug in the stomach.

The suspension form of this medication should be shaken well just before measuring each dose. The contents tend to settle at the bottom of the bottle, so it is necessary to shake the container to distribute the ingredients evenly and equalize the doses. Each dose should then be measured carefully with a specially designed 5-ml measuring spoon. An ordinary kitchen teaspoon is not accurate enough.

Dicloxacillin works best when the level of medicine in your bloodstream is kept constant. It is best, therefore, to take the doses at evenly spaced intervals day and night. For example, if you are taking four doses a day, the doses should be spaced six hours apart.

If you miss a dose of this medication, take the missed dose immediately. However, if you do not remember to take the missed dose until it is almost time for your next dose, take it; space the following dose about halfway through the regular interval between doses; then return to your regular schedule. Try not to skip any doses.

It is important for you to continue to take this medication for the entire time prescribed by your doctor (usually seven to 14 days), even if the symptoms of your infection disappear before the end of that period. If you stop taking the drug too soon, bacteria are given a chance to continue growing, and the infection could recur.

SIDE EFFECTS

Minor. Diarrhea, heartburn, nausea, or vomiting. These side effects should disappear as your body adjusts to this particular drug.

Major. Tell your doctor about any side effects that are persistent or particularly bothersome. IT IS ESPECIALLY IMPORTANT TO TELL YOUR DOCTOR about bloating, chills, cough, darkened tongue, difficulty in breathing, fever, irritation of the mouth, muscle aches, rash, rectal or vaginal itching, severe diarrhea, or sore throat. In addition, if the symptoms of your infection seem to be getting worse rather than improving, you should contact your doctor.

INTERACTIONS

Dicloxacillin interacts with other types of medications:

1. Probenecid can increase the blood concentrations and side effects of this medication.

2. Dicloxacillin may decrease the effectiveness of oral contraceptives (birth control pills), and pregnancy could result. You should, therefore, use a different or additional form of birth control while taking this medication. Discuss this with your doctor.

BE SURE TO TELL YOUR DOCTOR about any medications you are currently taking, especially any of those listed above.

WARNINGS

• Tell your doctor about unusual or allergic reactions you have had to any medications, especially to dicloxacillin or penicillins, or to cephalosporin antibiotics, penicillamine, or griseofulvin.

• Tell your doctor if you now have or if you have ever had kidney disease, asthma, or allergies.
• This medication has been prescribed for your current infection only. Another infection later on, or one that someone else has, may require a different medicine. You should not give your medicine to other people or use it for other infections, unless your doctor specifically directs you to do so.
• Diabetics taking dicloxacillin should know that this drug can cause interference with a Clinitest urine glucose test. To avoid this problem while taking dicloxacillin, you should switch to Clinistix or Tes-Tape to test your urine for sugar.
• Be sure to tell your doctor if you are pregnant. Although dicloxacillin appears to be safe to take during pregnancy, extensive studies in humans have not been conducted. Also, tell your doctor if you are breast-feeding an infant. Small amounts of this medication pass into breast milk and may temporarily alter the bacterial balance in the intestinal tract of the nursing infant, resulting in episodes of diarrhea.

---

dicyclomine

BRAND NAMES (Manufacturers)
Bentyl (Lakeside)
Byclomine (Major)
dicyclomine hydrochloride (various manufacturers)
Di-Spaz (Vortech)
TYPE OF DRUG
Antispasmodic
INGREDIENT
dicyclomine
DOSAGE FORMS
Tablets (20 mg)
Capsules (10 mg and 20 mg)
Oral liquid (10 mg per 5-ml spoonful)
STORAGE
Dicyclomine tablets, capsules, and oral liquid should be stored at room temperature in tightly closed containers. This medication should never be frozen.

USES

Dicyclomine is used to treat gastrointestinal tract disorders and irritable bowel syndrome. Dicyclomine acts directly on the muscles of the gastrointestinal tract to decrease tone and slow their activity.

TREATMENT

Dicyclomine can be taken before or after meals. Consult your doctor for specific recommendations.

Antacids and antidiarrheal medicines may prevent absorption of this drug; therefore, at least one hour should separate doses of dicyclomine and these medications.

Measure the liquid form of dicyclomine carefully with a specially designed 5-ml measuring spoon. An ordinary kitchen teaspoon is not accurate enough. You can then dilute the oral liquid in other liquids to mask its taste.

If you miss a dose of this medication, do not take the missed dose at all; just return to your regular dosing schedule. Do not double the next dose.

SIDE EFFECTS

Minor. Bloating; blurred vision; confusion; constipation; dizziness; drowsiness; dry mouth, throat, and nose; headache; increased sensitivity to light; insomnia; loss of taste; nausea; nervousness; decreased sweating; vomiting; or weakness. These side effects should disappear as your body adjusts to the medication.

If you are constipated, increase the amount of fiber in your diet (fresh fruits and vegetables, salads, bran, and whole-grain breads), get more exercise, and drink more water or other fluids (unless your doctor directs you to do otherwise).

Chew sugarless gum or suck on ice chips or a piece of hard candy to reduce mouth dryness.

Wear sunglasses if your eyes become sensitive to light.

To avoid dizziness or light-headedness when you stand, contract and relax the muscles of your legs for a few moments before rising. Do this by pushing one foot against the floor while raising the other foot slightly, alternating feet so that you are "pumping" your legs in a pedaling motion.

Major. Be sure to tell your doctor about any side effects that are persistent or particularly bothersome. IT IS ESPECIALLY IMPORTANT TO TELL YOUR DOCTOR about difficulty in urinating, fever, hallucinations, impotence, palpitations, rash, short-term memory loss, or sore throat.

INTERACTIONS

Dicyclomine interacts with several other types of medications:

1. It can cause extreme drowsiness when combined with central nervous system depressants (such as alcohol, antihistamines, barbiturates, benzodiazepine tranquilizers, muscle relaxants, narcotics, pain medications, and phenothiazine tranquilizers) or with tricyclic antidepressants.
2. Amantadine, antihistamines, haloperidol, monoamine oxidase (MAO) inhibitors, phenothiazine tranquilizers, procainamide, quinidine, and tricyclic antidepressants can increase the side effects of dicyclomine.

BE SURE TO TELL YOUR DOCTOR about any medications you are currently taking.

WARNINGS

• Be sure to tell your doctor about unusual or allergic reactions you have had to any medications, especially to dicyclomine.
• Tell your doctor if you have ever had glaucoma; heart disease; hiatal hernia; high blood pressure; kidney, liver, or thyroid disease; myasthenia gravis; obstructed bladder; obstructed intestine; enlarged prostate gland; ulcerative colitis; or internal bleeding.
• If this medication makes you dizzy or drowsy or blurs your vision, do not take part in any activity that requires alertness, such as driving an automobile or operating potentially dangerous equipment or machinery. Be careful on stairs, and avoid getting up suddenly from a lying or sitting position.
• This drug can decrease sweating and heat release from the body. Avoid taking hot baths, showers, or saunas.

Also, do not exercise in hot weather to avoid getting overheated.
• Before having surgery or other medical or dental treatment, be sure to tell your doctor or dentist you are taking this drug.
• Tell your doctor if you are pregnant. Although this drug appears to be safe during pregnancy, extensive studies in humans have not been conducted. Also, tell your doctor if you are breast-feeding an infant. Small amounts of dicyclomine pass into breast milk.

---

digoxin

BRAND NAMES (Manufacturers)
digoxin (various manufacturers)
Lanoxicaps (Burroughs Wellcome)
Lanoxin (Burroughs Wellcome)
TYPE OF DRUG
Cardiac glycoside
INGREDIENT
digoxin
DOSAGE FORMS
Tablets (0.125 mg, 0.25 mg, and 0.5 mg)
Capsules (0.05 mg, 0.1 mg, and 0.2 mg)
Pediatric elixir (0.05 mg per ml, with 10% alcohol)
STORAGE
Digoxin tablets, capsules, and pediatric elixir should be stored at room temperature in tightly closed, light-resistant containers. This medication should never be frozen.

USES

Digoxin is used to treat heart arrhythmias and congestive heart failure. It works directly on the muscle of the heart to strengthen the heartbeat and improve heart rhythm and contraction.

TREATMENT

To avoid stomach irritation, take digoxin with water or with food. Try to get in the habit of taking it at the same time every day.

Measure the dose of the pediatric elixir carefully with the dropper provided. An ordinary kitchen teaspoon is not accurate enough.

Antacids decrease the absorption of digoxin from the gastrointestinal tract. Therefore, if you are taking both digoxin and an antacid, the dose of digoxin should be taken one hour before or two hours after a dose of antacids.

Try not to miss any doses of this medication. If you do miss a dose, take the missed dose as soon as possible, unless it is almost time for the next dose. In that case, do not take the missed dose at all; just return to your regular dosing schedule. Do not double the next dose. If you miss more than two doses of digoxin, you should contact your doctor.

Digoxin does not cure congestive heart failure, but it will help to control the condition as long as you continue to take the medication.

SIDE EFFECTS

Minor. Apathy, diarrhea, drowsiness, headache, muscle weakness, or tiredness. These side effects should disappear as your body adjusts to the medication.
Major. Tell your doctor about any side effects that are persistent or particularly bothersome. IT IS ESPECIALLY IMPORTANT TO TELL YOUR DOCTOR about disorientation, enlarged and painful breasts (in both sexes), hallucinations, loss of appetite, mental depression, nausea, palpitations, severe abdominal pain, slowed heart rate, visual disturbances (such as blurred or yellow vision), or vomiting.

INTERACTIONS

Digoxin interacts with several other types of medications (interactions may vary depending upon the dose of digoxin being used):
1. Penicillamine, antiseizure medications, rifampin, aminoglutethimide, and levodopa can decrease the blood levels and, therefore, the effectiveness of digoxin.
2. Erythromycin, amiodarone, captopril, benzodiazepine tranquilizers, flecainide, tetracycline, hydroxychloroquine, ibuprofen, indomethacin, verapamil, nifedipine, diltiazem, quinidine, quinine, and spironolactone can increase the blood levels of digoxin, which can lead to an increase in side effects.
3. Thyroid hormone, propylthiouracil, and methimazole can change the dosage requirements of digoxin.
4. Antacids, kaolin-pectin, sulfasalazine, aminosalicylic acid, metoclopramide, antineoplastic agents (anticancer drugs), neomycin, colestipol, and cholestyramine can decrease the absorption of digoxin from the gastrointestinal tract, decreasing its effectiveness.
5. Calcium, tolbutamide, and reserpine can increase the side effects of digoxin.
6. Diuretics (water pills) and adrenocorticosteroids (cortisonelike medications) can cause hypokalemia (low blood levels of potassium).

BE SURE TO TELL YOUR DOCTOR about any medications you are currently taking, especially those listed above.

WARNINGS

• Tell your doctor about unusual or allergic reactions you have had to any medications, especially to digoxin, digitoxin, or any other digitalis glycoside.
• Tell your doctor if you now have or if you have ever had kidney disease, lung disease, thyroid disease, hypokalemia (low blood levels of potassium), or hypercalcemia (high blood levels of calcium).
• The pharmacologic activity of the different brands of this drug varies widely—the tablets dissolve in the stomach and bowel at different rates and to varying degrees. It is important not to change brands of the drug without consulting your doctor.
• Meals high in bran fiber may reduce the absorption of digoxin from the gastrointestinal tract. Avoid these types of meals when taking your dose of medication.
• Your doctor may want you to take your pulse daily while you are using digoxin. Contact your doctor if your pulse becomes slower than what your doctor tells you is normal, or if it drops below 50 beats per minute.

• Before having surgery or any other medical or dental treatment, be sure to tell your doctor or dentist that you are taking this medication.
• Before taking any over-the-counter (nonprescription) asthma, allergy, cough, cold, sinus, or diet product, be sure to check with your doctor or pharmacist. Some of these drugs can increase the side effects of digoxin.
• Be sure to tell your doctor if you are pregnant. Although this drug appears to be safe during pregnancy, extensive studies in humans have not been conducted. In addition, the dosage of digoxin required to control your symptoms may change during pregnancy. Also, tell your doctor if you are breast-feeding an infant. Small amounts of digoxin pass into breast milk.

---

diltiazem

BRAND NAMES (Manufacturers)
Cardizem (Marion-Merrell Dow)
Cardizem CD (Marion-Merrell Dow)
Cardizem SR (Marion-Merrell Dow)
TYPE OF DRUG
Antianginal and antihypertensive
INGREDIENT
diltiazem
DOSAGE FORMS
Extended-release capsules (180 mg, 240 mg, and 300 mg)
Tablets (30 mg, 60 mg, 90 mg, and 120 mg)
Sustained-release capsules (60 mg, 90 mg, and 120 mg)
STORAGE
Diltiazem should be stored at room temperature in a tightly closed container.

USES

This medication is used to prevent the symptoms of angina. It belongs to a group of drugs known as calcium channel blockers. It is unclear exactly how it does so, but diltiazem dilates the blood vessels of the heart and increases the amount of oxygen that reaches the heart muscle. This drug is also prescribed to lower blood pressure in patients who have hypertension.

TREATMENT

If stomach irritation occurs, diltiazem can be taken either on an empty stomach or with meals, as directed by your doctor. The sustained-release and extended-release capsules should be swallowed whole; chewing, crushing, or crumbling them destroys their controlled-release activity and possibly increases the side effects.

In order to become accustomed to taking this medication, try to take it at the same times each day.

Although diltiazem does not relieve chest pain once the pain has begun, this medication can be used to prevent angina attacks.

If you miss a dose of this medication, take the missed dose as soon as possible, unless it is within four hours of the next scheduled dose. In that case, do not take the missed dose at all; just return to your regular dosing schedule. Do not double the next dose.

This medication does not cure angina, but it will help to control the condition as long as you continue to take it.

SIDE EFFECTS

Minor. Constipation, diarrhea, dizziness, drowsiness, headache, insomnia, light-headedness, nausea, nervousness, stomach upset, or vomiting. These side effects should disappear as your body adjusts to the medication.

This drug can increase your sensitivity to sunlight. Therefore, avoid prolonged exposure to sunlight and sunlamps. Wear protective clothing and sunglasses, and use an effective sunscreen.

If you feel dizzy or light-headed, sit or lie down for a while; get up slowly from a sitting or reclining position; and be careful on stairs. To avoid dizziness when you stand, relax and contract the muscles of your legs for a few moments before rising. Do this by pushing one foot against the floor while raising the other foot slightly, alternating feet so that you are "pumping" your legs in a pedaling motion.

To relieve constipation, increase the amount of fiber in your diet (fresh fruits and vegetables, salads, bran, and whole-grain breads), exercise, and drink more water (unless your doctor directs you to do otherwise).

Major. Tell your doctor about any side effects that are persistent or particularly bothersome. IT IS ESPECIALLY IMPORTANT TO TELL YOUR DOCTOR about confusion, depression, fainting, fatigue, flushing, fluid retention, hallucinations, palpitations, skin rash, tingling in the fingers or toes, unusual weakness, or yellowing of the eyes or skin.

INTERACTIONS

Diltiazem can interact with several other medications:
1. Diltiazem should be used cautiously with beta blockers (acebutolol, atenolol, betaxolol, carteolol, esmolol, labetalol, metoprolol, nadolol, penbutolol, propranolol, pindolol, and timolol), digitoxin, digoxin, or disopyramide. Side effects on the heart may be increased by the concurrent use of these medications.
2. Cimetidine can reduce the elimination of diltiazem from the body, increasing the risk of side effects.
3. Diltiazem can increase the blood concentrations of carbamazepine and cyclosporine, which can increase the risk of side effects.

BE SURE TO TELL YOUR DOCTOR about any medications you are currently taking, especially any listed above.

WARNINGS

• Tell your doctor about unusual or allergic reactions you have had to any medications, especially to diltiazem.
• Be sure to tell your doctor if you now have or if you have ever had bradycardia (slow heartbeat), heart block, heart failure, kidney disease, liver disease, low blood pressure, or sick sinus syndrome.
• If this drug makes you dizzy or drowsy, avoid taking part in any activity that requires alertness, such as driving a car or operating potentially dangerous equipment.

• To prevent fainting while taking this drug, avoid drinking large amounts of alcohol. Also, avoid prolonged standing and strenuous exercise in hot weather.
• Be sure to tell your doctor if you are pregnant. Extensive studies in pregnant women have not been conducted, but birth defects have been reported in the offspring of animals that received large doses of diltiazem during pregnancy. It is also known that diltiazem passes into breast milk. If you are breast-feeding an infant while being treated with this medication, tell your doctor. Unless directed to do otherwise, breast-feeding is not recommended at this time.

---

diphenhydramine

BRAND NAMES (Manufacturers)
AllerMax (Pfeiffer)
Belix* (Halsey)
Benadryl* (Parke-Davis)
Benadryl Kapseals (Parke-Davis)
Benylin Cough Syrup* (Parke-Davis)
Bydramine Cough Syrup* (Major)
Compoz* (Jeffrey Martin)
Diphen Cough Syrup* (My-K Lab)
diphenhydramine hydrochloride (various manufacturers)
Dormarex 2* (Republic)
Hydramine* (Goldline)
Nervine Nighttime Sleep Aid* (Miles)
Nordryl (Vortech)
Nytol* (Block)
Sleep-Eze 3* (Whitehall)
Sominex 2* (SmithKline Beecham)
Tusstat (Century)
Twilite* (Pfeiffer)
Unisom Nighttime Sleep Aid (Leeming)
*Available over-the-counter (without a prescription)

TYPE OF DRUG
Antihistamine and sedative/hypnotic

INGREDIENT
diphenhydramine

DOSAGE FORMS
Tablets (50 mg)
Capsules (25 mg and 50 mg)
Elixir (12.5 mg per 5-ml spoonful, with 14% alcohol)
Oral syrup (12.5 mg per 5-ml spoonful, with 5% alcohol)

STORAGE
Store at room temperature in a tightly closed container, away from heat and direct sunlight.

USES

Diphenhydramine belongs to a group of drugs known as antihistamines (antihistamines block the action of histamine, a chemical that is released by the body during an allergic reaction). It is, therefore, used to treat or prevent symptoms of allergy. It is also used to treat motion sickness and Parkinson's disease, and it is used as a nighttime sleeping aid and nonnarcotic cough suppressant.

TREATMENT

To avoid stomach upset, take diphenhydramine with food, milk, or water (unless your doctor directs you otherwise).

The elixir and oral syrup forms of this medication should be measured carefully with a specially designed 5-ml measuring spoon. An ordinary teaspoon is not accurate enough.

If you miss a dose of this medication, take the missed dose as soon as possible, unless it is almost time for your next dose. In that case, do not take the missed dose at all; just return to your regular dosing schedule. Do not double the next dose.

SIDE EFFECTS

Minor. Blurred vision; confusion; constipation; diarrhea; dizziness; dry mouth, throat, or nose; headache; irritability; loss of appetite; nausea; restlessness; stomach upset; or unusual increase in sweating. These side effects should disappear over time as your body adjusts to the medication.

This medication can cause increased sensitivity to sunlight. It is, therefore, important to avoid prolonged exposure to sunlight and sunlamps. Wear protective clothing and use an effective sunscreen.

If you are constipated, increase the amount of fiber in your diet (fresh fruits and vegetables, salads, bran, and whole-grain breads), exercise, and drink more water (unless your doctor tells you not to do so).

To reduce mouth dryness, chew sugarless gum or suck on ice chips or a piece of hard candy.

If you feel dizzy or light-headed, sit or lie down for a while; get up slowly from a sitting or reclining position; and be careful on stairs.

Major. Tell your doctor about any side effects that are persistent or particularly bothersome. IT IS ESPECIALLY IMPORTANT TO TELL YOUR DOCTOR about changes in menstruation, clumsiness, difficult or painful urination, feeling faint, flushing of the face, hallucinations, palpitations, ringing or buzzing in the ears, rash, seizures, shortness of breath, sleeping disorders, sore throat or fever, tightness in the chest, unusual bleeding or bruising, or unusual tiredness or weakness.

INTERACTIONS

Diphenhydramine interacts with several other types of medications:

1. Concurrent use of diphenhydramine with other central nervous system depressants (for example, alcohol, barbiturates, benzodiazepine tranquilizers, muscle relaxants, narcotics, pain medications, and phenothiazine tranquilizers) or with tricyclic antidepressants can cause extreme fatigue or drowsiness.

2. Monoamine oxidase (MAO) inhibitors (isocarboxazid, pargyline, phenelzine, and tranylcypromine) can increase the side effects of this medication. At least 14 days should separate the use of this drug and the use of an MAO inhibitor.

3. Diphenhydramine can also interfere with the activity of oral anticoagulants (blood thinners, such as warfarin) and decrease their effectiveness.

BE SURE TO TELL YOUR DOCTOR about any medications you are currently taking, especially any of those listed above.

WARNINGS

• Be sure to tell your doctor about unusual or allergic reactions you have had to any medications, especially to diphenhydramine or to any other antihistamine (such as astemizole, azatadine, brompheniramine, carbinoxamine, chlorpheniramine, clemastine, cyproheptadine, dexchlorpheniramine, dimenhydrinate, dimethindene, diphenylpyraline, doxylamine, hydroxyzine, phenindamine, promethazine, pyrilamine, terfenadine, trimeprazine, tripelennamine, and triprolidine).
• Tell your doctor if you now have or if you have ever had asthma, blood vessel disease, glaucoma, high blood pressure, kidney disease, peptic ulcers, enlarged prostate gland, or thyroid disease.
• Diphenhydramine can cause drowsiness or dizziness. Your ability to perform tasks that require alertness, such as driving an automobile or operating potentially dangerous equipment or machinery, may be decreased. Appropriate caution should, therefore, be taken.
• Be sure to tell your doctor if you are pregnant. The effects of this medication during pregnancy have not been thoroughly studied in humans. Also, be sure that you consult with your doctor if you are breast-feeding an infant. Small amounts of diphenhydramine pass into breast milk and may cause unusual excitement or irritability in nursing infants.

---

disopyramide

BRAND NAMES (Manufacturers)
disopyramide (various manufacturers)
Napamide (Major)
Norpace (Searle)
Norpace CR (Searle)
TYPE OF DRUG
Antiarrhythmic
INGREDIENT
disopyramide
DOSAGE FORMS
Capsules (100 mg and 150 mg)
Sustained-release capsules (100 mg and 150 mg)
STORAGE
Disopyramide capsules should be stored at room temperature in tightly closed containers.

USES

Disopyramide is used for the treatment of heart arrhythmias. It corrects irregular heartbeats and helps to achieve a more normal rhythm.

TREATMENT

Disopyramide can be taken with or without food. Check with your doctor for a recommendation.

Try to take disopyramide at the same time(s) each day. This medication works best if the amount of the drug in your bloodstream is kept at a constant level. It is best, therefore, to take this medication at evenly spaced intervals day and night. For example, if you are to take it three times per day, the doses should be spaced eight hours apart.

Try not to miss any doses of this medication. If you do miss a dose and remember within two hours, take the missed dose as soon as possible. If more than two hours have passed, do not take the missed dose; just wait for your next scheduled dose. Do not double the next dose.

SIDE EFFECTS

Minor. Abdominal pain; aches and pain; blurred vision; constipation; decreased sweating; diarrhea; dizziness; dry mouth, eyes, and throat; fatigue; gas; headache; impotence; loss of appetite; nausea; nervousness; or vomiting. These side effects should disappear as you adjust to the drug.

To relieve constipation, increase the amount of fiber in your diet (fresh fruits and vegetables, salads, bran, and whole-grain breads), get more exercise, and drink more water or other nonalcoholic, decaffeinated beverages (unless your doctor directs you to do otherwise).

If you feel dizzy or light-headed, sit or lie down for a while; get up slowly from a sitting or reclining position; and be careful on stairs.

To relieve mouth dryness, suck on ice chips or a piece of hard candy or chew sugarless gum.

"Artificial tears" eye drops may help to relieve eye dryness.

Major. Tell your doctor about any side effects that are persistent or particularly bothersome. IT IS ESPECIALLY IMPORTANT TO TELL YOUR DOCTOR about chest pain; depression; difficult or painful urination; enlarged, painful breasts (in both sexes); fainting; fever; muscle pain; muscle weakness; numbness or tingling sensations; palpitations; rash; shortness of breath; sore throat; swelling of the feet or ankles; weight gain; or yellowing of the eyes or skin.

INTERACTIONS

Disopyramide interacts with several other medications:
1. Phenytoin, rifampin, barbiturates, and glutethimide can decrease its effectiveness.
2. The combination of alcohol and disopyramide can lead to dizziness and hypoglycemia (low blood-sugar levels). You should, therefore, avoid drinking alcoholic beverages while you are taking this medication.
3. The concurrent use of disopyramide and beta blockers (acebutolol, atenolol, betaxolol, carteolol, esmolol, labetalol, metoprolol, nadolol, penbutolol, pindolol, propranolol, and timolol) can have additive negative effects on the heart.
4. Disopyramide may interact with verapamil.

Before starting to take disopyramide, BE SURE TO TELL YOUR DOCTOR about any medications you are currently taking, especially any of those medications listed above.

WARNINGS

• Tell your doctor about unusual or allergic reactions you have had to any medications, especially to disopyramide.
• Tell your doctor if you now have or if you have ever had glaucoma, hypoglycemia (low blood-sugar levels), hypokalemia (low blood potassium levels), kidney disease, liver disease, myasthenia gravis, urinary retention, or an enlarged prostate gland.
• If this drug makes you dizzy or drowsy or blurs your vision, do not take part in any activity that requires alertness, such as driving a car or operating potentially dangerous equipment.
• This medication can decrease sweating and heat release from the body. You should, therefore, avoid getting overheated by strenuous exercise in hot weather and should avoid taking hot baths, showers, and saunas.
• Before having surgery or any other medical or dental treatment, be sure to tell your doctor or dentist that you are taking this medication.
• Disopyramide can cause hypoglycemia. Symptoms of hypoglycemia include anxiety, chills, pale skin, headache, hunger, nausea, nervousness, shakiness, sweating, and weakness. If you experience this reaction, eat or drink something containing sugar, and CONTACT YOUR DOCTOR.
• Be sure to tell your doctor if you are pregnant. The effects of this medication during pregnancy have not been thoroughly studied in humans. It is known that disopyramide passes into breast milk. If you are breast-feeding an infant while being treated with this medication, tell your doctor. Unless directed to do otherwise, breast-feeding is not recommended during treatment with this medication.

---

disulfiram

BRAND NAMES (Manufacturers)
Antabuse (Wyeth-Ayerst)
disulfiram (various manufacturers)
TYPE OF DRUG
Antialcoholic
INGREDIENT
disulfiram
DOSAGE FORM
Tablets (250 mg and 500 mg)
STORAGE
Disulfiram should be stored at room temperature in a tightly closed, light-resistant container.

USES

Disulfiram is used as an aid to treat alcoholics who are strongly motivated to remain sober. Disulfiram blocks the breakdown of alcohol by the body, leading to an accumulation of the chemical acetaldehyde in the bloodstream. Buildup of acetaldehyde in the body can lead to a severe reaction after alcohol consumption. Alcohol must, therefore, be avoided to prevent this reaction.

TREATMENT

Disulfiram can be taken either on an empty stomach or with food or milk (as directed by your doctor). The tablets can also be crushed and mixed with beverages (nonalcoholic).

If you miss a dose of this medication, take the missed dose as soon as possible, unless it is almost time for the next dose. In that case, do not take the missed dose at all; just return to your regular dosing schedule. Do not double the next dose.

SIDE EFFECTS

Minor. Drowsiness, fatigue, headache, metallic or garlic-like aftertaste, and restlessness. These side effects should disappear as your body adjusts to the medication.
Major. Tell your doctor about any side effects that are persistent or particularly bothersome. IT IS ESPECIALLY IMPORTANT TO TELL YOUR DOCTOR about blurred vision, impotence, joint pain, mental disorders, skin rash, tingling sensations, or yellowing of the eyes or skin.

INTERACTIONS

Disulfiram interacts with several other types of medications:
1. It can increase the blood levels and side effects of diazepam, chlordiazepoxide, phenytoin, and oral anticoagulants (blood thinners, such as warfarin).
2. Concurrent use of disulfiram with isoniazid, antidepressants, metronidazole, or marijuana can lead to severe reactions.

BE SURE TO TELL YOUR DOCTOR about any medications you are currently taking, especially any of those listed above. Also, be sure to tell your doctor if you use marijuana.

WARNINGS

• Tell your doctor about unusual or allergic reactions you have had to any medications, especially to disulfiram, rubber, pesticides, or fungicides.
• Before starting to take this medication, be sure to tell your doctor if you have ever had brain damage, dermatitis, diabetes mellitus, epilepsy, heart disease, kidney disease, liver disease, mental disorders, or thyroid disease.
• It is important not to drink or to use any alcohol-containing preparations, medications, or foods (including beer, elixirs, tonics, wine, liquor, vinegar, sauces, after-shave lotions, liniments, or colognes) while taking this medication. Be sure to check the labels on any over-the-counter (nonprescription) products for their alcohol content, especially cough syrups, mouthwashes, and gargles.
• It is important that you understand the serious nature of the disulfiram-alcohol reaction. If you take disulfiram within 12 hours after ingesting alcohol or drink alcohol within two weeks after your last dose of disulfiram, you may experience blurred vision, chest pain, confusion, dizziness, fainting, flushing, headache, nausea, pounding heartbeat, sweating, vomiting, or weakness. The reaction usually occurs within five to ten minutes of drinking alcohol and can last from half an hour to two hours, depending on the dose of disulfiram and the quantity of alcohol ingested.

• If this drug makes you drowsy, do not take part in any activity that requires alertness, such as driving an automobile or operating potentially dangerous machinery or equipment. Also, be careful when going up and down stairs.

• Be sure to tell your doctor if you are pregnant. Birth defects have been reported in both animals and humans whose mothers received disulfiram during pregnancy. It must also be kept in mind that alcohol, even in small amounts, can cause a variety of birth defects when ingested during pregnancy. Also, tell your doctor if you are breast-feeding an infant. It is not known if disulfiram passes into breast milk.

---

doxazosin

BRAND NAME (Manufacturer)
Cardura (Roerig)
TYPE OF DRUG
Antihypertensive
INGREDIENT
doxazosin
DOSAGE FORM
Tablets (1 mg, 2 mg, 4 mg, and 8 mg)
STORAGE
Store doxazosin at room temperature in a tightly closed container.

USES

Doxazosin mesylate is used to treat high blood pressure. It relaxes the muscle tissue of the blood vessels, which in turn lowers blood pressure.

TREATMENT

The first dose of this medication may cause fainting, especially in the elderly.

If you miss a dose of this medication, take it as soon as possible, unless it is almost time for your next dose. In that case, do not take the missed dose at all; just wait until the next scheduled dose. Do not double the dose.

This medication does not cure high blood pressure, but it will help to control the condition as long as you continue to take it. In order to become accustomed to taking this medication, try to take it at the same time(s) each day.

SIDE EFFECTS

Minor. Breast pain, constipation, diarrhea, dizziness, drowsiness, edema, frequent urination, headache, itching, lack of energy, malaise, nasal congestion, nausea, nervousness, rash, sweating, or weight gain. These side effects should disappear as your body adjusts to the medication. TELL YOUR DOCTOR if skin reactions or other side effects persist or become bothersome.

To prevent constipation, increase the amount of fiber in your diet (fresh fruits and vegetables, salads, bran, and whole-grain breads), unless your doctor tells you otherwise.

To avoid dizziness or light-headedness when you stand, contract and relax the muscles of your legs for a few moments before rising. Do this by pushing one foot against the floor while raising the other foot slightly, alternating feet so that you are "pumping" your legs.

Major. Tell your doctor about any side effects that are persistent or particularly bothersome. IT IS ESPECIALLY IMPORTANT TO TELL YOUR DOCTOR about blurred vision; chest pain; difficulty breathing; difficulty urinating; edema; fever; flulike syndrome; heart rate disturbance; nose bleeds; palpitations; persistent malaise/fatigue; postural effects (dizziness, light-headedness, vertigo leading to reductions in blood pressure or fainting); or ringing in the ears.

INTERACTIONS

Doxazosin has been known interact with other types of medications:

1. The combination of doxazosin and alcohol or verapamil can bring about a severe drop in blood pressure and cause fainting.

2. The severity and duration of the blood-pressure-lowering effects of the initial dose of doxazosin may be enhanced by a beta blocker.

BE SURE TO TELL YOUR DOCTOR about any medications you are currently taking, especially those listed above.

WARNINGS

• Tell your doctor about unusual or allergic reactions you have had to any medications, especially to doxazosin, prazosin, or terazosin.

• Before starting to take this medication, be sure to tell your doctor if you now have or if you have ever had angina (chest pain) or any kind of kidney disease or liver disease.

• Because initial therapy with this drug may cause dizziness or fainting, your doctor will probably start you on a low dosage and increase the dosage gradually.

• If this drug makes you dizzy or drowsy or blurs your vision, do not take part in any activity that requires alertness, such as driving a car or operating potentially dangerous machinery.

• In order to avoid dizziness or fainting while taking this drug, try not to stand for long periods of time, avoid drinking excess amounts of alcohol, and try not to get overheated (avoid exercising strenuously in hot weather and taking hot baths, showers, and saunas).

• Before taking any over-the-counter (nonprescription) sinus, allergy, asthma, cough, cold, or diet preparations, check with your doctor or pharmacist. Some of these products can increase blood pressure.

• Do not stop taking this medication unless you first check with your doctor. If you stop taking this drug, you may experience a rise in blood pressure. Your doctor may want to decrease your dose gradually.

• Be sure to tell your doctor if you are pregnant. Although the drug appears to be safe, there have been only limited studies in pregnant women. Also, tell your doctor if you are breast-feeding an infant; doxazosin should be used with caution in nursing women.

doxycycline

BRAND NAMES (Manufacturers)
Doryx (Parke-Davis)
Doxy-Caps (Edwards)
Doxychel Hyclate (Rachelle)
doxycycline (various manufacturers)
Vibramycin Hyclate (Pfizer)
Vibra Tabs (Pfizer)
TYPE OF DRUG
Tetracycline antibiotic
INGREDIENT
doxycycline
DOSAGE FORMS
Tablets (50 mg and 100 mg)
Capsules (50 mg and 100 mg)
Capsules, coated pellets (100 mg)
Oral suspension (25 mg per 5-ml spoonful)
Oral syrup (50 mg per 5-ml spoonful)
STORAGE
Doxycycline tablets, capsules, oral suspension, and oral syrup should be stored at room temperature in tightly closed, light-resistant containers. Any unused portion of the suspension should be discarded after 14 days because the drug loses its potency after that period. This medication should never be frozen.

USES

Doxycycline is used to treat a wide variety of bacterial infections and to prevent or treat traveler's diarrhea. It acts by inhibiting the growth of bacteria.

Doxycycline kills susceptible bacteria, but it is not effective against viruses or fungi.

TREATMENT

To avoid stomach upset, you can take this drug with food (unless your doctor directs you to do otherwise).

The suspension should be shaken well just before measuring each dose. The contents tend to settle on the bottom of the bottle, so it is necessary to shake the container to distribute the ingredients evenly and equalize the doses. Each dose of the oral suspension or oral syrup should be measured carefully with a specially designed 5-ml measuring spoon. An ordinary teaspoon is not accurate.

Do not mix the oral syrup form of this drug with other substances unless so directed by your doctor.

Doxycycline works best when the level of medicine in your bloodstream is kept constant. It is best, therefore, to take the doses at evenly spaced intervals day and night. For example, if you are to take two doses a day, the doses should be spaced 12 hours apart.

If you miss a dose of this medication, take the missed dose immediately. However, if you do not remember to take the missed dose until it is almost time for your next dose, take it; space the following dose about halfway through the regular interval between doses; then return to your regular dosing schedule. Try not to skip any doses.

It is very important that you take this drug for the entire time prescribed, even if the symptoms disappear before the end of that period. If you stop taking the drug too soon, resistant bacteria can continue to grow, and the infection could recur.

SIDE EFFECTS

Minor. Diarrhea, discoloration of the nails, dizziness, loss of appetite, nausea, stomach cramps and upset, or vomiting. These side effects should disappear as your body adjusts to the medication.

Doxycycline can increase your sensitivity to sunlight. You should, therefore, try to avoid prolonged exposure to sunlight and sunlamps. Wear protective clothing and sunglasses, and use an effective sunscreen.

Major. Tell your doctor about any side effects that are persistent or particularly bothersome. IT IS ESPECIALLY IMPORTANT TO TELL YOUR DOCTOR about darkened tongue, difficulty in breathing, joint pain, mouth irritation, rash, rectal or vaginal itching, sore throat and fever, unusual bleeding or bruising, or yellowing of the eyes or skin. Also, if your symptoms of infection seem to be getting worse rather than improving, you should contact your doctor.

INTERACTIONS

Doxycycline interacts with other types of medications:

1. It can increase the absorption of digoxin, which may lead to digoxin toxicity.

2. The gastrointestinal side effects (nausea, vomiting, stomach upset) of theophylline may be increased by doxycycline.

3. The dosage of oral anticoagulants (blood thinners, such as warfarin) may need to be adjusted when this medication is started.

4. Doxycycline may decrease the effectiveness of oral contraceptives (birth control pills), and pregnancy could result. You should, therefore, use a different or additional form of birth control while taking doxycycline. Discuss this with your doctor.

5. Barbiturates, carbamazepine, phenytoin, and antacids can lower the blood levels of doxycycline, decreasing its effectiveness.

6. Iron can bind to doxycycline in the gastrointestinal tract, which can decrease its absorption and, therefore, its effectiveness.

BE SURE TO TELL YOUR DOCTOR about any medications you are currently taking, especially any of those listed above.

WARNINGS

• Tell your doctor about any unusual or allergic reactions you have or ever have had to any medications, especially to doxycycline, oxytetracycline, tetracycline, or minocycline.

• Tell your doctor if you now have or if you have ever had kidney or liver disease.

• Doxycycline can affect tests for syphilis; if you are also being treated for this disease, tell your doctor you are taking this medication.

• Make sure that your prescription for this medication is marked with the drug's expiration date. The drug should be discarded after the expiration date. If doxycycline is used after it has expired, serious side effects (especially to the kidneys) could result.

• This medication has been prescribed for your current infection only. Another infection later on, or one that someone else has, may require a different medicine. You should not give your medicine to other people or use it for other infections, unless your doctor specifically directs you to do so.
• Be sure to tell your doctor if you are pregnant or if you are breast-feeding an infant. Doxycycline should not be used during pregnancy and breast-feeding. It crosses the placenta and passes into breast milk. This drug can cause permanent discoloration of the teeth and can inhibit tooth and bone growth if used during their development. This drug should not be used by children less than eight years.

---

enalapril

BRAND NAME (Manufacturer)
Vasotec (Merck Sharp & Dohme)
TYPE OF DRUG
Antihypertensive
INGREDIENT
enalapril
DOSAGE FORM
Tablets (2.5 mg, 5 mg, 10 mg, and 20 mg)
STORAGE
Store enalapril at room temperature in a tightly closed container.

USES

Enalapril is used to treat high blood pressure. It is a vasodilator (it widens the blood vessels) that acts by blocking the production of chemicals that may be responsible for constricting or narrowing the blood vessels.

TREATMENT

Enalapril can be taken either on an empty stomach or with food if it causes stomach irritation. To become accustomed to taking this medication, try to take it at the same time(s) every day.

It may be several weeks before you notice the full effects of this medication.

If you miss a dose of enalapril, take the missed dose as soon as possible, unless it is almost time for the next dose. In that case, do not take the missed dose at all; just wait until the next scheduled dose. Do not double the dose.

Enalapril does not cure high blood pressure, but it will help to control the condition as long as you continue to take the medication.

SIDE EFFECTS

Minor. Abdominal pain, cough, diarrhea, dizziness, drowsiness, fatigue, headache, heartburn, insomnia, nausea, nervousness, sweating, or vomiting. These side effects should disappear as your body adjusts to the medication.

To avoid dizziness when you stand, contract and relax the muscles of your legs for a few moments before rising. Do this by alternately pushing one foot against the floor while lifting the other foot slightly.

Major. Tell your doctor about any side effects that are persistent or particularly bothersome. IT IS ESPECIALLY IMPORTANT TO TELL YOUR DOCTOR about chest pain; difficulty in breathing; fainting; fever; itching; lightheadedness (especially during the first few days); muscle cramps; palpitations; rash; sore throat; swelling of the face, eyes, lips, or tongue; tingling in the fingers or toes; or yellowing of the eyes or skin.

INTERACTIONS

Enalapril interacts with several other types of medications:

1. Diuretics (water pills) and other antihypertensive medications can cause an excessive drop in blood pressure when they are combined with enalapril (especially with the first dose).

2. The combination of enalapril with spironolactone, triamterene, amiloride, potassium supplements, or salt substitutes can lead to hyperkalemia (dangerously high levels of potassium in the bloodstream).

Before starting to take enalapril, BE SURE TO TELL YOUR DOCTOR about any medications you are currently taking, especially any of those listed above.

WARNINGS

• Tell your doctor about unusual or allergic reactions you have had to any medications, especially to enalapril.
• Tell your doctor if you now have or if you have ever had blood disorders, heart failure, renal disease, or systemic lupus erythematosus.
• Excessive perspiration, dehydration, or prolonged vomiting or diarrhea can lead to an excessive drop in blood pressure while you are taking this medication. Contact your doctor if you have any of these symptoms.
• Before having surgery or other medical or dental treatment, tell your doctor or dentist you are taking this drug.
• If this drug makes you dizzy or drowsy, do not take part in any activity that requires alertness, such as driving a car or operating potentially dangerous equipment.
• If you have high blood pressure, do not take any over-the-counter (nonprescription) medications for weight control or for asthma, sinus, cough, cold, or allergy problems unless you first check with your doctor.
• Be sure to tell your doctor if you are pregnant. Drugs in the same class as enalapril have been shown to cause birth defects, including kidney damage, low blood pressure, improper skull development, and death, when taken in the second and third trimesters. Also, tell your doctor if you are breast-feeding an infant. It is not yet known if enalapril passes into human breast milk.

---

ergotamine

BRAND NAMES (Manufacturers)
Ergostat (Parke-Davis)
Medihaler Ergotamine (3M)

TYPE OF DRUG
Antimigraine (vasoconstrictor)
INGREDIENT
ergotamine
DOSAGE FORMS
Sublingual tablets (2 mg)
Aerosol (0.36 mg per spray)
STORAGE
This medication should be stored at room temperature in tightly closed, light-resistant containers.

The container of the aerosol is pressurized; it should, therefore, never be punctured, burned, or broken. It should also be stored away from heat and out of direct sunlight.

USES

This medication is used to treat migraine and cluster headaches. These headaches are thought to be caused by an increase in the diameter of the blood vessels in the head, which results in more blood flow, greater pressure, and pain. Ergotamine is a vasoconstrictor; it acts by constricting (narrowing) the blood vessels.

TREATMENT

Take this medication as soon as you notice your migraine headache symptoms. If you wait until the headache is severe, the drug takes longer to work and may not be as effective.

After you take either of these forms of ergotamine, you should try to lie down in a quiet, dark room for at least two hours (in order to help the medication work). The drug usually takes effect in 30 to 60 minutes.

It is very important that you understand how often you can repeat a dose of this medication during an attack (usually every 30 to 60 minutes for the sublingual tablets, and every five minutes for the aerosol spray) and the maximum amount of medication you can take per day (usually three sublingual tablets or six inhalations). Five is generally the maximum number of sublingual tablets and 15 is about the maximum number of inhalations that can be taken in any one-week period. CHECK WITH YOUR DOCTOR if you have any questions.

The sublingual tablets should be placed under your tongue. DO NOT swallow these tablets—they are more efficiently absorbed through the lining of the mouth than from the gastrointestinal tract. Try not to eat, drink, chew, or smoke while the tablet is dissolving.

The aerosol form of this medication comes packaged with instructions for use. Read the directions carefully; if you have any questions, check with your doctor or pharmacist. The aerosol can should be shaken well just before each dose is sprayed. The contents tend to settle on the bottom of the container, so it should be shaken to disperse the medication and equalize the doses. The container provides about 60 measured sprays.

If you are on prolonged treatment with this drug and you miss a dose, take it as soon as you remember. Wait four hours to take the next dose. It is very important that you consult your doctor before you discontinue using this drug. Your doctor may want to reduce your dosage gradually.

SIDE EFFECTS

Minor. Diarrhea, dizziness, headache, nausea, vomiting, or sensation of cold hands and feet with MILD numbness or tingling. These side effects should disappear as your body adjusts to the medication.

The aerosol form of ergotamine can cause hoarseness or throat irritation. Gargling or rinsing your mouth out with water after taking the dose may help prevent this side effect.

Major. Tell your doctor about any side effects that are persistent or particularly bothersome. IT IS ESPECIALLY IMPORTANT TO TELL YOUR DOCTOR about chest pain; coldness, numbness, pain, tingling, or dark discoloration of the fingers or toes; confusion; fluid retention; itching; localized swelling; muscle pain; severe abdominal pain and swelling; or unusual weakness.

INTERACTIONS

Ergotamine interacts with several other types of medications:

1. Ergotamine interacts with amphetamines, ephedrine, epinephrine (adrenaline), pseudoephedrine, erythromycin, and troleandomycin. Such combinations can lead to increases in blood pressure or increased risk of adverse reaction to ergotamine.

2. Do not drink alcoholic beverages while you are taking this medication. Since alcohol dilates (widens) the blood vessels (which are already dilated during migraine headaches), drinking will only make your headache worse.

3. Nicotine and cocaine decrease the effectiveness of ergotamine and, therefore, make the headache worse.

4. The caffeine in tea, coffee, and cola drinks also interacts with this medication. It may actually help to relieve your headache.

BE SURE TO TELL YOUR DOCTOR about any medications or substances you are currently taking or using, especially any of those listed above.

WARNINGS

- Tell your doctor about unusual or allergic reactions you have had to any medications, especially to ergotamine or other ergot alkaloids (such as ergonovine or bromocriptine).
- Before starting to take this medication, be sure to tell your doctor if you now have or if you have ever had heart or blood-vessel disease, high blood pressure, infections, kidney disease, liver disease, or thyroid disease.
- Avoid any foods to which you are allergic.
- If this drug makes you dizzy or drowsy, do not take part in any activity that requires alertness, such as driving a car or operating potentially dangerous equipment.
- Try to avoid exposure to cold. Since this drug acts by constricting blood vessels throughout the body, your fingers and toes may become especially sensitive.
- Elderly patients are more sensitive to the effects of ergotamine. Consult your doctor if the side effects become bothersome.
- This medication should not be taken for longer periods or in higher doses than recommended by your doctor. Extended use of this drug can lead to serious side effects.

In addition, tolerance can develop—higher doses would be required to obtain the same beneficial effects (at the same time increasing the risk of side effects).
• Be sure to tell your doctor if you are pregnant. Ergotamine can cause contractions of the uterus, which can harm the developing fetus. This drug should not be used during pregnancy. Also, tell your doctor if you are breastfeeding an infant. Ergotamine passes into breast milk and may cause vomiting, diarrhea, or convulsions in the nursing infant.

MONEY-SAVING TIP

Save the inhaler piece from the aerosol container. Refill units, which are less expensive, are available at most pharmacies.

erythromycin

BRAND NAMES (Manufacturers)

E.E.S. 200 Liquid (Abbott)
E.E.S. 400 Filmtab (Abbott)
E-Mycin (Boots)
Eramycin (Wesley)
Eryc (Parke-Davis)
EryPed (Abbott)
Ery-Tab (Abbott)
Erythrocin Stearate Filmtabs (Abbott)
Erythromycin Base (Abbott)
Ilosone (Dista)
Ilosone Pulvules (Dista)
PCE Dispertab (Abbott)
Robimycin (Robins)
Wyamycin S (Wyeth)

TYPE OF DRUG

Antibiotic

INGREDIENT

erythromycin

DOSAGE FORMS

Tablets (250 mg, 333 mg, and 500 mg)
Chewable tablets (200 mg)
Enteric-coated tablets (250 mg, 333 mg, and 500 mg)
Film-coated tablets (250 mg, 400 mg, and 500 mg)
Polymer-coated tablets (333 mg)
Capsules (250 mg)
Oral drops (100 mg per 2.5 ml)
Oral suspension (125 mg, 200 mg, 250 mg, and 400 mg per 5-ml spoonful)

STORAGE

Erythromycin tablets and capsules should be stored at room temperature in tightly closed, light-resistant containers. Erythromycin oral drops and oral suspension should be stored in the refrigerator in tightly closed, light-resistant containers. Any unused portion of the liquid forms should be discarded after 14 days. Erythromycin ethylsuccinate liquid does not need to be refrigerated; however, refrigeration helps to preserve the taste. This medication should never be frozen.

USES

Erythromycin is used to treat a wide variety of bacterial infections, including infections of the middle ear and the respiratory tract. It is also used to treat infections in persons who are allergic to penicillin. It acts by preventing the bacteria from growing. It is not effective against viruses, parasites, or fungi.

TREATMENT

In order to prevent stomach upset, erythromycin coated tablets and erythromycin estolate or ethylsuccinate can be taken with food or milk. Other erythromycin products should be taken with a full glass of water, preferably on an empty stomach, one hour before or two hours after a meal.

The liquid forms should be taken undiluted.

Each dose of the oral drops should be measured carefully with the dropper provided.

The oral suspension form of this medication should be shaken well just before measuring each dose. The contents tend to settle on the bottom of the bottle, so it is necessary to shake the container to distribute the ingredients evenly and equalize the doses. Each dose should then be measured carefully with a specially designed 5-ml measuring spoon. An ordinary kitchen teaspoon is not accurate enough.

In order to prevent gastrointestinal side effects, the coated tablets and capsules should be swallowed whole; do not break, chew, or crush these products.

Erythromycin works best when the level of medicine in your bloodstream is kept constant. It is best, therefore, to take the doses at evenly spaced intervals day and night. For example, if you are to take four doses a day, the doses should be spaced six hours apart.

If you miss a dose of this medication, take the missed dose immediately. However, if you do not remember to take the missed dose until it is almost time for your next dose, take it; space the following dose about halfway through the regular interval between doses; then return to your regular schedule. Try not to skip any doses.

It is important to continue to take this medication for the entire time prescribed by your doctor (usually seven to 14 days), even if the symptoms disappear before the end of that period. If you stop taking this drug too soon, the infection could recur.

SIDE EFFECTS

Minor. Abdominal cramps, diarrhea, fatigue, irritation of the mouth, loss of appetite, nausea, sore tongue, or vomiting. These side effects should disappear as your body adjusts to the medication.

Major. Tell your doctor about any side effects that are persistent or particularly bothersome. IT IS ESPECIALLY IMPORTANT TO TELL YOUR DOCTOR about fever, hearing loss, hives, rash, rectal or vaginal itching, or yellowing of the eyes or skin. If your symptoms of infection seem to be getting worse rather than improving, you should contact your doctor.

INTERACTIONS

1. Erythromycin can decrease the elimination of aminophylline, oxtriphylline, theophylline, digoxin, oral anti-

coagulants (blood thinners, such as warfarin), and carbamazepine from the body, which can lead to serious side effects.
2. Therapy with erythromycin may increase the effects of methylprednisolone.
BE SURE TO TELL YOUR DOCTOR about any medications you are currently taking, especially any listed above.

WARNINGS

• Tell your doctor about unusual or allergic reactions you have had to any medications, especially to erythromycin.
• Be sure to tell your doctor if you have ever had liver disease.
• This drug has been prescribed for your current infection only. Another infection later on, or one that someone else has, may require a different medication altogether. Do not give your medicine to other people or use it for other infections, unless your doctor specifically directs you to.
• Before having surgery or any other medical or dental treatment, be sure to tell your doctor or dentist that you are taking erythromycin.
• Not all erythromycin products are chemically equivalent. However, they all produce the same therapeutic effect. Discuss with your doctor or pharmacist which forms of erythromycin are appropriate for you, and then choose the least expensive product among those recommended.
• Some of these products contain the color additive FD&C Yellow No. 5 (tartrazine), which can cause allergic-type reactions (difficulty in breathing, rash, fainting) in certain susceptible individuals.
• Be sure to tell your doctor if you are pregnant. Although erythromycin appears to be safe during pregnancy, extensive studies in humans have not been conducted. Also, tell your doctor if you are breast-feeding an infant. Small amounts of this medication pass into breast milk and may temporarily alter the bacterial balance in the intestinal tract of the nursing infant, resulting in diarrhea.

---

fenfluramine

BRAND NAME (MANUFACTURER)
Pondimin (Robins)
TYPE OF DRUG
Anorectic
INGREDIENT
fenfluramine
DOSAGE FORM
Tablets (20 mg)
STORAGE
Fenfluramine should be stored at room temperature in a tightly closed, light-resistant container.

USES

Fenfluramine is used as an appetite suppressant during the first few weeks of dieting to help establish new eating habits. This medication is thought to relieve hunger by altering nerve impulses to the appetite control center in the brain. Its effectiveness lasts only for short periods (three to 12 weeks).

TREATMENT

You can take fenfluramine with a full glass of water, one hour before meals (unless your doctor directs you to do otherwise).

If you miss a dose of this medication, take the missed dose as soon as possible, unless it is almost time for your next dose. In that case, do not take the missed dose at all; just return to your regular dosing schedule. Do not double the next dose

SIDE EFFECTS

Minor. Blurred vision, constipation, diarrhea, dizziness, dry mouth, euphoria, fatigue, frequent urination, headache, insomnia, irritability, nausea, nervousness, restlessness, stomach pain, sweating, unpleasant taste in the mouth, or vomiting. These side effects should disappear as your body adjusts to the medication.

Dry mouth can be relieved by sucking on ice chips or a piece of hard candy or by chewing sugarless gum.

In order to prevent constipation, increase the amount of fiber in your diet (fresh fruits and vegetables, salads, bran, and whole-grain breads), exercise, and drink more water (unless your doctor tells you not to do so).
Major. Tell your doctor about any side effects that are persistent or particularly bothersome. IT IS ESPECIALLY IMPORTANT TO TELL YOUR DOCTOR about changes in sexual desire, chest pain, difficulty in urinating, enlarged breasts (in both sexes), fever, hair loss, headaches, impotence, increased blood pressure, menstrual irregularities, mental depression, mood changes, mouth sores, muscle pains, nosebleeds, palpitations, rash, sore throat, or tremors.

INTERACTIONS

Fenfluramine anorectic medication interacts with several other types of medications:
1. Concurrent use of it with central nervous system depressants (such as alcohol, antihistamines, barbiturates, muscle relaxants, narcotics, pain medications, and phenothiazine tranquilizers) or with tricyclic antidepressants can cause extreme drowsiness.
2. Fenfluramine may alter insulin and oral antidiabetic medication dosage requirements in diabetic patients.
3. The blood-pressure-lowering effects of antihypertensive medications, especially guanethidine, reserpine, methyldopa, and diuretics (water pills), may be increased by this medication.
4. Use of fenfluramine within 14 days of a monoamine oxidase (MAO) inhibitor (isocarboxazid, pargyline, phenelzine, tranylcypromine) can result in high blood pressure and other side effects.

BE SURE TO TELL YOUR DOCTOR about any medications you are currently taking.

WARNINGS

• Tell your doctor about unusual or allergic reactions you have had to any medications, especially to fenfluramine or other appetite suppressants (such as benzphetamine, phendimetrazine, diethylpropion, phenmetrazine, mazindol, and phentermine), or to epinephrine, norepinephrine, ephedrine, amphetamines, dextroamphetamine, phenylephrine, phenylpropanolamine, pseudoephedrine, albuterol, metaproterenol, or terbutaline.

• Tell your doctor if you have a history of drug abuse or alcoholism or if you have ever had angina, diabetes mellitus, emotional disturbances, glaucoma, heart or cardiovascular disease, high blood pressure, thyroid disease, epilepsy, or mental depression.

• Fenfluramine can mask the symptoms of extreme fatigue and can cause dizziness or light-headedness. Your ability to perform tasks that require alertness, such as driving a car or operating potentially dangerous equipment, may be decreased during therapy with this medication. Appropriate caution should also be taken when going up and down stairs.

• Before having surgery or any other medical or dental treatment, be sure to tell your doctor or dentist that you are taking this medication.

• Fenfluramine is related to amphetamine and may be habit-forming when taken for long periods of time (both physical and psychological dependence can occur). You should, therefore, not increase the dosage of this medication or take it for longer than 12 weeks, unless you first consult your doctor. It is also important that you not stop taking this medication abruptly. Fatigue, sleep disorders, mental depression, nausea, vomiting, stomach cramps, or pain could occur. Your doctor may want to decrease your dosage gradually in order to prevent these side effects.

• Fenfluramine can alter blood sugar levels in diabetic patients. Therefore, it is important to note that if you are diabetic and starting to take this medication, you should carefully monitor your blood or urine glucose levels for the first several days.

• Be sure to tell your doctor if you are pregnant. Although side effects in humans have not been studied, some of the appetite suppressants have been shown to cause side effects in the fetuses of animals that received large doses during pregnancy. Also, tell your doctor if you are breastfeeding an infant. It is not known at this time whether this medication passes into breast milk or poses a danger to a nursing infant.

---

fluconazole

BRAND NAME (Manufacturer)
Diflucan (Roerig)
TYPE OF DRUG
Antifungal Agent
INGREDIENT
fluconazole
DOSAGE FORMS
Tablets (50 mg, 100 mg, and 200 mg)
Oral suspension (50 mg and 200 mg per 5-ml spoonful)

STORAGE
The tablet form of this medication should be stored in a tightly closed container at room temperature, away from heat and direct sunlight. The suspension form should be stored in the refrigerator. Any unused portion of the oral suspension should be discarded after 14 days because it loses its potency after that time. This medication should be protected from freezing.

USES

Fluconazole is used to treat fungal infections of the mouth, throat, urinary tract, kidney, and liver. It is also used to treat pneumonia or meningitis caused by fungus. This medication acts by severely injuring the cell walls of the infecting fungus, thereby preventing them from growing and multiplying. Fluconazole is effective against susceptible fungus but does not kill bacteria, viruses, or parasites.

TREATMENT

This medication should be taken exactly as prescribed by your doctor, even if your symptoms improve. If you stop taking this medication too soon, resistant fungi are given a chance to grow and the infection may recur. You may have to take fluconazole for an extended period of time to completely cure the infection.

The contents of the suspension form of fluconazole tend to settle on the bottom of the bottle. Thus it is necessary to shake the container well immediately before each dose in order to distribute the ingredients evenly and to equalize the doses. Each dose should be carefully measured using a specially designed 5-ml measuring spoon. An ordinary kitchen spoon is not accurate enough.

If you miss a dose and remember within a few hours, take the missed dose and resume your regular schedule. If many hours have passed, take the missed dose as soon as you remember. Space the following dose halfway through the regular interval between doses, then return to your regular schedule. Try not to skip any doses.

SIDE EFFECTS

Minor. Abdominal pain or cramps, diarrhea, nausea, vomiting, dizziness, headache, skin rash, or itching.
Major. Tell your doctor about any side effects that are persistent or particularly bothersome. IT IS ESPECIALLY IMPORTANT TO TELL YOUR DOCTOR if you notice any yellowing of the skin or eyes, dark urine, or pale stools.

INTERACTIONS

Fluconazole interacts with several other types of drugs:
1. Fluconazole may increase the effectiveness of oral anticoagulants (blood thinners, such as warfarin), phenytoin, cyclosporine, and oral antidiabetic agents.
2. The effectiveness of fluconazole may be decreased when given together with rifampin.

BE SURE TO TELL YOUR DOCTOR about any medications you are currently taking, especially any of those listed above.

WARNINGS

• Tell your doctor about any reactions you have had to any medications, especially to fluconazole.

• Tell your doctor if you now have or if you have ever had liver disease.
• This drug should not be taken if you are pregnant or breast-feeding an infant. Be sure to tell your doctor if you are pregnant or breast-feeding.

---

fluoxetine

BRAND NAME (Manufacturer)
Prozac (Dista)
TYPE OF DRUG
Cyclic antidepressant
INGREDIENT
fluoxetine
DOSAGE FORMS
Capsules (20 mg)
Liquid (20 mg per 5 ml spoonful)
STORAGE
Store at room temperature in a tightly closed container. Do not store in the bathroom. Heat or moisture can cause this medicine to break down.

USES

Fluoxetine is used to treat the symptoms of mental depression. It increases the concentration of certain chemicals called neurotransmitters necessary for nerve transmission in the brain.

TREATMENT

This medication should be taken exactly as prescribed by your doctor. In order to avoid stomach irritation, you can take fluoxetine with food or with a full glass of water (unless your doctor directs you to do otherwise).

The effects of therapy with this medication may not become apparent for one to three weeks.

If you miss a dose of this medicine, it is not necessary to make up the missed dose. Skip that dose and continue at the next scheduled time. You should never take a double dose to make up for one you missed.

SIDE EFFECTS

Minor. Agitation, change in vision, changes in taste, constipation, decreased appetite, decreased mental concentration, decreased sex drive, diarrhea, dizziness, drowsiness, dry mouth, rapid heartbeat, flushing, frequent urination, headache, increased sweating, nausea, stomach cramps, stuffy nose, vomiting, or weight gain or loss.

Dry mouth can be relieved by chewing sugarless gum or sucking on hard candy.

To relieve constipation, increase the amount of fiber in your diet (fresh fruits and vegetables, salads, bran, and whole-grain breads), exercise, and drink more water (unless your doctor directs you to do otherwise).

To avoid dizziness or light-headedness when you stand, contract and relax the muscles of your legs for a few moments before rising.

Major. Tell your doctor about any side effects that are persistent or particularly bothersome. IT IS ESPECIALLY IMPORTANT TO TELL YOUR DOCTOR about anxiety, chills or fever, convulsions (seizures), enlarged lymph glands (swelling under the jaw, in armpits, or in the groin area), difficulty in breathing, joint or muscle pain, skin rash or hives, or swelling of the feet or lower legs.

INTERACTIONS

Fluoxetine interacts with a number of other types of drugs:
1. Extreme drowsiness can occur when this medicine is taken with central nervous system depressants (such as alcohol, antihistamines, barbiturates, benzodiazepine tranquilizers, muscle relaxants, narcotics, pain medications, phenothiazine tranquilizers, and sleeping medications) or with other antidepressants.
2. Fluoxetine may increase the effects of anticoagulants (blood thinners, such as warfarin) and certain heart medications (such as digitoxin).
3. Serious side effects may occur if a monoamine oxidase (MAO) inhibitor (such as furazolidone, isocarboxazid, pargyline, phenelzine, procarbazine, or tranylcypromine) is taken with fluoxetine. At least 14 days should separate the use of fluoxetine and the use of an MAO inhibitor.
4. Fluoxetine can increase agitation, restlessness, and stomach irritation when taken along with tryptophan.

Before starting to take fluoxetine, BE SURE TO TELL YOUR DOCTOR about any medications you are currently taking, especially any of those listed above.

WARNINGS

• Tell your doctor immediately if you develop a skin rash or hives while taking this medication, or if you have ever had an allergic reaction to fluoxetine.
• Tell your doctor if you have allergies to any substance; such as foods, sulfites, or other preservatives or dyes.
• Before starting to take this medication, be sure to tell your doctor if you have a history of alcoholism or if you have ever had a heart attack, asthma, circulatory disease, difficulty in urinating, electroshock therapy, enlarged prostate gland, epilepsy, glaucoma, high blood pressure, intestinal problems, liver or kidney disease, mental illness, stomach problems, or thyroid disease.
• If this drug makes you dizzy or drowsy, do not take part in any activity that requires alertness, such as driving a car or operating potentially dangerous equipment.
• Do not stop taking this drug suddenly. Abruptly stopping it can cause nausea, headache, stomach upset, or a worsening of your condition. Your doctor may want to reduce the dosage gradually.
• The elderly may be at increased risk for side effects. Use this drug cautiously, and report any mental status changes to your doctor immediately.
• The effects of this medication may persist for as long as five weeks after you stop taking it, so continue to observe all precautions during that period.
• Be sure to tell your doctor if you are pregnant. Although birth defects have not been documented in animal studies, it is not known if fluoxetine is safe during human pregnancy. It is also not known if fluoxetine passes into breast milk, so be sure to tell your doctor if you are breast-feeding an infant.

furosemide

BRAND NAMES (Manufacturers)
furosemide (various manufacturers)
Lasix (Hoechst-Roussel)
Luramide (Major)
TYPE OF DRUG
Diuretic (water pill) and antihypertensive
INGREDIENT
furosemide
DOSAGE FORMS
Tablets (20 mg, 40 mg, 80 mg, and 200 mg)
Oral solution (10 mg per ml, and 40 mg per 5 ml, with 0.02%, 0.2%, or 11.5% alcohol)
STORAGE
Furosemide tablets should be stored at room temperature in a tightly closed, light-resistant container. The oral solution should be stored in the refrigerator in a tightly closed, light-resistant container. While furosemide in the solution form should be kept cold, this medication should never be frozen.

USES

Furosemide is prescribed to treat high blood pressure. It is also used to reduce fluid accumulation in the body caused by conditions such as heart failure, cirrhosis of the liver, kidney disease, and the long-term use of some medications. Furosemide reduces fluid accumulation by increasing the elimination of sodium and water through the kidneys.

TREATMENT

To decrease stomach irritation, you can take furosemide with a glass of milk or with a meal (unless your doctor directs you to do otherwise). Try to take it at the same time every day. Avoid taking a dose after 6:00 P.M.—this will prevent you from having to get up during the night to urinate.

This medication does not cure high blood pressure, but it will help to control the condition, as long as you continue to take it.

If you miss a dose of this medication, take it as soon as possible, unless it is almost time for the next dose. In that case, do not take the missed dose at all; just wait until the next scheduled dose. Do not double the dose.

SIDE EFFECTS

Minor. Blurred vision, constipation, cramping, diarrhea, dizziness, headache, itching, loss of appetite, muscle spasms, nausea, sore mouth, stomach upset, vomiting, and weakness. As your body adjusts to the medication, these side effects should disappear.

This medication will cause an increase in the amount of urine or in your frequency of urination when you first begin to take it. It may also cause an unusual feeling of tiredness. These effects should subside.

Furosemide can cause increased sensitivity to sunlight. It is therefore important to avoid prolonged exposure to sunlight and sunlamps. Wear protective clothing and use an effective sunscreen.

To avoid dizziness and light-headedness when you stand, contract and relax the muscles of your legs for a few moments before rising. Do this by pushing one foot against the floor while raising the other foot slightly, alternating feet so that you are "pumping" your legs in a pedaling motion.

Major. Tell your doctor about any side effects that are persistent or bothersome. IT IS ESPECIALLY IMPORTANT TO TELL YOUR DOCTOR about confusion, difficulty in breathing, dry mouth, fainting, increased thirst, joint pains, loss of appetite, mood changes, muscle cramps, palpitations, rash, ringing in the ears, severe abdominal pain, sore throat, tingling in the fingers or toes, unusual bleeding or bruising, or yellowing of the eyes or skin.

INTERACTIONS

Furosemide interacts with several other drugs:

1. It can increase the side effects of alcohol, barbiturates, narcotics, cephalosporin antibiotics, chloral hydrate, cortisonelike steroids (such as cortisone, dexamethasone, hydrocortisone, prednisone, and prednisolone), digoxin, digitalis, lithium, amphotericin B, clofibrate, aspirin, and theophylline.

2. The effectiveness of antigout medications, insulin, and oral antidiabetic medications may be decreased by furosemide.

3. Phenytoin can decrease the absorption and effectiveness of furosemide.

4. Indomethacin can decrease the diuretic effects of furosemide.

Before taking furosemide, BE SURE TO TELL YOUR DOCTOR if you are taking any of the medicines listed above.

WARNINGS

• Tell your doctor about unusual or allergic reactions you have had to any medications, especially to diuretics, oral antidiabetic medicines, or sulfonamide antibiotics.

• Tell your doctor if you now have, or if you have ever had, kidney disease or problems with urination; diabetes mellitus; gout; liver disease; asthma; pancreatic disease; or systemic lupus erythematosus (SLE).

• Furosemide can cause potassium loss. Signs of potassium loss include dry mouth, thirst, weakness, muscle pain or cramps, nausea, and vomiting. If you experience any of these symptoms, call your doctor. Your doctor may want to have blood tests performed periodically in order to monitor your blood-potassium levels. To help avoid potassium loss, take this medication with a glass of fresh or frozen orange juice or cranberry juice, or eat a banana every day. The use of a salt substitute also helps to prevent potassium loss. Do not change your diet, however, before discussing it with your doctor. Too much potassium may also be dangerous.

• Before having any kind of surgery or other medical or dental treatment, be sure to tell your doctor or dentist that you are taking furosemide.

• To avoid dizziness, light-headedness, or fainting, get up from a sitting or lying position slowly; and avoid standing for long periods of time. You should also avoid strenuous exercise and prolonged exposure to hot weather.

• While taking this medication, limit your intake of alcoholic beverages in order to prevent dizziness.
• If you have high blood pressure, do not take any over-the-counter (nonprescription) medications for weight control; or for cough, cold, asthma, allergy, or sinus problems; unless you first check with your doctor.
• To prevent severe water loss (dehydration) while taking this drug, check with your doctor if you have any illness that causes severe nausea, vomiting, or diarrhea.
• This medication can raise blood-sugar levels in diabetic patients. Therefore, blood sugar should be monitored carefully with blood or urine tests when treatment with this medication is started.
• Be sure to tell your doctor if you are pregnant. This drug crosses the placenta. Although studies in humans have not been completed, adverse effects have been observed on the fetuses of animals who received large doses of this drug during pregnancy. Also, tell your doctor if you are breast-feeding an infant. Small amounts of furosemide pass into breast milk.

---

gemfibrozil

BRAND NAMES (Manufacturers)
gemfibrozil (various manufacturers)
Lopid (Parke-Davis)
TYPE OF DRUG
Antihyperlipidemic (lipid-lowering drug)
INGREDIENT
gemfibrozil
DOSAGE FORM
Tablets (600 mg)
STORAGE
This medication should be stored at room temperature in a tightly closed container.

USES

Gemfibrozil is used to treat hyperlipidemia (high blood-fat levels) in patients who have not responded to diet, weight reduction, exercise, and control of blood sugar. It is not clear how gemfibrozil lowers blood-lipid levels, but it is thought to decrease the body's production of certain fats.

TREATMENT

In order to maximize its effectiveness, gemfibrozil should be taken 30 minutes before meals.

If you miss a dose of this medication, take the missed dose of gemfibrozil as soon as possible, unless it is almost time for the next dose. In that case, do not take the missed dose; just return to your regular dosing schedule. Do not double the dose.

SIDE EFFECTS

Minor. Constipation, diarrhea, dizziness, dry mouth, gas, headache, insomnia, loss of appetite, nausea, and stomach upset. These side effects should disappear in several days, as your body adjusts to the medication.

To relieve constipation, increase the amount of fiber in your diet (bran, salads, fresh fruits and vegetables, and whole-grain breads), exercise, and drink more water (unless your doctor directs you to do otherwise).

If you feel dizzy, sit or lie down a while; get up slowly from a sitting or lying position; and be careful on stairs.

To help relieve mouth dryness, chew sugarless gum or suck on ice chips.

Major. Tell your doctor about any side effects that are persistent or particularly bothersome. IT IS ESPECIALLY IMPORTANT TO TELL YOUR DOCTOR about back pain, blurred vision, fatigue, muscle cramps, rash, swollen or painful joints, tingling sensations, or yellowing of the eyes or skin.

INTERACTIONS

Gemfibrozil can increase the effects of oral anticoagulants (blood thinners, such as warfarin), which can lead to bleeding complications.

BE SURE TO TELL YOUR DOCTOR if you are already taking a medication of this type.

WARNINGS

• Tell your doctor about unusual or allergic reactions you have had to any medications, especially to gemfibrozil.
• Before starting to take this medication, be sure to tell your doctor if you now have, or if you have ever had, biliary disorders; gallstones or gallbladder disease; kidney disease; or liver disease.
• If this drug makes you dizzy or or otherwise interferes with your vision, do not take part in activities that require mental alertness, such as driving an automobile or operating any potentially dangerous machinery or equipment.
• Do not stop taking this medication unless you first check with your doctor. Stopping the drug abruptly may lead to a rapid increase in blood-lipid (fats) and cholesterol levels. Your doctor may therefore want to start you on a special diet or another medication when gemfibrozil is discontinued.
• Large doses of gemfibrozil administered to animals for prolonged periods of time have been associated with benign and malignant cancers. This association has not been observed in humans.
• Be sure to tell your doctor if you are pregnant. Although gemfibrozil appears to be safe during pregnancy, extensive studies in humans have not yet been completed. Also, tell your doctor if you are breast-feeding an infant. It is not known whether or not gemfibrozil passes into breast milk.

---

glipizide

BRAND NAME (Manufacturer)
Glucotrol (Roerig)
TYPE OF DRUG
Oral antidiabetic

INGREDIENT
glipizide
DOSAGE FORM
Tablets (5 mg and 10 mg)
STORAGE
This medication should be stored at room temperature in a tightly closed container.

USES

Glipizide is used for the treatment of diabetes mellitus (sugar diabetes), which appears in adulthood and cannot be managed by control of diet alone. This type of diabetes is known as non-insulin-dependent diabetes (sometimes called maturity-onset or Type II diabetes). Glipizide lowers blood-sugar levels by increasing the release of insulin from the pancreas.

TREATMENT

This medication should be taken on an empty stomach 30 minutes before a meal (unless your doctor directs you to do otherwise).

It is important to try not to miss any doses of this medication. If you do miss a dose, take it as soon as possible, unless it is almost time for the next dose. In that case, do not take the missed dose at all; just return to your regular dosing schedule. Do not double the next dose. Tell your doctor if you feel any side effects from missing a dose of this drug.

Diabetics who are taking oral antidiabetic medication may need to be switched to insulin if they develop diabetic coma, have a severe infection, are scheduled for major surgery, or become pregnant.

SIDE EFFECTS

Minor. Diarrhea, headache, heartburn, loss of appetite, nausea, stomach pain, stomach discomfort, or vomiting. These side effects usually go away during treatment, as your body adjusts to the medicine.

Glipizide may increase your sensitivity to sunlight. It is therefore important to use caution during exposure to the sun. Use an effective sunscreen and avoid exposure to sunlamps.

Major. If any side effects are persistent or particularly bothersome, it is important to notify your doctor. IT IS ESPECIALLY IMPORTANT TO TELL YOUR DOCTOR about dark urine, fatigue, itching of the skin, light-colored stools, rash, sore throat and fever, unusual bleeding or bruising, or yellowing of the eyes or skin.

INTERACTIONS

Glipizide interacts with a number of other medications:
1. Chloramphenicol, guanethidine, insulin, monoamine oxidase (MAO) inhibitors, oxyphenbutazone, oxytetracycline, phenylbutazone, probenecid, aspirin or other salicylates, and sulfonamide antibiotics, when combined with glipizide, can lower blood-sugar levels—sometimes to dangerously low levels.
2. Thyroid hormones; dextrothyroxine; epinephrine; phenytoin; thiazide diuretics (water pills); and cortisonelike medications (such as dexamethasone, hydrocortisone, prednisone), combined with glipizide, can actually increase blood-sugar levels—just what you are trying to avoid.
3. Anti-diabetic medications can increase the effects of warfarin, which can lead to bleeding complications.
4. Beta-blocking medications (atenolol, metoprolol, nadolol, pindolol, propranolol, and timolol), combined with glipizide, can result in either high or low blood-sugar levels. Beta blockers can also mask the symptoms of low blood sugar, which can be dangerous.

BE SURE TO TELL YOUR DOCTOR if you are already taking any of the medications listed above.

WARNINGS

• It is important to tell your doctor if you have ever had any unusual or allergic reaction to this medicine or to any sulfa medication, including sulfonamide antibiotics, diuretics (water pills), or other oral antidiabetic medications.
• It is also important to tell your doctor if you now have, or if you have ever had, kidney disease, liver disease, severe infection, or thyroid disease.
• Avoid drinking alcoholic beverages while taking this medication (unless otherwise directed by your doctor). Some patients who take this medicine suffer nausea, vomiting, dizziness, stomach pain, pounding headache, sweating, and redness of the face and skin when they drink alcohol. Also, large amounts of alcohol can lower blood sugar to dangerously low levels.
• Follow the special diet that your doctor gave you. This is an important part of controlling your blood sugar and is necessary in order for this medicine to work properly.
• Be sure to tell your doctor or dentist that you are taking this medicine before having any kind of surgery or other medical or dental treatment.
• Test for sugar in your urine as directed by your doctor. It is a convenient way to determine whether or not your diabetes is being controlled by this medicine.
• Eat or drink something containing sugar right away if you experience any symptoms of low blood sugar (such as anxiety, chills, cold sweats, cool or pale skin, drowsiness, excessive hunger, headache, nausea, nervousness, rapid heartbeat, shakiness, or unusual tiredness or weakness). It is also important that your family and friends know the symptoms of low blood sugar and what to do if they observe any of these symptoms in you.
• Check with your doctor as soon as possible—even if these symptoms are corrected by the sugar. The blood-sugar-lowering effects of this medicine can last for hours, and the symptoms may return during this period. Good sources of sugar are orange juice, corn syrup, honey, sugar cubes, and table sugar. You are at greatest risk of developing low blood sugar if you skip or delay meals, exercise more than usual, cannot eat because of nausea or vomiting, or drink large amounts of alcohol.
• Be sure to tell your doctor if you are pregnant. Studies have not yet been completed in humans, but studies in animals have shown that this medicine can cause birth defects. Also, tell your doctor if you are breast-feeding an infant. Small amounts of glipizide pass into breast milk.

haloperidol

BRAND NAMES (Manufacturers)
Haldol (McNeil CPC)
haloperidol (various manufacturers)
TYPE OF DRUG
Antipsychotic
INGREDIENT
haloperidol
DOSAGE FORMS
Tablets (0.5 mg, 1 mg, 2 mg, 5 mg, 10 mg, and 20 mg)
Oral concentrate (2 mg per ml)
STORAGE
Haloperidol tablets and oral concentrate should be stored at room temperature in a tightly closed, light-resistant container. This medication should not be refrigerated and should never be frozen.

USES

Haloperidol is prescribed to treat the symptoms of certain types of mental illness, such as the emotional symptoms of psychosis, the manic phase of manic-depressive illness, Tourette's syndrome, and severe behavioral problems in children. This drug is thought to relieve symptoms of mental illness by blocking certain chemicals involved with nerve transmission in the brain.

TREATMENT

To avoid stomach irritation, you can take haloperidol tablets with a meal or with a glass of water or milk (unless your doctor directs you to do otherwise).

The oral-concentrate form of this drug should be measured carefully with the dropper provided, then added to four ounces (1/2 cup) or more of water, milk, or a cola-free, caffeine-free carbonated beverage or to applesauce or pudding immediately prior to administration. To prevent possible loss of effectiveness, haloperidol should not be diluted with tea, coffee, caffeine-containing beverages, or apple juice.

If you miss a dose of this medication and remember within six hours, take the missed dose as soon as possible, then return to your regular schedule. If more than six hours have passed, however, skip the missed dose and return to your regular dosing schedule. Do not double the next dose unless your doctor directs you to do so.

The full effects of haloperidol may not become apparent for two weeks after you start to take it.

SIDE EFFECTS

Minor. Blurred vision, constipation, decreased or increased sweating, diarrhea, dizziness, drooling, drowsiness, dry mouth, fatigue, headache, heartburn, jitteriness, loss of appetite, menstrual irregularities, nausea, restlessness, sleep disorders, vomiting, or weakness. As your body adjusts to the medication, these side effects should disappear.

This medication can cause increased sensitivity to sunlight. It is, therefore, important to avoid prolonged exposure to sunlight and sunlamps. Wear protective clothing and use an effective sunscreen.

If you are constipated, increase the amount of fiber in your diet (fresh fruits and vegetables, salads, bran, and whole-grain breads), exercise, and drink more water (unless your doctor directs you to do otherwise).

To reduce mouth dryness, chew sugarless gum or suck on ice chips or a piece of hard candy.

To avoid dizziness or light-headedness when you stand, contract and relax the muscles of your legs for a few moments before rising. Do this by pushing one foot against the floor while raising the other foot slightly, alternating feet so that you are "pumping" your legs in a pedaling motion.

Major. Tell your doctor about any side effects that are persistent or particularly bothersome. IT IS ESPECIALLY IMPORTANT TO TELL YOUR DOCTOR about aching joints and muscles; breast enlargement (in both sexes); chest pain; confusion; convulsions; difficulty in breathing or swallowing; difficulty in urinating; fainting; fever; fluid retention; hair loss; hallucinations; impotence; involuntary movements of the mouth, face, neck, tongue, or limbs; mouth sores; palpitations; skin darkening; skin rash; sore throat; tremors; unusual bleeding or bruising; visual disturbances; or yellowing of the eyes or skin (called jaundice).

INTERACTIONS

Haloperidol interacts with several other drugs:
1. It can cause extreme drowsiness when combined with alcohol or other central nervous system depressants (such as antihistamines, barbiturates, benzodiazepine tranquilizers, muscle relaxants, narcotics, and pain medications) or with tricyclic antidepressants.
2. This drug can lessen the effectiveness of guanethidine and anticonvulsants (antiseizure medications).
3. Haloperidol may increase the side effects of epinephrine, lithium, and methyldopa.

Before starting to take haloperidol, BE SURE TO TELL YOUR DOCTOR about any medications you are currently taking, especially any of those listed above.

WARNINGS

• Tell your doctor about unusual or allergic reactions you have had to any medications, especially to haloperidol or to any other drugs that are used to treat mental illness.
• Tell your doctor if you now have or if you have ever had any blood disorders, blockage of the urinary tract, drug-induced depression, enlarged prostate gland, epilepsy, glaucoma, heart or circulatory disease, kidney disease, liver disease, lung disease, mental depression, Parkinson's disease, peptic ulcers, or thyroid disease.
• Avoid drinking alcoholic beverages while taking this medication in order to prevent oversedation.
• If this medication makes you dizzy or drowsy, do not take part in any activity that requires alertness, such as driving a car or operating potentially dangerous machinery. Be careful on stairs, and avoid getting up suddenly from a lying or sitting position.

• Prior to having surgery or any other medical or dental treatment, be sure to tell your doctor or dentist that you are taking this medication.
• Some of the side effects caused by this drug can be prevented by taking an antiparkinsonism drug. Discuss this with your doctor.
• This medication can decrease sweating and heat release from the body. You should, therefore, avoid getting overheated by strenuous exercise in hot weather and should avoid taking hot baths, showers, and saunas.
• Do not stop taking this medication suddenly. If the drug is stopped abruptly, you may experience nausea, vomiting, stomach upset, headache, increased heart rate, insomnia, tremors, or a worsening of your condition. Your doctor may want to reduce the dosage gradually.
• The elderly may be at increased risk for side effects. Watch closely for side effects or other changes, especially in mental status after taking haloperidol and report them to your doctor.
• If you are planning to have a myelogram or any other procedure in which dye is injected into the spinal cord, tell your doctor that you are taking this medication.
• Avoid spilling the oral-concentrate form of this medication on your skin or clothing; it can cause redness and irritation of the skin.
• While taking haloperidol, do not take any over-the-counter (nonprescription) medications for weight control or for cough, cold, allergy, asthma, or sinus problems unless you first check with your doctor. The combination of these medications may cause high blood pressure.
• Haloperidol has the potential to cause a permanent movement disorder called tardive dyskinesia. It is important to discuss this with your doctor and to report any unusual or uncontrolled body movements.
• Some haloperidol formulations contain the color additive FD&C Yellow No. 5 (tartrazine), which can cause allergic-type reactions (rash, shortness of breath, fainting) in certain susceptible individuals.
• Be sure to tell your doctor if you are pregnant. A few cases of limb malformations have occurred in infants whose mothers had received haloperidol in combination with several other drugs during the first three months of pregnancy. Whether haloperidol was the cause is still not known. Also, tell your doctor if you are breast-feeding an infant. Small amounts of haloperidol pass into breast milk.

---

heparin

BRAND NAMES (MANUFACTURERS)
Calciparine (American Critical Care)
heparin sodium (various manufacturers)
Liquaemin (Organon)
TYPE OF DRUG
Anticoagulant
INGREDIENT
heparin
DOSAGE FORM
Injection solution obtained from beef lung or pig intestine (various concentrations)
STORAGE
Heparin should be stored at room temperature. DO NOT FREEZE. The solution should not be used if it is discolored or if it has particles floating in it.

USES

Heparin decreases the clotting ability of the blood. It doses not dissolve blood clots, but it does prevent clots that are already formed from becoming larger and causing more serious problems. It also prevents the formation of new clots.

This medication is used for the treatment of clotting disorders in the legs, lungs, or brain. It is also used to prevent clotting during surgery of dialysis. In low doses, heparin has also been used to prevent clots from forming in patients who must remain in bed for prolonged periods of time.

TREATMENT

Heparin is given by injection either directly into a vein or under the layers of the skin. If you are using these injections at home, it is important that you use the correct amount of heparin on a regular schedule to obtain the best results without causing serious bleeding.

If you miss a dose of this medication, inject as soon as possible, unless it is almost time for your next dose. In that case, do not inject the missed dose at all; just return to your regular dosing schedule. Do not double the next dose. Doubling the dose may cause bleeding.

SIDE EFFECTS

Minor. None
Major. Back or rib pain or unusual hair loss (can occur after six months of therapy); abdominal pain; backaches; black, tarry stools, bleeding from the gums; blood in the urine or stools; bruising; chest pains; chills; collection of blood under the skin; coughing up blood or coffee–ground–like material; difficulty in breathing; dizziness; fever; frequent or persistent erection; heavy bleeding or oozing from cuts or wounds; heavy or unexpected menstrual bleeding; joint pains; pain at the injection site; pain or blue discoloration of the skin of the hands or feet; rash; severe headache; sloughing of the skin; or tingling in the hands or feet. If you notice any of these effects, CONTACT YOUR DOCTOR IMMEDIATELY.

INTERACTIONS

Heparin interacts with several types of drugs, including warfarin, aspirin, anti–inflammatory medications (such as diflunisal, fenoprofen, ibuprofen, indomethacin, ketoprofen, naproxen, piroxicam, sulindac, suprofen, and tolmetin), sulfinpyrazone, adrenocorticosteroids (such as cortisone), ethacrynic acid, dipyridamole, hydroxychloroquine, methimazole, and propylthiouracil. These medications may cause bleeding problems when taken with heparin. SO BE SURE TO TELL YOUR DOCTOR if you are already taking any of them. Also, TELL YOUR DOCTOR about any other medications you are currently taking.

WARNINGS

- Tell your doctor about unusual or allergic reactions you have had to any medications or foods, especially to heparin or to beef or pork products.
- Tell your doctor if you now have or if you have ever had bleeding problems, colitis, diabetes, high blood pressure, kidney disease, liver disease, or stomach ulcers, or if you have had an intrauterine device (IUD) inserted. Also, TELL YOUR DOCTOR if you have had any recent falls, or blows to the body, medical or dental surgery, or spinal anesthesia.
- Before having surgery or any other medical or dental treatment, BE SURE TO TELL YOUR DOCTOR OR DENTIST that you are taking this medication.
- In order to prevent bleeding problems while taking this medication, it is important that you avoid sports and other activities that may cause you to become injured.
- To avoid gum bleeding, use a soft toothbrush. Take special care while shaving. An electric shaver may be safer than a razor blade.
- Avoid taking any product that contains aspirin while using this medication, because aspirin also decreases your clotting ability. Taking the two drugs together can lead to bleeding problems. Check the labels of all the medications you take to see if they contain aspirin.
- Be sure to tell your doctor if you are pregnant. Heparin does not cross the placenta, but it may cause bleeding problems in the mother, especially in the later months of pregnancy. Heparin does not pass into breast milk, but it can cause severe bone problems in a nursing mother.

---

hydralazine

BRAND NAMES (Manufacturers)
Apresoline (Ciba)
hydralazine hydrochloride (various manufacturers)
TYPE OF DRUG
Antihypertensive
INGREDIENT
hydralazine
DOSAGE FORM
Tablets (10 mg, 25 mg, 50 mg, and 100 mg)
STORAGE
Hydralazine tablets should be stored at room temperature in a tightly closed, light-resistant container.

USES

This medication is used to treat high blood pressure or heart failure. Hydralazine is a vasodilator that directly relaxes the muscle of the blood vessels and allows the blood to flow at a lower force, which causes a lowering of blood pressure.

TREATMENT

In order to avoid stomach irritation while you are taking this medication, you can take your dose of hydralazine with food or with a glass of water or milk. To become accustomed to taking this medication, try to take it at the same time(s) each day. It may take up to two weeks before the full effects of this medication are observed.

Try not to miss any doses of this medication. If you do miss a dose, take the missed dose as soon as possible, unless it is almost time for the next dose. In that case, do not take the missed dose at all; just return to your regular dosing schedule. Do not double the next dose.

Hydralazine does not cure high blood pressure, but it will help to control the condition as long as you continue to take the medication.

SIDE EFFECTS

Minor. Constipation, diarrhea, dizziness, drowsiness, flushing, headache, light-headedness, loss of appetite, muscle cramps, nasal congestion, nausea, or vomiting. These minor side effects should disappear as your body adjusts to therapy with this medication.

To relieve constipation, increase the amount of fiber in your diet (fresh fruits and vegetables, salads, bran, and whole-grain breads), exercise, and drink more water or other fluids (unless your doctor directs you to do otherwise).

If you feel dizzy or light-headed, sit or lie down for a while; get up slowly from a sitting or reclining position; and be careful on stairs. To avoid dizziness or light-headedness when you stand, contract and relax the muscles of your legs for a few moments before rising. Do this by pushing one foot against the floor while raising the other foot slightly, alternating feet so that you are "pumping" your legs in a pedaling motion.

Major. Tell your doctor about any side effects that are persistent or particularly bothersome. IT IS ESPECIALLY IMPORTANT TO TELL YOUR DOCTOR about anxiety, chest pain, confusion, cramping, depression, difficulty in urinating, fever, itching, numbness or tingling in the fingers or toes, palpitations, rapid weight gain (three to five pounds within a week), rash, shortness of breath, sore throat, tenderness in the joints and muscles, tiredness, unusual bleeding or bruising, or yellowing of the eyes or skin.

INTERACTIONS

Hydralazine interacts with several other types of drugs:

1. The combination of alcohol and hydralazine can lead to dizziness and fainting. You should, therefore, avoid drinking alcoholic beverages while on this drug.

2. Used within 14 days of a monoamine oxidase (MAO) inhibitor, hydralazine can cause severe reactions.

Before you start to take hydralazine, BE SURE TO TELL YOUR DOCTOR about any medications you are currently taking, especially an MAO inhibitor.

WARNINGS

- Tell your doctor about any unusual or allergic reactions you have had to any medications, especially to hydralazine.
- Tell your doctor if you have ever had angina, heart disease, stroke, a heart attack, or kidney disease.
- To avoid dizziness or fainting, try not to stand for long periods of time, and avoid drinking alcohol. You should also try not to get overheated (avoid hot baths, showers, saunas, and strenuous exercise in hot weather).

• If this drug makes you dizzy or drowsy, avoid taking part in any activities that require alertness, such as driving a car or operating potentially dangerous machinery.
• Before having surgery or any other medical or dental treatment, be sure to tell your doctor or dentist that you are taking this medication.
• Do not take any over-the-counter (nonprescription) allergy, asthma, sinus, cough, cold, or diet products unless you first consult your doctor or pharmacist. The combination of these medications with hydralazine may cause an increase in blood pressure.
• Some hydralazine formulations contain the color additive FD&C Yellow No. 5 (tartrazine), which can cause allergic-type reactions (rash, shortness of breath, fainting) in certain susceptible individuals.
• Do not stop taking this medication until you check with your doctor. If this drug is stopped abruptly, you could experience a sudden rise in blood pressure and other complications. Your doctor may, therefore, want to decrease your dosage gradually.
• Be sure to tell your doctor if you are pregnant. Although studies in humans have not been conducted, hydralazine crosses the placenta, and studies have shown that it causes birth defects in the offspring of animals that received large doses of it during pregnancy. Also, tell your doctor if you are breast-feeding an infant. It is not known whether hydralazine passes into breast milk.

hydrochlorothiazide

BRAND NAMES (Manufacturers)
Aquazide-H (Jones Medical)
Diaqua (Mallard)
Esidrix (Ciba)
hydrochlorothiazide (various manufacturers)
Hydro-Chlor (Vortech)
Hydro-D (Halsey)
HydroDIURIL (Merck Sharp & Dohme)
Hydromal (Hauck)
Hydro-T (Major)
Mictrin (EconoMed)
Oretic (Abbott)
TYPE OF DRUG
Diuretic and antihypertensive
INGREDIENT
hydrochlorothiazide
DOSAGE FORMS
Tablets (25 mg, 50 mg, and 100 mg)
Oral solution (50 mg per 5-ml spoonful)
Intensol oral solution (100 mg per ml)
STORAGE
This medication should be stored at room temperature in a tightly closed container.

USES

Hydrochlorothiazide is prescribed to treat high blood pressure (hypertension). It is also used to reduce fluid accumulation in the body caused by conditions such as heart failure, cirrhosis of the liver, kidney disease, and the long-term use of some medications. This medication reduces body fluid accumulation by increasing the elimination of salt and water through the kidneys.

TREATMENT

To decrease stomach irritation, you can take this medication with a glass of milk or with a meal (unless your doctor directs you to do otherwise). Each dose of the oral solution should be measured carefully with the dropper provided (Intensol solution) or a specially designed 5-ml measuring spoon. An ordinary kitchen teaspoon is not accurate enough. Try to take it at the same time every day. Avoid taking a dose after 6:00 P.M.; otherwise, you may have to get up during the night to urinate.

If you miss a dose of this medication, take the missed dose as soon as possible, unless it is almost time for the next dose. In that case, do not take the missed dose at all; just wait until the next scheduled dose. Do not double the dose.

This drug does not cure high blood pressure.

SIDE EFFECTS

Minor. Constipation, cramps, diarrhea, dizziness, drowsiness, headache, heartburn, loss of appetite, restlessness, or upset stomach. As your body adjusts to the medication, these side effects should disappear.

This drug can cause increased sensitivity to sunlight. Therefore, avoid prolonged exposure to sunlight and sunlamps. Wear protective clothing and use an effective sunscreen.

To relieve constipation, increase the amount of fiber in your diet (fresh fruits and vegetables, salads, bran, and whole-grain breads) and exercise more (unless your doctor directs you to do otherwise).

To avoid dizziness or light-headedness when you stand, contract and relax the muscles of your legs for a few moments before rising. Do this by pushing one foot against the floor while raising the other foot slightly, alternating feet so that you are "pumping" your legs in a pedaling motion.

Major. Tell your doctor about any side effects you experience that are persistent or particularly bothersome. IT IS ESPECIALLY IMPORTANT TO TELL YOUR DOCTOR about blurred vision, confusion, difficulty in breathing, dry mouth, excessive thirst, excessive weakness, fever, itching, joint pain, mood changes, muscle pain or spasms, nausea, palpitations, skin rash, sore throat, tingling in the fingers or toes, vomiting, or yellowing of the eyes or skin.

INTERACTIONS

Hydrochlorothiazide interacts with certain other drugs:
1. It can decrease the effectiveness of oral anticoagulants, antigout medications, insulin, oral antidiabetic medicines, and methenamine.
2. Fenfluramine can increase the blood-pressure-lowering effects of hydrochlorothiazide (which can be dangerous).
3. Indomethacin can decrease the blood-pressure-lowering effects of hydrochlorothiazide, thereby counteracting the desired effects.

4. Cholestyramine and colestipol decrease the absorption of this medication from the gastrointestinal tract. Hydrochlorothiazide should, therefore, be taken one hour before or four hours after a dose of cholestyramine or colestipol (if you have also been prescribed one of these medications).
5. Hydrochlorothiazide may increase the side effects of amphotericin B, calcium, cortisone and cortisonelike steroids (such as dexamethasone, hydrocortisone, prednisone, or prednisolone), digoxin, digitalis, lithium, and vitamin D.

BE SURE TO TELL YOUR DOCTOR about any medications you are currently taking, especially any of those listed above.

WARNINGS

- Be sure to tell your doctor about unusual or allergic reactions you have had to any medications, especially to hydrochlorothiazide or other sulfa medications, including other diuretics, oral antidiabetic medications, and sulfonamide antibiotics.
- Be sure to tell your doctor if you now have or if you have ever had kidney disease or problems with urination, diabetes mellitus, gout, liver disease, asthma, pancreatic disease, or systemic lupus erythematosus.
- Hydrochlorothiazide can cause potassium loss. Signs of potassium loss include dry mouth, thirst, weakness, muscle pain or cramps, nausea, and vomiting. If you experience any of these symptoms, it is important that you call your doctor. To help avoid potassium loss, take this medication with a glass of fresh or frozen orange or cranberry juice, or eat a banana every day. The use of a salt substitute also helps to prevent potassium loss. Do not change your diet or use a salt substitute, however, before discussing it with your doctor. Too much potassium can also be dangerous. Your doctor may want you to have blood tests performed periodically in order to monitor your potassium levels while you are taking this drug.
- Limit your intake of alcoholic beverages while taking this medication to prevent dizziness and light-headedness.
- Becoming overheated can be hazardous while you are taking this medication. Avoid strenuous exercise in hot weather and do not take hot baths, showers, or saunas.
- If you have high blood pressure, do not take any over-the-counter (nonprescription) medications for weight control or for allergy, asthma, cough, cold, or sinus problems unless your doctor directs you to do so.
- To prevent dehydration (severe water loss) while taking this medication, check with your doctor if you have any illness that causes severe or continuous nausea, vomiting, or diarrhea.
- This medication can raise blood-sugar levels in diabetic patients. Therefore, blood sugar should be carefully monitored by blood or urine tests when this medication is being taken.
- Before having surgery or any other medical or dental treatment, be sure to tell your doctor or dentist that you are taking this medication.
- Be certain to inform your doctor if you are pregnant. Hydrochlorothiazide can cross the placenta and may cause adverse effects on the developing fetus. Also, tell your doctor if you are breast-feeding an infant. Although problems in humans have not been reported, small amounts of this medication can pass into breast milk, so caution is warranted.

---

hydrocortisone

BRAND NAMES (Manufacturers)
Cortef (Upjohn)
hydrocortisone (various manufacturers)
Hydrocortone (Merck Sharp & Dohme)
TYPE OF DRUG
Adrenocorticosteroid hormone
INGREDIENT
hydrocortisone (cortisol)
DOSAGE FORMS
Tablets (5 mg, 10 mg, and 20 mg)
Oral suspension (10 mg per 5-ml spoonful)
STORAGE
Store at room temperature in a tightly closed container. Systemic hydrocortisone should not be refrigerated, and it should never be frozen.

USES

Your adrenal glands naturally produce certain cortisonelike chemicals. These chemicals are involved in various regulatory processes in the body (such as those involving fluid balance, temperature, and reaction to inflammation). Hydrocortisone belongs to a group of drugs known as adrenocorticosteroids (or cortisonelike medications). It is used to treat a variety of disorders, including endocrine (hormonal) and rheumatic disorders; asthma; blood diseases; certain cancers; eye disorders; gastrointestinal disturbances, such as ulcerative colitis; respiratory diseases; and inflammations such as arthritis, dermatitis, poison ivy, and other allergic conditions. How this medication acts to relieve these disorders is not completely understood.

TREATMENT

In order to prevent stomach irritation, you can take hydrocortisone with food or milk.

If you are taking only one dose of this medication each day, try to take it before 9:00 A.M. This mimics the normal hormonal production in your body.

The oral suspension form of this medication should be shaken well just before measuring each dose. The contents tend to settle on the bottom of the bottle, so it is necessary to shake the container to distribute the ingredients evenly and equalize the doses. Each dose should then be measured carefully with a specially designed 5-ml measuring spoon. An ordinary kitchen teaspoon is not accurate enough.

It is important to try not to miss any doses of hydrocortisone. However, if you do miss a dose of this medication, follow these guidelines:
1. If you are taking hydrocortisone more than once a day, take the missed dose as soon as possible, then return to

your regular schedule. If it is already time for the next dose, double the dose.
2. If you are taking this medication once a day, take the dose you missed as soon as possible, unless you don't remember until the next day. In that case, do not take the missed dose at all; just follow your regular schedule. Do not double the next dose.
3. If you are taking this drug every other day, take the missed dose as soon as you remember. If you missed the scheduled dose by a whole day, take it when you remember and then skip a day before you take the next dose. Do not double the dose.

If you miss more than one dose of hydrocortisone, CONTACT YOUR DOCTOR.

SIDE EFFECTS

Minor. Dizziness, false sense of well-being, increased appetite, increased sweating, indigestion, menstrual irregularities, nausea, reddening and swelling of the skin on the face, restlessness, sleep disorders, or weight gain. These side effects should disappear as your body adjusts to the medication.

To help avoid potassium loss while using systemic hydrocortisone, take your dose of medication with a glass of fresh or frozen orange juice, or eat a banana each day. The use of a salt substitute also helps to prevent potassium loss. Check with your doctor before changing your diet or using a salt substitute.

Major. Tell your doctor about any side effects that are persistent or particularly bothersome. IT IS ESPECIALLY IMPORTANT TO TELL YOUR DOCTOR about abdominal (area around and above the waist) enlargement; acne or other skin problems; back or rib pain; bloody or black, tarry stools; blurred vision; convulsions; eye pain; fever and sore throat; growth impairment (in children); headaches; slow healing of wounds; increased thirst and urination; mental depression; mood changes; muscle wasting; muscle weakness; nightmares; rapid weight gain (three to five pounds within a week); rash; red lines across the abdomen; severe abdominal pain; shortness of breath; thinning of the skin; unusual bleeding or bruising; or unusual weakness.

INTERACTIONS

The systemic form of hydrocortisone interacts with several other types of medications:
1. Alcohol, aspirin, and anti-inflammatory medications (such as diclofenac, diflunisal, flurbiprofen, ibuprofen, indomethacin, ketoprofen, mefenamic acid, meclofenamate, naproxen, piroxicam, sulindac, and tolmetin) aggravate the stomach problems that are common with use of this medication.
2. The dosage of oral anticoagulants (blood thinners, such as warfarin), oral antidiabetic drugs, or insulin may need to be adjusted when this medication is started or stopped.
3. The loss of potassium caused by hydrocortisone can lead to serious side effects in individuals taking digoxin. Also, thiazide diuretics (water pills) can increase the potassium loss caused by hydrocortisone.
4. Phenobarbital, phenytoin, rifampin, and ephedrine can increase the elimination of hydrocortisone from the body, thereby decreasing its effectiveness.
5. Oral contraceptives (birth control pills) and estrogen-containing drugs may decrease the elimination of this drug from the body, which can lead to an increase in side effects.
6. Hydrocortisone can increase the elimination of aspirin and isoniazid from the body, thereby decreasing the effectiveness of these two medications.
7. Cholestyramine and colestipol can chemically bind with this medication in the stomach and gastrointestinal tract, preventing its absorption and decreasing its effectiveness.

BE SURE TO TELL YOUR DOCTOR about any medications you are currently taking, especially any of those listed above.

WARNINGS

- Tell your doctor about unusual or allergic reactions you have had to any medications, especially to hydrocortisone or other adrenocorticosteroids (such as betamethasone, cortisone, dexamethasone, fluocinolone, methylprednisolone, prednisolone, prednisone, and triamcinolone).
- Tell your doctor if you now have or if you have ever had bone disease, diabetes mellitus, emotional instability, glaucoma, fungal infections, heart disease, high blood pressure, high cholesterol levels, myasthenia gravis, peptic ulcers, osteoporosis, thyroid disease, tuberculosis, ulcerative colitis, kidney disease, or liver disease.
- If you are using this medication for longer than a week, you may need to receive higher dosages if you are subjected to stress, such as serious infections, injury, or surgery. Discuss this with your doctor.
- If you have been taking this drug for more than a week, do not stop taking it suddenly. If it is stopped suddenly, you may experience abdominal or back pain, dizziness, fainting, fever, muscle or joint pain, nausea, vomiting, shortness of breath, or extreme weakness. Your doctor may, therefore, want to reduce the dosage gradually. Never increase the dosage or take the drug for longer than the prescribed time, unless you first consult your doctor.
- While you are taking this drug, you should not be vaccinated or immunized. This medication decreases the effectiveness of vaccines and can lead to overwhelming infection if a live-virus vaccine is administered.
- Before having surgery or any other medical or dental treatment, be sure to tell your doctor or dentist that you are taking this medication.
- Because this drug can cause glaucoma and cataracts with long-term use, your doctor may want you to have your eyes examined by an ophthalmologist periodically during treatment.
- If you are taking this medication for prolonged periods, you should wear or carry an identification card or notice that clearly states that you are taking an adrenocorticosteroid medication.
- This medication can raise blood-sugar levels in diabetic patients. Blood-sugar levels should, therefore, be monitored carefully with blood or urine tests.
- Be sure to tell your doctor if you are pregnant. This drug crosses the placenta. Although studies in humans have not been conducted, birth defects have been ob-

served in the offspring of animals that were given large doses of this drug during pregnancy. Also, tell your doctor if you are breast-feeding an infant. Small amounts of this drug pass into breast milk and may cause growth suppression or a decrease in natural adrenocorticosteroid hormone production in the nursing infant.

---

hydroxyzine

BRAND NAMES (Manufacturers)
Anxanil (EconoMed)
Atarax (Roerig)
hydroxyzine hydrochloride (various manufacturers)
hydroxyzine pamoate (various manufacturers)
Vistaril (Pfizer)
TYPE OF DRUG
Antihistamine and sedative/hypnotic
INGREDIENT
hydroxyzine
DOSAGE FORMS
Tablets (10 mg, 25 mg, 50 mg, and 100 mg)
Capsules (25 mg, 50 mg, and 100 mg)
Oral solution (10 mg per 5-ml spoonful, with 0.5% alcohol)
Oral suspension (25 mg per 5-ml spoonful)
STORAGE
Hydroxyzine tablets, capsules, oral solution, and oral suspension should be stored at room temperature in tightly closed, light-resistant containers. This medication should never be frozen.

USES

Hydroxyzine belongs to a group of drugs known as antihistamines (antihistamines block the action of histamine, which is a chemical that is released by the body during an allergic reaction). This medication is used to treat or prevent symptoms associated with allergies. It is also used as a sleeping aid and to relieve the symptoms of anxiety and tension.

TREATMENT

To avoid stomach upset, you can take hydroxyzine with food or with a full glass of milk or water (unless your doctor directs you to do otherwise).

The oral suspension form of this medication should be shaken well just before measuring each dose. The contents tend to settle on the bottom of the bottle, so it is necessary to shake the container to distribute the ingredients evenly and equalize the doses. Each dose of the oral solution or oral suspension should be measured carefully with a specially designed 5-ml measuring spoon. An ordinary kitchen teaspoon is not accurate enough for medical purposes.

If you miss a dose of this medication, take the missed dose as soon as possible, unless it is almost time for your next dose. In that case, don't take the missed dose at all; just return to your regular dosing schedule. Do not double the next dose.

SIDE EFFECTS

Minor. Drowsiness or dry mouth. These side effects should disappear as your body gets accustomed to the medication.

Dry mouth can be relieved by chewing sugarless gum or by sucking on ice chips or a piece of hard candy.

Major. Tell your doctor about any side effects that are persistent or particularly bothersome. IT IS ESPECIALLY IMPORTANT TO TELL YOUR DOCTOR about convulsions, feeling faint, irritability, mental confusion, rash, or trembling or shakiness.

INTERACTIONS

Hydroxyzine can interact with other types of drugs: Concurrent use of it with other central nervous system depressants (such as alcohol, barbiturates, benzodiazepine tranquilizers, muscle relaxants, narcotics, pain medications, and phenothiazine tranquilizers) or with tricyclic antidepressants can cause extreme drowsiness.

BE SURE TO TELL YOUR DOCTOR about any medications you are currently taking, especially any listed above.

WARNINGS

- Tell your doctor about allergic or unusual reactions you have had to medications, especially to hydroxyzine or to any other antihistamines (such as azatadine, brompheniramine, carbinoxamine, chlorpheniramine, clemastine, cyproheptadine, dexchlorpheniramine, dimenhydrinate, dimethindene, diphenhydramine, diphenylpyraline, doxylamine, promethazine, pyrilamine, trimeprazine, tripelennamine, and triprolidine).
- Hydroxyzine can cause drowsiness or dizziness. Your ability to perform tasks that require alertness, such as driving a car or operating potentially dangerous machinery, may be decreased. Appropriate caution should, therefore, be taken.
- Elderly patients may be more sensitive to side effects, especially drowsiness, confusion, and irritability. Report any such effects to your doctor.
- Be sure to tell your doctor if you are pregnant. The effects of this medication during pregnancy have not been thoroughly studied in humans. Also, tell your doctor if you are breast-feeding an infant. Small amounts of hydroxyzine pass into breast milk.

---

ibuprofen

BRAND NAMES (Manufacturers)
Aches-N-Pain* (Lederle)
Advil* (Whitehall)
Advil Children's (Wyeth-Ayerst)
Genpril* (Goldline)
Haltran* (Roberts)
Ibuprin* (Thompson Medical)
ibuprofen (various manufacturers)
Medipren* (McNeil CPC)
Midol 200* (Glenbrook)

Motrin (Upjohn)
Motrin IB* (Upjohn)
Nuprin* (Bristol-Myers)
Pamprin-IB* (Chattem)
PediaProfen (McNeil CPC)
Rufen (Boots)
Trendar* (Whitehall)
*Available over-the-counter (without a prescription) as 200-mg tablets.

TYPE OF DRUG
Nonsteroidal anti-inflammatory analgesic

INGREDIENT
ibuprofen

DOSAGE FORMS
Tablets (200 mg, 300 mg, 400 mg, 600 mg, and 800 mg)
Oral suspension (100 mg per 5-ml spoonful)

STORAGE
Store in a tightly closed, light-resistent container at room temperature. This medication should never be frozen.

USES
Ibuprofen is used to treat the inflammation (pain, swelling, stiffness) of certain types of arthritis, gout, bursitis, and tendinitis. It is also used to treat painful menstruation. Ibuprofen has been shown to block production of prostaglandins, which may trigger pain.

TREATMENT
You should take this medication on an empty stomach 30 to 60 minutes before meals or two hours after meals, so that it gets into your bloodstream quickly. However, to decrease stomach irritation, your doctor may want you to take the medication with food or antacids.

The oral suspension form of this medication should be shaken well just before measuring each dose. The contents tend to settle on the bottom of the bottle, so it is necessary to shake the container to distribute the ingredients evenly and equalize the doses. Each dose of the oral syrup or oral suspension should be measured carefully with a specially designed 5-ml measuring spoon. An ordinary kitchen teaspoon is not accurate enough.

If you are taking ibuprofen to relieve arthritis, you must take it regularly as directed by your doctor. It may take up to two weeks before you feel the full effects of this medication. Ibuprofen does not cure arthritis, but it will help to control the condition as long as you continue to take it.

It is important to take ibuprofen on schedule and not to miss any doses. If you do miss a dose, take it as soon as possible, unless it is almost time for your next dose. In that case, don't take the missed dose at all; return to your regular dosing schedule. Do not double the next dose.

SIDE EFFECTS
Minor. Bloating, constipation, diarrhea, difficulty in sleeping, dizziness, drowsiness, headache, heartburn, indigestion, light-headedness, loss of appetite, nausea, nervousness, soreness of the mouth, unusual sweating, or vomiting. As your body adjusts to the drug, these side effects should disappear.

To relieve constipation, increase the amount of fiber in your diet (fresh fruits and vegetables, salads, bran, and whole-grain breads), exercise, and drink more water (unless your doctor directs you to do otherwise).

If you become dizzy or light-headed, sit or lie down for a while; get up slowly from a sitting or reclining position; and be careful on stairs.

Major. If you experience any side effects that are persistent or particularly bothersome, you should report them to your doctor. IT IS ESPECIALLY IMPORTANT TO TELL YOUR DOCTOR about bloody or black, tarry stools; blurred vision; confusion; depression; difficult or painful urination; palpitations; a problem with hearing; ringing or buzzing in your ears; skin rash, hives, or itching; stomach pain; swelling of the feet; tightness in the chest; unexplained sore throat and fever; unusual bleeding or bruising; unusual fatigue or weakness; unusual weight gain; wheezing or difficulty in breathing; or yellowing of the eyes or skin.

INTERACTIONS
Ibuprofen interacts with several other types of medications:

1. Anticoagulants (blood thinners, such as warfarin) can lead to an increase in bleeding complications.
2. Aspirin, other salicylates, and other anti-inflammatory medications can increase stomach irritation. Aspirin may also decrease the effectiveness of ibuprofen.
3. Ibuprofen can interact with diuretics (water pills).
4. Probenecid may increase blood levels of ibuprofen, which may increase the risk of side effects.
5. The action of beta blockers may be decreased by this drug.

BE SURE TO TELL YOUR DOCTOR about any medications you are currently taking, especially any listed above.

WARNINGS
• Before you start to take this medication, it is important to tell your doctor if you have ever had unusual or allergic reactions to ibuprofen, or to any of the other chemically related drugs (aspirin, other salicylates, diclofenac, diflunisal, fenoprofen, flurbiprofen, indomethacin, ketoprofen, meclofenamate, mefenamic acid, naproxen, oxyphenbutazone, phenylbutazone, piroxicam, sulindac, or tolmetin).
• Tell your doctor if you now have or if you have ever had bleeding problems, colitis, stomach ulcers or other stomach problems, epilepsy, heart disease, high blood pressure, asthma, kidney disease, liver disease, mental illness, or Parkinson's disease.
• If ibuprofen makes you dizzy or drowsy, do not take part in any activity that requires alertness.
• Because this drug can prolong bleeding time, tell your doctor or dentist you are taking this drug before having surgery or other medical or dental treatment.
• Stomach problems are more likely to occur if you take aspirin regularly or drink alcohol while being treated with this medication. These should, therefore, be avoided (unless your doctor directs you to do otherwise).
• The elderly may be at increased risk for experiencing side effects of this drug.
• Be sure to tell your doctor if you are pregnant. This type of medication can cause unwanted effects to the

heart or blood flow of the fetus. Studies in animals have also shown that this type of medicine, if taken late in pregnancy, may increase the length of pregnancy, prolong labor, or cause other problems during delivery. Also, tell your doctor if you are breast-feeding an infant. Small amounts of ibuprofen can pass into breast milk.

---

imipramine

BRAND NAMES (Manufacturers)
imipramine hydrochloride (various manufacturers)
Janimine (Abbott)
Tipramine (Major)
Tofranil (Geigy)
Tofranil-PM (Geigy)
TYPE OF DRUG
Tricyclic antidepressant
INGREDIENT
imipramine
DOSAGE FORMS
Tablets (10 mg, 25 mg, and 50 mg)
Capsules (75 mg, 100 mg, 125 mg, and 150 mg)
STORAGE
Store at room temperature in a tightly closed container.

USES

Imipramine is used to relieve the symptoms of mental depression. This medication belongs to a group of drugs referred to as tricyclic antidepressants. These medicines are thought to relieve depression by increasing the concentration of certain chemicals necessary for nerve transmission in the brain. This medication is also used to treat enuresis (bed-wetting) in children six to 12 years of age.

TREATMENT

Imipramine should be taken exactly as your doctor prescribes. It can be taken with water or with food to lessen the chance of stomach irritation, unless your doctor tells you to do otherwise.

If you miss a dose of this medication, take the missed dose as soon as possible, then return to your regular dosing schedule. If, however, the dose you missed was a once-a-day bedtime dose, do not take that dose in the morning; check with your doctor instead. If the dose is taken in the morning, it may cause unwanted side effects.

The effects of therapy with this medication may not become apparent for two or three weeks.

SIDE EFFECTS

Minor. Agitation, anxiety, blurred vision, confusion, constipation, cramps, diarrhea, dizziness, drowsiness, dry mouth, fatigue, heartburn, insomnia, loss of appetite, nausea, peculiar tastes in the mouth, restlessness, sweating, vomiting, weakness, or weight gain or loss. As you adjust to the medication, these side effects should disappear.

This drug may cause increased sensitivity to sunlight. Therefore, avoid prolonged exposure to sunlight and sunlamps. Wear protective clothing, and use an effective sunscreen.

Dry mouth caused by therapy with this medication can be relieved by chewing sugarless gum or by sucking on ice chips or a piece of hard candy.

To relieve constipation, increase the amount of fiber in your diet (fresh fruits and vegetables, salads, bran, and whole-grain breads). You can also increase your exercise and drink more water (unless your doctor directs you to do otherwise).

To avoid dizziness or light-headedness when you stand, contract and relax the muscles of your legs for a few moments before rising. Do this by pushing one foot against the floor while raising the other foot slightly, alternating feet so that you are "pumping" your legs in a pedaling motion.

Major. Tell your doctor about any side effects that are persistent or particularly bothersome. IT IS ESPECIALLY IMPORTANT TO TELL YOUR DOCTOR about chest pains, convulsions, difficulty in urinating, enlarged or painful breasts (in both sexes), fainting, fever, fluid retention, hair loss, hallucinations, headaches, impotence, mood changes, mouth sores, nervousness, nightmares, numbness in the fingers or toes, palpitations, ringing in the ears, seizures, skin rash, sleep disorders, sore throat, tremors, uncoordinated movements or balance problems, unusual bleeding or bruising, or yellowing of the eyes or skin.

INTERACTIONS

Imipramine interacts with a number of other types of medications:

1. Extreme drowsiness can occur when this medicine is taken with central nervous system depressants (such as alcohol, antihistamines, barbiturates, benzodiazepine tranquilizers, muscle relaxants, narcotics, pain medications, phenothiazine tranquilizers, and sleeping medications) or with other tricyclic antidepressants.

2. Imipramine may decrease the effectiveness of antiseizure medications. Imipramine may also possibly block the blood-pressure-lowering effects of clonidine and guanethidine.

3. Oral contraceptives (birth control pills) and estrogen-containing drugs can increase the side effects and reduce the effectiveness of the tricyclic antidepressants (including imipramine).

4. Cimetidine can decrease the breakdown of imipramine in the body, thus increasing the possibility of side effects.

5. Tricyclic antidepressants may increase the side effects of thyroid medication and of over-the-counter (nonprescription) cough, cold, allergy, asthma, sinus, and diet medications.

6. The concurrent use of tricyclic antidepressants and monoamine oxidase (MAO) inhibitors should be avoided, because the combination may result in fever, convulsions, or high blood pressure. At least 14 days should separate the use of this drug and the use of an MAO inhibitor.

BE SURE TO TELL YOUR DOCTOR about any medications you are currently taking.

WARNINGS

• Tell your doctor if you have had unusual or allergic reactions to any medications, especially to imipramine or

any of the other tricyclic antidepressants (such as amitriptyline, doxepin, trimipramine, amoxapine, protriptyline, desipramine, maprotiline, and nortriptyline).
• Tell your doctor if you have a history of alcoholism or if you have ever had asthma, high blood pressure, liver or kidney disease, heart disease, a heart attack, circulatory disease, stomach problems, intestinal problems, difficulty in urinating, enlarged prostate gland, epilepsy, glaucoma, thyroid disease, mental illness, or electroshock therapy.
• If the use of imipramine makes you dizzy or drowsy, do not take part in any activity that requires alertness, such as driving a car or operating potentially dangerous machinery.
• Before having surgery or any other medical or dental treatment, tell your doctor or dentist you are taking this drug.
• Do not stop taking this drug suddenly. Stopping it abruptly can cause nausea, headache, stomach upset, fatigue, or a worsening of your condition. Your doctor may want to reduce the dosage gradually.
• The effects of this medication may last as long as seven days after you stop taking it, so continue to observe all precautions during that period.
• Some of these products contain the color additive FD&C Yellow No. 5 (tartrazine), which can cause allergic-type reactions (skin rash, fainting, difficulty in breathing) in certain susceptible individuals.
• The elderly may be at increased risk for experiencing side effects. Report any such effects, especially dizziness, drowsiness, dry mouth, difficulty urinating, or mental confusion to your doctor.
• Be sure to tell your doctor if you are pregnant. Adverse effects have been observed in the fetuses of animals that were given large doses of this drug during pregnancy. Also, tell your doctor if you are breast-feeding an infant. Small amounts of this drug can pass into breast milk and may cause unwanted effects in nursing infants.

indomethacin

BRAND NAMES (Manufacturers)
Indocin (Merck Sharp & Dohme)
Indocin SR (Merck Sharp & Dohme)
indomethacin (various manufacturers)
TYPE OF DRUG
Nonsteroidal anti-inflammatory analgesic
INGREDIENT
indomethacin
DOSAGE FORMS
Capsules (25 mg and 50 mg)
Extended-release capsules (75 mg)
Oral suspension (25 mg per 5-ml spoonful, with 1% alcohol)
Rectal suppositories (50 mg)
STORAGE
Indomethacin capsules, oral suspension, and rectal suppositories should be stored in closed containers at room temperature away from heat and direct sunlight. The rectal suppositories can also be stored safely in the refrigerator.

USES

Indomethacin is used to treat the inflammation (pain, swelling, and stiffness) of certain types of arthritis, gout, bursitis, and tendinitis. Indomethacin has been shown to block the production of certain body chemicals, called prostaglandins, that may trigger pain. However, it is not yet fully understood how indomethacin works.

TREATMENT

You should take this drug immediately after meals or with food, in order to reduce stomach irritation. Ask your doctor if you can take indomethacin with an antacid.

Do not chew or crush the extended-release capsules; they should be swallowed whole. Breaking the capsule would release the medication all at once—defeating the purpose of the extended-release dosage form.

The suspension form of this medication should be shaken well just before measuring each dose. The contents tend to settle on the bottom of the bottle, so it is necessary to shake the container to distribute the ingredients evenly and equalize the doses. Each dose should be measured carefully with a specially designed 5-ml measuring spoon. An ordinary kitchen teaspoon is not accurate enough.

To use the rectal suppository form of this medication, remove the foil wrapper, and moisten the suppository with water. If the suppository is too soft to insert, refrigerate it for 30 minutes or run cold water over it before removing the foil wrapper. Lie on your left side with your right knee bent. Push the suppository into the rectum, pointed end first. Lie still for a few minutes. Try to avoid having a bowel movement for at least one hour after medicating.

It is important to take indomethacin on schedule and not to miss any doses. If you do miss a dose, take the missed dose as soon as possible, unless more than an hour has passed. In that case, do not take the missed dose at all; just return to your regular dosing schedule. Do not double the next dose.

This drug does not cure arthritis, but will help to control the condition as long as you continue to take it. It may take up to four weeks before you feel the full benefits of this medication.

SIDE EFFECTS

Minor. Bloating, constipation, diarrhea, difficulty in sleeping, dizziness, drowsiness, headache, heartburn, indigestion, light-headedness, loss of appetite, nausea, nervousness, soreness of the mouth, unusual sweating, or vomiting. As you adjust to the drug, the side effects should disappear.

To relieve constipation, increase the amount of fiber in your diet (fresh fruits and vegetables, salads, bran, and whole-grain breads), exercise, and drink more water (unless your doctor directs you to do otherwise).

If you become dizzy, sit or lie down for a while; get up slowly from a sitting or reclining position; and be careful on stairs.

Major. Tell your doctor about any side effects that are persistent or particularly bothersome. IT IS ESPECIALLY IMPORTANT TO TELL YOUR DOCTOR about bloody or black, tarry stools; blurred vision; confusion; depression; difficult or painful urination; palpitations; a problem with hearing; ringing or buzzing in the ears; skin rash, hives, or itching; stomach pain; swelling of the feet; rectal irritation; tightness in the chest; unexplained sore throat and fever; unusual bleeding or bruising; unusual fatigue or weakness; unusual weight gain; wheezing or difficulty in breathing; or yellowing of the eyes or skin.

INTERACTIONS

Indomethacin interacts with several other types of drugs:

1. Use of anticoagulants (blood thinners, such as warfarin) can lead to an increase in bleeding complications.

2. Anti-inflammatory medications such as aspirin, salicylates, and diflunisal can cause increased stomach irritation when used while taking this drug.

3. Indomethacin can decrease the elimination of lithium from the body, possibly resulting in lithium toxicity.

4. Indomethacin may interfere with the blood-pressure-lowering effects of captopril, enalapril, or beta-blocking medications (acebutolol, atenolol, betaxolol, carteolol, esmolol, labetalol, metoprolol, nadolol, penbutolol, pindolol, propranolol, timolol).

5. Indomethacin can interfere with the diuretic effects of furosemide and thiazide-type diuretics (water pills).

6. Indomethacin can alter the effects of the potassium-sparing diuretics (such as amiloride, spironolactone, or triamterene).

7. The concurrent use of triamterene and indomethacin can result in kidney problems.

8. Probenecid can increase the amount of indomethacin in the bloodstream when both drugs are being taken.

BE SURE TO TELL YOUR DOCTOR about any medications you are currently taking, especially those listed above.

WARNINGS

- Tell your doctor if you have ever had unusual or allergic reactions to any medications, especially to indomethacin or any chemically related drugs.
- Before taking indomethacin, tell your doctor if you now have or if you have ever had bleeding problems, colitis, stomach ulcers or other stomach problems, epilepsy, heart disease, high blood pressure, asthma, kidney disease, liver disease, mental illness, or Parkinson's disease.
- If indomethacin makes you dizzy or drowsy, do not take part in any activity that requires alertness, such as driving a car or operating potentially dangerous machinery.
- If you will be taking this medication for a long period of time, your doctor may want to have your eyes examined periodically by an ophthalmologist. Some visual problems have been known to occur with long-term indomethacin use. Your doctor might want to keep a careful watch for these.
- Stomach problems are more likely to occur if you take aspirin regularly or drink alcohol while being treated with this medication. These should therefore be avoided (unless your doctor directs you to do otherwise).
- The elderly may be at increased risk for experiencing side effects of this drug.
- Be sure to tell your doctor if you are pregnant. Studies in animals have shown that indomethacin can cause unwanted effects in offspring, including lower birth weights, slower development of bones, nerve damage, and heart damage. If taken late in pregnancy, the drug can also prolong labor. Studies in humans have not been conducted. Also, tell your doctor if you are breast-feeding. Small amounts of indomethacin can pass into breast milk, so caution is warranted.

---

insulin

BRAND NAMES (Manufacturers)

Humulin L (Lilly)
Humulin N (Lilly)
Humulin R (Lilly)
Iletin I (Lilly)
Iletin II (Lilly)
Insulatard NPH (Novo Nordisk)
Mixtard (Novo Nordisk)
Novolin (Novo Nordisk)
Velosulin (Novo Nordisk)

TYPE OF DRUG

Antidiabetic

INGREDIENT

insulin

DOSAGE FORMS

Injectable (all types) (100 units/ml)
Injectable (regular) (100 units/ml, 500 units/ml)
This drug is available only as an injectable (if swallowed, it is destroyed by stomach acid). Various types of insulin provide different times of onset and durations of action (see below).

Insulin type	Onset of action (in hours)	Duration of action (in hours)
Regular insulin	½	6
Insulin zinc suspension, prompt (Semilente)	1½	14
Isophane insulin (NPH)	1	24
Insulin zinc suspension (Lente)	1	24
Protamine zinc insulin (PZI)	6	36
Insulin zinc suspension, extended (Ultralente)	6	36

STORAGE

After opening, keep most forms (except 500 units/ml strength) at room temperature if used in six months. Refrigerate unopened vials of insulin, but never freeze this medication.

USES

Insulin is a hormone that is normally produced by the pancreas; it functions in the regulation of blood-sugar levels. This medication is used to treat diabetes mellitus (sugar diabetes) a disorder that results from an inability of the pancreas to produce enough insulin. Injectable insulin is used only to treat those patients whose blood-sugar levels cannot be controlled by diet or by oral antidiabetic medications.

TREATMENT

Your doctor, nurse, dietitian, or pharmacist will show you how to inject insulin, using a specially marked hypodermic syringe. This medication is packaged with printed instructions that should be carefully followed.

You may prefer to use presterilized disposable needles and syringes, which are used once and then discarded. If you use a glass syringe and metal needle, you must sterilize them before reuse.

Make sure that the insulin you are using is exactly the kind your doctor ordered and that its expiration date has not passed.

Do not shake the bottle; tip it gently, end to end, to mix. ALWAYS CHECK THE DOSE in the syringe at least twice before injecting it.

Clean the site of the injection thoroughly with an antiseptic, such as rubbing alcohol.

Change the site of the injection daily, and avoid injecting cold insulin.

NEVER use a vial of insulin if there are any signs of lumps in it.

Make your insulin injection a regular part of your schedule, so that you do not miss any doses. Ask your doctor what to do if you have to take a dose later than the scheduled time.

SIDE EFFECTS

Minor. Insulin can cause redness and rash at the site of injection. Try to rotate injection sites in order to avoid this reaction.

Major. Be sure to tell your doctor about any side effects that are persistent or particularly bothersome. IT IS ESPECIALLY IMPORTANT TO TELL YOUR DOCTOR about palpitations, fainting, shortness of breath, skin rash, or sweating.

Too much insulin can cause hypoglycemia (low blood sugar), which can lead to anxiety, chills, cold sweats, drowsiness, fast heart rate, headache, loss of consciousness, nausea, nervousness, tremors, unusual hunger, or unusual weakness. If you experience these symptoms, you should eat a quick source of sugar (such as table sugar, orange juice, honey, or a nondiet cola). You should also make it a point to tell your doctor that you have had this reaction.

Too little insulin can cause symptoms of hyperglycemia (high blood sugar), such as confusion, drowsiness, dry skin, fatigue, flushing, frequent urination, fruit-like breath odor, loss of appetite, or rapid breathing. If you experience any of these symptoms, contact your doctor; he or she may want to modify your dosing schedule or change your insulin dosage.

INTERACTIONS

Insulin can be expected to interact with several other types of medications:

1. Insulin can increase the side effects of digoxin on the heart.

2. Oral contraceptives (birth control pills), adrenocorticosteroids (cortisonelike medicines), danazol, dextrothyroxine, furosemide, ethacrynic acid, thyroid hormone, thiazide diuretics (water pills), phenytoin, or nicotine can increase insulin requirements.

3. Monoamine oxidase (MAO) inhibitors, phenylbutazone, fenfluramine, guanethidine, disopyramide, sulfinpyrazone, tetracycline, alcohol, anabolic steroids, or large doses of aspirin can increase the effects of insulin, leading to hypoglycemia.

4. Beta blockers (acebutolol, atenolol, betaxolol, carteolol, esmolol, labetalol, metoprolol, nadolol, penbutolol, pindolol, propranolol, timolol) may prolong the effects of insulin and mask the signs of hypoglycemia.

BE SURE TO TELL YOUR DOCTOR about any medications you are currently taking, especially any of those listed above.

WARNINGS

- Tell your doctor about unusual or allergic reactions you have had to any medications, especially to insulin.
- Before starting to take this medication, be sure to tell your doctor if you now have or if you have ever had high fevers, infections, kidney disease, liver disease, thyroid disease, or severe nausea and vomiting.
- If your doctor prescribes two types of insulin to achieve better glucose control and recommends mixing the insulin into one syringe, always draw the regular insulin (clear) into the syringe first.
- Some insulin mixtures won't interact with each other for some time. Others react quickly and require immediate injection. Consult your doctor or pharmacist.
- Make sure that your friends and family are aware of the symptoms of an insulin reaction and know what to do should they observe any of the symptoms in you.
- Carry a card or wear a bracelet that identifies you as a diabetic.
- Always have insulin and syringes available.
- When traveling, always carry an ample supply of your diabetic needs and, if possible, a prescription for insulin and syringes. Carry insulin and syringes on your person; baggage can be lost, delayed, or stolen.
- Do not store insulin in your car's glove compartment.
- To avoid the possibility of hypoglycemia (low blood-sugar levels), you should eat on a regular schedule and should avoid skipping meals.
- Before having surgery or other medical or dental treatment, tell your doctor or dentist you are taking insulin.
- Check with your doctor or pharmacist before taking any over-the-counter (nonprescription) cough, cold, diet, allergy, asthma, or sinus medications. Some of these products affect blood-sugar levels.
- If you become ill, it is possible your insulin requirements may change. Consult your doctor.
- Be sure to tell your doctor if you are pregnant. Insulin dosing requirements often change during pregnancy.

isoniazid

BRAND NAMES (Manufacturers)
isoniazid (various manufacturers)
Izonid (Major)
Laniazid (Lannett)
TYPE OF DRUG
Antitubercular
INGREDIENT
isoniazid
DOSAGE FORMS
Tablets (100 mg and 300 mg)
Oral syrup (50 mg per 5-ml spoonful)
STORAGE
Store at room temperature in a tightly closed, light-resistant container. This medication should never be frozen.

USES

Isoniazid is used to prevent and treat tuberculosis. It acts by severely injuring the cell structure of tuberculosis bacteria, thereby preventing them from growing and multiplying.

TREATMENT

In order to avoid stomach irritation, you can take isoniazid with food or a full glass of water or milk (unless your doctor directs you to do otherwise).

Antacids prevent the absorption of isoniazid from the gastrointestinal tract, so they should not be taken within an hour of a dose of isoniazid.

Each dose of the oral syrup should be measured carefully with a specially designed 5-ml measuring spoon. An ordinary kitchen teaspoon is not accurate enough for medical purposes.

It is important to continue to take this medication for the entire time prescribed by your doctor, even if your symptoms disappear before the end of that period. If you stop taking the drug too soon, your infection could recur.

It is common for therapy to last for at least six months and, at times, for as long as two years.

Try not to miss any doses of this medication. If you do miss a dose, take the missed dose as soon as possible, unless it is almost time for the next dose. In that case, do not take the missed dose at all; just return to your regular dosing schedule. Do not double the next dose.

SIDE EFFECTS

Minor. Abdominal pain, dizziness, heartburn, nausea, or vomiting. These side effects should disappear as your body adjusts to the medication.

If you feel dizzy, sit or lie down for a while; get up slowly from a sitting or reclining position; and be careful on stairs.

Major. Tell your doctor about any side effects that are persistent or particularly bothersome. IT IS ESPECIALLY IMPORTANT TO TELL YOUR DOCTOR about blurred vision, breast enlargement (in both sexes), chills, darkening of the urine, eye pain, fever, malaise, memory impairment, numbness or tingling in the fingers or toes, rash, unusual bleeding or bruising, vision changes, weakness, or yellowing of the eyes or skin.

Your doctor may want to prescribe vitamin B_6 (pyridoxine) to prevent the numbness and tingling. However, do not take vitamin B_6 without consulting your doctor.

INTERACTIONS

Isoniazid interacts with several other medications:
1. Concurrent use of isoniazid and alcohol can lead to decreased effectiveness of isoniazid and increased side effects on the liver.
2. The combination of isoniazid and cycloserine can result in dizziness or drowsiness.
3. The combination of isoniazid and disulfiram can lead to dizziness, loss of coordination, irritable disposition, and insomnia.
4. Isoniazid can decrease the breakdown of phenytoin and carbamazepine in the body, which can lead to an increase in side effects from phenytoin and carbamazepine.
5. Isoniazid can decrease the effectiveness of ketoconazole.
6. In combination, rifampin and isoniazid can increase the risk of liver damage. However, this is a commonly prescribed combination.
7. The effectiveness of isoniazid may be decreased by adrenocorticosteroids (cortisonelike medicines).
8. The side effects of benzodiazepine tranquilizers or meperidine may be increased by isoniazid.

BE SURE TO TELL YOUR DOCTOR about any medications you are currently taking, especially those listed above.

WARNINGS

• Tell your doctor about unusual or allergic reactions you have had to any medications, especially to isoniazid, ethionamide, pyrazinamide, or niacin (vitamin B_3).
• Before starting to take this medication, be sure to tell your doctor if you have a history of alcoholism or if you now have or ever had kidney disease, liver disease, or seizures.
• If this drug makes you dizzy, avoid tasks that require alertness, such as driving a car.
• Your doctor may want you to have periodic eye examinations while taking this medication, especially if you begin to have vision side effects.
• Isoniazid can interact with several foods (skipjack fish, tuna, yeast extracts, sauerkraut juice, sausages, and certain cheeses), leading to severe reactions. You should, therefore, avoid eating these foods while being treated with isoniazid.
• Diabetics using Clinitest urine glucose tests may get erroneously high sugar readings while they are taking isoniazid. Temporarily changing to Clinistix or Tes-Tape urine tests avoids this problem.
• Be sure to tell your doctor if you are pregnant. Although isoniazid appears to be safe during pregnancy, it does cross the placenta. Extensive studies in pregnant women have not been conducted. Also, tell your doctor if you are breast-feeding an infant. Small amounts of isoniazid pass into breast milk.

levodopa

BRAND NAMES (Manufacturers)
Dopar (Roberts)
Larodopa (Roche)
TYPE OF DRUG
Antiparkinsonism agent
INGREDIENT
levodopa
DOSAGE FORMS
Tablets (100 mg, 250 mg, and 500 mg)
Capsules (100 mg, 250 mg, and 500 mg)
STORAGE
Levodopa tablets and capsules should be stored at room temperature in tightly closed, light-resistant containers.

USES

Levodopa is used to treat the symptoms of Parkinson's disease. It is converted in the body to dopamine, a chemical in the brain that is diminished in patients with Parkinson's disease.

TREATMENT

In order to avoid stomach irritation, you can take levodopa with food or with a full glass of milk or water (unless your doctor directs you to do otherwise).

You may not observe significant benefit from this drug for two to three weeks after starting to take it.

If you miss a dose, take the missed dose as soon as possible, unless it is within two hours of the next scheduled dose. In that case, do not take the missed dose at all; just return to your regular dosing schedule. Do not double the next dose.

SIDE EFFECTS

Minor. Abdominal pain, anxiety, bitter taste in the mouth, constipation, diarrhea, dizziness, dry mouth, fatigue, flushing, gas, headache, hiccups, hoarseness, increased hand tremors, increased sexual interest, increased sweating, insomnia, loss of appetite, nausea, offensive body odor, salivation, vision changes, vomiting, weakness, or weight gain. These side effects may disappear as your body adjusts to the medication.

Levodopa can cause a darkening of your urine or sweat. This is a harmless effect.

To relieve constipation, increase the amount of fiber in your diet (fresh fruits and vegetables, salads, bran, and whole-grain breads), drink more water, and exercise (unless your doctor directs you to do otherwise).

If you feel dizzy, sit or lie down for a while; get up slowly from a sitting or reclining position; and be careful on stairs.

To relieve mouth dryness, chew sugarless gum or suck on ice chips or a piece of hard candy.

Major. Tell your doctor about any side effects that are persistent or particularly bothersome. IT IS ESPECIALLY IMPORTANT TO TELL YOUR DOCTOR about bloody or black, tarry stools; confusion; convulsions; depression; fainting; false sense of well-being; loss of coordination; loss of hair; nightmares; painful erection; palpitations; rapid weight gain (three to five pounds within a week); skin rash; visual disturbances; uncontrolled movements; or unusual weakness.

INTERACTIONS

Levodopa interacts with several other types of medications:

1. The dosage of antihypertensive drugs may require adjustment when levodopa is started.
2. The effectiveness of levodopa may be decreased by benzodiazepine tranquilizers, phenothiazine tranquilizers, haloperidol, thiothixene, phenytoin, papaverine, and reserpine.
3. Methyldopa can increase or decrease the side effects of therapy with levodopa.
4. Use of levodopa and a monoamine oxidase (MAO) inhibitor within 14 days of each other can lead to severe side effects.
5. Levodopa can increase the side effects of tricyclic antidepressants, ephedrine, and amphetamines.
6. Antacids may alter the absorption of levodopa from the gastrointestinal tract.
7. Pyridoxine (vitamin B_6) can decrease the effectiveness of levodopa.

BE SURE TO TELL YOUR DOCTOR about any medications you are taking, especially those listed above.

WARNINGS

• Tell your doctor about unusual or allergic reactions you have had to any medications, especially to levodopa.
• Before starting to take this medication, be sure to tell your doctor if you now have or if you have ever had asthma, diabetes mellitus, difficulty in urinating, epilepsy, glaucoma, heart disease, hormone disorders, kidney disease, liver disease, lung disease, melanoma (a type of skin cancer), mental disorders, or peptic ulcers.
• Some of these products contain the color additive FD&C Yellow No. 5 (tartrazine), which can cause allergic-type symptoms (difficulty in breathing, faintness, or rash) in certain susceptible individuals.
• If levodopa makes you dizzy or blurs your vision, avoid activities that require mental alertness, such as driving a car or operating potentially dangerous machinery.
• Notify your doctor if you start to experience any uncontrolled movements of the limbs or face while taking this medication.
• Before having surgery or any other medical or dental treatment, be sure to tell your doctor or dentist that you are taking this medication.
• Levodopa can cause erroneous readings of urine glucose and ketone tests. Diabetic patients should not change their medication dosage unless they first check with their doctor.
• Pyridoxine (vitamin B_6) can decrease the effectiveness of levodopa. Persons taking levodopa should avoid taking this vitamin and should avoid foods rich in pyridoxine (including beans, bacon, avocados, liver, dry skim milk, oatmeal, sweet potatoes, peas, and tuna).
• Be sure to tell your doctor if you are pregnant. Although levodopa appears to be safe in humans, birth defects have been reported in the offspring of animals that were administered large doses during pregnancy. Also, tell your

doctor if you are breast-feeding an infant. Levodopa passes into breast milk and can cause side effects in nursing infants.

---

lithium

BRAND NAMES (Manufacturers)
Cibalith-S (Ciba)
Eskalith (SmithKline Beecham)
Eskalith CR (SmithKline Beecham)
Lithane (Miles)
lithium carbonate (various manufacturers)
lithium citrate (various manufacturers)
Lithobid (Ciba)
Lithonate (Solvay)
Lithotabs (Solvay)
TYPE OF DRUG
Antimanic (mood stabilizer)
INGREDIENT
lithium
DOSAGE FORMS
Tablets (300 mg)
Extended-release tablets (300 mg and 450 mg)
Capsules (150 mg, 300 mg, and 600 mg)
Syrup (300 mg per 5-ml spoonful, with 0.3% alcohol)
STORAGE
Lithium tablets, capsules, and syrup should be stored at room temperature away from heat and direct sunlight. The medication should not be refrigerated, and the syrup form should not be frozen. Do not store the medication in the bathroom cabinet, because moisture may cause the breakdown of lithium. Do not keep these medications beyond the expiration date.

USES

Lithium is a medication used to treat manic-depressive illness by controlling the manic (excited) phase of the illness and by reducing the frequency and severity of depression. Manic-depressive patients often experience unstable emotions ranging from excitement to hostility to depression. The mechanism of the mood-stabilizing effect of lithium is unknown, but it appears to work on the central nervous system to control emotions.

TREATMENT

Lithium should be taken exactly as directed by your doctor. The effectiveness of this medication depends upon the amount of lithium in your bloodstream. Therefore, the medication should be taken every day at regularly spaced intervals in order to keep a constant amount of lithium in your bloodstream.

The syrup form must be measured carefully with a specially designed 5-ml measuring spoon. An ordinary kitchen teaspoon is not accurate enough for therapeutic purposes.

If you miss a dose of this medication, take it as soon as possible. However, if it is within two hours (six hours for extended-release tablets) of your next scheduled dose, skip the missed dose and return to your regular schedule. Do not take more than one dose at a time.

If you are taking the long-acting or slow-release form of lithium, swallow the tablet or capsule whole. Do not break, crush, or chew before swallowing.

An improvement in your condition may not be seen for several weeks after you start this drug.

SIDE EFFECTS

Minor. Acne, bloating, diarrhea, drowsiness, increased frequency of urination, increased thirst, nausea, trembling of the hands, weight gain, or weakness or tiredness. These side effects should disappear as your body adjusts to this medication.

Major. Blurred vision, clumsiness, confusion, convulsions, difficulty in breathing, dizziness, fainting, palpitations, severe trembling, and slurred speech are possible effects of too much drug in the bloodstream. Dry, rough skin; hair loss; hoarseness; swelling of the feet or lower legs; swelling of the neck; unusual sensitivity to the cold; unusual tiredness; or unusual weight gain may be the result of low thyroid function caused by the medication. CHECK WITH YOUR DOCTOR IMMEDIATELY if any of these side effects appear.

INTERACTIONS

Lithium interacts with a number of other types of medications:

1. Aminophylline, caffeine, verapamil, acetazolamide, sodium bicarbonate, dyphylline, oxtriphylline, and theophylline can increase the elimination of lithium from the body, thus decreasing its effectiveness.
2. Diuretics (water pills), especially hydrochlorothiazide, chlorothiazide, chlorthalidone, triamterene and hydrochlorothiazide combination, and furosemide may cause lithium toxicity by delaying lithium's elimination.
3. Captopril, chlorpromazine and other phenothiazine tranquilizers, ibuprofen, indomethacin, naproxen, and piroxicam can also slow lithium elimination.
4. Lithium can increase the side effects of haloperidol and other medications for mental illness.
5. Phenytoin, methyldopa, carbamazepine, and tetracycline can increase the side effects of lithium.
6. Drinking large amounts of caffeine-containing coffees, teas, or colas may reduce the effectiveness of lithium by increasing its elimination from the body through the urine.

BE SURE TO TELL YOUR DOCTOR about any medications you are currently taking, especially any of those listed above.

WARNINGS

- Tell your doctor about unusual or allergic reactions you have had to any medications, especially to lithium.
- Tell your doctor if you now have or if you have ever had diabetes mellitus, epilepsy, heart disease, kidney disease, Parkinson's disease, or thyroid disease.
- Elderly patients may be more sensitive to lithium's side effects.
- In order to maintain a constant level of lithium in your bloodstream, it is important to drink two to three quarts of water or other fluids each day and not to change the

amount of salt in your diet, unless your doctor specifically directs you to do so.

• The loss of large amounts of body fluid (from prolonged vomiting or diarrhea or from heavy sweating due to hot weather, fever, exercise, saunas, or hot baths) can result in increased lithium levels in the blood, which can lead to an increase in side effects.

• The toxic dose of lithium is very close to the therapeutic dose, so it is extremely important to follow your correct dosing schedule. Diarrhea, drowsiness, lack of coordination, muscular weakness, and vomiting may be signs of toxicity. If these symptoms occur for any length of time or begin shortly after taking a dose, be sure to inform your doctor.

• Lithium is not recommended for use during pregnancy, especially during the first three months, because of possible effects on the thyroid and heart of the developing fetus. Also, tell your doctor if you are breast-feeding. Lithium also passes into breast milk and may cause side effects in the nursing infant.

• If this drug makes you drowsy or dizzy, do not take part in any activities that require alertness, such as driving a car or operating potentially dangerous machinery.

---

loperamide

BRAND NAME (Manufacturer)
Imodium (Janssen)
TYPE OF DRUG
Antidiarrheal
INGREDIENT
loperamide
DOSAGE FORMS
Capsules (2 mg)
Oral liquid (1 mg per 5-ml spoonful)*
*Available over-the-counter (without a prescription)
STORAGE
Loperamide capsules and liquid should be stored at room temperature in tightly closed containers. This medication should never be frozen.

USES

Loperamide is used to treat acute and chronic diarrhea and to reduce the volume of discharge in patients who have ileostomies. It acts by slowing the movement of the gastrointestinal tract and decreasing the passage of water and other substances into the bowel.

TREATMENT

In order to avoid stomach upset, you can take loperamide with food or with a full glass of water or milk.

If you miss a dose of this medication, do not take the missed dose at all; just return to your regular dosing schedule. Do not double the next dose.

SIDE EFFECTS

Minor. Constipation, dizziness, drowsiness, dry mouth, fatigue, loss of appetite, nausea, or vomiting. These effects should disappear over time as your body adjusts to the drug.

To relieve constipation, exercise and drink more water (unless your doctor directs you to do otherwise).

To reduce mouth dryness, chew sugarless gum or suck on ice chips or a piece of hard candy.

If you feel dizzy or light-headed, sit or lie down for a while; get up from a sitting or lying position slowly; and be careful on stairs.

Major. Tell your doctor about any side effects that are persistent or particularly bothersome. IT IS ESPECIALLY IMPORTANT TO TELL YOUR DOCTOR about abdominal bloating or pain, fever, rash, or sore throat.

INTERACTIONS

Loperamide should not interact with any other drugs.

WARNINGS

• Tell your doctor about unusual or allergic reactions you have had to any medications.

• Tell your doctor if you now have or if you have ever had colitis, diarrhea caused by infectious organisms, drug-induced diarrhea, liver disease, dehydration, or conditions in which constipation must be avoided (such as hemorrhoids, diverticulitis, heart or blood vessel disorders, or blood clotting disorders).

• If this drug makes you dizzy or drowsy, do not take part in any activity that requires alertness.

• Before having surgery or any other medical or dental treatment, be sure to tell your doctor or dentist that you are taking this medication.

• Check with your doctor if your diarrhea does not subside within three days. Unless prescribed otherwise, do not take this drug for more than ten days at a time.

• While taking this medication, drink lots of fluids to replace those lost because of diarrhea.

• Be sure to tell your doctor if you are pregnant. The effects of this medication during pregnancy have not been thoroughly studied in humans. Also, tell your doctor if you are breast-feeding an infant. It is not known whether loperamide passes into breast milk.

---

lorazepam

BRAND NAMES (Manufacturers)
Ativan (Wyeth)
lorazepam (various manufacturers)
TYPE OF DRUG
Benzodiazepine sedative/hypnotic
INGREDIENT
lorazepam
DOSAGE FORMS
Tablets (0.5 mg, 1 mg, and 2 mg)
Oral solution (2 mg/ml)
STORAGE
This medication should be stored at room temperature in a tightly closed, light-resistant container. It should not be refrigerated.

USES

Lorazepam is prescribed to treat symptoms of anxiety and anxiety associated with depression. It is not clear exactly how this medicine works, but it may relieve anxiety by acting as a depressant of the central nervous system (brain and spinal cord). This medication is currently used by many people to relieve nervousness. It is effective for this purpose for short periods, but it is important to try to remove the cause of the anxiety as well.

TREATMENT

Lorazepam should be taken exactly as your doctor directs. It can be taken with food or a full glass of water if stomach upset occurs. Do not take this medication with a dose of antacids, since they may slow its absorption from the gastrointestinal tract.

If you are taking this medication regularly and you miss a dose, take the missed dose immediately if you remember within an hour. If more than an hour has passed, skip the dose you missed and wait for the next scheduled dose. Do not double the dose.

SIDE EFFECTS

Minor. Bitter taste in the mouth, constipation, diarrhea, dizziness, drowsiness (after a night's sleep), dry mouth, fatigue, flushing, headache, heartburn, excessive salivation, loss of appetite, nausea, nervousness, sweating, or vomiting. As your body adjusts to the medication, these side effects should disappear.

To relieve constipation, increase the amount of fiber in your diet (fresh fruits and vegetables, salads, bran, and whole-grain breads), exercise, and drink more water (unless your doctor directs you to do otherwise).

Dry mouth can be relieved by chewing sugarless gum or by sucking on ice chips.

If you feel dizzy, sit or lie down for a while; get up slowly from a sitting or reclining position; and be careful on stairs.

Major. Tell your doctor about any side effects that are persistent or particularly bothersome. IT IS ESPECIALLY IMPORTANT TO TELL YOUR DOCTOR about blurred or double vision, chest pain, depression, difficulty in urinating, fainting, falling, fever, joint pain, hallucinations, memory problems, mouth sores, nightmares, palpitations, rash, shortness of breath, slurred speech, sore throat, uncoordinated movements, unusual excitement, unusual tiredness, or yellowing of the eyes or skin.

INTERACTIONS

Lorazepam interacts with several other types of medications:

1. To prevent oversedation, this drug should not be taken with alcohol, other sedative drugs, or central nervous system depressants (such as antihistamines, barbiturates, muscle relaxants, pain medicines, narcotics, medicines for seizures, and phenothiazine tranquilizers) or with antidepressants.

2. This medication may decrease the effectiveness of carbamazepine, levodopa, and oral anticoagulants (blood thinners) and may increase the effects of phenytoin.

3. Disulfiram, cimetidine, and isoniazid can increase the blood levels of lorazepam, leading to toxic effects.

4. Concurrent use of rifampin may decrease the effectiveness of lorazepam.

BE SURE TO TELL YOUR DOCTOR about any medications you are currently taking, especially any listed above.

WARNINGS

• Tell your doctor about unusual or allergic reactions you have had to any medications, especially to lorazepam or other benzodiazepine tranquilizers (such as alprazolam, chlordiazepoxide, clorazepate, diazepam, flurazepam, halazepam, midazolam, oxazepam, prazepam, temazepam, and triazolam).

• Tell your doctor if you now have or if you have ever had liver disease, kidney disease, epilepsy, lung disease, myasthenia gravis, porphyria, mental depression, or mental illness.

• This medicine can cause drowsiness. Avoid tasks that require alertness, such as driving a car or using potentially dangerous machinery.

• This medication has the potential for abuse and must be used with caution. Tolerance may develop quickly; do not increase the dosage without first consulting your doctor. It is also important not to stop this drug suddenly if you have been taking it in large amounts or if you have used it for several weeks. Your doctor may want to reduce the dosage gradually.

• This is a safe drug when used properly. When it is combined with other sedative drugs or alcohol, however, serious side effects can develop.

• Be sure to tell your doctor if you are pregnant. This medicine may increase the chance of birth defects if it is taken during the first three months of pregnancy. In addition, too much use of this medicine during the last six months of pregnancy may cause the fetus to become dependent on it, resulting in withdrawal side effects in the newborn. Also, use of this drug during the last weeks of pregnancy may cause drowsiness, slowed heartbeat, and breathing difficulties in the newborn. Tell your doctor if you are breast-feeding. This drug can pass into the breast milk and cause drowsiness, slowed heartbeat, and breathing difficulties in the nursing infant.

lovastatin

BRAND NAME (Manufacturer)
Mevacor (Merck Sharp & Dohme)
TYPE OF DRUG
Antihyperlipidemic (lipid-lowering drug)
INGREDIENT
lovastatin
DOSAGE FORM
Tablets (10 mg, 20 mg, and 40 mg)
STORAGE
This medication should be stored at room temperature in a tightly closed, light-resistant container. Exposure to heat or moisture may cause this drug to break down chemically.

USES

Lovastatin is used to treat hyperlipidemia (high blood-fat levels). It is prescribed in conjunction with nondrug therapies, such as diet modification and regular exercise, in an attempt to regulate lipid and cholesterol levels.

Lovastatin chemically interferes with an enzyme in the body that is responsible for synthesizing cholesterol. This decreases the LDL (low-density lipoprotein) type of cholesterol, which deposits cholesterol in the arteries and has been associated with coronary heart disease and atherosclerosis.

TREATMENT

This medication should be taken exactly as prescribed by your doctor. If you are to take the drug once a day, it is best to take the drug in the evening. Lovastatin can be taken with meals or a full glass of water if stomach upset occurs.

While using this medication, try to develop a set schedule for taking it. If you miss a dose and remember within a few hours, take the missed dose and resume your regular schedule. If many hours have passed, skip the dose you missed and then take your next dose as scheduled. Do not double the dose.

SIDE EFFECTS

Minor. Abdominal pain or cramps, constipation, diarrhea, gas, nausea, or stomach pain. These effects may be relieved by taking lovastatin with a meal, adding fiber to your diet, or using mild stool softeners.

Major. Tell your doctor about any side effects that are persistent or particularly bothersome. IT IS ESPECIALLY IMPORTANT TO TELL YOUR DOCTOR about blurred vision (or any other visual changes or difficulties) or muscle pain or tenderness, especially if it is associated with malaise (a general feeling of being unwell) or significant fever.

INTERACTIONS

There do not appear to be any significant drug interactions with this medication. However, you should make sure your doctor knows all the medications you are currently taking.

WARNINGS

- Tell your doctor about unusual or allergic reactions you have had to any medications.
- Tell your doctor if you have ever had liver disease, heart disease, stroke, or any disorders of the digestive tract.
- In preliminary studies with lovastatin, some patients were found to develop eye-related problems during treatment. Although these findings are inconclusive, and it has not yet been determined whether lovastatin is involved in such occurrences, it is advisable to have regular checkups with your ophthalmologist and inform him or her of your use of this drug so appropriate precautions can be taken.
- This drug should not be taken if you are pregnant or breast-feeding an infant.

meperidine

BRAND NAMES (Manufacturers)
Demerol (Winthrop-Breon)
meperidine hydrochloride (various manufacturers)
TYPE OF DRUG
Analgesic
INGREDIENT
meperidine
DOSAGE FORMS
Tablets (50 mg and 100 mg)
Syrup (50 mg per 5-ml spoonful)
STORAGE
Store at room temperature in a tightly closed, light-resistant container. This medication should not be refrigerated and should never be frozen.

USES

Meperidine is a narcotic analgesic (pain reliever) that acts directly on the central nervous system (brain and spinal cord). It is used to relieve moderate to severe pain.

TREATMENT

In order to avoid stomach upset, you can take meperidine with food or milk. It works most effectively if you take it at the onset of pain, rather than waiting until the pain becomes intense.

Measure the syrup form of this medication carefully with a specially designed 5-ml measuring spoon. An ordinary kitchen teaspoon is not accurate enough. Each dose of the syrup should be diluted in four ounces (half a glass) of water in order to avoid the numbness of the mouth and throat that this medication can cause.

If you are taking this medication on a regular schedule and you miss a dose, take the missed dose as soon as possible, unless it is almost time for your next dose. In that case, do not take the missed dose at all; just return to your regular dosing schedule. Do not double the next dose.

SIDE EFFECTS

Minor. Constipation, dizziness, drowsiness, dry mouth, false sense of well-being, flushing, light-headedness, loss of appetite, nausea, rash, or sweating. These side effects should disappear as your body adjusts to the medication.

If you are constipated, increase the amount of fiber in your diet (fresh fruits and vegetables, salads, bran, and whole-grain breads). You can also increase your exercise and drink more water (unless your doctor directs you to do otherwise).

Chew sugarless gum or suck on ice chips or a piece of hard candy to reduce mouth dryness associated with the use of this medication.

If you feel dizzy or light-headed, sit or lie down for a while; get up from a sitting or lying position slowly; and be careful on stairs.

Major. Tell your doctor about any side effects that are persistent or particularly bothersome. IT IS ESPECIALLY IMPORTANT TO TELL YOUR DOCTOR about anxiety, breathing difficulties, excitability, fatigue, painful or difficult urination, restlessness, sore throat and fever, tremors, or weakness.

INTERACTIONS

Meperidine interacts with several other types of medications:

1. Concurrent use of this medication with other central nervous system depressants (such as alcohol, antihistamines, barbiturates, benzodiazepine tranquilizers, muscle relaxants, and phenothiazine tranquilizers) or with tricyclic antidepressants can cause extreme drowsiness.

2. A monoamine oxidase (MAO) inhibitor taken within 14 days of this medication can lead to unpredictable and severe side effects.

3. The combination of cimetidine and meperidine can cause confusion, disorientation, and shortness of breath.

BE SURE TO TELL YOUR DOCTOR about any medications you are currently taking, especially any listed above.

WARNINGS

• Tell your doctor about unusual or allergic reactions you have had to any drugs, especially to meperidine or to any other narcotic analgesic (such as codeine, hydrocodone, hydromorphone, methadone, morphine, oxycodone, and propoxyphene).

• Tell your doctor if you now have or if you have ever had acute abdominal conditions, asthma, brain disease, colitis, epilepsy, gallstones or gallbladder disease, head injuries, heart disease, kidney disease, liver disease, lung disease, mental illness, emotional disorders, enlarged prostate gland, thyroid disease, or urethral stricture.

• If this drug makes you dizzy or drowsy, do not take part in any activity that requires alertness, such as driving a car or operating potentially dangerous machinery. Take special care going up and down stairs.

• Before having surgery or any other medical or dental treatment, tell your doctor or dentist that you are taking this drug.

• Meperidine has the potential for abuse and must be used with caution. Usually, it should not be taken on a regular schedule for longer than ten days (unless your doctor directs you to do so). Tolerance develops quickly; do not increase the dosage or stop taking the drug abruptly unless you first consult your doctor. If you have been taking large amounts of this medication or have been taking it for a long period of time, you may experience withdrawal symptoms (muscle aches, diarrhea, gooseflesh, runny nose, nausea, vomiting, shivering, trembling, stomach cramps, sleep disorders, irritability, weakness, excessive yawning, or sweating) when you stop taking it. Your doctor may, therefore, want to reduce your dosage gradually.

• Tell your doctor if you are pregnant. The effects of this drug during the early stages of pregnancy have not been thoroughly studied in humans. However, the use of meperidine regularly in large doses during the later stages of pregnancy can result in addiction of the fetus. Also, tell your doctor if you are breast-feeding. Small amounts of this drug may pass into breast milk and cause excessive drowsiness in the nursing infant.

---

metaproterenol

BRAND NAMES (Manufacturers)
Alupent (Boehringer Ingelheim)
Metaprel (Sandoz)

TYPE OF DRUG
Bronchiodilator

INGREDIENT
metaproterenol

DOSAGE FORMS
Tablets (10 mg and 20 mg)
Oral syrup (10 mg per 5-ml spoonful)
Inhalation aerosol (each spray delivers 0.65 mg)
Solution for nebulization (0.4%, 0.6%, and 5%)

STORAGE
Metaproterenol tablets and oral syrup should be stored at room temperature in tightly closed, light-resistant containers. The solution for nebulization should be stored in the refrigerator. The inhalation aerosol should be stored at room temperature away from excessive heat—the contents are pressurized, and the container can explode if heated. Metaproterenol syrup and solution should not be used if they turn brown or contain particles.

USES

Metaproterenol is used to relieve wheezing and shortness of breath caused by lung diseases such as asthma, bronchitis, and emphysema. This drug acts directly on the muscles of the bronchi (breathing tubes) to relieve bronchospasm (muscle contractions of the bronchi), thereby allowing air to move to and from the lungs.

TREATMENT

In order to lessen stomach upset, you can take metaproterenol tablets or oral syrup with food (unless your doctor directs you to do otherwise).

The oral syrup form of this medication should be measured carefully with a specially designed 5-ml measuring spoon. An ordinary kitchen teaspoon is not accurate enough.

The inhalation aerosol form of this medication is usually packaged along with an instruction sheet. Read the directions carefully before using this medication. The container should be shaken well just before each use. The contents tend to settle on the bottom, so it is necessary to shake the container in order to distribute the ingredients evenly and equalize the doses. If more than one inhalation is necessary, wait at least one full minute between doses, so that you receive the full therapeutic benefit of the first dose.

If you miss a dose of this medication and remember within an hour, take it; then follow your regular schedule for the next dose. If you miss the dose by more than an hour or so, just wait until the next scheduled dose. Do not double the dose.

If you are also using an aerosol corticosteroid (such as beclomethasone, dexamethasone, or triamcinolone), use the metaproterenol inhalation first and wait about five minutes before using the corticosteroid inhalation (unless otherwise directed by your doctor). This will allow the corticosteroid inhalation to better reach your lungs.

SIDE EFFECTS

Minor. Anxiety, dizziness, headache, flushing, irritability, insomnia, loss of appetite, muscle cramps, nausea, nervousness, restlessness, sweating, vomiting, weakness, or dryness or irritation of the mouth or throat (from the inhalation aerosol). These side effects should disappear as your body adjusts to the medication.

To help prevent dryness and irritation of the mouth or throat, rinse your mouth with water after each dose of the inhalation aerosol.

In order to avoid difficulty in falling asleep, check with your doctor to see if you can take the last dose of this medication several hours before bedtime each day.

If you feel dizzy, sit or lie down for a while; get up from a sitting or lying position slowly; and be careful on stairs.

Major. Tell your doctor about any side effects that are persistent or particularly bothersome. IT IS ESPECIALLY IMPORTANT TO TELL YOUR DOCTOR about chest pain, difficult breathing, difficult or painful urination, palpitations, rash, or tremors.

INTERACTIONS

Metaproterenol interacts with several other types of medications:

1. Beta blockers (acebutolol, atenolol, betaxolol, carteolol, esmolol, labetalol, metoprolol, nadolol, penbutolol, pindolol, propranolol, timolol) antagonize (act against) this medication, decreasing its effectiveness.

2. Monoamine oxidase (MAO) inhibitors, tricyclic antidepressants, antihistamines, levothyroxine, and over-the-counter (nonprescription) cough, cold, allergy, asthma, diet, and sinus medications may increase the side effects of metaproterenol. At least 14 days should separate the use of this drug and the use of an MAO inhibitor.

3. There may be a change in the dosage requirements of insulin or oral antidiabetic medications when metaproterenol is started.

4. The blood-pressure-lowering effects of guanethidine may be decreased by this medication.

5. The use of metaproterenol with other bronchodilator drugs (either oral or inhaled) can have additive side effects. Discuss this with your doctor.

BE SURE TO TELL YOUR DOCTOR about any medications you are currently taking, especially any of the medications that are listed above.

WARNINGS

• Tell your doctor about unusual or allergic reactions you have had, especially to metaproterenol or any related drug (such as albuterol, amphetamines, ephedrine, epinephrine, isoproterenol, norepinephrine, phenylephrine, phenylpropanolamine, pseudoephedrine, and terbutaline).

• Tell your doctor if you now have or if you have ever had diabetes, glaucoma, high blood pressure, epilepsy, heart disease, enlarged prostate gland, or thyroid disease.

• This medication can cause dizziness. Your ability to perform tasks that require alertness, such as driving a car or operating potentially dangerous machinery, may be decreased. Appropriate caution should, therefore, be taken.

• Before having surgery or any other medical or dental treatment, be sure to tell your doctor or dentist that you are taking this medication.

• Do not exceed the recommended dosage of this medication. Excessive use may lead to an increase in side effects or a loss of effectiveness.

• Try to avoid contact of the aerosol with your eyes.

• Do not puncture, break, or burn the aerosol container. The contents are under pressure and may explode.

• Contact your doctor if you do not respond to the usual dose of this medication. It may be a sign of worsening asthma, which may require additional therapy.

• Be sure to tell your doctor if you are pregnant. The effects of this medication during pregnancy have not been thoroughly studied in humans. Also, tell your doctor if you are breast-feeding an infant. It is not known whether this drug passes into breast milk.

---

methotrexate

BRAND NAMES (Manufacturers)

Methotrexate (Lederle)
Rheumatrex Dose Pack (Lederle)

TYPE OF DRUG

Antineoplastic (anticancer drug), antipsoriatic

INGREDIENT

methotrexate

DOSAGE FORM

Tablets (2.5 mg)

STORAGE

Methotrexate should be stored at room temperature in a tightly closed container.

USES

Methotrexate is used to treat certain types of cancer and severe psoriasis. It works by slowing the growth rate of rapidly proliferating cells.

TREATMENT

In order to avoid stomach irritation, you can take methotrexate with food or with a full glass of water or milk (unless your doctor directs you to do otherwise).

Try not to miss any doses of this medication. If you do miss a dose, take the missed dose as soon as possible, unless it is almost time for the next dose. In that case, do not take the missed dose at all; just return to your regular dosing schedule. Do not double the next dose. If you miss more than two doses , CONTACT YOUR DOCTOR.

SIDE EFFECTS

Minor. Abdominal distress, fatigue, loss of appetite, nasal congestion, nausea, or vomiting. These side effects should disappear as your body adjusts to the medication. Methotrexate also causes hair loss, which is reversible when the medication is stopped.

This medication can increase your sensitivity to sunlight. You should, therefore, try to avoid prolonged exposure to sunlight and sunlamps. Wear protective clothing and sunglasses, and use an effective sunscreen.

Major. Tell your doctor about any side effects that are persistent or particularly bothersome. IT IS ESPECIALLY IMPORTANT TO TELL YOUR DOCTOR about back pain, blurred vision, convulsions, diarrhea, difficult or painful urination, drowsiness, fever, headache, itching, menstrual changes, mouth sores, rash, severe abdominal pain, skin color changes, unusual bleeding or bruising, or yellowing of the eyes or skin.

INTERACTIONS

Methotrexate interacts with several other types of medications:

1. Concurrent use of alcohol and methotrexate can lead to an increased risk of liver damage.

2. Methotrexate can block the effectiveness of antigout medications.

3. Phenylbutazone, probenecid, phenytoin, tetracycline, aspirin, chloramphenicol, salicylates, naproxen, ketoprofen, and sulfonamide antibiotics can increase the blood levels of methotrexate, which can lead to an increase in serious side effects.

4. Methotrexate can increase the effects of the blood thinner warfarin, which can lead to bleeding complications.

5. Folic acid vitamins may decrease the effect of this medication.

Before starting to take methotrexate, BE SURE TO TELL YOUR DOCTOR about any medications you are currently taking, especially any of those medications listed above.

WARNINGS

• Tell your doctor about unusual or allergic reactions you have ever had to any medications, especially to methotrexate.

• Before starting to take this medication, be sure to tell your doctor if you now have or if you have ever had blood disorders, gout, infection, kidney disease, liver disease, or inflammation of the gastrointestinal tract.

• If this drug makes you dizzy or drowsy, be careful going up and down stairs, and do not take part in any activity that requires alertness, such as driving a car or operating potentially dangerous machinery.

• While you are taking methotrexate, you should drink plenty of fluids so that you urinate often (unless your doctor directs you to do otherwise). This helps prevent kidney and bladder problems during therapy.

• You should not be immunized or vaccinated while taking methotrexate. The vaccination or immunization will not be effective and may lead to an infection if a live-virus vaccine is used.

• Methotrexate is a potent medication that can cause serious side effects. Your doctor will, therefore, want to monitor your therapy carefully with blood tests.

• It is important to tell your doctor if you are pregnant. Methotrexate has been shown to cause birth defects or death of the fetus. Effective contraception should be used during treatment and for at least eight weeks after treatment is stopped. Also, tell your doctor if you are breast-feeding an infant. Methotrexate passes into breast milk and can cause side effects in nursing infants.

---

methylprednisolone

BRAND NAMES (Manufacturers)
Medrol (Upjohn)
methylprednisolone (various manufacturers)
TYPE OF DRUG
Adrenocorticosteroid hormone
INGREDIENT
methylprednisolone
DOSAGE FORM
Tablets (2 mg, 4 mg, 8 mg, 16 mg, 24 mg, and 32 mg)
STORAGE
Store at room temperature in a tightly closed container.

USES

Your adrenal glands naturally produce certain cortisonelike chemicals. These chemicals are involved in various regulatory processes in the body (such as those involving fluid balance, temperature, and reactions to inflammation). Methylprednisolone belongs to a group of drugs known as adrenocorticosteroids (or cortisone-like medications). It is used to treat a variety of disorders, including endocrine and rheumatic disorders; asthma; blood diseases; certain cancers; eye disorders; gastrointestinal disturbances, such as ulcerative colitis; respiratory diseases; and inflammations, such as arthritis, dermatitis, and poison ivy. How this drug acts to relieve these disorders is not completely understood.

TREATMENT

In order to prevent stomach irritation, you can take methylprednisolone with food or milk.

If you are taking only one dose of this medication each day, try to take it before 9:00 A.M. This will mimic the body's normal production of this type of chemical.

It is important to try not to miss any doses of methylprednisolone. However, if you do miss a dose of this medication, follow these guidelines:

1. If you are taking this medication more than once a day, take the missed dose as soon as possible and return to your regular schedule. If it is already time for the next dose, double the dose.

2. If you are taking this medication once a day, take the dose you missed as soon as possible, unless you don't remember until the next day. In that case, do not take the missed dose at all; just follow your regular schedule. Do not double the next dose.

3. If you are taking this drug every other day, take it as soon as you remember. If you missed the scheduled time by a whole day, take it when you remember, and then skip a day before you take the next dose. Do not double the dose.

If you miss more than one dose, CONTACT YOUR DOCTOR IMMEDIATELY.

SIDE EFFECTS

Minor. Dizziness, false sense of well-being, increased appetite, increased susceptibility to infections, increased sweating, indigestion, menstrual irregularities, nausea, reddening of the skin on the face, restlessness, sleep disorders, or weight gain. These side effects should disappear as your body adjusts to the medication.

Major. Tell your doctor about any side effects that are persistent or particularly bothersome. IT IS ESPECIALLY IMPORTANT TO TELL YOUR DOCTOR about abdominal enlargement; abdominal pain; acne or other skin problems; back or rib pain; bloody or black, tarry stools; blurred vision; convulsions; eye pain; fever and sore throat; growth impairment (in children); headaches; impaired healing of wounds; increased thirst and urination; mental depression; mood changes; muscle wasting; muscle weakness; nightmares; rapid weight gain (three to five pounds within a week); rash; shortness of breath; thinning of the skin; unusual bleeding or bruising; and unusual weakness.

INTERACTIONS

Methylprednisolone interacts with several other types of medications:

1. Alcohol, aspirin, and anti-inflammatory medications (diclofenac, diflunisal, fenoprofen, flurbiprofen, ibuprofen, indomethacin, ketoprofen, mefenamic acid, meclofenamate, naproxen, piroxicam, sulindac, or tolmetin) aggravate the stomach problems that are common with use of this medication.

2. The dosage of oral anticoagulants (blood thinners, such as warfarin), oral antidiabetic medications, or insulin may need to be altered when this therapy with systemic methylprednisolone is started or stopped.

3. The loss of potassium caused by methylprednisolone can lead to serious side effects in individuals taking digoxin. Thiazide diuretics (water pills) can increase the potassium loss caused by methylprednisolone.

4. Phenobarbital, phenytoin, rifampin, and ephedrine can increase the elimination of methylprednisolone from the body, thereby decreasing its effectiveness.

5. Oral contraceptives (birth control pills) and estrogen-containing drugs may decrease the elimination of this medication from the body, which can lead to an increase in side effects.

6. Methylprednisolone can increase the elimination of aspirin and isoniazid, thereby decreasing the effectiveness of these two medications.

7. Cholestyramine and colestipol can prevent this medication's absorption.

BE SURE TO TELL YOUR DOCTOR about any medications you are currently taking, especially any of those listed above.

WARNINGS

• Tell your doctor about reactions you have had to any medications, especially to methylprednisolone or other adrenocorticosteroids (such as betamethasone, cortisone, dexamethasone, hydrocortisone, paramethasone, prednisolone, prednisone, and triamcinolone).

• Tell your doctor if you now have or if you have ever had bone disease, diabetes mellitus, emotional instability, glaucoma, fungal infections, heart disease, high blood pressure, high cholesterol levels, myasthenia gravis, peptic ulcers, osteoporosis, thyroid disease, tuberculosis, ulcerative colitis, kidney disease, or liver disease.

• To help avoid potassium loss while using this drug, take your dose with a glass of fresh or frozen orange juice or eat a banana each day. The use of a salt substitute also helps to prevent potassium loss. Check with your doctor before using a salt substitute.

• If you are using this medication for longer than a week, you may need to have your dosage adjusted if you are subjected to stress, such as serious infections, injury, or surgery. Discuss this with your doctor.

• If you have been taking this drug for more than a week, do not stop taking it suddenly. If it is stopped suddenly, you may experience abdominal or back pain, dizziness, fainting, fever, muscle or joint pain, nausea, vomiting, shortness of breath, or extreme weakness. Your doctor may, therefore, want to reduce the dosage gradually. Never increase the dosage or take the drug for longer than the prescribed time, unless you first consult your doctor.

• While you are taking methylprednisolone, you should not be vaccinated or immunized. This medication decreases the effectiveness of vaccines and can lead to overwhelming infection if a live-virus vaccine is administered.

• Before having surgery or medical or dental treatment, be sure to tell your doctor or dentist about this drug.

• Because this drug can cause glaucoma and cataracts with long-term use, your doctor may want you to have your eyes examined by an ophthalmologist periodically during treatment.

• If you are taking this medication for prolonged periods, you should wear or carry a notice or identification card stating that you are taking an adrenocorticosteroid.

• This medication can raise blood-sugar levels in diabetic patients. Blood-sugar levels should, therefore, be monitored carefully with blood or urine tests when this medication is being taken.

• Some of these products contain the color additive FD&C Yellow No. 5 (tartrazine), which can cause allergic-type reactions in certain susceptible individuals.

• Be sure to tell your doctor if you are pregnant. This drug crosses the placenta. Although studies in humans have not been conducted, birth defects have been observed in the fetuses of animals that were given large doses of this type of drug during pregnancy. Also, tell your doctor if you are breast-feeding an infant. Small amounts of methylprednisolone are known to pass into breast milk and may cause growth suppression or a decrease in natural adrenocorticosteroid production in the nursing infant.

---

metoclopramide

BRAND NAMES (Manufacturers)

Maxolon (SmithKline Beecham)
metoclopramide (various manufacturers)

Octamide (Adria)
Reglan (Robins)

TYPE OF DRUG

Dopamine antagonist and antiemetic

INGREDIENT

metoclopramide

DOSAGE FORMS

Tablets (5 mg and 10 mg)
Oral concentrate (10 mg per 5-ml spoonful)
Oral syrup (5 mg per 5-ml spoonful)

STORAGE

Metoclopramide tablets and oral syrup should be stored at room temperature in tightly closed containers. Do not freeze the syrup form of this medication.

USES

This medication is used to relieve the symptoms associated with diabetic gastric stasis or gastric reflux and to prevent nausea and vomiting. Metoclopramide acts directly on the vomiting center in the brain to prevent nausea and vomiting. It also increases the movement of the stomach and intestines.

TREATMENT

To obtain the best results from treatment, you should take metoclopramide tablets or syrup 30 minutes before a meal and at bedtime.

Each dose of the syrup should be measured carefully with a specially designed 5-ml measuring spoon. An ordinary kitchen teaspoon is not accurate enough.

If you miss a dose of this medication, take the missed dose as soon as possible, unless it is almost time for the next dose. In that case, do not take the missed dose at all; just return to your regular dosing schedule. Do not double the next dose.

SIDE EFFECTS

Minor. Diarrhea, dizziness, drowsiness, dry mouth, fatigue, headache, insomnia, nausea, restlessness, or weakness. These side effects should disappear as your body adjusts to the medication.

If you feel dizzy or light-headed, sit or lie down for a while; stand up slowly; and be careful on stairs.

To relieve mouth dryness, chew sugarless gum or suck on ice chips or a piece of hard candy.

Major. Tell your doctor about any side effects that are persistent or particularly bothersome. IT IS ESPECIALLY IMPORTANT TO TELL YOUR DOCTOR about anxiety; confusion; depression; disorientation; involuntary movements of the eyes, face, or limbs; muscle spasms; rash; or trembling of the hands.

INTERACTIONS

Metoclopramide interacts with several types of drugs:

1. Concurrent use of metoclopramide with other central nervous system depressants (such as alcohol, antihistamines, barbiturates, muscle relaxants, narcotics, pain medications, phenothiazine tranquilizers, benzodiazepine tranquilizers, and sleeping medications) or with tricyclic antidepressants can cause extreme drowsiness.

2. Narcotic analgesics may block the effectiveness of metoclopramide.

3. Metoclopramide can block the effectiveness of bromocriptine. It can also decrease the absorption of cimetidine and digoxin from the gastrointestinal tract, decreasing their effectiveness.

4. Metoclopramide can increase the absorption of acetaminophen, tetracycline, levodopa, and alcohol.

5. Diabetic patients should know that dosage requirements of insulin may change when metoclopramide is being taken.

Before starting to take metoclopramide, BE SURE TO TELL YOUR DOCTOR about any medications you are currently taking, especially any of those drugs that are listed above.

WARNINGS

• Tell your doctor about unusual or allergic reactions you have had to any medications, especially to metoclopramide, procaine, or procainamide.

• Before starting to take metoclopramide, be sure to tell your doctor if you now have or if you have ever had epilepsy, kidney disease, liver disease, intestinal bleeding or blockage, Parkinson's disease, or pheochromocytoma.

• If this drug makes you dizzy or drowsy, do not take part in any activities that require mental alertness, such as driving an automobile or operating potentially dangerous machinery or equipement.

• Be sure to tell your doctor if you are pregnant. Extensive studies in women during pregnancy have not been conducted. Also, tell your doctor if you are breast-feeding an infant. Metoclopramide passes into breast milk.

---

metoprolol

BRAND NAME (Manufacturer)

Lopressor (Geigy)

TYPE OF DRUG

Beta-adrenergic blocking agent

INGREDIENT

metoprolol

DOSAGE FORM

Tablets (50 mg and 100 mg)

STORAGE

Metoprolol should be stored at room temperature in a tightly closed, light-resistant container.

USES

Metoprolol is used to treat high blood pressure and angina (chest pain) and to prevent additional heart attacks in heart attack patients. Metoprolol belongs to a group of medicines known as beta-adrenergic blocking agents or, as they are more commonly known, beta blockers. These drugs work by controlling nerve impulses along certain nerve pathways.

TREATMENT

Metoprolol can be taken with a glass of water, with meals, immediately following meals, or on an empty stomach, depending on your doctor's instructions. Try to take the medication at the same time(s) each day.

Try not to miss any doses of this medicine. If you do miss a dose of the medication, take the missed dose as soon as possible. However, if the next scheduled dose is within eight hours (if you are taking this medicine only once a day) or within four hours (if you are taking this medicine more than once a day), do not take the missed dose of the medication at all; just return to your regular dosing schedule. Do not double the next dose of the medication.

It is important to remember that metoprolol does not cure high blood pressure, but it will help to control the condition as long as you continue to take it.

SIDE EFFECTS

Minor. Anxiety; cold hands or feet (due to decreased blood circulation to the skin, fingers, and toes); constipation; decreased sexual ability; diarrhea; difficulty in sleeping; drowsiness; dryness of the eyes, mouth, and skin; headache; nausea; nervousness; stomach discomfort; tiredness; or weakness. These side effects should disappear during treatment, as your body adjusts to the medicine.

If you are extra-sensitive to the cold, be sure to dress warmly during cold weather.

To relieve constipation, increase the amount of fiber in your diet (fresh fruits and vegetables, salads, bran, and whole-grain breads) and exercise more (unless your doctor directs you to do otherwise).

Plain, nonmedicated eye drops (artificial tears) may help to relieve eye dryness.

Chew sugarless gum or suck on ice chips or a piece of hard candy to relieve mouth or throat dryness.

Major. Tell your doctor about any side effects that you are experiencing that are persistent or particularly bothersome. IT IS ESPECIALLY IMPORTANT TO TELL YOUR DOCTOR about breathing difficulty or wheezing, confusion, dizziness, fever and sore throat, hair loss, hallucinations, light-headedness, mental depression, nightmares, numbness or tingling of the fingers or toes, rapid weight gain (three to five pounds within a week), reduced alertness, skin rash, swelling, or any unusual bleeding or bruising.

INTERACTIONS

Metoprolol interacts with several other types of medications:

1. Indomethacin, aspirin, or other salicylates may decrease the blood-pressure-lowering effects of beta blockers.
2. Concurrent use of beta blockers and calcium channel blockers or disopyramide can lead to heart failure or very low blood pressure.
3. Cimetidine and oral contraceptives (birth control pills) can increase the blood concentrations of metoprolol, which can result in greater side effects.
4. Alcohol, barbiturates, and rifampin can decrease the effectiveness of metoprolol.
5. Side effects may be increased if beta blockers are taken with clonidine, digoxin, epinephrine, phenylephrine, phenylpropanolamine, phenothiazine tranquilizers, prazosin, or monoamine oxidase (MAO) inhibitors. At least 14 days should separate the use of a beta blocker and the use of an MAO inhibitor.
6. Beta blockers may antagonize (work against) the effects of theophylline, aminophylline, albuterol, isoproterenol, metaproterenol, and terbutaline.
7. Beta blockers can also interact with insulin or oral antidiabetic agents, raising or lowering blood-sugar levels and masking the symptoms of low blood sugar.
8. The action of beta blockers may be increased if they are used with chlorpromazine, furosemide, or hydralazine, which may have a negative effect.

BE SURE TO TELL YOUR DOCTOR about any medications you are currently taking, especially any listed above.

WARNINGS

• Tell your doctor if you have ever had unusual or allergic reactions to any drugs, especially to metoprolol or any other beta blocker (acebutolol, atenolol, carteolol, esmolol, labetalol, nadolol, penbutolol, pindolol, propranolol, or timolol).

• Tell your doctor if you now have or have ever had allergies, asthma, hay fever, eczema, slow heartbeat, bronchitis, diabetes mellitus, emphysema, heart or blood-vessel disease, kidney disease, liver disease, thyroid disease, or poor circulation in the fingers or toes.

• You may want to check your pulse while taking this medication. If your pulse is much slower than your usual rate (or if it is less than 50 beats per minute), check with your doctor. A pulse rate that is too slow may cause circulation problems.

• This medicine may affect your body's response to exercise. Make sure you discuss with your doctor a safe amount of exercise for your medical condition.

• It is important that you do not stop taking this medicine without first checking with your doctor. Some conditions may become worse when the medicine is stopped suddenly, and the danger of a heart attack is increased in some patients. Your doctor may want you to reduce gradually the amount of medicine you take before stopping completely to minimize the potential risks. Make sure that you have enough medicine on hand to last through vacations, holidays, and weekends.

• Before having surgery or any other medical or dental treatment, tell your doctor or dentist that you are taking metoprolol.

• Metoprolol can cause dizziness, drowsiness, light-headedness, or decreased alertness. Exercise caution while driving a car or using any potentially dangerous machinery.

• While taking this medicine, do not use any over-the-counter (nonprescription) allergy, asthma, cough, cold, sinus, or diet preparation without first checking with your pharmacist or doctor. Some of these medicines can result in high blood pressure when taken at the same time as a beta blocker.

• Be sure to tell your doctor if you are pregnant. Animal studies have shown that some beta blockers, when used in very high doses, can cause problems in pregnancy. Adequate studies have not been conducted in humans, but there has been some association between beta blockers used during pregnancy and low birth weight, as well as breathing problems and slow heart rate in newborn infants. However, other reports have shown no effects on newborn infants. Also, tell your doctor if you are breast-feeding an infant. Although this medicine has not been shown to cause problems in breast-fed infants, some of the medicine may pass into breast milk, so caution is warranted.

---

metronidazole

BRAND NAMES (Manufacturers)
Flagyl (Searle)
MetroGel (Curatek)
metronidazole (various manufacturers)
Protostat (Ortho)
TYPE OF DRUG
Antibiotic and antiparasitic
INGREDIENT
metronidazole
DOSAGE FORMS
Tablets (250 mg and 500 mg)
Topical gel (0.75%)
STORAGE
Metronidazole should be stored at room temperature in a tightly closed, light-resistant container. The topical gel form of this medication should never be frozen.

USES

Metronidazole is used to treat a wide variety of infections, including infections of the vagina, urinary tract, lower respiratory tract, bones, joints, intestinal tract, and skin. It is also used topically to treat acne rosacea. It acts by killing bacteria or parasites.

TREATMENT

In order to avoid stomach irritation, you should take metronidazole with food or with a full glass of water or milk (unless your doctor directs you to do otherwise).

Metronidazole works best when the level of medicine in your bloodstream is kept constant. It is best, therefore, to take the doses at evenly spaced intervals day and night. For example, if you are to take three doses a day, the doses should be spaced eight hours apart.

Try not to miss any doses of this medication. If you do miss a dose, take the missed dose as soon as possible, unless it is almost time for the next dose. In that case, do not take the missed dose at all; just return to your regular dosing schedule. Do not double the next dose.

It is important to continue to take this medication for the entire time prescribed by your doctor (usually seven to 14 days), even if the symptoms disappear before the end of that period. If you stop taking the drug too soon, resistant bacteria and parasites are given a chance to continue growing, and the infection could recur.

SIDE EFFECTS

Minor. Abdominal cramps, constipation, decreased sexual interest, diarrhea, dizziness, dry mouth, headache, insomnia, irritability, joint pain, loss of appetite, metallic taste in the mouth, nasal congestion, nausea, restlessness, or vomiting. These side effects should disappear as your body adjusts to the medication.

To relieve constipation, increase the amount of fiber in your diet (fresh fruits and vegetables, salads, bran, and whole-grain breads), exercise, and drink more water (unless your doctor directs you to do otherwise).

If you feel dizzy, sit or lie down for a while; get up slowly from a sitting or lying position; and be careful on stairs.

To relieve mouth dryness, chew sugarless gum or suck on ice chips or a piece of hard candy.

Major. Tell your doctor about any side effects that are persistent or particularly bothersome. IT IS ESPECIALLY IMPORTANT TO TELL YOUR DOCTOR about confusion, convulsions, flushing, hives, itching, joint pain, loss of bladder control, mouth sores, numbness or tingling in the fingers or toes, rash, sense of pressure inside your abdomen, unexplained sore throat and fever, or unusual weakness. Also, if your symptoms of infection seem to be getting worse rather than improving, you should contact your doctor.

INTERACTIONS

Metronidazole interacts with several other types of medications:

1. Concurrent use of alcohol and metronidazole can lead to a severe reaction (abdominal cramps, nausea, vomiting, headache, and flushing), the severity of which is dependent upon the amount of alcohol ingested.
2. Concurrent use of disulfiram and metronidazole can lead to confusion.
3. The effects of oral anticoagulants (blood thinners, such as warfarin) may be increased by metronidazole, which can lead to bleeding complications.
4. Barbiturates can increase the breakdown of metronidazole, which can decrease its effectiveness.
5. Cimetidine can decrease the breakdown of metronidazole, which can increase the chance of side effects.

BE SURE TO TELL YOUR DOCTOR about any medications you are currently taking, especially any of those listed above.

WARNINGS

• Tell your doctor about unusual or allergic reactions you have had to any medications.
• Before starting to take this medication, be sure to tell your doctor if you now have or if you have ever had blood disorders, a central nervous system (brain or spinal cord) disease, or liver disease.
• When metronidazole is used to treat a vaginal infection, sexual partners should receive concurrent therapy in order to prevent reinfection. In addition, sexual intercourse should be avoided or condoms should be used until treatment is completed.
• This medication has been prescribed for your current infection only. Another infection later on, or one that someone else has, may require different drug therapy. Therefore, you should not give your medicine to other people or use it for other infections, unless your doctor specifically directs you to do so.

• If this drug makes you dizzy, avoid tasks that require alertness, such as driving a car or operating potentially dangerous machinery.
• Before having surgery or any other medical or dental treatment, be sure to tell your doctor or dentist that you are taking this medication.
• Be sure to tell your doctor if you are pregnant. Although metronidazole appears to be safe, it does cross the placenta, and extensive studies in pregnant women have not been conducted. Also, tell your doctor if you are breast-feeding an infant. Metronidazole passes into breast milk.

---

morphine

BRAND NAMES (Manufacturers)
morphine sulfate (various manufacturers)
MS Contin (Purdue-Frederick)
MSIR (Purdue-Frederick)
Oramorph SR (Roxane)
RMS (Upsher-Smith)
Roxanol (Roxane)
Roxanol SR (Roxane)
TYPE OF DRUG
Analgesic
INGREDIENT
morphine
DOSAGE FORMS
Capsules (15 mg and 30 mg)
Tablets (15 mg and 30 mg)
Sustained-release tablets (15 mg, 30 mg, 60 mg, and 100 mg)
Oral solution (10 mg and 20 mg per 5-ml spoonful, with 10% alcohol; 20 mg per ml; 100 mg per 5-ml spoonful)
Rectal suppositories (5 mg, 10 mg, 20 mg, and 30 mg)
STORAGE
Morphine tablets and oral solution should be stored at room temperature in tightly closed, light-resistant containers. The rectal suppositories should be stored in the refrigerator.

USES

Morphine is a narcotic analgesic that acts directly on the central nervous system (brain and spinal cord). It is used to relieve moderate to severe pain.

TREATMENT

In order to avoid stomach upset, you can take morphine with food or milk. This medication works most effectively if you take it at the onset of pain, rather than waiting until the pain becomes intense.

The solution form of this medication can be mixed with fruit juices to improve the taste. Measure each dose carefully with a specially designed 5-ml measuring spoon or with the dropper provided. An ordinary kitchen teaspoon is not accurate enough.

The sustained-release tablets should be swallowed whole. Chewing, crushing, or crumbling the tablets destroys their sustained-release activity and possibly increases the side effects.

To use the suppository form of this medication, remove the foil wrapper and moisten the suppository with water (if the suppository is too soft to insert, refrigerate it for half an hour or run cold water over it before removing the wrapper). Lie on your left side with your right knee bent. Push the suppository into the rectum, pointed end first. Lie still for a few minutes. Try to avoid having a bowel movement for at least an hour (to give the medication time to be absorbed).

If you are taking this drug on a regular schedule and you miss a dose, take the missed dose as soon as possible, unless it is almost time for your next dose. In that case, do not take the missed dose at all; just return to your regular dosing schedule. Do not double the next dose.

SIDE EFFECTS

Minor. Constipation, dizziness, drowsiness, dry mouth, false sense of well-being, flushing, light-headedness, loss of appetite, nausea, rash, or sweating. These side effects should disappear as your body adjusts to the medication.

If you are constipated, increase the amount of fiber in your diet (fresh fruits and vegetables, salads, bran, and whole-grain breads), exercise, and drink more water (unless your doctor directs you to do otherwise).

Chew sugarless gum or suck on ice chips to reduce mouth dryness.

If you feel dizzy or light-headed, sit or lie down for a while; get up from a sitting or lying position slowly; and be careful on stairs.

Major. Tell your doctor about any side effects that are persistent or particularly bothersome. IT IS ESPECIALLY IMPORTANT TO TELL YOUR DOCTOR about anxiety, difficulty in breathing, excitation, fainting, fatigue, painful or difficult urination, palpitations, restlessness, sore throat and fever, tremors, or weakness.

INTERACTIONS

Morphine will interact with several other types of medications:

1. Concurrent use of it with other central nervous system depressants (such as alcohol, antihistamines, barbiturates, benzodiazepine tranquilizers, muscle relaxants, and phenothiazine tranquilizers) or with tricyclic antidepressants can cause extreme drowsiness.
2. A monoamine oxidase (MAO) inhibitor taken within 14 days of this medication can lead to unpredictable and severe side effects.
3. The depressant effects of morphine can be dangerously increased by chloral hydrate, glutethimide, beta blockers, and furazolidone.
4. The combination of cimetidine and morphine can cause confusion, disorientation, and shortness of breath.

BE SURE TO TELL YOUR DOCTOR about any medications you are currently taking, especially any of those listed above.

WARNINGS

• Tell your doctor about unusual or allergic reactions you have had to any medications, especially to morphine or to other narcotic analgesics (such as codeine, hydrocodone, hydromorphone, meperidine, methadone, oxycodone, and propoxyphene).

• Tell your doctor if you now have or if you have ever had acute abdominal conditions, asthma, brain disease, colitis, epilepsy, gallstones or gallbladder disease, head injuries, heart disease, kidney disease, liver disease, lung disease, mental illness, emotional disorders, enlarged prostate gland, thyroid disease, or urethral stricture.

• If this drug makes you dizzy or drowsy, do not take part in any activity that requires attentiveness or alertness, such as driving a car or operating potentially dangerous machinery.

• Before having surgery or any other medical or dental treatment, be sure to tell your doctor or dentist that you are taking this medication.

• Morphine has the potential for abuse and must be used with caution. Usually, it should not be taken for longer than ten days (unless your doctor directs you to do so). Tolerance develops quickly; do not increase the dosage or stop taking the drug abruptly, unless you first consult your doctor. If you have been taking large amounts of this drug, or if you have been taking it for long periods of time, you may experience a withdrawal reaction (muscle aches, diarrhea, gooseflesh, runny nose, nausea, vomiting, shivering, trembling, stomach cramps, sleep disorders, irritability, weakness, excessive yawning, or sweating) when you stop taking it. Your doctor may, therefore, want to reduce the dosage gradually.

• Be sure to tell your doctor if you are pregnant. The effects of this medication during the early stages of pregnancy have not been thoroughly studied in humans. However, regular use of morphine in large doses during the later stages of pregnancy can result in addiction of the fetus, leading to withdrawal symptoms (irritability, excessive crying, tremors, fever, vomiting, diarrhea, sneezing, or excessive yawning) at birth. Also, tell your doctor if you are breast-feeding an infant. Small amounts of this medication may pass into breast milk and cause excessive drowsiness in the nursing infant.

---

naproxen

BRAND NAMES (Manufacturers)

Aleve* (Procter & Gamble)
Anaprox (Syntex)
Anaprox DS (Syntex)
Naprosyn (Syntex)
* Available over-the-counter (without a prescription)

TYPE OF DRUG

Nonsteroidal anti-inflammatory analgesic

INGREDIENT

naproxen (Naprosyn)
naproxen as the sodium salt (Aleve and Anaprox)

DOSAGE FORMS

Tablets (225 mg [Aleve]; 250 mg, 375 mg, and 500 mg [Naprosyn]; 275 mg and 550 mg [Anaprox])
Oral suspension (125 mg per 5-ml spoonful [Naprosyn])

STORAGE

This medication should be stored in a tightly closed container at room temperature, away from heat and direct sunlight.

USES

Naproxen is used to treat the inflammation (pain, swelling, and stiffness) of certain types of arthritis, gout, bursitis, and tendinitis. Naproxen is also used to treat painful menstruation. Naproxen has been shown to block the production of certain body chemicals, called prostaglandins, that may trigger pain. However, it is not yet fully understood how naproxen works.

TREATMENT

You should take this medication on an empty stomach 30 to 60 minutes before meals or two hours after meals, so that it gets into your bloodstream quickly. However, to decrease stomach irritation, your doctor may want you to take the medicine with food or antacids.

It is important to take naproxen on schedule and not to miss any doses. If you do miss a dose, take it as soon as possible, unless it is almost time for your next dose. In that case, do not take the missed dose at all; just return to your regular dosing schedule. Do not double the next dose.

If you are taking naproxen to relieve arthritis, you must take it regularly, as directed by your doctor. It may take up to four weeks before you feel the full benefits of this medication. This medication does not cure arthritis, but it will help to relieve the condition as long as you continue to take it.

SIDE EFFECTS

Minor. Bloating, constipation, diarrhea, difficulty in sleeping, dizziness, drowsiness, headache, heartburn, indigestion, light-headedness, loss of appetite, nausea, nervousness, soreness of the mouth, unusual sweating, and vomiting. As your body adjusts to the medication, these side effects should disappear.

To relieve constipation, increase the amount of fiber in your diet (fresh fruits and vegetables, salads, bran, and whole-grain breads), exercise, and drink more water (unless your doctor directs you to do otherwise).

If you become dizzy, sit or lie down for a while; get up slowly from a sitting or reclining position; and be careful on stairs.

Major. Tell your doctor about any side effects that are persistent or particularly bothersome. IT IS ESPECIALLY IMPORTANT TO TELL YOUR DOCTOR about bloody or black, tarry stools; blurred vision; confusion; depression; palpitations; ringing or buzzing in the ears or a problem with hearing; shortness of breath or wheezing; skin rash, hives, or itching; stomach pain; sudden decrease in amount of urine; swelling of the feet; tightness in the chest; unexplained sore throat and fever; unusual bleeding or bruising; unusual fatigue or weakness; unusual weight gain; or yellowing of the eyes or skin.

INTERACTIONS

Naproxen interacts with several other types of medications:

1. Concurrent use of anticoagulants (blood thinners, such as warfarin) can lead to an increase in bleeding complications.
2. Aspirin, salicylates, or other anti-inflammatory medications can cause increased stomach irritation when used concurrently with naproxen.
3. Naproxen can decrease the elimination of lithium and methotrexate from the body, resulting in possible toxicity from these medications.
4. Naproxen may interfere with the blood-pressure-lowering effects of beta-blocking medications (such as acebutolol, atenolol, betaxolol, carteolol, esmolol, labetalol, metoprolol, nadolol, penbutolol, pindolol, propranolol, and timolol).
5. This medication can also interfere with the diuretic effects of furosemide and thiazide-type diuretics.
6. Probenecid can increase the amount of naproxen in the bloodstream when both drugs are being taken.

Before starting to take this medication, BE SURE TO TELL YOUR DOCTOR about any medications you are currently taking, especially any of those medications listed above.

WARNINGS

• Before you take this medication, it is important to tell your doctor if you have ever had unusual or allergic reactions to any medications, especially to naproxen or any of the other chemically related drugs (including aspirin, other salicylates, carprofen, diclofenac, diflunisal, fenoprofen, flurbiprofen, indomethacin, ketoprofen, meclofenamate, mefenamic acid, oxyphenbutazone, phenylbutazone, piroxicam, sulindac, or tolmetin).
• Before taking this medication, it is important to tell your doctor if you now have or if you have ever had bleeding problems, colitis, stomach ulcers or other stomach problems, asthma, epilepsy, heart disease, high blood pressure, kidney disease, liver disease, mental illness, or Parkinson's disease.
• If naproxen makes you dizzy or drowsy, do not take part in any activity that requires alertness, such as driving a car or operating potentially dangerous machinery.
• Because this drug can prolong your bleeding time, it is important to tell your doctor or dentist that you are taking this drug before having surgery or any other medical or dental treatment.
• Stomach problems are more likely to occur if you take aspirin regularly or drink alcohol while being treated with this medication. You should avoid taking frequent doses of aspirin or drinking alcohol while undergoing treatment with this medication (unless your doctor tells you otherwise).
• Be sure to tell your doctor if you are pregnant. Naproxen analgesic may cause unwanted effects on the heart or blood flow of the fetus. Studies in animals have shown that taking naproxen late in pregnancy may increase the length of pregnancy, prolong labor, or cause other problems during delivery. Also, be sure to tell your doctor if you are currently breast-feeding an infant. Small amounts of this medication have been shown to pass into breast milk.

---

nifedipine

BRAND NAMES (Manufacturers)
Adalat (Miles)
Procardia (Pfizer)
Procardia XL (Pfizer)
TYPE OF DRUG
Antianginal
INGREDIENT
nifedipine
DOSAGE FORMS
Capsules (10 mg and 20 mg)
Substained-release tablets (30 mg, 60 mg, and 90 mg)
STORAGE
Nifedipine capsules should be stored at room temperature in a tightly closed, light-resistant container.

USES

This medication is used to treat various types of angina (chest pain). Nifedipine belongs to a group of drugs known as calcium channel blockers. By blocking calcium, nifedipine relaxes the blood vessels of the heart and reduces the oxygen needs of the heart muscle.

TREATMENT

Nifedipine should be taken on an empty stomach with a full glass of water one hour before or two hours after a meal (unless your doctor directs you to do otherwise). These capsules should be swallowed whole.

If you miss a dose of this medication, take the missed dose as soon as possible, unless it is within two hours of your next scheduled dose. In that case, do not take the missed dose at all; just return to your regular dosing schedule. Do not double the next dose.

SIDE EFFECTS

Minor. Bloating, cough, dizziness, flushing, gas, giddiness, headache, heartburn, heat sensation, nasal congestion, nausea, nervousness, sleep disturbances, sweating, or weakness. These side effects should disappear as your body adjusts to the medication.

If you feel dizzy or light-headed, sit or lie down for a while; get up slowly from a sitting or reclining position; and be careful on stairs. To avoid dizziness or light-headedness when you stand, contract and relax the muscles of your legs for a few moments before rising. Do this by pushing one foot against the floor while raising the other foot slightly, alternating feet so that you are "pumping" your legs in a pedaling motion.
Major. Tell your doctor about any side effects that are persistent or particularly bothersome. IT IS ESPECIALLY IMPORTANT TO TELL YOUR DOCTOR about blurred vision, chills, confusion, difficulty in breathing, fainting, fever, fluid retention, impotence, mood changes, muscle cramps, palpitations, rash, sore throat, or tremors.

INTERACTIONS

Nifedipine interacts with several other types of medications:

1. Nifedipine can increase the active blood levels of digoxin, warfarin, phenytoin, and quinine, which can lead to an increase in side effects.
2. The combination of nifedipine and beta blockers (acebutolol, atenolol, betaxolol, carteolol, esmolol, labetalol, metoprolol, nadolol, penbutolol, pindolol, propranolol, or timolol) can lead to a severe drop in blood pressure.
3. Nifedipine can lower quinidine blood levels, which can decrease its effectiveness.
4. Cimetidine can decrease the breakdown of nifedipine in the body, which can increase the risk of side effects.

Before starting to take nifedipine, BE SURE TO TELL YOUR DOCTOR about any medications you are currently taking, especially any of those listed above.

WARNINGS

- Tell your doctor about unusual or allergic reactions you have had to any medications, especially to nifedipine.
- Tell your doctor if you have ever had heart disease, kidney disease, low blood pressure, or liver disease.
- If this drug makes you dizzy or drowsy, do not take part in any activity that requires alertness, such as driving a car or operating potentially dangerous machinery.
- Before having surgery or any other medical or dental treatment, tell your doctor or dentist you are taking this drug.
- Do not stop taking this medication unless you first consult your doctor. Stopping this medication abruptly may lead to severe chest pain. Your doctor may, therefore, want to decrease your dosage gradually.
- It is important sure to tell your doctor if you are pregnant. Nifedipine has been shown to cause birth defects in the offspring of animals that received large doses of it during pregnancy. This medication has not been studied in pregnant women. Also, tell your doctor if you are breast-feeding an infant. It is not known whether nifedipine passes into breast milk.

---

nitroglycerin

BRAND NAMES (Manufacturers)
Nitrogard (Forest)
nitroglycerin (various manufacturers)
Nitroglyn (Kenwood)
Nitrong (Winthrop)
Nitrostat (Parke-Davis)
Nitro-Time (Time-Caps Labs)
TYPE OF DRUG
Antianginal
INGREDIENT
nitroglycerin
DOSAGE FORMS
Sustained-release tablets (2.6 mg and 6.5 mg)
Sustained-release capsules (2.5 mg, 6.5 mg, 9 mg, and 13 mg)
Sublingual tablets (0.15 mg, 0.3 mg, 0.4 mg, and 0.6 mg)
Buccal tablets, controlled release (1 mg, 2 mg, and 3 mg)
Oral spray (0.4 mg per dose)
STORAGE
Nitroglycerin tablets, capsules, and oral spray should be stored in a tightly capped bottle in a cool, dry place.

The sublingual tablets should be kept in their original glass container. A small, temporary supply of tablets can also be stored in a stainless-steel container that is now available. The pendant-type container, which can be worn around your neck, is a convenient storage place for an emergency supply. Never store them in the refrigerator or the bathroom medicine cabinet, because the drug may lose its potency.

USES

This medication is used to treat angina (chest pain). Nitroglycerin is a vasodilator, which relaxes the muscles of the blood vessels, causing an increase in the oxygen supply to the heart.

The oral tablets and capsules do not act quickly; they are used to prevent chest pain. The sublingual tablets and oral spray act quickly and can be used to relieve chest pain after it has started.

TREATMENT

You should take the sustained-release tablets or capsules with a full glass of water on an empty stomach one hour before or two hours after a meal. The tablets and capsules should be swallowed whole. Chewing, crushing, or breaking them destroys their sustained-release activity and possibly increases the side effects.

NEVER chew or swallow the sublingual or buccal tablets. The sublingual tablet and oral spray forms of the drug are absorbed directly through the lining of the mouth. The sublingual tablet should be allowed to dissolve under the tongue or against the cheek.

To use the spray, remove the plastic cover on the container. Then, without shaking the container, spray the medication onto or under the tongue. Try not to inhale the spray. Close your mouth after each spray, and try to avoid swallowing right away. Nitroglycerin spray loses its effectiveness if it is swallowed.

Take one tablet or one or two spray doses at the first sign of chest pain. Sit down while you are waiting for the medicine to take effect. Do not eat, drink, or smoke while nitroglycerin is in your mouth. Try not to swallow while nitroglycerin is dissolving, and do not rinse your mouth afterward. Sublingual nitroglycerin or nitroglycerin spray should start working in one to three minutes. If there is no relief, take another tablet in five minutes. IF YOU TAKE THREE TABLETS OR THREE SPRAY DOSES WITHOUT ANY SIGN OF IMPROVEMENT, CALL A DOCTOR IMMEDIATELY OR GO TO A HOSPITAL EMERGENCY ROOM. As a preventive measure, take a nitroglycerin sublingual tablet or a spray dose five or ten minutes before heavy exercise, exposure to high altitudes or extreme cold, or any other potentially stressful situation. Be sure to carry some nitroglycerin sublingual tablets or oral spray with you at ALL times.

The buccal tablet should be placed between the upper lip and the gum on either side of the front teeth or between the cheek and the gum. The tablet is held in place by a sticky gel seal that develops once the tablet is in contact with saliva. If you wear dentures, the tablet can be placed anywhere between the cheek and the gum. Avoid drinking hot liquids or touching the tablet with your tongue. This can cause the tablet to dissolve faster and could increase the risk of side effects. If the buccal tablet is swallowed by mistake, replace it with another tablet. Nitroglycerin buccal tablets lose their effectiveness when swallowed. Try not to take the buccal tablet at bedtime in order to avoid inadvertently swallowing and choking on the tablet while you are sleeping.

If you miss a dose of the sustained-release tablets or capsules, take the missed dose as soon as possible, unless it is more than halfway through the interval between doses. In that case, do not take the missed dose at all; just return to your regular dosing schedule. Do not double the next dose.

SIDE EFFECTS

Minor. Dizziness, flushing of the face, headache, lightheadedness, nausea, vomiting, or weakness. These side effects should disappear as your body adjusts to the medication.

If you feel dizzy or light-headed, sit or lie down for a while; get up slowly from a sitting or reclining position; and be careful on stairs. To avoid dizziness or light-headedness when you stand, contract and relax the muscles of your legs for a few moments before rising. Do this by pushing one foot against the floor while raising the other foot slightly, alternating feet so that you are "pumping" your legs in a pedaling motion.

Acetaminophen may help to relieve headaches caused by this medication.

Major. Tell your doctor about any side effects that are persistent or particularly bothersome. IT IS ESPECIALLY IMPORTANT TO TELL YOUR DOCTOR about diarrhea, fainting, palpitations, rash, or sweating.

INTERACTIONS

Nitroglycerin can interact with other types of medications:

1. The combination of alcohol and nitroglycerin can lead to dizziness and fainting.

2. Nitroglycerin can increase the side effects of the tricyclic antidepressants.

Before starting to take nitroglycerin, BE SURE TO TELL YOUR DOCTOR about any medications you are currently taking, especially tricyclic antidepressants (such as imipramine, desipramine, amitriptyline, and doxepin).

WARNINGS

• Tell your doctor about unusual or allergic reactions you have had to any medications, especially to nitroglycerin or isosorbide dinitrate.
• Before starting to take this medication, be sure to tell your doctor if you now have or if you have ever had anemia, glaucoma, a head injury, low blood pressure, or thyroid disease or if you have recently had a heart attack.
• If this drug makes you dizzy or light-headed, do not take part in any activity that requires alertness, such as driving a car or operating potentially dangerous machinery.
• Before surgery or other medical or dental treatment, tell your doctor or dentist you are taking this drug.
• Tolerance may develop to this medication within one to three months. If it seems to lose its effectiveness, contact your doctor.
• You should not discontinue use of nitroglycerin (if you have been taking it on a regular basis) unless you first consult your doctor. Stopping the drug abruptly may lead to further chest pain. Your doctor may, therefore, want to decrease your dosage gradually.
• If you have frequent diarrhea, you may not be absorbing the sustained-release form of this medication. Discuss this with your doctor.
• While taking this medication, do not take any over-the-counter (nonprescription) asthma, allergy, sinus, cough, cold, or diet preparations unless you first check with your doctor or pharmacist. Some of these drugs decrease the effectiveness of nitroglycerin.
• The cotton plug should be removed when the bottle is first opened; it should not be replaced. The cotton plug absorbs some of the medication, decreasing its potency.
• Nitroglycerin is highly flammable. Do not use it in places where it might be ignited.
• Be sure to tell your doctor if you are pregnant. Although the systemic form of nitroglycerin appears to be safe, extensive studies in pregnant women have not been conducted. Also, tell your doctor if you are breast-feeding an infant. It is not known whether nitroglycerin passes into breast milk.

---

ofloxacin

BRAND NAME (Manufacturer)
Floxin (McNeil)
TYPE OF DRUG
Quinolone antibiotic
INGREDIENT
ofloxacin
DOSAGE FORM
Tablets (200 mg, 300 mg, and 400 mg)
STORAGE
This medication should be stored in a tightly closed container at room temperature, away from heat and direct sunlight.

USES

Ofloxacin is an antibiotic that is used to treat skin and bone infections as well as infections of the gastrointestinal and urinary tracts. It is also used to treat pneumonia. Ofloxacin acts by severely injuring the cell walls of the infecting bacteria, thereby preventing them from growing and multiplying. This medication kills susceptible bacteria, but it is not effective against viruses, parasites, or fungi.

TREATMENT

Ofloxacin should be taken exactly as prescribed by your doctor, even if your symptoms improve. If you stop taking this drug too soon, resistant bacteria are given the chance to grow and the infection may recur. Ofloxacin is usually taken twice a day for seven to 14 days, although it may be given for longer periods of time. This medication can be taken with meals or a full glass of water if stomach upset occurs.

If you miss a dose of ofloxacin, take the missed dose as soon as possible. If it is almost time for your next dose, take the missed dose and space the following dose halfway through the regular interval between doses, then return to your regular schedule. Try not to skip any doses.

SIDE EFFECTS

Minor. Abdominal pain, diarrhea, dizziness, light-headedness, nausea, or vomiting. These side effects should disappear as your body adjusts to the drug.

Major. Tell your doctor about any side effects that are persistent or particularly bothersome. IT IS ESPECIALLY IMPORTANT TO TELL YOUR DOCTOR about agitation, headache, restlessness, severe diarrhea (which may be watery or contain blood or pus), or skin rash. If your symptoms of infection seem to be getting worse rather than improving, contact your doctor.

INTERACTIONS

Ofloxacin interacts with several other types of medications:

1. Probenecid can increase the blood concentrations of this drug.

2. Ofloxacin may increase the effects of theophylline or oral anticoagulants.

3. Ofloxacin may make you more susceptible to the effects of caffeine (anxiety, insomnia, palpitations). The use of large amounts of coffee, tea, or other caffeine-containing products should be avoided when taking this medication.

BE SURE TO TELL YOUR DOCTOR about any medications you are currently taking.

WARNINGS

• Tell your doctor about any unusual or allergic reactions you have had to any medications, especially to ofloxacin or ciprofloxacin.

• Tell your doctor if you now have or if you have ever had liver disease, kidney disease, or epilepsy.

• Avoid taking antacids within four hours of taking a dose of this medication.

• Be sure to tell your doctor if you are pregnant. Studies in pregnant women have not been conducted. However, lameness has occurred in the mature offspring of animals that received large doses of ofloxacin during pregnancy. Also, tell your doctor if you are breast-feeding an infant. It is not yet known if ofloxacin can be passed into breast milk.

---

omeprazole

BRAND NAME (Manufacturer)
Prilosec (MSD)

TYPE OF DRUG
Gastric-acid-secretion inhibitor

INGREDIENT
omeprazole

DOSAGE FORM
Delayed-release capsules (20 mg)

STORAGE
Omeprazole should be stored at room temperature in a tightly closed container.

USES

Omeprazole is prescribed to treat peptic ulcer disease, gastroesophageal reflux, and hypersecretory syndromes. This medication suppresses stomach-acid secretion.

TREATMENT

Omeprazole capsules should not be opened, chewed, or crushed. They should be taken with a glass of water on an empty stomach. It is best to take the dose one hour before meals or two hours after meals.

Try to take the medication at the same time(s) each day. If you miss a dose of the medication, take the missed dose as soon as possible, then return to your regular dosing schedule. If it is almost time for the next dose, however, skip the one you missed and return to your regular schedule. Do not double the next dose of the medication (unless your doctor directs you to do so).

It is important that you take this medication for as long as prescribed by your doctor.

SIDE EFFECTS

Minor. Abdominal pain, burning sensation in mouth, constipation, diarrhea, dizziness, dry mouth, fatigue, headache, or palpitations.

To relieve constipation while you are being treated with this medication, increase the amount of fiber in your diet (fresh fruits and vegetables, salads, bran, and whole-grain breads), exercise, and drink more water (unless your doctor directs you to do otherwise).

To avoid dizziness when you stand, contract and relax the muscles of your legs for a few moments before rising. Do this by pushing one foot against the floor while raising the other foot slightly, alternating feet so that you are "pumping" your legs in a pedaling motion.

To relieve dry mouth, chew sugarless gum or suck on ice chips or a piece of hard candy.

Major. Tell your doctor about any side effects that are persistent or particularly bothersome. IT IS ESPECIALLY IMPORTANT TO TELL YOUR DOCTOR about itching, numbness or tingling of fingers or toes, rash, or yellowing of the eyes and skin.

INTERACTIONS

Omeprazole may increase the effects of diazepam, warfarin, and phenytoin.

BE SURE TO TELL YOUR DOCTOR about any medications you are currently taking, especially any of the ones listed above.

WARNINGS

• Be sure to tell your doctor about unusual reactions you have had to any drugs, especially to omeprazole.

• Tell your doctor if you now have or if you have ever had thyroid disease, liver disease, Addison's disease, or Cushing's disease.
• This medication may cause dizziness and light-headedness, so use caution while driving a car or operating potentially dangerous equipment.
• Long-term and high-dose treatment with omeprazole has been associated with higher incidences of gastric tumors. Consult your doctor if you need to take high doses of omeprazole for a long time.
• Be sure to tell your doctor if you are pregnant. Adequate human studies have not been conducted with omeprazole. Also, be sure to tell your doctor if you are breast-feeding an infant.

---

paroxetine

BRAND NAME (Manufacturer)
Paxil (SmithKline Beecham)
TYPE OF DRUG
Cyclic antidepressant
INGREDIENT
paroxetine
DOSAGE FORM
Tablets (20 mg and 30 mg)
STORAGE
This medication should be stored in a tightly closed container at room temperature, away from heat and direct sunlight. Do not store in the bathroom. Heat or moisture can cause this medicine to break down.

USES

Paroxetine is used to treat the symptoms of mental depression. It increases the concentration of certain chemicals that are necessary for nerve transmission in the brain.

TREATMENT

This medication should be taken exactly as prescribed by your doctor. In order to avoid stomach irritation, take paroxetine with food or a full glass of water (unless your doctor directs you to do otherwise).

The effects of treatment with this medication may not become apparent for one to three weeks.

If you miss a dose of this medicine, it is not necessary to make up the missed dose. Skip that dose and continue at the next scheduled time. You should never take a double dose to make up for the one you missed.

SIDE EFFECTS

Minor. Agitation, changes in taste, constipation, decreased concentration, decreased sex drive, diarrhea, dizziness, drowsiness, dry mouth, fast heartbeat, flushing, frequent urination, headache, increased sweating, loss of appetite, nausea, stuffy nose, vision changes, weight gain or loss.

Dry mouth can be relieved by chewing sugarless gum or sucking on hard candy.

To relieve constipation, increase the amount of fiber in your diet (fresh fruits and vegetables, salads, bran, and whole-grain breads), exercise, and drink more water or other fluids (unless your doctor directs you to do otherwise).

To avoid dizziness when you stand, contract and relax the muscles in your legs for a few moments before rising to your feet.

Major. Tell your doctor about any side effects you experience that are persistent or particularly bothersome. IT IS ESPECIALLY IMPORTANT TO TELL YOUR DOCTOR about anxiety, chills or fever, convulsions (seizures), enlarged lymph glands (swelling under the jaw, in the armpits, or in the groin area), difficulty in breathing, joint or muscle pain, skin rash or hives, or swelling of the feet or lower legs.

INTERACTIONS

Paroxetine will interact with several other types of medications:

1. Extreme drowsiness can occur when this medication is taken with other central nervous system depressants (such as alcohol, antihistamines, barbiturates, benzodiazepine tranquilizers, muscle relaxants, narcotics, pain medications, phenothiazine tranquilizers, and sleeping medications) or with other antidepressants.

2. Paroxetine may increase the effects of oral anticoagulants (blood thinners, such as warfarin) and certain heart medications (such as digoxin).

3. Serious side effects may occur if a monoamine oxidase (MAO) inhibitor (such as furazolidone, isocarboxazid, pargyline, phenelzine, procarbazine, or tranylcypromine) is taken with paroxetine. At least 14 days should separate the use of paroxetine and the use of an MAO inhibitor.

4. Paroxetine can increase agitation, restlessness, and stomach irritation when taken with tryptophan.

Before taking paroxetine, BE SURE TO TELL YOUR DOCTOR about any medication you are taking, especially any of those listed above.

WARNINGS

• Tell your doctor immediately if you develop a skin rash or have hives while taking this medication or if you have ever had a reaction to paroxetine before.
• Tell your doctor if you have a history of alcoholism, if you ever had a heart attack, asthma, circulatory disease, difficulty in urinating, electroshock therapy, enlarged prostate gland, epilepsy, glaucoma, high blood pressure, intestinal problems, liver or kidney disease, mental illness, or thyroid disease.
• If this medication makes you drowsy or dizzy, do not take part in any activity that requires mental alertness, such as driving a car or operating dangerous equipment.
• Do not stop taking this medication suddenly. Abruptly stopping it can cause nausea, headache, stomach upset, or a worsening of your condition. Your doctor may want to reduce the dose gradually.
• Elderly individuals may be at greater risk for side effects. Use this drug cautiously and report any mental-status changes to your doctor immediately.
• The effects of this medication may be present for as long as five weeks after you stop taking it, so continue to observe all precautions during this period.

• Be sure to tell your doctor if you are pregnant. Although birth defects have not been documented in animal studies, it is not known if paroxetine is safe during pregnancy. It is not known if paroxetine passes into breast milk, so tell your doctor if you are breast-feeding an infant.

---

penicillin VK

BRAND NAMES (Manufacturers)
Beepen-VK (SmithKline Beecham)
Betapen-VK (Apothecon)
Ledercillin VK (Lederle)
penicillin VK (various manufacturers)
Pen-Vee K (Wyeth-Ayerst)
Robicillin VK (Robins)
Uticillin VK (Upjohn)
V-Cillin K (Lilly)
Veetids (Bristol-Myers Squibb)

TYPE OF DRUG
Penicillin antibiotic

INGREDIENT
penicillin potassium phenoxymethyl

DOSAGE FORMS
Tablets (125 mg, 250 mg, and 500 mg)
Oral solution (125 mg and 250 mg per 5-ml spoonful)

STORAGE
Penicillin VK tablets should be stored at room temperature in a tightly closed container. The oral solution should be stored in the refrigerator in a tightly closed container. Any unused portion of the solution should be discarded after 14 days because the drug loses its potency after that time. This medication should never be frozen.

USES

Penicillin VK is used to treat a wide variety of bacterial infections, including infections of the middle ear, the respiratory tract, and the urinary tract. It acts by severely injuring the cell membranes of infecting bacteria, thereby preventing them from growing and multiplying. Penicillin VK kills susceptible bacteria, but it is not effective against viruses, parasites, or fungi.

TREATMENT

Penicillin VK should be taken on an empty stomach or with a glass of water one hour before or two hours after a meal. This medication should never be taken with fruit juices or carbonated beverages because the acidity of these drinks destroys the drug in the stomach.

The oral solution should be measured carefully with a specially designed 5-ml measuring spoon. An ordinary kitchen teaspoon is not accurate enough.

Penicillin VK works best when the level of medicine in your bloodstream is kept constant. It is best, therefore, to take the doses at evenly spaced intervals day and night. For example, if you are taking four doses a day, the doses should be spaced six hours apart.

If you miss a dose of this medication, take the missed dose immediately. However, if you do not remember to take the missed dose until it is almost time for the next dose, take it; space the following dose about halfway through the regular interval between doses; then return to your regular dosing schedule. Try not to skip any doses.

It is important to continue to take this medication for the entire time prescribed by your doctor (usually a period of up to seven to 14 days), even if the symptoms of infection disappear before the end of that time. If you stop taking the drug too soon, resistant bacteria are given a chance to continue growing, and the infection could recur.

SIDE EFFECTS

Minor. Diarrhea, heartburn, nausea, or vomiting. These side effects should disappear as your body adjusts to the drug.

Major. Tell your doctor about any side effects that are persistent or particularly bothersome. IT IS ESPECIALLY IMPORTANT TO TELL YOUR DOCTOR about bloating, chills, cough, darkened tongue, difficulty in breathing, fever, irritation of the mouth, muscle aches, rash, rectal or vaginal itching, severe diarrhea, or sore throat. If the infection seems to be getting worse rather than improving, you should contact your physician.

INTERACTIONS

Penicillin VK will interact with several other types of medications:

1. Probenecid can increase the blood concentrations of this medication.

2. Oral neomycin may decrease the absorption of penicillin from the gastrointestinal tract.

3. Penicillin VK may decrease the effectiveness of oral contraceptives (birth control pills), and pregnancy could result. You should, therefore, use a different or additional form of birth control while taking this medication. Discuss this with your doctor.

BE SURE TO TELL YOUR DOCTOR about any medications you are currently taking, especially any of those listed above.

WARNINGS

• Tell your doctor about unusual or allergic reactions you have had to any medications, especially to penicillin or other penicillin antibiotics (such as ampicillin and amoxicillin), cephalosporin antibiotics, penicillamine, or griseofulvin.

• Tell your doctor if you now have or if you have ever had kidney disease, asthma, or allergies.

• This medication has been prescribed for your current infection only. Another infection later on, or one that someone else has, may require a different medicine. You should not give your medicine to other people or use it for other infections, unless your doctor specifically directs you to do so.

• Diabetics taking penicillin should know that this drug can cause a false-positive sugar reaction with a Clinitest urine glucose test. To avoid this problem while taking penicillin, you should switch to Clinistix or Tes-Tape to test your urine for sugar.

• Be sure to tell your doctor if you are pregnant. Although penicillin appears to be safe during pregnancy, extensive studies in humans have not been conducted. Also, tell your doctor if you are breast-feeding an infant. Small amounts of this medication pass into breast milk and may temporarily alter the bacterial balance in the intestinal tract of a nursing infant, resulting in diarrhea.

---

prazosin

BRAND NAMES (Manufacturers)
Minipress (Pfizer)
prazosin (various manufacturers)
TYPE OF DRUG
Antihypertensive
INGREDIENT
prazosin
DOSAGE FORM
Capsules (1 mg, 2 mg, 5 mg, and 10 mg)
STORAGE
Prazosin capsules should be stored at room temperature in a tightly closed, light-resistant container. This medication should not be refrigerated.

USES

Prazosin is used to treat high blood pressure. It is a vasodilator that relaxes the muscle tissue of the blood vessels, which in turn lowers blood pressure.

TREATMENT

To avoid stomach irritation, you can take prazosin with food or with a full glass of water or milk. In order to become accustomed to taking this medication, try to take it at the same time(s) each day. The first dose of this medication can cause fainting. Therefore, it is often recommended that this dose be taken at bedtime.

If you miss a dose of this medication, take the missed dose as soon as possible, unless it is almost time for the next dose. In that case, do not take the missed dose at all; just return to your regular dosing schedule. Do not double the next dose.

Prazosin does not cure high blood pressure, but it will help to control the condition as long as you continue to take the medication.

The effects of this medication may not become apparent for two weeks.

SIDE EFFECTS

Minor. Abdominal pain, constipation, diarrhea, dizziness, drowsiness, dry mouth, frequent urination, headache, impotence, nasal congestion, nausea, nervousness, sweating, tiredness, vomiting, or weakness. These side effects should disappear as your body adjusts to the medication.

To relieve constipation, increase the amount of fiber in your diet (fresh fruits and vegetables, salads, bran, and whole-grain breads), exercise, and drink more water (unless your doctor directs you to do otherwise).

To relieve mouth dryness, chew sugarless gum or suck on ice chips or a piece of hard candy.

If you feel dizzy or light-headed, sit or lie down for a while; get up slowly from a sitting or reclining position; and be careful on stairs. To avoid dizziness or light-headedness when you stand, contract and relax the muscles of your legs for a few moments before rising. Do this by pushing one foot against the floor while raising the other foot slightly, alternating feet so that you are "pumping" your legs in a pedaling motion.

Major. Tell your doctor about any side effects that are persistent or particularly bothersome. IT IS ESPECIALLY IMPORTANT TO TELL YOUR DOCTOR about blurred vision; chest pain; constant erection; depression; difficulty in breathing; difficulty in urinating; fainting; hallucinations; itching; loss of hair; nosebleeds; palpitations; rapid weight gain (three to five pounds within a week); rash; ringing in the ears; swelling of the feet, legs, or ankles; or tingling of the fingers or toes.

INTERACTIONS

Prazosin may possibly interact with other types of medications:

1. The combination of prazosin and alcohol or verapamil can lead to a severe drop in blood pressure and fainting.

2. The severity and duration of the blood-pressure-lowering effects of the first dose of prazosin may be enhanced by a beta blocker.

BE SURE TO TELL YOUR DOCTOR about any medications you are currently taking, especially those listed above.

WARNINGS

- Tell your doctor about unusual or allergic reactions you have had to any medications, especially to prazosin or terazosin.
- Before starting to take this medication, be sure to tell your doctor if you now have or if you have ever had angina (chest pain) or kidney disease.
- Because initial therapy with this drug may cause dizziness or fainting, your doctor will probably start you on a low dosage and increase the dosage gradually.
- If this drug makes you dizzy or drowsy or blurs your vision, do not take part in any activity that requires alertness, such as driving a car or operating potentially dangerous machinery.
- In order to avoid dizziness or fainting while taking this drug, try not to stand for long periods of time, avoid drinking excessive amounts of alcohol, and try not to get overheated (avoid exercising strenuously in hot weather and taking hot baths, showers, or saunas).
- Before taking any over-the-counter (nonprescription) sinus, allergy, asthma, cough, cold, or diet preparations, check with your doctor or pharmacist. Some of these products can cause an increase in blood pressure.
- Do not stop taking this medication unless you first check with your doctor. If you stop taking this drug you may experience a rise in blood pressure. Your doctor may, therefore, want to decrease your dosage gradually.
- Be sure to tell your doctor if you are pregnant. Although this drug appears to be safe, there have been only limited studies in pregnant women. Also, tell your doctor if you are breast-feeding an infant.

prednisone

BRAND NAMES (Manufacturers)
Deltasone (Upjohn)
Liquid Pred (Muro)
Meticorten (Schering)
Orasone (Solvay)
Panasol-S (Seatrace)
Prednicen-M (Central)
prednisone (various manufacturers)
TYPE OF DRUG
Adrenocorticosteroid hormone
INGREDIENT
prednisone
DOSAGE FORMS
Tablets (1 mg, 2.5 mg, 5 mg, 10 mg, 20 mg, 25 mg, and 50 mg)
Oral syrup (5 mg per 5-ml spoonful, with 5% alcohol)
Oral solution (5 mg per 5-ml spoonful, with 5% alcohol)
Oral intensol solution (5 mg per ml, with 30% alcohol)
STORAGE
Prednisone should be stored at room temperature (never frozen) in a tightly closed container.

USES

Your adrenal glands naturally produce certain cortisonelike chemicals. These chemicals are involved in various regulatory processes in the body (such as those involving fluid balance, temperature, and reaction to inflammation). Prednisone belongs to a group of drugs known as adrenocorticosteroids (or cortisonelike medications). It is used to treat a variety of disorders, including endocrine and rheumatic disorders; asthma; blood diseases; certain cancers; eye disorders; gastrointestinal disturbances, such as ulcerative colitis; respiratory diseases; and inflammations, such as arthritis, dermatitis, and poison ivy. How this drug acts to relieve these disorders is not completely understood.

TREATMENT

In order to prevent stomach irritation, you can take prednisone with food or milk.

If you are taking only one dose of this medication each day, try to take it before 9:00 A.M.

The oral syrup or solution form of this medication should be measured carefully with a specially designed dropper (intensol solution) or 5-ml measuring spoon. An ordinary kitchen teaspoon is not accurate enough for therapeutic purposes.

It is important to try not to miss any doses of prednisone. However, if you do miss a dose, follow these guidelines:

1. If you are taking it more than once a day, take the missed dose as soon as possible and return to your regular dosing schedule. If it is already time for the next dose, double it.
2. If you are taking this medication once a day, take the dose you missed as soon as possible, unless you don't remember until the next day. In that case, do not take the missed dose at all; just follow your regular dosing schedule. Do not double the next dose.
3. If you are taking this drug every other day, take it when you remember. If you missed the scheduled dose by a whole day, take it; then skip a day before you take the next dose. Do not double the dose.

If you miss more than one dose of prednisone, CONTACT YOUR DOCTOR.

SIDE EFFECTS

Minor. Dizziness, false sense of well-being, increased appetite, increased sweating, indigestion, menstrual irregularities, nausea, reddening of the skin on the face, restlessness, sleep disorders, or weight gain. These side effects should disappear as your body adjusts to the medication.

Major. Tell your doctor about any side effects that are persistent or particularly bothersome. IT IS ESPECIALLY IMPORTANT TO TELL YOUR DOCTOR about abdominal enlargement; abdominal pain; acne or other skin problems; back or rib pain; bloody or black, tarry stools; blurred vision; convulsions; eye pain; fever and sore throat; growth impairment (in children); headaches; impaired healing of wounds; increased thirst and urination; mental depression; mood changes; muscle wasting or weakness; rapid weight gain (three to five pounds within a week); rash; shortness of breath; thinning of the skin; unusual bruising or bleeding; or unusual feeling of weakness.

INTERACTIONS

Prednisone interacts with several other types of medications:

1. Alcohol, aspirin, and anti-inflammatory medications (such as diclofenac diflunisal, fenoprofen, flurbiprofen, ibuprofen, indomethacin, ketoprofen, meclofenamate, mefenamic acid, naproxen, piroxicam, sulindac, or tolmetin) aggravate the stomach problems that are common with this drug.
2. The dosage of oral anticoagulants (blood thinners, such as warfarin), oral antidiabetic drugs, or insulin may need to be adjusted when this medication is being taken.
3. The loss of potassium caused by prednisone can lead to serious side effects in individuals taking digoxin.
4. Thiazide diuretics (water pills) can increase the potassium loss caused by this medication.
5. Phenobarbital, phenytoin, rifampin, and ephedrine can increase the elimination of prednisone from the body, thereby decreasing its effectiveness.
6. Oral contraceptives (birth control pills) and estrogen-containing drugs may decrease the elimination of this drug from the body, which can lead to an increase in side effects.
7. Prednisone can increase the elimination of aspirin and isoniazid, decreasing the effectiveness of these two drugs.
8. Cholestyramine and colestipol can chemically bind this medication in the stomach and gastrointestinal tract, preventing its absorption.

BE SURE TO TELL YOUR DOCTOR about any medications you are currently taking.

WARNINGS

• Tell your doctor about unusual or allergic reactions you have had to any medications, especially to prednisone or other adrenocorticosteroids (such as betamethasone, cortisone, dexamethasone, hydrocortisone, methylprednisolone, prednisolone, and triamcinolone).
• Tell your doctor if you now have or if you have ever had bone disease, diabetes mellitus, emotional instability, glaucoma, fungal infections, heart disease, high blood pressure, high cholesterol levels, kidney disease, liver disease, myasthenia gravis, peptic ulcers, osteoporosis, thyroid disease, tuberculosis, or ulcerative colitis.
• To help avoid potassium loss while using this drug, take your dose with a glass of fresh or frozen orange juice or eat a banana each day. The use of a salt substitute also helps prevent potassium loss. Check with your doctor before making any dietary changes.
• If you are using this medication for longer than a week, you may need to have your dosage adjusted if you are subjected to stress, such as serious infections, injury, or surgery.
• If you have been taking this drug for more than a week, do not stop taking it suddenly. If it is stopped abruptly, you may experience abdominal or back pain, dizziness, fainting, fever, muscle or joint pain, nausea, vomiting, shortness of breath, or extreme weakness. Your doctor may therefore want to reduce the dosage gradually. Never increase the dosage or take the drug for longer than the prescribed time unless you first consult your doctor.
• While you are taking this drug, you should not be vaccinated or immunized. This medication decreases the effectiveness of vaccines and can lead to overwhelming infection if a live-virus vaccine is administered.
• Before surgery or other medical or dental treatment, tell your doctor or dentist you are taking this drug.
• Because this drug can cause glaucoma and cataracts with long-term use, your doctor may want you to have your eyes examined by an ophthalmologist.
• If you are taking this medication for prolonged periods, you should wear or carry an identification card or notice stating that you are taking an adrenocorticosteroid.
• This drug can raise blood-sugar levels in diabetic patients. Blood sugar should, therefore, be monitored carefully with blood or urine tests when this drug is started.
• Be sure to tell your doctor if you are pregnant. Birth defects have been observed in the fetuses of animals that were given large doses of this drug during pregnancy. Also, tell your doctor if you are breast-feeding an infant. It has been shown that small amounts of this drug pass into breast milk and may cause growth suppression or other problems in the nursing infant.

---

probenecid

BRAND NAMES (Manufacturers)
Benemid (Merck Sharp & Dohme)
Probalan (Lannett)
probenecid (various manufacturers)

TYPE OF DRUG
Uricosuric (antigout preparation)

INGREDIENT
probenecid

DOSAGE FORM
Tablets (500 mg)

STORAGE
Probenecid should be stored at room temperature in a tightly closed container. This medication should not be refrigerated.

USES

Probenecid is used to prevent gout attacks. It increases the elimination of uric acid (the chemical responsible for the symptoms of gout) through the kidneys. Probenecid is also occasionally used in combination with penicillin or ampicillin to increase the length of time that the antibiotics remain in the bloodstream.

TREATMENT

In order to avoid stomach irritation, you may take probenecid with a full glass of water or milk. You should also drink at least ten to 12 full eight-ounce glasses of liquids (not alcoholic beverages) each day to prevent formation of uric acid kidney stones.

If you miss a dose of this medication, take the missed dose as soon as possible, unless it is almost time for the next dose. In that case, do not take the missed dose at all; just return to your regular dosing schedule. Do not double the next dose.

SIDE EFFECTS

Minor. Dizziness, frequent urination, headache, loss of appetite, nausea, rash, sore gums, or vomiting. These side effects should disappear as your body adjusts to the medication.

If you feel dizzy, sit or lie down for a while; get up slowly from a sitting or reclining position; and be careful on stairs.

Major. Tell your doctor about any side effects you are experiencing that are persistent or particularly bothersome. TELL YOUR DOCTOR about fatigue, fever, flushing, lower back pain, painful or difficult urination, sore throat, unusual bleeding or bruising, or yellowing of the eyes or skin.

INTERACTIONS

Probenecid can be expected to interact with several other types of medications:

1. Aspirin and pyrazinamide antagonize (act against) the antigout effects of probenecid.

2. The blood levels of methotrexate, sulfonamide antibiotics, nitrofurantoin, oral antidiabetic medicines, ketoprofen, naproxen, indomethacin, rifampin, sulindac, dapsone, and clofibrate can be increased by probenecid, which can lead to an increase in the incidence and intensity of side effects.

3. Alcohol, chlorthalidone, ethacrynic acid, furosemide, or thiazide diuretics (water pills) can increase blood uric acid levels, which can decrease the effectiveness of probenecid.

Before starting to take probenecid, BE SURE TO TELL YOUR DOCTOR about any medications you are taking, especially any of those listed above.

WARNINGS

• Tell your doctor about unusual or allergic reactions you have had to any medications, especially to probenecid.

• Before starting to take probenecid, be sure to tell your doctor if you now have or if you have ever had blood diseases, diabetes mellitus, glucose-6-phosphate dehydrogenase (G6PD) deficiency, kidney stones, peptic ulcers, or porphyria.

• Diabetics using Clinitest urine glucose tests may get erroneously high readings of blood-sugar levels while they are taking this drug. Temporarily changing to Clinistix or Tes-Tape urine tests will avoid this problem.

• If probenecid makes you dizzy, do not take part in any activity that requires alertness, such as driving a car or operating potentially dangerous machinery.

• Avoid taking large amounts of vitamin C while on probenecid. Vitamin C can increase the risk of kidney stone formation.

• Probenecid is not effective during an attack of gout. It is used to prevent attacks.

• Tell your doctor if you are pregnant. Although probenecid appears to be safe, it does cross the placenta. Extensive studies in pregnant women have not been conducted. Also, tell your doctor if you are breast-feeding an infant. It is not known whether probenecid passes into breast milk.

---

procainamide

BRAND NAMES (Manufacturers)

procainamide hydrochloride (various manufacturers)
Procan-SR (Parke-Davis)
Promine (Major)
Pronestyl (Princeton)
Rhythmin (Sidmak)

TYPE OF DRUG

Antiarrhythmic

INGREDIENT

procainamide

DOSAGE FORMS

Tablets (250 mg, 375 mg, and 500 mg)
Sustained-release tablets (250 mg, 500 mg, 750 mg, and 1,000 mg)
Capsules (250 mg, 375 mg, and 500 mg)

STORAGE

Procainamide tablets and capsules should be stored in tightly closed containers in a cool, dry place. Exposure to moisture causes deterioration of this medication.

USES

Procainamide is used to treat heart arrhythmias. It corrects irregular heartbeats to achieve a more normal rhythm.

TREATMENT

To increase absorption, take procainamide with a full glass of water on an empty stomach one hour before or two hours after a meal. However, if this medication upsets your stomach, ask your doctor if you can take it with food or milk.

Try to take it at the same time(s) each day. Procainamide works best when the amount of drug in your bloodstream is kept at a constant level. This medication should, therefore, be taken at evenly spaced intervals day and night. For example, if you are to take this medication four times per day, the doses should be spaced six hours apart.

The sustained-release tablets should be swallowed whole. Breaking, chewing, or crushing these tablets destroys their sustained-release activity and possibly increases the side effects.

If you miss a dose of this medication and remember within two hours, take the missed dose immediately. If more than two hours have passed (four hours for the sustained-release tablets), do not take the missed dose; just return to your regular dosing schedule. Do not double the next dose.

SIDE EFFECTS

Minor. Bitter taste in the mouth, diarrhea, dizziness, dry mouth, loss of appetite, nausea, stomach upset, or vomiting. These side effects should disappear as your body adjusts to the medication.

If you feel dizzy, sit or lie down for a while; get up slowly from a sitting or reclining position; and be careful on stairs.

To relieve mouth dryness, chew sugarless gum or suck on ice chips or a piece of hard candy.

Major. Tell your doctor about any side effects that are persistent or bothersome. IT IS ESPECIALLY IMPORTANT TO TELL YOUR DOCTOR about chest pain, chills, confusion, depression, fainting, fatigue, fever, giddiness, hallucinations, itching, joint pain, palpitations, rash, sore throat, unusual bleeding or bruising, or weakness.

INTERACTIONS

Procainamide interacts with several other types of medications:

1. The combination of digoxin and procainamide can lead to an increase in side effects to the heart.

2. Procainamide can block the effectiveness of neostigmine, pyridostigmine, and prostigmine.

3. Cimetidine, ranitidine, and amiodarone can increase the blood levels of procainamide, which can lead to an increase in side effects.

Before starting to take procainamide, TELL YOUR DOCTOR about any medications you are currently taking.

WARNINGS

• Tell your doctor about unusual or allergic reactions you have had to any medications, especially to procainamide, procaine, lidocaine, benzocaine, or tetracaine.

• Before starting this medication, be sure to tell your doctor if you now have or if you have ever had asthma, heart block, kidney disease, liver disease, myasthenia gravis, or systemic lupus erythematosus.

• If this drug makes you dizzy, do not take part in any activity that requires alertness, such as driving a car or operating potentially dangerous machinery.
• Before having surgery or any other medical or dental treatment, be sure to tell your doctor or dentist that you are taking this medication.
• Do not stop taking this drug without first consulting your doctor. Stopping procainamide abruptly may cause a serious change in the activity of your heart. Your doctor may therefore want to reduce your dosage gradually.
• If you are taking Procan-SR and you occasionally notice something in your stool that looks like a tablet, it does not mean that the drug is not being absorbed. The drug is "held" in a wax core designed to release the medication slowly. The wax core is eliminated in the stool after the drug has been absorbed.
• Some of these products contain the color additive FD&C Yellow No. 5 (tartrazine), which can cause allergic-type symptoms (rash, shortness of breath, fainting) in certain susceptible individuals.
• Be sure to tell your doctor if you are pregnant. Although this drug appears to be safe, extensive studies in pregnant women have not been conducted. Also, tell your doctor if you are breast-feeding an infant. It is not known whether procainamide passes into breast milk.

---

prochlorperazine

BRAND NAMES (Manufacturers)
Compazine (SmithKline Beecham)
Compazine Spansules (SmithKline Beecham)
prochlorperazine maleate (various manufacturers)
TYPE OF DRUG
Phenothiazine tranquilizer and antiemetic
INGREDIENT
prochlorperazine
DOSAGE FORMS
Tablets (5 mg, 10 mg, and 25 mg)
Sustained-release capsules (10 mg, 15 mg, and 30 mg)
Suppositories (2.5 mg, 5 mg, and 25 mg)
Oral syrup (5 mg per 5-ml spoonful)
STORAGE
The tablet and capsule forms of this medication should be stored at room temperature in tightly closed, light-resistant containers. The oral syrup and suppository forms may be stored in the refrigerator in tightly closed, light-resistant containers.

If the oral syrup turns slightly yellow, the medicine is still effective and can be used. However, if the syrup changes color markedly or has particles floating in it, it should not be used; rather, it should be discarded down the sink. Prochlorperazine should never be frozen.

USES

Prochlorperazine is prescribed to treat the symptoms of certain types of mental illness, such as the emotional symptoms of psychosis, the manic phase of manic-depressive illness, and severe behavioral problems in children. This medication is thought to relieve the symptoms of mental illness by blocking certain chemicals involved with nerve transmission in the brain. Prochlorperazine is also frequently used to treat nausea and vomiting (this medication works at the vomiting center in the brain to relieve nausea and vomiting).

TREATMENT

To avoid stomach irritation, you can take the tablet or capsule form of this medication with a meal or with a glass of water or milk (unless your doctor directs you to do otherwise).

Antacids and antidiarrheal medicines may decrease the absorption of this medication from the gastrointestinal tract. Therefore, at least one hour should separate doses of one of these medicines and prochlorperazine.

The sustained-release capsules should be swallowed whole; do not crush, break, or open them. Breaking the capsules releases the medication all at once, destroying their sustained-release activity.

Measure the oral syrup carefully with a specially designed 5-ml measuring spoon. An ordinary kitchen teaspoon is not accurate enough.

To use the suppository form, remove the foil wrapper (if the suppository is too soft to insert, refrigerate it for half an hour or run cold water over it before removing the wrapper), and moisten the suppository with water. Lie on your left side with your right knee bent. Push the suppository into the rectum, pointed end first. Lie still for a few minutes. Try to avoid having a bowel movement for at least an hour (to give the medication time to be absorbed).

If you miss a dose of this medication, take the missed dose as soon as possible, unless it is almost time for your next dose. In that case, do not take the missed dose at all; just return to your regular schedule. Do not double the dose (unless your doctor directs you to do so).

The full effects of this medication for the control of emotional or mental symptoms may not become apparent for two weeks after you start to take it.

SIDE EFFECTS

Minor. Blurred vision, constipation, decreased sweating, diarrhea, dizziness, drooling, drowsiness, dry mouth, fatigue, jitteriness, menstrual irregularities, nasal congestion, restlessness, vomiting, or weight gain. As your body adjusts to the medication, these side effects should disappear.

Prochlorperazine can also cause discoloration of the urine to red, pink, or red-brown. This is a harmless effect.

This medication can cause increased sensitivity to sunlight. It is, therefore, important to avoid prolonged exposure to sunlight and sunlamps. Wear protective clothing and sunglasses, and use an effective sunscreen.

If you are constipated, increase the amount of fiber in your diet (fresh fruits and vegetables, salads, bran, and whole-grain breads), exercise, and drink more water (unless your doctor directs you to do otherwise).

Chew sugarless gum or suck on ice chips or a piece of hard candy to reduce mouth dryness.

To avoid dizziness or light-headedness when you stand, contract and relax the muscles of your legs for a few moments before rising. Do this by pushing one foot against the floor while raising the other foot slightly, alternating feet so that you are "pumping" your legs in a pedaling motion.

Major. Tell your doctor about any side effects that are persistent or particularly bothersome. IT IS ESPECIALLY IMPORTANT TO TELL YOUR DOCTOR about unusual bleeding or bruising; breast enlargement (in both sexes); chest pain; convulsions; darkened skin; difficulty in swallowing or breathing; fainting; fever; impotence; involuntary movements of the face, mouth, jaw, or tongue; palpitations; rash; sleep disorders; sore throat; tremors; uncoordinated movements; visual disturbances; or yellowing of the eyes or skin.

INTERACTIONS

Prochlorperazine interacts with several other types of medications:

1. It can cause drowsiness when combined with alcohol or central nervous system depressants (drugs that slow the activity of the brain and spinal cord), such as barbiturates, benzodiazepine tranquilizers, muscle relaxants, narcotics, and pain medications, or with tricyclic antidepressants.

2. Prochlorperazine can decrease the effectiveness of amphetamines, guanethidine, anticonvulsants, and levodopa.

3. The side effects of epinephrine, monoamine oxidase (MAO) inhibitors, propranolol, phenytoin, and tricyclic antidepressants may be increased by this medication. At least 14 days should separate the use of this drug and the use of an MAO inhibitor.

4. Lithium may increase the side effects and decrease the effectiveness of this medication.

5. Thiazide diuretics can enhance the blood-pressure-lowering side effects of prochlorperazine.

Before starting to take prochlorperazine, BE SURE TO TELL YOUR DOCTOR about any medications you are currently taking.

WARNINGS

• Tell your doctor about unusual reactions you have had to any drugs, especially to the medication prochlorperazine or other phenothiazine tranquilizers (such as chlorpromazine, fluphen-azine, mesoridazine, perphenazine, promazine, thiorid-azine, trifluoperazine, and triflupromazine) or to loxapine.

• Tell your doctor if you have a history of alcoholism or if you now have or have ever had any blood disease, bone marrow disease, brain disease, breast cancer, blockage in the urinary or digestive tracts, drug-induced depression, epilepsy, high or low blood pressure, diabetes mellitus, glaucoma, heart or circulatory disease, liver disease, lung disease, Parkinson's disease, peptic ulcers, or an enlarged prostate gland.

• Tell your doctor about any recent exposure to a pesticide or an insecticide. Prochlorperazine may increase the side effects from the exposure.

• To prevent oversedation, avoid drinking alcoholic beverages while taking this medication.

• If this medication makes you dizzy or drowsy, do not take part in any activity that requires alertness, such as driving a car or operating potentially dangerous machinery. Be careful on stairs, and avoid getting up suddenly from a lying or sitting position.

• Prior to having surgery or any other medical or dental treatment, be sure to tell your doctor or dentist that you are taking this medication.

• Some of the side effects caused by this drug can be prevented by taking an antiparkinsonism drug.

• This medication can decrease sweating and heat release from the body. You should therefore try not to get overheated (avoid exercising strenuously in hot weather, and avoid taking hot baths, showers, or saunas).

• Do not stop taking prochlorperazine suddenly if you have been taking it for a prolonged period. If the drug is stopped abruptly, you may experience nausea, vomiting, stomach upset, headache, increased heart rate, insomnia, tremors, or a worsening of your condition. Your doctor may therefore want to reduce the dosage gradually.

• If you are planning to have a myelogram, or any other procedure in which dye will be injected into your spinal cord, tell your doctor that you are taking this medication.

• Avoid spilling the oral syrup form on your skin; it may cause redness and irritation.

• While taking this medication, do not take any over-the-counter (nonprescription) medications for weight control or for cough, cold, allergy, asthma, or sinus problems unless you first check with your doctor. The combination of these medications with prochlorperazine may cause high blood pressure.

• Be sure to tell your doctor if you are pregnant. Although there are reports of safe use of this drug during pregnancy, there are also reports of liver disease and tremors in newborn infants whose mothers received this type of medication close to term. Also, tell your doctor if you are breast-feeding an infant.

---

propranolol

BRAND NAMES (Manufacturers)

Inderal (Wyeth-Ayerst)
Inderal LA (Wyeth-Ayerst)
propranolol (various manufacturers)

TYPE OF DRUG

Beta-adrenergic blocking agent

INGREDIENT

propranolol

DOSAGE FORMS

Tablets (10 mg, 20 mg, 40 mg, 60 mg, 80 mg, and 90 mg)
Extended-release capsules (60 mg, 80 mg, 120 mg, and 160 mg)
Oral solution (20 mg and 40 mg per 5-ml spoonful)
Oral concentrated solution (80 mg per ml)

STORAGE

Store at room temperature in a tightly closed, light-resistant container. The solutions should never be frozen.

USES

Propranolol is used to treat high blood pressure, angina pectoris (chest pain), and irregular heartbeats. It is also useful in preventing migraine headaches and preventing additional heart attacks in heart attack patients. Propranolol belongs to a group of medicines known as beta-adrenergic blocking agents or, more commonly, beta blockers. These drugs work by controlling nerve impulses along certain nerve pathways.

TREATMENT

Propranolol can be taken with a glass of water, with meals, immediately following meals, or on an empty stomach (depending on your doctor's instructions). Try to take the medication at the same time(s) each day.

The extended-release capsules should be swallowed whole. Do not chew or crush them. Breaking the capsule releases the medication all at once—defeating the purpose of extended-release capsules.

The oral solution should be measured with a specially designed 5-ml measuring spoon.

The oral-concentrated solution must be mixed in four ounces (1/2 cup) of water, juice, or soda before drinking. The cup should be refilled with more of the liquid, which must be drunk to ensure that the entire dose is taken. This form may also be mixed with applesauce or pudding.

It is important to remember that propranolol does not cure high blood pressure, but it will help control the condition as long as you continue to take it.

Try not to miss any doses of this medicine. If you do miss a dose, take the missed dose as soon as possible, unless it is within eight hours (if you are taking this medicine only once a day) or within four hours (if you are taking this medicine more than once a day) of your next scheduled dose. In that case, do not take the missed dose at all; just return to your regular dosing schedule. Do not double the next dose of the medication.

SIDE EFFECTS

Minor. Anxiety; constipation; decreased sexual ability; diarrhea; difficulty in sleeping; drowsiness; dryness of the eyes, mouth, and skin; headache; nausea; nervousness; stomach discomfort; tiredness; or weakness. These side effects should disappear with time.

To relieve constipation, increase the amount of fiber in your diet (fresh fruits and vegetables, salads, bran, and whole-grain breads) and drink more water (unless your doctor directs you to do otherwise).

If you are extra-sensitive to the cold, be sure to dress warmly during cold weather.

Plain, nonmedicated eye drops (artificial tears) may help to relieve eye dryness.

Sucking on ice chips or chewing sugarless gum helps to relieve mouth and throat dryness.

Major. Tell your doctor about any side effects you experience that are persistent or particularly bothersome. IT IS ESPECIALLY IMPORTANT TO TELL YOUR DOCTOR about breathing difficulty or wheezing, cold hands or feet (due to decreased blood circulation to skin, fingers, and toes), confusion, depression, dizziness, hair loss, hallucinations, light-headedness, nightmares, numbness or tingling of the fingers or toes, rapid weight gain (three to five pounds within a week), reduced alertness, swelling, sore throat and fever, skin rash, or unusual bleeding or bruising.

INTERACTIONS

Propranolol interacts with a number of other types of medications:

1. Indomethacin, aspirin, or other salicylates lessen the blood-pressure-lowering effects of beta blockers.

2. Concurrent use of beta blockers and calcium channel blockers (diltiazem, nifedipine, or verapamil) or disopyramide can lead to heart failure or very low blood pressure.

3. Cimetidine and oral contraceptives (birth control pills) can increase the blood concentrations of propranolol, which can result in greater side effects.

4. Side effects may also be increased when beta blockers are taken with clonidine, digoxin, epinephrine, phenylephrine, phenylpropanolamine, phenothiazine tranquilizers, prazosin, reserpine, or monoamine oxidase (MAO) inhibitors. At least 14 days should separate the use of a beta blocker and an MAO inhibitor.

5. Barbiturates, alcohol, and rifampin can increase the breakdown of propranolol in the body, which can lead to a decrease in its effectiveness.

6. Beta blockers may antagonize (work against) the effects of theophylline, aminophylline, albuterol, isoproterenol, metaproterenol, and terbutaline.

7. Beta blockers can also interact with insulin or oral antidiabetic agents, raising or lowering blood-sugar levels or masking the symptoms of low blood sugar.

8. The action of beta blockers may be excessively increased if they are used with chlorpromazine, furosemide, or hydralazine.

BE SURE TO TELL YOUR DOCTOR about any medications you are currently taking, especially any of those listed above.

WARNINGS

- Before starting to take this medication, it is important to tell your doctor if you have ever had unusual or allergic reactions to any beta blocker (acebutolol, atenolol, betaxolol, carteolol, esmolol, labetalol, metoprolol, nadolol, penbutolol, pindolol, propranolol, or timolol).
- Tell your doctor if you now have or if you have ever had allergies, asthma, hay fever, eczema, slow heartbeat, bronchitis, diabetes mellitus, emphysema, heart or blood-vessel disease, kidney disease, liver disease, thyroid disease, or poor circulation in the fingers or toes.
- You may want to check your pulse while taking this medication. If your pulse is much slower than your usual rate (or if it is less than 50 beats per minute), check with your doctor. A pulse rate that is too slow may cause circulation problems.
- This medicine may affect your body's response to exercise. Make sure you ask your doctor what an appropriate amount of exercise would be for you, taking into account your medical condition.
- It is important that you do not stop taking this medicine without first checking with your doctor. Some conditions may become worse when the medicine is stopped suddenly, and the danger of a heart attack is increased in some patients. Your doctor may want you to gradually reduce the amount you take before stopping completely. Make sure that you have enough on hand to last through vacations, holidays, and weekends.

• Before having surgery or any other medical or dental treatment, tell your physician or dentist that you are taking this medicine. Often, this medication will be discontinued 48 hours prior to any major surgery.
• Propranolol can cause dizziness, drowsiness, lightheadedness, and decreased alertness. Use caution while driving a car or operating dangerous machinery. Be especially careful when going up or down stairs.
• While taking this medicine, do not use any over-the-counter (nonprescription) allergy, asthma, cough, cold, sinus, or diet preparations without first checking with your pharmacist or doctor. The combination of these medicines with a beta blocker can result in high blood pressure.
• Be sure to tell your doctor if you are pregnant. Animal studies have shown that some beta blockers can cause problems in pregnancy when used at very high doses. Adequate studies have not been done in humans, but there has been some association between use of beta blockers during pregnancy and low birth weight, as well as breathing problems and slow heart rate in newborn infants. However, other reports have shown no effects in newborn infants. Also, tell your doctor if you are breast-feeding an infant. Although this medicine has not been shown to cause problems in breast-fed infants, some of the medicine may pass into breast milk.

---

ranitidine

BRAND NAMES (Manufacturers)
Zantac (Glaxo)
Zantac (Roche)
TYPE OF DRUG
Gastric-acid-secretion inhibitor (decreases stomach acid)
INGREDIENT
ranitidine
DOSAGE FORMS
Tablets (150 mg and 300 mg)
Oral syrup (15 mg per ml)
STORAGE
Ranitidine should be stored at room temperature in a tightly closed, light-resistant container.

USES

Ranitidine is used to treat duodenal and gastric ulcers. It is also used in the long-term treatment of excessive stomach acid secretion, in the prevention of recurrent ulcers, and in the treatment of reflex esophagitis (inflammation of the esophagus). Ranitidine works by blocking the effects of histamine on the stomach, thereby reducing stomach-acid secretion.

TREATMENT

You can take ranitidine either on an empty stomach or with food or milk.

Antacids can block the absorption of ranitidine. If you are taking antacids as well as ranitidine, at least one hour should separate doses of the two medications.

If you miss a dose of this medication, take the missed dose as soon as possible, unless it is almost time for the next dose. In that case, do not take the missed dose at all; just return to your regular dosing schedule. Do not double the next dose.

SIDE EFFECTS

Minor. Constipation, diarrhea, dizziness, headache, nausea, or stomach upset. These side effects should disappear as your body adjusts to the medication.

To relieve constipation, exercise and drink more water (unless your doctor directs you to do otherwise).

If you feel dizzy while taking this medication, sit or lie down for a while.

Major. Tell your doctor about any side effects that are persistent or particularly bothersome. IT IS ESPECIALLY IMPORTANT TO TELL YOUR DOCTOR about confusion, decreased sexual ability, unusual bleeding or bruising, or weakness.

INTERACTIONS

Ranitidine can interact with other types of medications:
1. Ranitidine may increase the blood-sugar-lowering effects of glipizide.
2. Ranitidine can decrease the elimination of the blood-thinner warfarin from the body, which can increase the risk of bleeding complications.
3. Ranitidine can increase blood levels of procainamide.
4. Ranitidine may cause a false-positive result with the Multistix urine protein test.

BE SURE TO TELL YOUR DOCTOR about any medications you are currently taking, especially any listed above.

WARNINGS

• Tell your doctor about unusual or allergic reactions you have had to any medications, especially to ranitidine.
• Tell your doctor if you now have or if you have ever had kidney or liver disease.
• Ranitidine should be taken continuously for as long as your doctor prescribes. To do otherwise may result in ineffective therapy.
• Cigarette smoking may block the beneficial effects of ranitidine.
• If this drug makes you dizzy, do not take part in any activity that requires alertness.
• Be sure to tell your doctor if you are pregnant. Ranitidine appears to be safe during pregnancy; however, extensive testing has not been conducted. Also, tell your doctor if you are breast-feeding an infant. Small amounts of ranitidine pass into breast mlk.

---

rifampin

BRAND NAMES (Manufacturers)
Rifadin (Marion Merrell Dow)
Rimactane (Ciba)

TYPE OF DRUG
Antibiotic
INGREDIENT
rifampin
DOSAGE FORM
Capsules (150 mg and 300 mg)
STORAGE
Rifampin should be stored at room temperature in a tightly closed, light-resistant container.

USES

Rifampin is an antibiotic that is used to treat tuberculosis and to prevent meningococcal meningitis. Rifampin works by preventing the growth and multiplication of susceptible bacteria. Rifampin, however, is not effective against viruses, parasites, or fungi.

TREATMENT

Rifampin should be taken with a full glass of water on an empty stomach one hour before or two hours after a meal. If this medication causes stomach irritation, however, check with your doctor to see if you can take it with food.

Try not to miss any doses of this medication. If you do miss a dose, take the missed dose as soon as possible, unless it is almost time for your next dose. In that case, do not take the missed dose at all; just return to your regular dosing schedule. Do not double your next dose of rifampin.

Continue to take this medication for the entire time prescribed by your doctor (which may be months to years), even if the symptoms disappear before the end of that period. If you stop taking the drug too soon, resistant bacteria will continue to grow, and your infection could recur.

SIDE EFFECTS

Minor. Diarrhea, dizziness, drowsiness, gas, headache, heartburn, loss of appetite, nausea, stomach irritation, or vomiting. These side effects should disappear as your body adjusts to the medication.

If you feel dizzy, sit or lie down for a while; get up slowly from a sitting or reclining position; and be careful on stairs.

Major. Tell your doctor about any side effects that are persistent or particularly bothersome. IT IS ESPECIALLY IMPORTANT TO TELL YOUR DOCTOR about confusion, difficult or painful urination, fatigue, fever, flushing, itching, muscle weakness, numbness, skin rash, uncoordinated movements, visual disturbances, or yellowing of the eyes or skin. Also, if your symptoms of infection seem to be worsening rather than improving, tell your doctor.

INTERACTIONS

Rifampin interacts with several other types of medications:

1. Concurrent use with paminosalicylic acid may decrease the blood levels and effectiveness of rifampin.

2. Rifampin can decrease the blood levels and effectiveness of metoprolol, propranolol, verapamil, aminophylline, theophylline, oxtriphylline, quinidine, adrenocorticosteroids (cortisonelike medicines), progestins, clofibrate, methadone, oral anticoagulants (blood thinners, such as warfarin), oral antidiabetic medicines, barbiturates, benzodiazepine tranquilizers, dapsone, digitoxin, and trimethoprim.

3. Concurrent use of rifampin with alcohol or isoniazid can lead to an increased risk of liver damage.

4. Rifampin may decrease the effectiveness of oral contraceptives (birth control pills), and pregnancy could result. You should use a different or additional form of birth control while taking rifampin. Discuss available options with your doctor.

BE SURE TO TELL YOUR DOCTOR about any medications you are currently taking.

WARNINGS

- Tell your doctor about unusual or allergic reactions you have had to any medications, especially to rifampin.
- Before starting to take this medication, be sure to tell your doctor if you have a history of alcoholism or liver disease.
- Rifampin has been prescribed for your current infection only. Another infection later on, or one that someone else has, may require a different medicine. You should not give your medicine to other people or use it for other infections, unless your doctor specifically directs you to do so.
- If this drug makes you dizzy or drowsy, do not take part in any activity that requires alertness, such as driving a car or operating potentially dangerous machinery.
- Rifampin can cause reddish-orange to reddish-brown discoloration of your urine, feces, saliva, sputum, sweat, and tears. This is a harmless effect. The drug may also permanently discolor soft contact lenses. You might want to stop wearing them while you are taking this medication. Discuss this with your ophthalmologist.
- Do not stop taking this medication unless you first check with your doctor. Stopping the drug and restarting it at a later time can lead to an increase in side effects.
- Be sure to tell your doctor if you are pregnant. Although rifampin appears to be safe in humans, birth defects have been reported in the offspring of animals that received large doses of the drug during pregnancy. Also, tell your doctor if you are breast-feeding an infant. Small amounts of rifampin pass into breast milk.

---

simvastatin

BRAND NAME (Manufacturer)
Zocor (Merck Sharp & Dohme)
TYPE OF DRUG
Antihyperlipidemic (lipid-lowering drug)
INGREDIENT
simvastatin
DOSAGE FORM
Tablets (5 mg, 10 mg, 20 mg, and 40 mg)
STORAGE
This medication should be stored in a tightly closed container at room temperature, away from heat and di-

rect sunlight. Simvastatin tablets should not be refrigerated.

USES

Simvastatin is used to treat hyperlipidemia (high blood-fat levels). It may be prescribed with nondrug therapies such as diet control and exercise in an attempt to regulate lipid and cholesterol levels. Simvastatin chemically interferes with an enzyme in the body that is responsible for synthesizing cholesterol. This enzyme blockade decreases the LDL (low-density lipoprotein) type of cholesterol, which has been associated with coronary artery disease and atherosclerosis.

TREATMENT

This medication should be taken exactly as prescribed by your doctor. If you are to take simvastatin once a day, it is best to take the drug in the evening. Simvastatin can be taken with meals or with a full glass of water if stomach upset occurs.

While using this medication, try to develop a set schedule for taking it. If you miss a dose and remember within a few hours, take the missed dose and resume your regular schedule. If many hours have passed, skip the dose you missed and then take your next dose as scheduled. Do not double the dose.

SIDE EFFECTS

Minor. Abdominal pain or cramps, constipation, diarrhea, gas, nausea, or stomach pain. These effects may be relieved by taking simvastatin with a meal, adding fiber to your diet, or using mild stool softeners.

Major. Tell your doctor about any side effects that are persistent or particularly bothersome. IT IS ESPECIALLY IMPORTANT TO TELL YOUR DOCTOR about blurred vision (or any other visual changes or difficulties), or muscle pain or tenderness, especially with malaise or fever.

INTERACTIONS

1. Simvastatin may increase the effectiveness of oral anticoagulants (blood thinners, such as warfarin) and digoxin.

2. Because of the risk of severe myopathy (muscle weakness), the combined use of simvastatin with gemfibrozil or clofibrate should generally be avoided.

3. Cyclosporine, erythromycin, nicotinic acid, or niacin may increase the side effects of simvastatin and should be used with extreme caution.

BE SURE TO TELL YOUR DOCTOR about any medications you are taking, especially any of those listed above.

WARNINGS

• Tell your doctor about unusual or allergic reactions you have had to any medications.

• Be sure that you tell your doctor if you have ever had liver disease, heart disease, stroke, or disorders of the digestive tract.

• Patients taking another drug in this same class developed eye-related problems during treatment. It is advisable to have regular checkups with your ophthalmologist, who should be informed of your use of this drug.

• This drug should not be taken if you are pregnant. Serious side effects have been reported in the offspring of animals given this drug during pregnancy. Also, be sure to tell your doctor if you are breast-feeding an infant. This drug should not be used while breast-feeding.

---

sucralfate

BRAND NAME (Manufacturer)
Carafate (Marion Merrel Dow)
TYPE OF DRUG
Antiulcer
INGREDIENT
sucralfate
DOSAGE FORM
Tablets (1 g)
STORAGE
Sucralfate should be stored at room temperature in a tightly closed container. This medication should not be refrigerated.

USES

Sucralfate is used for the short-term treatment of ulcers. This medication binds to the surface of the ulcer, thereby protecting it from stomach acid and promoting healing.

TREATMENT

In order to obtain maximum benefit from this drug, you should swallow it whole with a full glass of water. Take it on an empty stomach one hour before or two hours after a meal and at bedtime. Do not take antacids within 30 minutes before or one hour after taking your prescribed dose of sucralfate.

Continue to take sucralfate for the full length of time prescribed by your doctor, even if your symptoms disappear. Your ulcer may not yet be healed. However, do not take it for more than eight weeks without your doctor's authorization.

If you miss a dose of this medication, take the missed dose as soon as possible, unless it is almost time for the next dose. In that case, do not take the missed dose at all; just return to your regular dosing schedule. Do not double the next dose.

SIDE EFFECTS

Minor. Back pain, constipation, diarrhea, dizziness, drowsiness, dry mouth, indigestion, nausea, or stomach pain. These side effects should disappear as your body adjusts to the medication.

To relieve constipation, exercise and drink more water (unless your doctor directs you to do otherwise).

If you feel dizzy, sit or lie down for a while; get up slowly from a sitting or reclining position; and be careful on stairs.

To relieve mouth dryness, chew sugarless gum or suck on ice chips or a piece of hard candy.

Major. Tell your doctor about any side effects that are persistent or particularly bothersome. IT IS ESPECIALLY IMPORTANT TO TELL YOUR DOCTOR about itching or rash. Also, if your condition does not improve or seems to be getting worse, you should contact your doctor.

INTERACTIONS

1. Sucralfate may prevent the absorption of tetracycline, digoxin, phenytoin, ranitidine, and fat-soluble vitamins (vitamins A, D, E, and K) from the gastrointestinal tract. At least one hour should separate doses of any of these medications and sucralfate.

2. Sucralfate may increase stomach absorption of ciprofloxacin and norfloxacin. At least two hours should separate doses of these medications and sucralfate.

BE SURE TO TELL YOUR DOCTOR about any medications you are taking, especially any listed above.

WARNINGS

• Tell your doctor about unusual or allergic reactions you have had to any medications, especially to sucralfate.

• Tell your doctor if you now have or if you have ever had kidney disease.

• If sucralfate makes you dizzy or drowsy, do not take part in any activity that requires mental alertness, such as driving an automobile or operating potentially dangerous machinery or equipment.

• Be sure to tell your doctor if you are pregnant. Although sucralfate appears to be safe to use during gestation, extensive studies in pregnant women have not been conducted. Also, tell your doctor if you are breast-feeding an infant. It is not known whether sucralfate passes into breast milk.

---

sulfasalazine

BRAND NAMES (Manufacturers)

Azaline (Major)
Azulfidine (Kabi Pharmacia)
Azulfidine EN-tabs (Kabi Pharmacia)
sulfasalazine (various manufacturers)

TYPE OF DRUG

Sulfonamide and anti-inflammatory

INGREDIENT

sulfasalazine

DOSAGE FORMS

Tablets (500 mg)
Enteric-coated tablets (500 mg)

STORAGE

Store at room temperature in a tightly closed, light-resistant container. This drug should not be refrigerated.

USES

This medication is used to treat inflammatory bowel disease (regional enteritis or ulcerative colitis). In the intestine, sulfasalazine is converted to 5-aminosalicylic acid, an aspirin-like drug, which acts to relieve inflammation.

TREATMENT

In order to avoid stomach irritation while you are being treated with this medication, you should take your doses with a full glass of water, with food, or after meals (unless your doctor directs you to do otherwise).

The enteric-coated tablets should be swallowed whole. The enteric coating is added to lessen stomach irritation. Chewing, breaking, or crushing these tablets destroys the coating.

If you miss a dose of this medication, take the missed dose as soon as possible, unless it is almost time for the next dose. In that case, do not take the missed dose at all; just return to your regular dosing schedule. Do not double the next dose.

SIDE EFFECTS

Minor. Diarrhea, dizziness, drowsiness, insomnia, loss of appetite, mild headache, nausea, stomach upset, or vomiting. These side effects should disappear as your body adjusts to the drug.

This medication can increase your sensitivity to sunlight. Avoid prolonged exposure to sunlight and sunlamps. Wear protective clothing and use a sunscreen. However, a sunscreen containing para-aminobenzoic acid (PABA) interferes with this drug and should not be used.

Sulfasalazine can discolor contact lenses. You may want to stop wearing them while taking this medication. Discuss this with your ophthalmologist.

Sulfasalazine can cause your urine to change to an orange-yellow color. This is a harmless effect.

If you feel dizzy, sit or lie down for a while; get up slowly from a sitting or reclining position; and be careful on stairs.

Major. Tell your doctor about any side effects that are persistent or particularly bothersome. IT IS ESPECIALLY IMPORTANT TO TELL YOUR DOCTOR about blood in the urine, convulsions, depression, difficulty in swallowing, difficult or painful urination, fatigue, fever, hallucinations, hearing loss, itching, joint pain, lower back pain, mouth sores, pale skin, rash or peeling skin, ringing in the ears, severe headache, sore throat, swelling of the front part of the neck, tingling sensations, unusual bleeding or bruising, or yellowing of the eyes or skin.

INTERACTIONS

Sulfasalazine interacts with several other types of drugs:

1. It can increase the side effects of oral anticoagulants (blood thinners, such as warfarin), oral antidiabetic agents, methotrexate, aspirin, and phenytoin.

2. The blood levels and effectiveness of digoxin and folic acid are decreased by concurrent use of sulfasalazine.

3. Probenecid, oxyphenbutazone, phenylbutazone, methenamine, and sulfinpyrazone can increase the blood levels and side effects of sulfasalazine.

BE SURE TO TELL YOUR DOCTOR about any medications you are currently taking, especially any listed above.

WARNINGS

• Tell your doctor about unusual or allergic reactions you have had to any medications, especially to sulfasalazine, aspirin or other salicylates, or any sulfa drug (diuretics, oral antidiabetic medications, sulfonamide antibiotics, oral antiglaucoma medication, acetazolamide, sulfoxone, dapsone).

• Before starting to take this medication, BE SURE TO TELL YOUR DOCTOR if you now have or if you have ever had blood disorders, blockage of the urinary tract or intestine, glucose-6-phosphate dehydrogenase (G6PD) deficiency, kidney disease, liver disease, or porphyria.

• To help prevent the formation of kidney stones, try to drink at least eight to 12 glasses of water or fruit juice each day while you are taking this medication (unless your doctor directs you to do otherwise).

• Before having surgery or other medical or dental treatment, tell your doctor or dentist that you are taking this drug.

• If your condition does not improve within a month or two after starting to take sulfasalazine, check with your doctor. It may be necessary to change your medication.

• Be sure to tell your doctor if you are pregnant. Although sulfasalazine appears to be safe during most of pregnancy, extensive studies in humans have not been conducted. There is also concern that if this drug is taken during the ninth month of pregnancy, it may cause liver or brain disorders in the infant. Also, tell your doctor if you are breast-feeding an infant. Small amounts of sulfasalazine pass into breast milk.

---

terazosin

BRAND NAME (Manufacturer)
Hytrin (Abbott)
TYPE OF DRUG
Antihypertensive
INGREDIENT
terazosin
DOSAGE FORM
Tablets (1 mg, 2 mg, 5 mg, and 10 mg)
STORAGE
Terazosin tablets should be stored at room temperature in a tightly closed, light-resistant container.

USES

Terazosin is used to treat high blood pressure. It relaxes the muscle tissue of the blood vessels, which in turn lowers blood pressure.

Terazosin is also used to reduce urinary obstruction and relieve the symptoms associated with symptomatic benign prostatic hyperplasia (BPH). The drug can effectively relieve the hesitancy, terminal dribbling of urine, and sensation of incomplete bladder emptying often associated with this condition.

TREATMENT

The first dose of this medication may cause fainting, especially in the elderly.

If you miss a dose of this medication, take it as soon as possible, unless it is almost time for your next dose. In that case, do not take the missed dose at all; just wait until the next scheduled dose. Do not double the dose.

This medication does not cure high blood pressure, but it will help to control the condition as long as you continue to take it. In order to become accustomed to taking this medication, try to take it at the same time(s) each day.

A minimum of four to six weeks may be needed to see a response from the medication.

SIDE EFFECTS

Minor. Cold symptoms, constipation, diarrhea, dizziness, drowsiness, dry mouth, fluid retention, frequent urination, headache, itching, lack of energy, malaise, nasal congestion, nausea, nervousness, rash, sweating, or weight gain. These side effects should disappear as your body adjusts to the medication.

To prevent constipation, increase the amount of fiber in your diet (fresh fruits and vegetables, salads, bran, and whole-grain breads), unless your doctor tells you otherwise.

To avoid dizziness or light-headedness when you stand, contract and relax the muscles of your legs for a few moments before rising. Do this by pushing one foot against the floor while raising the other foot slightly, alternating feet so that you are "pumping" your legs.

Major. Tell your doctor about any side effects that are persistent or particularly bothersome. IT IS ESPECIALLY IMPORTANT TO TELL YOUR DOCTOR about blurred vision, chest pain, difficulty breathing, difficulty urinating, fever, flulike symptoms, heart-rate disturbance, impotence, nose bleeds, palpitations, persistent malaise or fatigue, postural effects (dizziness, light-headedness, vertigo leading to reductions in blood pressure or fainting), ringing in the ears, or swelling.

INTERACTIONS

Terazosin has been known to interact with certain other types of medications:

1. The combination of terazosin and alcohol or verapamil can lead to a severe drop in blood pressure and fainting.

2. The severity and duration of the blood-pressure-lowering effects of the initial dose of terazosin may be enhanced by a beta blocker.

BE SURE TO TELL YOUR DOCTOR about any medications you are currently taking, especially those listed above.

WARNINGS

• Tell your doctor about unusual or allergic reactions you have had to any medications, especially to terazosin, prazosin, or doxazosin.

• Before starting to take this medication, BE SURE TO TELL YOUR DOCTOR if you now have or if you have ever had angina (chest pain), kidney disease, or liver disease.

• Because initial therapy with this drug may cause dizziness or fainting, your doctor will probably start you on a low dosage and increase the dosage gradually.

• If this drug makes you dizzy or drowsy or blurs your vision, do not take part in any activity that requires alertness, such as driving a car or operating potentially dangerous machinery.

• In order to avoid dizziness or fainting while taking this drug, try not to stand for long periods of time, avoid drinking excess amounts of alcohol, and try not to get overheated (avoid exercising strenuously in hot weather and taking hot baths, showers, or saunas).

• Before taking any over-the-counter (nonprescription) sinus, allergy, asthma, cough, cold, or diet preparations, check with your doctor or pharmacist. Some of these products can cause an increase in blood pressure.

• Terazosin is only indicated for hypertension and benign prostatic hyperplasia (BPH). This agent is not for symptoms or conditions that appear to be similar to BPH, such as cancer of the prostate.

• Do not stop taking this medication unless you first check with your doctor. If you stop taking this drug, you may experience a rise in blood pressure. Your doctor may want to decrease your dose gradually.

• Be sure to tell your doctor if you are pregnant. Although the drug appears to be safe, there have been only limited studies in pregnant women. Also, tell your doctor if you are breast-feeding an infant; terazosin should be used with caution in nursing women.

---

terfenadine

BRAND NAME (Manufacturer)
Seldane (Marion Merrell Dow)

TYPE OF DRUG
Antihistamine

INGREDIENT
terfenadine

DOSAGE FORM
Tablets (60 mg)

STORAGE
Terfenadine should be stored at room temperature in a tightly closed container. The tablets should not be exposed to high temperatures (above 104°F), direct sunlight, or moisture during storage.

USES

Terfenadine is used to treat the symptoms of allergic response, including sneezing, runny nose, itching, and tearing. This medication belongs to a group of drugs known as antihistamines, which act by blocking the action of histamine, a chemical that is released by the body during an allergic reaction.

TREATMENT

Terfenadine can be taken either on an empty stomach or with food or milk (unless your doctor directs otherwise).

Terfenadine should be taken only as needed to control the symptoms of allergy.

If you miss a dose of this medication and you are taking it on a regular schedule, take the missed dose as soon as possible, unless it is almost time for your next dose. In that case, do not take the missed dose at all; just return to your regular dosing schedule. Do not double the next dose.

SIDE EFFECTS

Minor. Abdominal pain; cough; dizziness; drowsiness; dry mouth, nose, or throat; fatigue; headache; increased appetite; insomnia; nausea; nervousness; nosebleeds; sore throat; sweating; vomiting; or weakness. These side effects should disappear as your body adjusts to this medication.

To reduce mouth dryness, chew sugarless gum or suck on ice chips or hard candy.

If you feel dizzy or light-headed, sit or lie down for a while; get up slowly from a sitting or reclining position; and be careful on stairs.

Major. Tell your doctor about any side effects that are persistent or particularly bothersome. IT IS ESPECIALLY IMPORTANT TO TELL YOUR DOCTOR about depression, hair loss, itching, menstrual disorders, muscle or bone pain, nightmares, palpitations, shortness of breath, tingling of your fingers or toes, tremors, urinary frequency, visual disturbances, or yellowing of the skin or eyes.

Hypotension (low blood pressure), palpitations, and dizziness could reflect undetected ventricular arrhythmias. In some patients, cardiac arrest and irregular heartbeat have been preceded by episodes of fainting.

INTERACTIONS

Terfenadine interacts with the following medications:

1. The combination of terfenadine and ketoconazole or itraconazole can result in serious adverse effects.

2. The combination of terfenadine and certain antibiotics, such as erythromycin and troleandomycin, can also result in serious adverse effects.

BE SURE TO TELL YOUR DOCTOR about any medications you are currently taking, especially any listed above.

WARNINGS

• Tell your doctor about unusual or allergic reactions you have had to any medications, especially to terfenadine.

• Before starting terfenadine, tell your doctor if you now have or if you have ever had asthma.

• Terfenadine causes less drowsiness than other antihistamines. However, until you see how it affects you, be cautious about performing tasks that require alertness, such as driving a car or operating potentially dangerous machinery.

• Be sure to tell your doctor if you are pregnant. This drug's safety in human pregnancy has not been established. Also, tell your doctor if you are breast-feeding. The effects of terfenadine on nursing infants are not yet known.

• Be sure to take only the dose recommended by your doctor. DO NOT EXCEED THE PRESCRIBED DOSE.

• Before starting terfenadine, tell your doctor if you now have or if you have ever had high blood pressure, heart disease, or arrhythmias.

• Before starting terfenadine, tell you doctor if you now have or if you have ever had liver disease.

• Following high doses of terfenadine, serious cardiovascular adverse effects (QT interval prolongation, arrhythmias, cardiac arrest, and death) have been observed.

---

tetracycline

BRAND NAMES (Manufacturers)
Achromycin V (Lederle)
Nor-Tet (Vortech)
Panmycin (Upjohn)
Robitet Robicaps (Robins)
Sumycin (Bristol-Myers Squibb)
Tetracap (Circle)
tetracycline hydrochloride (various manufacturers)
Tetracyn (Pfizer)
Tetralan (Lannett)
Tetram (Dunhall)

TYPE OF DRUG
Tetracycline antibiotic

INGREDIENT
tetracycline

DOSAGE FORMS
Tablets (250 mg and 500 mg)
Capsules (100 mg, 250 mg, and 500 mg)
Oral suspension (125 mg per 5-ml spoonful)

STORAGE
Tetracycline tablets, capsules, and oral suspension should be stored at room temperature in tightly closed, light-resistant containers. Any unused portion of the suspension should be discarded after 14 days because the drug loses its potency after that period. Discard any medication that is outdated or no longer needed. This medication should never be frozen.

USES

Tetracycline is used to treat acne (bacteria may be partly responsible for the development of acne lesions) and a wide variety of bacterial infections. It acts by inhibiting the growth of bacteria. Tetracycline kills susceptible bacteria, but it is not effective against viruses or fungi.

TREATMENT

Ideally, this medication should be taken on an empty stomach one hour before or two hours after a meal. It should be taken with a full glass of water in order to avoid irritating the throat or esophagus (swallowing tube). If this drug causes stomach upset, however, you can take it with food (unless your doctor directs you otherwise).

Avoid consuming dairy products (milk, cheese, etc.) within two hours of any dose of this drug. Avoid taking antacids and laxatives that contain aluminum, calcium, or magnesium within an hour or two of a dose. Avoid taking any medication containing iron within three hours of a dose. These products, including vitamins, chemically bind tetracycline in the stomach and gastrointestinal tract, preventing the drug from being absorbed into the body.

The oral suspension form of this medication should be shaken well just before measuring each dose. The contents tend to settle on the bottom of the bottle, so it is necessary to shake the container to distribute the ingredients evenly and equalize the doses. Each dose should then be measured carefully with a specially designed 5-ml measuring spoon. An ordinary kitchen teaspoon is not accurate enough. The oral suspension form of this medication should not be mixed with any other substance, unless your doctor says so.

Tetracycline works best when the level of medicine in your bloodstream is kept constant. It is best, therefore, to take the doses at evenly spaced intervals day and night. For example, if you are to take four doses a day, the doses should be spaced six hours apart.

If you miss a dose of this medication, take the missed dose immediately. However, if you do not remember to take the missed dose until it is almost time for your next dose, take it; space the following dose about halfway through the regular interval between doses; and then return to your regular dosing schedule.

It is important to continue to take this medication for the entire time prescribed by your doctor, even if the symptoms disappear before the end of that period. If you stop taking the drug too soon, resistant bacteria can continue growing, and the infection could recur.

SIDE EFFECTS

Minor. Diarrhea, discoloration of the nails, dizziness, loss of appetite, nausea, stomach cramps and upset, or vomiting. These side effects should disappear as your body adjusts to the medication.

Tetracycline can increase your sensitivity to sunlight. You should, therefore, avoid prolonged exposure to sunlight or sunlamps. Wear protective clothing and sunglasses, and use an effective sunscreen.

Major. Tell your doctor about any side effects that are persistent or particularly bothersome. IT IS ESPECIALLY IMPORTANT TO TELL YOUR DOCTOR about darkened tongue, difficulty in breathing, joint pain, mouth irritation, rash, rectal or vaginal itching, sore throat and fever, unusual bleeding or bruising, or yellowing of the eyes or skin. Also, if your symptoms of infection seem to be getting worse rather than improving, you should contact your doctor.

INTERACTIONS

Tetracycline interacts with other types of medications:

1. It can increase the absorption of digoxin, which may lead to digoxin toxicity.

2. The gastrointestinal side effects (nausea, vomiting, or stomach upset) of theophylline may be increased by tetracycline.

3. The dosage of oral anticoagulants (blood thinners, such as warfarin) may need to be adjusted when this medication is started.

4. Tetracycline may decrease the effectiveness of oral contraceptives (birth control pills), and pregnancy could result. You should, therefore, use a different or additional form of birth control while taking tetracycline. Discuss this with your doctor.

BE SURE TO TELL YOUR DOCTOR about any medications that you are currently taking, especially any of the medications that are listed above.

WARNINGS

- Tell your doctor about unusual or allergic reactions you have had to any medications, especially to tetracycline or to oxytetracycline, doxycycline, or minocycline.
- Tell your doctor if you now have or if you have ever had kidney or liver disease.
- Tetracycline can affect tests for syphilis; tell your doctor you are taking this drug if you are being treated for syphilis.
- Make sure that your prescription for this drug is marked with the expiration date. The drug should be discarded after the expiration date. If tetracycline is used after it has expired, serious side effects (especially to the kidneys) could result.
- This medication has been prescribed for your current infection only. Another infection later on, or one that someone else has, may require a different medicine. You should not give your medicine to other people or use it for other infections unless your doctor specifically directs you to do so.
- Be sure to tell your doctor if you are pregnant or if you are breast-feeding. Tetracycline crosses the placenta and passes into breast milk. If used during tooth development, this drug can cause permanent tooth discoloration. It can also inhibit tooth and bone growth in the fetus. It should not be used in pregnant or nursing women, infants, or children less than eight years of age.

---

theophylline

BRAND NAMES (Manufacturers)

Accurbron (Merrell Dow)
Aerolate (Fleming)
Aquaphyllin (Ferndale)
Asmalix (Century)
Bronkodyl (Breon)
Constant-T (Geigy)
Elixomin (Cenci)
Elixophyllin (Berlex)
Lanophyllin (Lannett)
Quibron-T (Mead Johnson)
Respbid (Boehringer Ingelheim)
Slo-bid Gyrocaps (Rorer)
Slo-Phyllin (Rorer)
Somophyllin-T (Fisons)
Sustaire (Pfipharmics)
Theobid (Glaxo)
Theochron (Forest)
Theoclear (Central)
Theo-Dur (Key)
Theolair (Riker)
theophylline (various manufacturers)
Theospan (Laser)
Theostat (Laser)
Theo-24 (Searle)
Theovent (Schering)
Uniphyl (Purdue Frederick)

TYPE OF DRUG

Bronchodilator

INGREDIENT

theophylline

DOSAGE FORMS

Tablets (100 mg, 125 mg, 200 mg, 250 mg, and 300 mg)
Capsules (100 mg, 125 mg, 200 mg, 300 mg, and 400 mg)
Sustained-release tablets and capsules (50 mg, 60 mg, 65 mg, 75 mg, 100 mg, 125 mg, 130 mg, 200 mg, 250 mg, 260 mg, 300 mg, 400 mg, 450 mg, and 500 mg)
Oral liquid (80 mg per 15-ml spoonful, some with alcohol of varying amounts, including 1%, 7.5%, and 20%)
Oral suspension (300 mg per 15-ml spoonful)

STORAGE

Theophylline tablets, capsules, liquid, and suspension should be stored at room temperature. It should also be kept in tightly closed, light-resistant containers. This medication should never be frozen. Discard any outdated medication.

USES

Theophylline is prescribed to treat breathing problems (wheezing and shortness of breath) caused by asthma, bronchitis, or emphysema. It relaxes the smooth muscle of the bronchial airways (breathing tubes), which opens the air passages to the lungs and allows air to move in and out more easily.

TREATMENT

Theophylline should be taken on an empty stomach 30 to 60 minutes before a meal or two hours after a meal. If this medication causes stomach irritation, however, you can take it with food or with a full glass of water or milk (unless your doctor directs you to do otherwise).

Antidiarrheal medications and some antacids prevent the absorption of theophylline into the bloodstream from the gastrointestinal tract. Therefore, at least one hour should separate doses of one of these medications and theophylline.

The sustained-release tablets and capsules should be swallowed whole. Chewing, crushing, or crumbling the tablets or capsules destroys their sustained-release activity and possibly increases the side effects. If the tablet is scored for breaking, you can break it along these lines. If the regular capsules are too large to swallow, they can be opened and the contents mixed with jam, jelly, or applesauce. The mixture should then be swallowed without chewing.

The theophylline sprinkle capsules can also be taken whole, or the capsule can be opened and the beads sprinkled on a spoonful of soft food, such as applesauce or pudding. The sprinkles should be swallowed immediately without chewing the beads. The contents of the capsule should not be subdivided in order to ensure equal doses.

If you are using the suspension form of this medication, the bottle should be shaken well just before measuring each dose. The contents tend to settle on the bottom of the bottle, so it is necessary to shake the container to distribute the medication evenly and equalize the doses. Each dose of the oral liquid or suspension should be measured carefully with a 5-ml measuring spoon or a dose cup designed for that purpose. Ordinary kitchen spoons are not accurate enough to ensure that you receive the proper dose.

Theophylline works best when the level of the medicine in your bloodstream is kept constant. It is best, therefore, to take it at evenly spaced intervals day and night. For example, if you are to take four doses a day, the doses should be spaced six hours apart. Try to take your medication at the same time(s) each day.

Try not to miss any doses of this medication. If you do miss a dose, take the missed dose as soon as possible, unless it is almost time for the next dose. In that case, do not take the missed dose at all; just return to your regular dosing schedule. Do not double the next dose.

SIDE EFFECTS

Minor. Diarrhea, dizziness, flushing, headache, heartburn, increased urination, insomnia, irritability, loss of appetite, nausea, nervousness, stomach pain, or vomiting. These side effects should disappear as your body adjusts to the medication.

If you feel dizzy or light-headed, sit or lie down for a while; get up slowly from a sitting or reclining position; and be careful on stairs.

Major. Tell your doctor about any side effects that are persistent or particularly bothersome. IT IS ESPECIALLY IMPORTANT TO TELL YOUR DOCTOR about black, tarry stools; confusion; convulsions; difficulty in breathing; fainting; muscle twitches; palpitations; rash; severe abdominal pain; or unusual weakness.

INTERACTIONS

Theophylline interacts with several other types of drugs:

1. It can increase the diuretic effect of furosemide.

2. Concurrent use of reserpine and theophylline can cause a rapid heart rate.

3. Beta blockers (acebutolol, atenolol, betaxolol, carteolol, esmolol, labetalol, metoprolol, nadolol, penbutolol, pindolol, propranolol, or timolol) can decrease the effectiveness of theophylline.

4. Theophylline can increase the side effects of over-the-counter (nonprescription) sinus, cough, cold, asthma, allergy, and diet products; digoxin; and oral anticoagulants (blood thinners, such as warfarin).

5. Theophylline can decrease the effectiveness of phenytoin and lithium.

6. Phenobarbital, carbamazepine, and rifampin can increase the elimination of theophylline from the body, decreasing its effectiveness.

7. Cimetidine, ciprofloxacin, erythromycin, norfloxacin, troleandomycin, oral contraceptives (birth control pills), allopurinol, and thiabendazole can decrease the elimination of theophylline from the body and increase its side effects.

8. Verapamil can cause an increase in the effects of theophylline.

Before you start to take this medication, BE SURE TO TELL YOUR DOCTOR about any medications you are currently taking, especially any of those listed above.

WARNINGS

• Tell your doctor about unusual or allergic reactions you have had to any medications, especially to theophylline, aminophylline, caffeine, dyphylline, oxtriphylline, or theobromine.

• Tell your doctor if you now have or if you have ever had an enlarged prostate gland, fibrocystic breast disease, heart disease, kidney disease, low or high blood pressure, liver disease, stomach ulcers, or thyroid disease.

• Cigarette or marijuana smoking may affect this drug's action. BE SURE TO TELL YOUR DOCTOR if you smoke. However, do not quit smoking without first informing your doctor.

• High fever, diarrhea, flu, and influenza vaccinations can affect the action of this drug. Therefore, be sure to tell your doctor if you experience any episodes of high fever or prolonged diarrhea while taking this drug. Before having any vaccinations, especially those to prevent the flu, BE SURE TO TELL YOUR DOCTOR that you are taking this medication.

• Avoid drinking large amounts of caffeine-containing beverages (coffee, cocoa, tea, or cola drinks), and avoid eating large amounts of chocolate. These products may increase the side effects of theophylline.

• Do not change your diet without first consulting your doctor. A high-protein, low-carbohydrate diet or charbroiled foods may affect the action of this drug.

• Before having surgery or any other medical or dental treatment, be sure to tell your doctor or dentist that you are taking this medication.

• Before taking any over-the-counter (nonprescription) asthma, allergy, cough, cold, sinus, or diet products, ask your doctor or pharmacist. These products may add to the side effects of theophylline.

• Do not change brands or dosage forms of this medication without your doctor's permission. If your medication refill looks different, check with your doctor.

• The elderly and young children may be more sensitive to the effects of theophylline.

• Your doctor may require you to have periodic blood tests to be sure your medication is working properly.

• Be sure to tell your doctor if you are pregnant. Although theophylline appears to be safe during pregnancy, extensive studies in humans have not been conducted. Also, tell your doctor if you are breast-feeding an infant. Small amounts of theophylline pass into breast milk and may cause irritability, or insomnia in nursing infants.

---

thioridazine

BRAND NAMES (Manufacturers)

Mellaril (Sandoz)

thioridazine hydrochloride (various manufacturers)

TYPE OF DRUG

Phenothiazine tranquilizer

INGREDIENT

thioridazine

DOSAGE FORMS

Tablets (10 mg, 15 mg, 25 mg, 50 mg, 100 mg, 150 mg, and 200 mg)

Oral concentrate (30 mg and 100 mg per ml, with 3% and 4.2% alcohol, respectively)

Oral suspension (25 mg and 100 mg per 5-ml spoonful)

STORAGE

The tablet form of this medication should be stored at room temperature in a tightly closed, light-resistant container. The oral concentrate and oral suspension forms of this medication should be stored in the refrigerator in tightly closed, light-resistant containers. If the oral concentrate or suspension turns slightly yellowish, the medication is still effective and can be used. However, if it changes color markedly or has particles floating in it, it should not be used; rather, it should be discarded down the sink. This medication should never be frozen.

USES

Thioridazine is prescribed to treat the symptoms of certain types of mental illness, such as emotional symptoms of psychosis, the manic phase of manic-depressive illness, and severe behavioral problems in children. It may also be used for moderate to marked depression or sleep disturbances in adults. This medication is thought to relieve the symptoms of mental illness by blocking certain chemicals involved with nerve transmission in the brain. Thioridazine may also be used to treat the symptoms of anxiety.

TREATMENT

In order to avoid stomach irritation, you can take this medication with a meal or with a glass of water or milk (unless your doctor directs you to do otherwise).

Antacids and antidiarrheal medicines may decrease the absorption of this medication from the gastrointestinal tract. Therefore, at least one hour should separate doses of one of these medicines and thioridazine.

The oral suspension form of this medication should be shaken well just before measuring each dose. The contents tend to settle on the bottom of the bottle, so it is necessary to shake the container to distribute the ingredients evenly and equalize the doses. Each dose should then be measured carefully with a specially designed 5-ml measuring spoon. An ordinary kitchen teaspoon is not accurate enough.

The oral-concentrate form of this medication should be measured carefully with the dropper provided, then added to four ounces (1/2 cup) or more of water, milk, or a carbonated beverage or to applesauce or pudding immediately prior to administration. To prevent possible loss of effectiveness, the medication should not be diluted in tea, coffee, or apple juice.

If you miss a dose of this medication, take the missed dose as soon as possible, unless it is almost time for your next dose. In that case, do not take the missed dose at all; just return to your regular dosing schedule. Do not double the next dose without your doctor's approval.

The full effects of this medication for the control of emotional or mental symptoms may not become apparent for at least two weeks after you start to take it.

SIDE EFFECTS

Minor. Blurred vision, constipation, decreased sweating, diarrhea, dizziness, drowsiness, dry mouth, fatigue, jitteriness, menstrual irregularities, nasal congestion, restlessness, vomiting, and weight gain. As your body adjusts to the medication, these side effects should disappear.

This medication can cause increased sensitivity to sunlight. It is, therefore, important to avoid prolonged exposure to sunlight and sunlamps. Wear protective clothing and sunglasses, and use an effective sunscreen.

Thioridazine can also cause discoloration of the urine to red, pink, or red-brown. This is a harmless effect.

If you are constipated, increase the amount of fiber in your diet (fresh fruits and vegetables, salads, bran, and whole-grain breads), exercise, and drink more water (unless your doctor directs you to do otherwise).

Chew sugarless gum or suck on ice chips or a piece of hard candy to reduce mouth dryness.

To avoid dizziness or light-headedness when you stand, contract and relax the muscles of your legs for a few moments before rising. Do this by pushing one foot against the floor while raising the other foot slightly, alternating feet so that you are "pumping" your legs in a pedaling motion.

Major. Tell your doctor about any side effects that are persistent or particularly bothersome. IT IS ESPECIALLY IMPORTANT TO TELL YOUR DOCTOR about breast enlargement (in both sexes); chest pain; convulsions; darkened skin; difficulty in swallowing or breathing; drooling; fainting; fever; impotence; involuntary movements of the face, mouth, jaw, or tongue; palpitations; rash; sleep disorders; sore throat; tremors; uncoordinated movements; unusual bleeding or bruising; visual disturbances; or yellowing of the eyes or skin.

INTERACTIONS

Thioridazine interacts with several other medications:

1. It can cause extreme drowsiness when combined with alcohol or other central nervous system depressants (drugs that slow the activity of the brain and spinal cord), such as barbiturates, benzodiazepine tranquilizers, muscle relaxants, narcotics, and pain medications, or with tricyclic antidepressants.

2. Thioridazine can decrease the effectiveness of amphetamines, guanethidine, anticonvulsants, and levodopa.

3. The side effects of epinephrine, monoamine oxidase (MAO) inhibitors, metoprolol, propranolol, phenytoin, and tricyclic antidepressants may be increased by this medication. At least 14 days should separate the use of this drug and the use of an MAO inhibitor.

4. Lithium may increase the side effects and decrease the effectiveness of this medication.

5. False-positive pregnancy tests may occur. If you think you may be pregnant, call your doctor.

BE SURE TO TELL YOUR DOCTOR about any medications you are currently taking, especially those listed above.

WARNINGS

• Tell your doctor about unusual or allergic reactions you have had to any medications, especially to thioridazine or any other phenothiazine tranquilizers (such as chlorpromazine, fluphenazine, mesoridazine, perphenazine, prochlorperazine, promazine, trifluoperazine, and triflupromazine) or to loxapine.

• Tell your doctor if you have a history of alcoholism or if you now have or have ever had any blood disease, bone marrow disease, brain disease, breast cancer, blockage in the urinary or digestive tracts, drug-induced depression, epilepsy, high or low blood pressure, diabetes mellitus, glaucoma, heart or circulatory disease, liver disease, lung disease, Parkinson's disease, peptic ulcers, or enlarged prostate gland.

• Tell your doctor about any recent exposure to a pesticide or an insecticide. Thioridazine may increase the side effects from the exposure.

• To prevent oversedation, avoid drinking alcoholic beverages while taking this medication.

• If this medication makes you dizzy or drowsy, do not take part in any activity that requires alertness, such as driving a car or operating potentially dangerous machinery. Be careful on stairs and avoid getting up suddenly from a lying or sitting position.

• Prior to having surgery or any other medical or dental treatment, be sure to tell your doctor or dentist that you are taking thioridazine.

• Some of the side effects caused by this drug can be prevented by taking an antiparkinsonism drug. Discuss this with your doctor.

• This medication can decrease sweating and heat release from the body. You should, therefore, try not to become overheated (avoid exercising strenuously in hot weather, and do not take hot baths, showers, and saunas).

• Do not stop taking this medication suddenly. If the drug is stopped abruptly, you may experience a number of withdrawal symptoms, such as nausea, vomiting, stomach upset, headache, increased heart rate, insomnia, and tremors, or a worsening of your condition. Your doctor may want to reduce the dosage gradually.

• If you are planning to have a myelogram, or any other procedure in which dye will be injected into your spinal cord, tell your doctor that you are taking this medication.

• Avoid getting the oral concentrate or suspension form of this medication on your skin; either may cause redness and irritation.

• While taking this medication, do not take any over-the-counter (nonprescription) drugs for weight control or for cough, cold, allergy, asthma, or sinus problems unless you first check with your doctor. Concurrent use of any of these drugs and thioridazine may cause high blood pressure.

• Your doctor may schedule regular office visits for your first few months of therapy with this medication in order to monitor your progress and possibly adjust your dosage.

• Your doctor may want to schedule you for an eye examination if you take thioridazine for longer than a year. Prolonged use of this drug can cause visual disturbances.

• Be sure to tell your doctor if you are pregnant. Small amounts of this medication cross the placenta. Although there are reports of safe use of this drug during pregnancy, there are also reports of liver disease and tremors in newborn infants whose mothers received this type of medication close to term. Also, tell your doctor if you are breast-feeding. Small amounts of this medication pass into breast milk and may cause unwanted effects in nursing infants.

---

triamcinolone

BRAND NAMES (Manufacturers)
Aristocort A (Fujisawa)
Kenacort (Bristol-Myers Squibb)
triamcinolone (various manufacturers)

TYPE OF DRUG
Adrenocorticosteroid hormone

INGREDIENT
triamcinolone

DOSAGE FORMS
Tablets (1 mg, 2 mg, 4 mg, and 8 mg)
Oral syrup (2 mg and 4 mg per 5-ml spoonful)

STORAGE
Triamcinolone tablets and oral syrup should be stored at room temperature in tightly closed containers. Discard any outdated medication or any medication that is no longer needed.

USES

Your adrenal glands naturally produce certain cortisonelike chemicals. These chemicals are involved in various processes in the body (such as maintenance of fluid balance, regulation of temperature, and reaction to inflammation). Triamcinolone belongs to a group of drugs known as adrenocorticosteroids (or cortisonelike medications). It is used to treat a variety of disorders, including endocrine and rheumatic disorders; asthma; blood diseases; certain cancers; eye disorders; gastrointestinal disturbances, such as ulcerative colitis; respiratory diseases; and inflammations such as arthritis, dermatitis, and poison ivy. How this drug acts to relieve these disorders is not completely understood.

TREATMENT

In order to prevent stomach irritation, you can take triamcinolone with food or milk (unless your doctor directs you to do otherwise).

To help avoid potassium loss while using this drug, take your dose with a glass of fresh or frozen orange juice, or eat a banana each day. The use of a salt substitute also helps prevent potassium loss. Check with your doctor.

If you are taking only one dose of this medication each day, try to take it before 9:00 A.M.

The oral syrup form of this medication should be measured carefully with a special 5-ml measuring spoon. An ordinary kitchen teaspoon is not accurate enough.

It is important to try not to miss any doses of triamcinolone. If you do miss a dose of this medication, follow these guidelines:

1. If you are taking it more than once a day, take the missed dose as soon as possible, and then return to your regular dosing schedule. If it is already time for the next dose, double the dose.

2. If you are taking this medication once a day, take the dose you missed as soon as possible, unless you do not remember until the next day. In that case, do not take the missed dose at all; just follow your regular dosing schedule. Do not double the next dose.
3. If you are taking this drug every other day, take it as soon as you remember. If you miss the dose by a whole day, take it when you remember, and then skip a day before you take the next dose. Do not double the dose.

If you miss more than one dose of triamcinolone, CONTACT YOUR DOCTOR.

SIDE EFFECTS

Minor. Dizziness, false sense of well-being, increased appetite, increased sweating, indigestion, nausea, reddening of the skin on the face, restlessness, sleep disorders, or weight gain. These side effects should disappear as your body adjusts to the medication.

Major. Tell your doctor about any side effects that are persistent or particularly bothersome. IT IS ESPECIALLY IMPORTANT TO TELL YOUR DOCTOR about abdominal enlargement; abdominal pain; acne or other skin problems; back or rib pain; bloody or black, tarry stools; blurred vision; convulsions; difficulty in breathing; eye pain; fatigue; fever and sore throat; filling out of the face; growth impairment (in children); headaches; impaired healing of wounds; increased thirst and urination; menstrual irregularities; mental depression; mood changes; muscle wasting or weakness; nightmares; rapid weight gain (three to five pounds within a week); rash; thinning of the skin; unusual bleeding or bruising; or unusual weakness.

INTERACTIONS

Triamcinolone interacts with several other types of medications:

1. Alcohol, aspirin, and anti-inflammatory medications (such as diflunisal, ibuprofen, indomethacin, ketoprofen, meclofenamate, mefenamic acid, naproxen, piroxicam, sulindac, and tolmetin) aggravate the stomach problems that are common with use of this medication.
2. There may be a change in the dosage requirements of oral anticoagulants, oral antidiabetic drugs, or insulin when this medication is started or stopped.
3. The loss of potassium caused by triamcinolone can lead to serious side effects in individuals taking digoxin.
4. Thiazide diuretics (water pills) can increase the potassium loss caused by triamcinolone.
5. Phenobarbital, phenytoin, rifampin, and ephedrine can increase the elimination of triamcinolone from the body, thereby decreasing its effectiveness.
6. Oral contraceptives (birth control pills) and estrogen-containing drugs may decrease the elimination of this drug from the body, which can lead to an increase in side effects.
7. Triamcinolone can increase the elimination of aspirin and isoniazid from the body, thereby decreasing the effectiveness of these two medications.
8. Cholestyramine and colestipol can chemically bind this medication in the stomach and gastrointestinal tract, preventing its absorption.

BE SURE TO TELL YOUR DOCTOR about any medications you are currently taking, especially any of those listed above.

WARNINGS

• Tell your doctor about unusual or allergic reactions you have had to any medications, especially to triamcinolone or other adrenocorticosteroids (such as betamethasone, cortisone, dexamethasone, hydrocortisone, methylprednisolone, paramethasone, prednisolone, and prednisone).

• Tell your doctor if you now have or if you have ever had bone disease, diabetes mellitus, emotional instability, fungal infections, glaucoma, heart disease, high blood pressure, high cholesterol levels, kidney disease, liver disease, myasthenia gravis, peptic ulcers, osteoporosis, thyroid disease, tuberculosis, or ulcerative colitis.

• If you are using this medication for longer than a week, you may need to receive higher doses if you are subjected to stress, such as serious infections, injury, or surgery. Discuss this with your doctor.

• If you have been taking this drug for more than a week, do not stop taking it suddenly. If it is stopped abruptly, you may experience abdominal or back pain, difficulty in breathing, dizziness, extreme weakness, fainting, fever, muscle or joint pain, nausea, or vomiting. Your doctor may, therefore, want to reduce the drug's dosage gradually. Never increase the dosage or take the drug for longer than the prescribed time, unless you first consult your doctor.

• While you are taking this drug, you should not be vaccinated or immunized. This medication decreases the effectiveness of vaccines and can lead to overwhelming infection if a live-virus vaccine is administered.

• Before having surgery or any other medical or dental treatment, be sure to tell your doctor or dentist that you are taking this medication.

• Because this drug can cause glaucoma and cataracts with long-term use, your doctor may want you to have your eyes examined by an ophthalmologist periodically.

• If you are taking this medication for prolonged periods, you should wear or carry an identification card or notice stating that you are taking an adrenocorticosteroid.

• This medication can raise blood-sugar levels in diabetic patients. Blood-sugar levels should, therefore, be monitored carefully with blood or urine tests when this medication is being taken.

• Some of these products contain the color additive FD&C Yellow No. 5 (tartrazine), which can cause allergic-type reactions (wheezing, rash, fainting, difficulty in breathing) in certain susceptible individuals.

• Be sure to tell your doctor if you are pregnant. This drug crosses the placenta, and its safety in human pregnancy is not established. Birth defects have been observed in the offspring of animals given large doses of this type of drug during pregnancy. Also, tell your doctor if you are breast-feeding. Small amounts of this drug pass into breast milk and may cause growth suppression or a decrease in natural adrenocorticosteroid production in the nursing infant.

triazolam

BRAND NAME (Manufacturer)
Halcion (Upjohn)
TYPE OF DRUG
Benzodiazepine sedative/hypnotic
INGREDIENT
triazolam
DOSAGE FORM
Tablets (0.125 mg and 0.25 mg)
STORAGE
This medication should be stored at room temperature in a tightly closed, light-resistant container.

USES

Triazolam is prescribed to treat insomnia, including problems with falling asleep, waking during the night, and early morning wakefulness. It is not clear exactly how this medicine works, but it may relieve insomnia by acting as a depressant of the central nervous system (brain and spinal cord).

TREATMENT

This medicine should be taken 30 to 60 minutes before bedtime. It can be taken with a full glass of water or with food if stomach upset occurs. Do not take this medication with a dose of antacid, since this may slow its absorption.

If you are taking this medication regularly and you miss a dose, take the missed dose immediately if you remember within an hour. If more than an hour has passed, skip the dose you missed and wait for the next scheduled dose. Do not double the dose.

SIDE EFFECTS

Minor. Bitter taste in mouth, constipation, diarrhea, dizziness, drowsiness (after a night's sleep), dry mouth, excessive salivation, fatigue, flushing, headache, heartburn, loss of appetite, nausea, nervousness, sweating, or vomiting. As your body adjusts to the medication, these should disappear.

To relieve constipation, increase the amount of fiber in your diet (fresh fruits and vegetables, salads, bran, and whole-grain breads), exercise, and drink more water (unless your doctor directs you to do otherwise).

Dry mouth can be relieved by chewing sugarless gum or by sucking on ice chips.

If you feel dizzy, sit or lie down for a while; get up slowly from a sitting or reclining position; and be careful on stairs.

Major. Tell your doctor about any side effects that are persistent or particularly bothersome. IT IS ESPECIALLY IMPORTANT TO TELL YOUR DOCTOR about blurred or double vision, chest pain, depression, difficulty in urinating, fainting, falling, fever, hallucinations, joint pain, mouth sores, nightmares, palpitations, rash, shortness of breath, slurred speech, sore throat, uncoordinated movements, unusual excitement, unusual tiredness, or yellowing of the eyes or skin.

INTERACTIONS

Triazolam interacts with a number of other types of medications:

1. To prevent oversedation, it should not be taken with alcohol, other sedative drugs, central nervous system depressants (such as antihistamines, barbiturates, muscle relaxants, pain medicines, narcotics, medicines for seizures, and phenothiazine tranquilizers), or with antidepressants.

2. Triazolam may decrease the effectiveness of carbamazepine, levodopa, and oral anticoagulants (blood thinners, such as warfarin) and may increase the side effects of phenytoin.

3. Disulfiram, oral contraceptives (birth control pills), isoniazid, and cimetidine can increase the blood levels of triazolam, which can lead to toxic effects.

4. Concurrent use of rifampin may decrease the effectiveness of triazolam.

BE SURE TO TELL YOUR DOCTOR about any medications you are currently taking, especially those listed above.

WARNINGS

- Tell your doctor about unusual or allergic reactions you have had to any medications, especially to triazolam or other benzodiazepine tranquilizers (such as alprazolam, chlordiazepoxide, clorazepate, diazepam, flurazepam, halazepam, lorazepam, prazepam, and temazepam).
- Tell your doctor if you now have or if you have ever had liver disease, kidney disease, epilepsy, lung disease, myasthenia gravis, porphyria, mental depression, or mental illness.
- This medicine can cause considerable drowsiness. Avoid tasks that require mental alertness, such as driving an automobile or operating potentially dangerous machinery or equipment.
- Triazolam has the potential for abuse and must be used with caution. Tolerance may develop quickly; do not increase the dosage unless you first consult your doctor. It is also important not to stop taking this drug suddenly if you have been taking it in large amounts or if you have used it for several weeks. Your doctor may want to reduce the dosage gradually.
- This is a safe drug when used properly. When it is combined with other sedative drugs or with alcohol, however, serious side effects can develop.
- Be sure to tell your doctor if you are pregnant. This type of medicine may increase the chance of birth defects if it is taken during the first three months of pregnancy. In addition, use of too much of this medicine during the last six months of pregnancy may lead to addiction of the fetus, resulting in withdrawal side effects in the newborn. Also, use of this medicine during the last weeks of pregnancy may cause excessive drowsiness, slowed heartbeat, and breathing difficulties in the infant. Tell your doctor if you are breast-feeding an infant. This medicine can pass into breast milk and cause unwanted side effects in nursing infants.

trimethoprim

BRAND NAMES (Manufacturers)
Proloprim (Burroughs Wellcome)
trimethoprim (various manufacturers)
Trimpex (Roche)
TYPE OF DRUG
Antibiotic
INGREDIENT
trimethoprim
DOSAGE FORM
Tablets (100 mg and 200 mg)
STORAGE
Trimethoprim should be stored in a dry place at room temperature in a tightly closed, light-resistant container.

USES

This antibiotic is used in the treatment of uncomplicated urinary tract infections. It acts by preventing production of the nutrients that are required for the growth of infecting bacteria. Trimethoprim kills a wide range of bacteria, but it is not effective against viruses or fungi.

TREATMENT

You can take trimethoprim tablets on an empty stomach or, to avoid stomach upset, with food or milk.

This medication works best when the level of the medicine in your urine is kept constant. It is best, therefore, to take the doses at evenly spaced intervals day and night. For example, if you are to take two doses a day, the doses should be spaced 12 hours apart.

If you miss a dose of this medication, take the missed dose immediately. However, if you do not remember to take the missed dose until it is almost time for your next dose and you are taking one dose a day, then space the missed dose and the following dose ten to 12 hours apart. Similarly, if you are taking two doses a day, space the missed dose and the following dose five to six hours apart. Then return to your regular dosing schedule. Try not to skip any doses.

It is important to continue to take this medication for the entire time prescribed by your doctor (usually seven to 14 days), even if the symptoms disappear before the end of that period.

SIDE EFFECTS

Minor. Abdominal pain, diarrhea, headache, loss of appetite, nausea, unusual taste in the mouth, or vomiting. These should disappear as your body adjusts to the drug.
Major. Tell your doctor about any side effects that are persistent or particularly bothersome. IT IS ESPECIALLY IMPORTANT TO TELL YOUR DOCTOR about itching, skin rash, sore throat and fever, swollen or inflamed tongue, unusual bleeding or bruising, unusual fatigue, or unusually pale skin. Also, if your symptoms seem to be getting worse rather than improving, contact your doctor.

INTERACTIONS

Trimethoprim will interact with several other types of medications:

1. Rifampin can increase the elimination of trimethoprim from the body and thus decrease its antibacterial effectiveness.
2. Concurrent use of trimethoprim with antineoplastic agents (anticancer drugs) can increase the risk of developing blood disorders.
3. Trimethoprim can decrease the elimination of phenytoin from the body and may, therefore, lead to an increase in the risk of side effects.

Before starting to take this medication, BE SURE TO TELL YOUR DOCTOR about any medications you are currently taking, especially any of those listed above.

WARNINGS

• Tell your doctor about unusual reactions you have to any medications, especially to trimethoprim.
• Tell your doctor if you now have or if you have ever had megaloblastic anemia (folate-deficiency anemia), kidney disease, or liver disease.
• This medication has been prescribed for your current infection only. Another infection later on, or one that a family member or friend has, may require a different medicine. You should not give your medicine to other people or use it for other infections, unless your doctor specifically directs you to do so.
• If there is no improvement in your condition several days after starting this medication, check with your doctor. Trimethoprim may not be effective.
• Before medical or dental treatment, be sure to tell your doctor or dentist that you are taking this drug.
• Be sure to tell your doctor if you are pregnant. Although there are reports of safe use of trimethoprim during pregnancy, extensive studies in humans have not been conducted. In addition, this medication has been shown to cause birth defects in the offspring of animals that received very large doses of it during pregnancy. Also, tell your doctor if you are breast-feeding an infant. Small amounts of the drug pass into breast milk, and there is a chance that it may cause anemia in the nursing infant.

verapamil

BRAND NAMES (Manufacturers)
Calan (Searle)
Calan SR (Searle)
Isoptin (Knoll)
Isoptin SR (Knoll)
verapamil (various manufacturers)
Verelan (Lederle)
TYPE OF DRUG
Antianginal (calcium channel blocker) and antihypertensive
INGREDIENT
verapamil
DOSAGE FORMS
Tablets (40 mg, 80 mg, and 120 mg)
Sustained-release tablets (120 mg, 180 mg, and 240 mg)
Sustained-release capsules (120 mg, 180 mg, and 240 mg)

STORAGE
Store this medication at room temperature in a tightly closed container. Do not refrigerate it.

USES

Verapamil is used to treat angina pectoris (chest pain) and high blood pressure. It belongs to a group of drugs known as calcium channel blockers. It is not clearly understood how verapamil works, but it is thought to increase the blood supply to the heart. It is also a vasodilator that relaxes the muscle tissue of the blood vessels, thereby lowering blood pressure.

TREATMENT

Verapamil can be taken either on an empty stomach or with meals, as directed by your doctor or pharmacist. The sustained-release tablets should not be crushed or chewed, but swallowed whole.

If you miss a dose of this medication, take the missed dose as soon as possible, unless it is almost time for the next dose. In that case, do not take the missed dose at all; just return to your regular dosing schedule. Do not double the next dose.

This medication does not cure high blood pressure, but it will help to control the condition as long as you continue to take it.

SIDE EFFECTS

Minor. Abdominal pain, blurred vision, constipation, dizziness, headache, muscle cramps, nausea, sleeplessness, or sweating. These side effects should disappear as your body adjusts to the medication.

To relieve constipation, increase the amount of fiber in your diet (fresh fruits and vegetables, salads, bran, and whole-grain breads), and drink more water (unless your doctor directs you to do otherwise).

Major. Tell your doctor about any side effects that are persistent or particularly bothersome. IT IS ESPECIALLY IMPORTANT TO TELL YOUR DOCTOR about changes in menstruation, confusion, depression, fainting, fatigue, hair loss, itching, loss of balance, palpitations, rapid weight gain (three to five pounds within a week), shortness of breath, swelling of the hands or feet, tremors, or unusual weakness.

INTERACTIONS

This drug will interact with a number of other types of medications:

1. The concurrent use of alcohol, quinidine, or prazosin and verapamil can cause a severe drop in blood pressure and result in fainting.

2. Beta blockers (acebutolol, atenolol, betaxolol, carteolol, esmolol, labetalol, metoprolol, nadolol, penbutolol, pindolol, propranolol, or timolol) and digoxin should be used cautiously with verapamil, because side effects to the heart may be increased.

3. Disopyramide should not be taken within 48 hours of verapamil; the combination of these medications could lead to heart failure.

4. Cimetidine can decrease the elimination of verapamil from the body, which can lead to an increased risk of side effects.

5. Sulfinpyrazone and rifampin can increase the elimination of verapamil from the body, which can lead to a decrease in its effectiveness.

6. Verapamil can cause an increase in the effects of the drug theophylline.

BE SURE TO TELL YOUR DOCTOR about any medications you are currently taking.

WARNINGS

- Tell your doctor about unusual or allergic reactions you have had to any medications, especially to verapamil.
- Before starting therapy with this medication, be sure that you inform your doctor if you have ever had any type of heart disease, kidney disease, liver disease, low blood pressure, or a slowed heartbeat.
- Your doctor may want you to check your pulse while you are taking this drug. If your heart rate drops below 50 beats per minute, contact your doctor.
- Verapamil is not effective for an attack of chest pain that has already started; this medication is only effective in preventing attacks from occurring.
- It is extremely important that you do not stop taking this medication without first consulting your doctor. Stopping abruptly may lead to a worsening of your chest pain. Your doctor may, therefore, want to reduce your dosage gradually or have you switch to another similar medication when verapamil is discontinued.
- In order to prevent dizziness or fainting while taking this medication, try not to stand for long periods of time, avoid drinking alcoholic beverages, and try not to become overheated (avoid exerting yourself or exercising strenuously in hot weather, and do not take hot baths, showers, and saunas).
- Be sure to tell your doctor if you are pregnant. Extensive studies in pregnant women have not been conducted. Also, be sure to tell your doctor if you are breast-feeding an infant. Small amounts of verapamil pass into breast milk and may cause unwanted side effects in the nursing infant.

---

warfarin

BRAND NAMES (Manufacturers)
Coumadin (DuPont)
Panwarfin (Abbott)
Sofarin (Lemmon)
warfarin sodium (various manufacturers)

TYPE OF DRUG
Anticoagulant

INGREDIENT
warfarin

DOSAGE FORM
Tablets (1 mg, 2 mg, 2.5 mg, 5 mg, 7.5 mg, and 10 mg)

STORAGE
Warfarin should be stored at room temperature in a tightly closed, light-resistant container. This medication should not be refrigerated.

USES

Warfarin is used to prevent blood-clot formation. It acts by decreasing the production of blood-clotting substances by the liver.

TREATMENT

You can take warfarin with a full glass of water. In order to become accustomed to taking this medication, try to take it at the same time each day.

If you miss a dose of this medication, take the missed dose as soon as possible, unless it is almost time for the next dose. In that case, do not take the missed dose at all; just return to your regular dosing schedule. Do not double the next dose of warfarin. If you miss more than two doses in a row of this medication, contact your doctor as soon as possible.

SIDE EFFECTS

Minor. Blurred vision, cramps, decreased appetite, diarrhea, or nausea. These side effects should disappear as your body adjusts to the medication. Warfarin may produce a red-orange discoloration of urine.

Major. Tell your doctor about any side effects that are persistent or particularly bothersome. IT IS ESPECIALLY IMPORTANT TO TELL YOUR DOCTOR about bloody or black, tarry stools; blood in sputum; fever; heavy bleeding from cuts; internal bleeding (signs of internal bleeding include abdominal pain or swelling and vomiting of blood or material that resembles coffee grounds); loss of hair; mouth sores; nausea; nosebleeds; rash; red urine; severe bruising; severe headache; swelling of joints; unusually heavy menstrual bleeding; or yellowing of the eyes or skin.

INTERACTIONS

Warfarin interacts with several other types of drugs:

1. Alcohol, allopurinol, amiodarone, anabolic steroids, antibiotics, chloral hydrate, chloramphenicol, chlorpropamide, cimetidine, clofibrate, danazol, disulfiram, erythromycin, glucagon, isoniazid, ketoconazole, methyldopa, methylphenidate, metronidazole, monoamine oxidase (MAO) inhibitors, nalidixic acid, phenylbutazone, propoxyphene, quinidine, quinine, salicylates, sulfamethoxazole and trimethoprim combination, sulfinpyrazone, sulfonamides, sulindac, tetracycline, thyroid hormones, and tolbutamide can increase the effects of warfarin, which can be dangerous.

2. Azathioprine, barbiturates, carbamazepine, cholestyramine, colestipol, estrogens, ethchlorvynol, griseofulvin, oral contraceptives (birth control pills), phenytoin, propylthiouracil, rifampin, sucralfate, and vitamin K can decrease the effectiveness of warfarin.

3. Adrenocorticosteroids (cortisonelike medications), anticancer drugs, aspirin, diflunisal, dipyridamole, fenoprofen, ibuprofen, indomethacin, oxyphenbutazone, phenylbutazone, potassium, quinidine, quinine, and salicylates can increase the bleeding complications of warfarin.

4. Warfarin can increase the side effects of oral antidiabetic agents and phenytoin.

5. Diuretics (water pills) may either increase the effects or decrease the effectiveness of warfarin. Be sure to ask your doctor about the safety of concurrent use of diuretics and warfarin.

Before starting to take warfarin, BE SURE TO TELL YOUR DOCTOR about any medications (both prescription and nonprescription) you are currently taking, especially any of those listed above.

WARNINGS

- Tell your doctor about unusual or allergic reactions you have had to any medications, especially to warfarin.
- Before starting to take this medication, BE SURE TO TELL YOUR DOCTOR if you now have or if you have ever had any condition for which bleeding is an added risk—an aneurysm, blood disorders, cancer, diabetes mellitus, congestive heart failure, edema, endocarditis, high blood pressure, indwelling catheters, intestinal infections, kidney or liver disease, malnutrition, menstrual difficulties, pericarditis, surgery, thyroid disease, tuberculosis, ulcers, vasculitis, or wounds and injuries.
- Before having surgery or any other medical or dental treatment, BE SURE TO TELL YOUR DOCTOR OR DENTIST that you are taking warfarin.
- Do not take any aspirin-containing products or any over-the-counter products while you are on warfarin, unless you first check with your doctor or pharmacist.
- Avoid any activity, such as a contact sport, that might lead to physical injury. Tell your doctor about any fall or blow that occurs. Warfarin can cause heavy bleeding from cuts.
- Use an electric razor while shaving to reduce the risk of cutting yourself, and be especially careful while brushing your teeth.
- Since factors such as travel, diet, the environment, and your general health can affect your body's response to warfarin, your dosage level should be carefully monitored by your doctor.
- Do not stop taking warfarin unless you first consult your doctor. If you stop taking this drug abruptly, you may experience blood clotting. Your doctor may, therefore, want to reduce your dosage gradually.
- Do not change brands of this medication without consulting your doctor.
- Some of these products contain the color additive FD&C Yellow No. 5 (tartrazine), which can cause allergic-type reactions in certain susceptible individuals.
- Be sure to tell your doctor if you are pregnant. Warfarin has been associated with birth defects and bleeding complications in fetuses. Also, tell your doctor if you are breast-feeding an infant.

INDEX